AIR & SURFACE TRANSPORT NURSES ASSOCIATION

PATIENT TRANSPORT

PRINCIPLES & PRACTICE

AIR & SURFACE TRANSPORT NURSES ASSOCIATION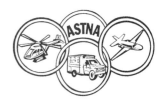

PATIENT TRANSPORT

PRINCIPLES & PRACTICE

SIXTH EDITION

Allen C. Wolfe Jr., MSN, CNS, APRN, CFRN, CCRN, CTRN, TCRN, CMTE, FAASTN
Senior Director of Education
Clinical Nurse Specialist
Life Link III
Minneapolis, Minnesota

Michael A. Frakes, APRN, FCCM, FAEN, FAASTN, FACHE
Chief Quality Officer and Director of Clinical Care
Boston MedFlight
Bedford, Massachusetts

B. Daniel Nayman, MBA, NRP, FP-C, CCP-C, CMTE
Vice President
Board of Directors
International College of Advanced Practice Paramedics
Washington, DC
Paramedic
Life Flight
Duke University Hospital System
Durham, North Carolina
Product Manager
Patient Care
ZOLL Data Systems
Broomfield, Colorado

ELSEVIER

Elsevier
3251 Riverport Lane
St. Louis, Missouri 63043

Content Strategist: Yvonne Alexopoulos
Content Development Specialist: Casey Potter
Publishing Services Manager: Deepthi Unni
Project Manager: Thoufiq Mohammed
Design Direction: Patrick Ferguson

Printed in India

Last digit is the print number: 9 8 7 6 5 4 3 2 1

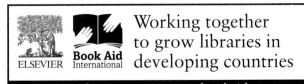

This book is dedicated to my Mom, my #1 cheerleader; my late Dad; my brothers, Timothy, Mike, and Zane; and my mentors for being inspiring people. Thanks to Dan Davis, MD, and David Olvera for collaboration on the HEAVEN criteria research which has become a standard across the country in airway management (this is a big deal!!!). To the clinicians I see at conferences who've told me that I was a role model for you, it brings me joy and makes me teary-eyed I was able to be that for you.

Thanks to the clinicians and leadership of Life Link III and FlightBridgeED in Minneapolis, my current employer, for their unwavering support in allowing me to develop and raise the standard for others within the industry.

In 1990, I was introduced to the air–ground transport industry at MedSTAR at the Washington Hospital Center in Washington, DC. After 20 years at that hospital and air program I obtained my Master's degree as a Critical Care Clinical Nurse Specialist. In 2010 I became Director of Education at the Air Methods Corporation (Denver, CO), the largest air medical company in the United States under one aviation certificate. Thanks to Rob Hamilton for enabling an African American man to hold one of the highest-profile positions in the industry. The visibility of qualified minority candidates matters.

This has been an amazing career and opportunity. I hope that my legacy in this industry lives on, and that I have moved clinical quality to a new level. This will be my last few years as an editor for ASTNA publications as I move toward retirement and a decreased role, and I hope that this will allow younger leaders to garner experience and guide the industry. It has been a pleasure to serve you.

Allen C. Wolfe Jr., MSN, CNS, APRN, CFRN, CCRN-K, CTRN, TCRN, CMTE, FAASTN

Thank you to the colleagues and mentors who continue to help me be a better transport nurse. I appreciate the work that ASTNA, Allen, and Danny put into this work, and the efforts of the multiprofession team of collaborators who worked on this book. I am proud to be able to dedicate my part of this book to Malisa, Charlie, and Gabriele, who support and inspire me every day; to the late Ray and Agnes Frakes, who taught me the value of books and language; and to the late Dr. Suzanne Wedel, for her visions of excellence and collaboration.

Michael A. Frakes, APRN, FCCM, FAEN, FAASTN, FACHE

My work on this book is dedicated to my wife, Angie, and my kids, Braydan and Amelia, for the love, support, and inspiration they give me. I want to thank Dr. Brent Myers, Billy and Christina Shelton, Sean Gibson, Dr. Brendan Berry, Joseph Zalkin, René Borghese, Donna York, Ryan Lewis, Phil Ward, Cory Oaks, Ryan Gapinski, Ryan Walter, Chris Hall, the late Cory Pittman, and the many other colleagues and mentors I have had in my life who have believed in me and pushed me to achieve more than I ever could have otherwise. Thank you to the ASTNA Board, Allen Wolfe, and Michael Frakes for allowing me to work on this project with them, and to the I-CAPP Board for allowing me to represent the organization on this project. To my Mom, Dad, and sisters (Trish, Rebecca, Kelli, and my late sister Jaime), thank you for always believing in me. It has been an honor to work with each of the authors, reviewers, and collaborators on this project and to have a small part in creating content that will improve the knowledge of clinicians and the lives of patients for years to come.

B. Daniel (Danny) Nayman, MBA, NRP, FP-C, CCP-C, CMTE

Contributors

Karen Arndt, RN, BSN, MS, CFRN, CMTE, FAASTN
Clinical Quality and Safety Nurse Specialist
UCHealth LifeLine
UCHealth
Aurora, Colorado

Tom L. Baldwin, NRP, MBA, CMTE
Vice President of Safety
Global Medical Response
Lewisville, Texas

Eric Bauer, MBA, FP-C, CCP-C, C-NPT, NRP, FAASTN(H)
President & Chief Executive Officer
FlightBridgeED
Bowling Green, Kentucky

Ami Bess, BSN, MBA-HCM, RNC-OB, RNC-EFM, CEN, CCRN, CFRN, FAASTN
Chief Flight Nurse
UCHealth LifeLine
UCHealth
Denver, Colorado

James C. Boomhower, MS(c), BS, FP-C, NR-P, C-NPT, CCISM
Lead Peer Support Coordinator/Critical Care Transport Specialist-Paramedic
Critical Care Transport
Boston MedFlight
Bedford, Massachusetts

Jason Boutwell
Operations Control Center Manager
Operations Control Center
Med-Trans Corp.
Lewisville, Texas

Arthur Broadstock, MD, FAWM
Clinical Instructor
Department of Emergency Medicine
University of Cincinnati Medical Center
Cincinnati, Ohio

Tyler Christifulli, AA, NRO, FP-C
Flight Paramedic
Clinical Services
Life Link III
Minneapolis, Minnesota

Patricia Frances Corbett, BSN
Director of Patient Safety
Clinical Services
Air Methods Corporation
Englewood, Colorado

Todd Denison, MAS, BS, NRP, FP-C, NPT-C
Director of Safety
Department of Safety
Boston MedFlight
Bedford, Massachusetts

Kelly Edwards, NRP, FP-C, MPA
Flight Paramedic
AirLife 12
Air Methods
Valdosta, Georgia
Past President
International Association of Flight and Critical Care Paramedics
Snellville, Georgia

Patrick Falvey, BSN, RN, EMT-P, CFRN
Lieutenant Colonel, Critical Care Nurse
Critical Care Aeromedical Transport (CCAT)
United States Air Force Nurse Corps
Cary, North Carolina
Critical Care Transport Nurse
Life Flight
Duke University Hospital
Durham, North Carolina

Michael J. Feldman, MD
Professor
Department of Surgery
Virginia Commonwealth University
Richmond, Virginia
Medical Director
Evans-Haynes Burn Center
Virginia Commonwealth University
Richmond, Virginia

Dana Flieger, MSN, RN, CCRN, CFRN, CEN
Critical Care/En Route Care Nurse
Naval Medical Center Camp Lejeune
United States Navy
Jacksonville, North Carolina

Brian Foster, BSAT, MTS, ATP, CFI, MEI, CFII
Vice President
Flight Operations
Global Medical Response
Lewisville, Texas

Michael A. Frakes, APRN, FCCM, FAEN, FAASTN, FACHE
Chief Quality Officer and Director of Clinical Care
Boston MedFlight
Bedford, Massachusetts

Robert L. Grabowski, DNP, MBA, APRN-CNP, AGACNP-BC, CPNP-AC, CEN, CCRN, CFRN, CMTE, EMT-P
Chief Flight Nurse Practitioner
Metro Life Flight
The MetroHealth System
Cleveland, Ohio
Captain
629th Forward Resuscitative Surgical Team
United States Army Reserve
Blacklick, Ohio
Special Faculty
The Dorothy Ebersbach Academic Center for Flight Nursing
Case Western Reserve University
Cleveland, Ohio

Casey Green, BSN, RN, CCRN-CMC, CTRN, CFRN, CEN, TCRN, CPEN, NRP
Registered Nurse
Critical Care Ground Transport
Procare Ambulance of Maryland
Rosedale, Maryland
Assistant Nurse Manager
Intensive Care Unit
Sinai Hospital of Baltimore
Baltimore, Maryland
Senior Nursing Adjunct Faculty
Nursing and Allied Health
Howard Community College
Columbia, Maryland

Robert Andrew Hamilton III, NREMT-P, MBA
Group President
Alliances
Global Medical Response
Lewisville, Texas

Sardis Harward, MD, MPH
Resident Physician
University of Cincinnati Medical Center
Department of Emergency Medicine
Cincinnati, Ohio

Krista Haugen, RN (BSN), MN, CMTE
National Director of Patient Safety
Clinical Practices
Global Medical Response
Lewisville, Texas

John B. Heffernan, BGS, ATP
Aviation Safety Consultant
Virginia Beach, Virginia

Reneé Semonin Holleran, FNP-BC, PhD, CEN, CCRN (Emeritus), CFRN and CTRN (Retired), FAEN
Nurse Practitioner
Anesthesia Chronic Pain
Veterans Health Administration
Salt Lake City, Utah
Former Chief Flight Nurse
University Air Care
University Hospital
Cincinnati, Ohio
Former Manager of Adult Transport
Intermountain Life Flight
Intermountain Health Care
Salt Lake City, Utah
Family Nurse Practitioner
Hope Free Clinic
Midvale, Utah

Jeffrey Maler, BSN, RN, CEN, CFRN, TCRN, LP, FP-C
EMS Director/Enroute Critical Care Nurse
Emergency Department
Brian D Allgood Army Community Hospital
Camp Humphreys, Armed Forces Pacific
San Antonio, Texas

Julius J. McAdams, BME, FP-C, CCP-C, NRP
Education Coordinator
AirLink/VitaLink
Novant Health
Wilmington, North Carolina

Jacob A. Miller, DNP, MBA, ACNP, ENP-C, CNS, NRP
Clinical Educator & Flight APRN
Air Care and Mobile Care
University of Cincinnati Medical Center
Cincinnati, Ohio

B. Daniel Nayman, MBA, NRP, FP-C, CCP-C, CMTE
Vice President
Board of Directors
International College of Advanced Practice Paramedics
Washington, DC
Paramedic
Life Flight
Duke University Hospital System
Durham, North Carolina
Product Manager
Patient Care
ZOLL Data Systems
Broomfield, Colorado

David J. Olvera, MBA, NRP, FP-C, CMTE
Research Services Assistant Manager
Hematology Clinical Trials Unit
University of Colorado Anschutz School of Medicine
Aurora, Colorado

Marin Peterson, DNP, APRN, CNP, CEN, CFRN
Life Link III
Minneapolis, Minnesota

Rhonda Reeder, BSN, MBA, MHA, RN, CEN, CFRN, CMTE, EMT-P
Site Surveyor
Accreditation
Commission on Accreditation of Medical Transport Systems
Anderson, South Carolina

Kevin Schitoskey, RN, MSN, CFRN, TCRN, CMTE
Director of Patient Safety and Medical Risk Management
Department of Clinical Safety
Med-Trans Corporation
Denton, Texas

Christopher P. Stevenson, MSN, AGACNP-BC, RN, CFRN
Nurse Practitioner/Flight Nurse
Evans-Haynes Burn Center
VCU Health
Richmond, Virginia

Charles F. Swearingen, BS, NRP, FP-C
Flight Paramedic
Helicopter Transport
University of Mississippi Medical Center
Jackson, Mississippi
CEO/Owner
MeduPros.com
Brandon, Mississippi

Christopher Taylor, PA-C, NRP
Paramedic/CME Instructor
Operations
Sunstar Paramedics
Largo, Florida
Physician Assistant
Center for Neurosurgical and Spine Care
BayCare Health System
Clearwater, Florida
Clinical Assistant Professor of Physician Assistant Medicine
College of Natural & Health Sciences
University of Tampa
Tampa, Florida

Kelly Tillotson, MD
Resident Physician
Emergency Medicine
University of Cincinnati
Cincinnati, Ohio

Kyle Williams, BSN, RN, EMT-P, CFRN, CEN
Regional Education Manager
Midwest Region
Air Methods Corporation
Greenwood Village, Colorado

Brian M. Wilson, MS, RN, CCRN, CFRN, NRP, DiMM, FAWM
Director of Quality, Performance Improvement, and Infection Prevention
Quality Improvement
Mass General Brigham Cooley Dickinson Hospital
Northampton, Massachusetts

Allen C. Wolfe Jr., MSN, CNS, APRN, CFRN, CCRN, CTRN, TCRN, CMTE, FAASTN
Senior Director of Education
Clinical Nurse Specialist
Life Link III
Minneapolis, Minnesota

Ryan Wyatt, NREMT-P, FP-C, TP-C
Ultrasound IV Program Coordinator
Emergency and Trauma
Banner University Medical Center
Oro Valley, Arizona

Donna York, DNP, RN, CMTE, CAFO, FAASTN
National Director RCM Business Development
Golden Hour A ZOLL Company
Carmel, Indiana
Coordinator
Safety Management Training Academy
Association of Air Medical Services
Alexandria, Virginia

Reviewers

Michael Austin, BAS, FP-C, CCP-C, NRP
Global Medical Response
Clermont, Florida

Jamie Eastman, MA, RN, NRP
Boston MedFlight
Boston, Massachusetts

Nicholas Fatolitis, BSN, RN, CEN, CFRN, EMT-P, FP-C
Med-Trans Corporation
Palm Harbor, Florida

Patricia Frances Corbett, BSN
Clinical Services
Air Methods Corporation
Englewood, Colorado

Katee Goff, NREMT, CFC
ThedaStar
Neenah, Wisconsin

Mark Larson, RN, BSN, MBA, EMTP
LifeStar
Lawrence, Kansas

Lorie J. Ledford, MSN, RN, CFRN, CTRN, CEN, TCRN, CPEN, CCRN
Native Air 8, Air Methods Corporation
Lake Havasu City, Arizona

Jennifer Liebman, MSL, CFRN, CMTE
Guardian Flight, LLC
South Jordan, Utah

Travis Mason, MBA, NRP, FP-C
Carilion Clinic Life-Guard
Roanoke, Virginia

Gene McCutcheon, RN, BSN, CEN, CFRN
MedSTAR Transport
Lanham, Maryland

Heather McLellan, MEd, BN, RN, CEN, CFRN, FAASTN
Critical Care Nursing
Mount Royal University
Calgary, Alberta, Canada

Sue L. Parrigin, MSN, CFRN, NRP
Global Medical Response
Waco, Texas

Marin Peterson, DNP, APRN, CNP, CEN, CFRN
Life Link III
Minneapolis, Minnesota

Craig Richardson, CFI, CFII
Med-Trans Corporation
Abilene, Kansas

Emily Roberts, MSN, RN, APRN, FNP-BC, ENP-C, CEN, CFRN, EMT-B
SCP Health
Knoxville, Tennessee

Joseph P. Santiago, MBA, MS, RN, CEN, CFRN, EMT-P, CMTE, CACO
Global Medical Response
Troy, New York

Michael Templeton, CertHE, FdSc, BSc Hons, DipROM RCSed
International SOS
Georgetown, Guyana

Jason C. Vest, BSN
Metro West Ambulance
Hillsboro, Oregon

John vonRosenberg, PhD, FP-C
Vidant Health
Eden, North Carolina

Ryan Walter, MBA, CEP, FP-C, IC
Air Methods
Phoenix, Arizona
Navy Reserve Medicine, US Navy Reserves
Gilbert, Arizona

Brian M. Wilson, MS, RN, CCRN, CFRN, NRP, DiMM, FAWM
Quality Improvement
Mass General Brigham Cooley Dickinson Hospital
Northampton, Massachusetts

Foreword

As we launch this sixth edition, we are pleased to collaborate with the leadership of the Air and Surface Transport Nurses Association (ASTNA), International College of Advanced Practice Paramedics (I-CAPP), International Association of Medical Transport Communication Specialists (IAMTCS), and National EMS Pilots Association (NEMSPA). This project has expanded in some areas to focus specifically on the care of the trauma patient in all modes of transport. A new volume, the first edition of *Patient Transport: Medical Critical Care*, will also be launched this year as a companion to this publication. Some chapters that were developed from a medically focused perspective in previous editions have been moved to the new volume, along with other all-new chapters related to medical critical care.

The appreciation we have for our editors, authors, and reviewers is unmeasurable. Without their commitment to improving patient care and their love of transport medicine, this text would not have become a reality. We offer a sincere and heartfelt "*Thank You!*" to them all for sharing with us their dedication and expertise.

Finally, to the reader: it is what each of you does every day to ensure excellence in patient care and the safe returns of our teammates and patients that makes all the difference. Thank you for your dedication!

Allen C. Wolfe Jr., MSN, CNS, APRN, CFRN, CCRN, CTRN, TCRN, CMTE, FAASTN
Michael A. Frakes, APRN, FCCM, FAEN, FAASTN, FACHE
B. Daniel Nayman, MBA, NRP, FP-C, CCP-C, CMTE

Preface

The Air and Surface Transport Nurses Association (ASTNA) recognized the need for a comprehensive textbook that provided a foundation for the art and science of transport nursing more than 20 years ago. We stand on the shoulders of giants: the first edition of this book (the "Brown Book") was edited by Genell Lee, and the second through fifth editions were edited by Reneé Semonin Holleran. The fourth edition won the American Journal of Nursing Book of the Year Award in 2011.

This edition welcomes Danny Nayman, Vice President of International College of Advanced Practice Paramedics (I-CAPP), to the editorial team, reflecting the collaboration and teamwork among providers that is inherent to transport care. This edition has been reviewed, updated, and expanded by a diverse team of providers, including nurses, physicians, and medics, all in support of the goal of comprehensive education reflective of the broad scope of knowledge and skills necessary for transport providers. Wherever applicable and whenever possible, this content aligns with the latest edition of the *Air and Surface Transport Nurses Association's Critical Care Transport Core Curriculum, Second Edition.*

Those familiar with previous editions of this book might also notice that there are some topics "missing." This is not because we've determined that content is unnecessary. It's just the opposite, in fact: we've created a second volume to give more information that is essential to transport care. In creating a second volume, *Patient Transport: Medical Critical Care, First Edition,* we also were able to allocate more space in this sixth edition for more in-depth discussions of issues of interest, such as updated evidence-based consensus guidelines or recommendations, and provider health

and well-being, including resilience, stress management, and other self-care practices. In addition to expanded discussion of issues like these, this sixth edition also brings the all-new Chapter 3, Aviation for Medical Personnel, which was conceived of through collaboration between veteran transport providers and those at the beginning stages of their career. We asked ourselves the question, "What do we know now about flight transport that we wish we had known on day 1 in the aircraft?" The result of those discussions is a full chapter in which providers collaborated with a veteran transport pilot to give you, the reader, a head start on discovering some of the idiosyncrasies, tips, and tricks about transport aircraft that can otherwise take a decades-long career in flight transport to learn. We are thrilled to bring this content to our sixth edition and we hope you find it as enlightening as we do.

Patient transport is a unique, multidisciplinary process. This text has been used for the past 20 years as one of the primary resources for patient transport all over the world. This edition again demonstrates why.

"You must be the change you wish to see in the world," so the saying goes. This will continue to be one of the major challenges we all face in today's world. Please use the wisdom of the authors in this book to inspire your practice . . . and the changes you wish to see in the world. And finally, we always invite you to share your unique insights with us.

Allen C. Wolfe Jr., MSN, CNS, APRN, CFRN, CCRN, CTRN, TCRN, CMTE, FAASTN
Michael A. Frakes, APRN, FCCM, FAEN, FAASTN, FACHE
B. Daniel Nayman, MBA, NRP, FP-C, CCP-C, CMTE

Acknowledgments

We are overwhelmed, humbled, and extremely grateful for the members of the transport community who contribute to the success of transporting patients from one location to another each day. From a distance, it may appear simple, but in reality, we know that transport is a complex operation involving multiple individuals and service lines within an organization—working together, these teams provide care of the highest clinical quality and safety to get transport patients from one place to another.

Special thanks to Nikole Goode for the industry guidance, Sarah Loiero for her tireless work and organization, and Casey Potter for helping us meet our goals for this sixth edition.

Allen C. Wolfe Jr., MSN, CNS, APRN, CFRN, CCRN, CTRN, TCRN, CMTE, FAASTN
Michael A. Frakes, APRN, FCCM, FAEN, FAASTN, FACHE
B. Daniel Nayman, MBA, NRP, FP-C, CCP-C, CMTE

Contents

SECTION I History and the Current Role of Air and Ground Transport Personnel

1 **History of Patient Transport, 1**
Stefan Becker, Reneé Semonin Holleran, and Kelly Edwards

2 **Members of the Transport Team and Preparation for Practice, 12**
Julius J. Mcadams

3 **Aviation for Medical Personnel, 24**
Jacob A. Miller

4 **Military Patient Transport, 38**
Jeffrey Maler

SECTION II General Principles of Practice

5 **Transport Physiology, 52**
Charles F. Swearingen

6 **Scene Operations and Safety, 68**
Casey Green and Marin Peterson

7 **Communications, 88**
Jason Boutwell, Brian Foster, and Robert Andrew Hamilton III

8 **Teamwork and Human Performance, 99**
Patrick Falvey and B. Daniel Nayman

9 **Patient Safety, 113**
Krista Haugen, Kevin Schitoskey, and Patricia Frances Corbett

10 **Operational Safety and Survival, 124**
Ami Bess and Karen Arndt

SECTION III Patient Care Principles

11 **Patient Assessment, 153**
Jacob A. Miller

12 **Airway Management, 185**
David J. Olvera and Michael A. Frakes

13 **Mechanical Ventilation, 209**
Eric Bauer

14 **Shock, 230**
Michael A. Frakes

SECTION IV Trauma

15 **General Principles of Trauma Management, 245**
Robert L. Grabowski

16 **Neurologic Trauma, 261**
Robert L. Grabowski

17 **Thoracoabdominal Trauma, 282**
Kyle Williams

18 **Musculoskeletal and Soft Tissue Trauma, 295**
Dana Flieger

19 **Burn Trauma, 307**
Christopher P. Stevenson and Michael J. Feldman

20 **Point-of-Care Ultrasound, 320**
Arthur Broadstock, Kelly Tillotson, Sardis Harward, Tyler Christifulli, and Ryan Wyatt

SECTION V Professional Issues

21 **Legal and Professional Issues in Critical Care Transport, 333**
Christopher Taylor

22 **Quality, 343**
Michael A. Frakes and Brian M. Wilson

23 **Accreditation for Air and Ground Medical Transport, 349**
Rhonda Reeder

24 **Mental Health and Wellness for the Provider, 355**
James C. Boomhower

25 **Post-Incident and Emergency Response Planning, 361**
Donna York, Krista Haugen, J. Heffernan, Tom Baldwin, and Todd Denison

Index, 372

1

History of Patient Transport

STEFAN BECKER, RENEÉ SEMONIN HOLLERAN, AND KELLY EDWARDS

Introduction

The history of patient transport started when the first injured or sick persons were carried, dragged, or otherwise moved to care providers. During the Middle Ages, the first systems began to be established for moving war casualties to care providers. These early methods saw little change until the late 18th century and beyond, when it was recognized that the rapid transport of injured soldiers reduced morbidity and mortality.

After the World Wars, there had been dramatic changes in patient transport in both military and civilian settings. The usefulness of airplanes, and later helicopters, for patient transport was realized in the 20th century and quickly spread. As these changes in the modality and the proliferation of transport took place, the training of care providers during transport was gaining attention. Patients were increasingly being transported in specialized vehicles with care providers trained beyond the basic requirements of ambulance crews.

Critical care transport is the term used to describe the most common level of patient transport service. Critical care patients have an acute, life-threatening medical condition that requires intervention and care typically beyond the scope and capability of advanced life-support care providers. As critical care transport has continued to grow, so have the requirements in education, training, and certification for the transport care providers.

This chapter will detail the pertinent history of critical care transport and its origins in patient transport. The second part of the chapter will examine the history of the main professions involved and the professional associations that are part of the critical care transport industry.

Origins of Patient Transport

The first documented record of moving injured patients to care providers was in the 11th century during the Crusades. The Knights of St. John treated and transported injured soldiers after learning first-aid techniques from Arab and Greek physicians. The impetus for providing care was likely both altruistic and monetary – any soldier who carried an injured comrade to medical treatment often received a small payment. Regardless, this may be the genesis of the first emergency medical transport and treatment providers. By the 1400s, rudimentary ambulance systems using carts were common for transporting injured soldiers after battle.[1-5]

Serious interest in resuscitation and care began in the 18th century. One of the first organized efforts to establish resuscitation systems started in 1767 in Amsterdam by a group of wealthy men called the Society for the Recovery of Drowned Persons. This group recommended the use of rapid transport of patients to hospitals capable of providing resuscitation care. These early groups were the first to conceive of a civilian patient transport, but little progress was made other than rudimentary stretchers and they were dependent on volunteers.[1-11]

In 1792 French surgeon Dominique Jean Larrey was dismayed by how long injured soldiers would lay on the battlefield before being evacuated for care. Dr. Larrey was convinced that many deaths could be prevented with timely evacuation from the battlefield, including evacuation during the battle. He designed different tow and four-wheeled carts that were more maneuverable for carrying injured soldiers. He called these carts the *ambulance volante* (the flying ambulance).

Larrey's design proved to be very successful for both transporting medical personnel to the battlefield to provide care and transporting injured soldiers from the battlefield to field hospitals. This was the first recorded use of a patient evacuation system to reduce the mortality and morbidity of injured soldiers. Dr. Larrey is credited with creating the first official military medical corps and a system for moving injured soldiers.[1-17]

Although some hospitals in Europe and England had a rudimentary stretcher service, something similar to a civilian ambulance service did not appear in London until 1832. A special carriage for cholera patients was used to transport them to the hospital for care. The *London Times* reported that the use of these carriages allowed the patient to receive definitive care quicker and could even allow for fewer hospitals that were further apart. Despite this initial innovation, patient transport via ambulance did not spread in the United Kingdom until the 1880s with the St. John Ambulance Association and a few towns adopting ambulance carriages.[1-17]

In the United States American surgeon Jonathan Letterman developed a plan for a medical treatment and evacuation system. This system became the US Ambulance Corps, and it used its own personnel, vehicles, and facilities. Instituted in 1862 at the Battle of Antietam, it was a resounding success and became enshrined in military doctrine. By 1917 the Ambulance Corps had evolved into the US Army Ambulance Service and had grown to include the utilization of trains, automobiles, and steamboats.[1-17]

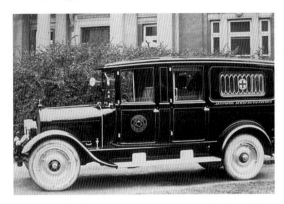

• **Figure 1.1** Early Ambulance Dispatched From Cincinnati Hospital to Transport Patients. (Courtesy University Hospital, Cincinnati, Ohio.)

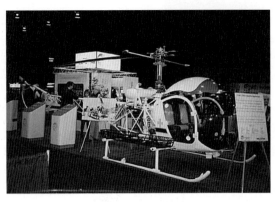

• **Figure 1.2** Helicopter Used to Transport Patients During the Korean War.

In 1865 Cincinnati Commercial Hospital started the first hospital-based ambulance service in the United States (Fig. 1.1). By 1869, Bellevue Hospital in New York City had established its own ambulance service staffed by hospital physicians. The rapidly increasing call volume for the Bellevue ambulance forced the hospital to begin staffing the ambulances with orderlies or staff with no medical training. As a result, mortality rates increased, and the focus shifted to the rapid transport of the patient to the hospital.[1-17]

By 1899, the Michael Reese Hospital in Chicago received the first motorized ambulance. This new ambulance was capable of an astounding top speed of 25 kilometers per hour (16 miles per hour) and promised smoother and quicker transport to the hospital. The motorized ambulance was quickly adopted by other hospital ambulance services.[1-17]

In 1905, the first motorized ambulance designed for military use, the Palliser Ambulance, which was named for Captain John Palliser of the Canadian Militia, came about. This unique design featured three wheels (one at the front and two at the rear) and was essentially a modified heavy tractor encased in bulletproof steel sheets. The British followed quickly behind the Canadians in introducing a limited number of automobile ambulances and commissioned several motorized ambulance vans based on a double-decker bus design.[1-17]

By 1909 the first mass-produced automobile-based ambulance designs began to appear. James Cunningham, Son and Company in Rochester, New York, designed the Model 774 automobile ambulance. Their design featured a 32-horsepower engine, electric headlights, pneumatic tires, room for an attendant, a suspended cot system, and even a large external gong as a warning device. This design was the culmination of the changing ideas of ambulance use for civilians, because ambulance crews had increasingly become centered on a driver and a patient care attendant.[1-17]

Following the World Wars (and the Korean War; Fig. 1.2), physicians had become increasingly interested in the quality of care provided to patients during transport. In 1946 the British National Health Services Act required local authorities to provide ambulances "where necessary," and ambulances were gradually adopted throughout the United Kingdom. Initially staffed by volunteers, professionals were introduced gradually. In 1964 British ambulances were retracted to provide care to patients and not just for patient transport. This was a result of an earlier horrific rail crash resulting in the death of 112 people with 340 injured, most of whom waited a considerable amount of time to receive care.[13]

Physicians in the rest of the world were similarly concerned with ambulances being able to provide care as well as transport patients. By the 1960s the work of Safar and Elam had demonstrated the benefit of resuscitation techniques (which would become cardiopulmonary resuscitation) outside of the hospital setting. In Ireland in 1966, a mobile coronary care ambulance was introduced that successfully used new pharmaceuticals and devices (such as the defibrillator). Similar advanced ambulances went into service throughout Europe and the United States soon afterward.[1-4]

The publication of the paper *Accidental Death and Disability: The Neglected Disease of Modern Society* by the National Institutes of Health in 1966 had a profound effect on emergency medical services in the United States.[14] This paper pushed for the Department of Transportation to set national standards for ambulances and emergency medical technicians, which was still largely unregulated. In 1969 President Lyndon Johnson's Committee on Highway Traffic Safety recommended the creation of a national certification agency to establish uniform standards for training and examination of personnel active in the delivery of emergency ambulance service. The first paramedic programs started in Miami in 1969, and other cities in the United States quickly followed. By the 1970s the Emergency Medical Service (EMS) started to resemble what it is today.

As the requirements and use of ambulances changed, there was the need for a new design. By the 1970s a standard car chassis was unable to carry the weight and meet the performance demands for ambulance use. Ambulance designers and manufacturers turned to the van and light truck chassis to solve this problem. The result was the first van-based ambulances, followed by truck chassis box-mounted–style ambulances. As ambulance use has changed and matured, ambulance design has also evolved to meet the technical, performance, safety, and human ergonomic requirements for emergency medical services.[1-17]

Origins of Air Medical Transport

There is a persistent myth that air transport of patients originated with the Prussian siege of Paris in 1870. This myth likely has its roots in Jules Verne's story *Robur le Conquerant*, published in 1866, which described rescuing shipwrecked sailors by balloon. There is no conclusive primary evidence that any patients were ever evacuated by balloon at the Siege of Paris; it was likely only a proposed plan that never came to fruition. Balloons were used during that battle to carry mail in and out of the city during the siege as well as some important military personnel and civilians, but not significantly injured personnel.[18-20]

In 1890 M. de Mooy, chief of the Dutch Medical Service, began to seriously pursue the concept of transporting injured patients by balloon. He proposed a method of suspending stretchers from balloons that could move patients out of the front line and to field hospitals further away. During this time, it was a radical departure from the traditional means of patient transport and met with resistance from critics. These first experiments in changing the traditional means of patient transport would not become a reality until aviation became more established.[18-20]

Fixed-Wing Transport

In December of 1903 the Wright brothers made their famous successful flight in Kill Devil Hills, North Carolina. This event marked the beginning of a new era of machine-powered aircraft flight. More important was the Wright brothers' continued success in developing better planes and showcasing them to the rest of the world at demonstrations in Europe and the United States.[18-22]

Soon medical personnel realized the potential of the airplane. In 1909 Captain George Grosman from the US Army Medical Corps and Lieutenant Albert Rhoades of the Coast Auxiliary Corps designed and constructed a plane to transport patients. The plane design required a physician to be the pilot and to sit next to the patient during the flight. Unfortunately, they were unsuccessful, and the plane crashed during the initial test flight. The US government put a halt on the project, but 3 years later, it would change its position.[18-22]

This change in position may be attributable to European experiments with airplanes and wounded soldier evacuation. In 1912 Emilie Raymond, a medical doctor and French senator, proposed using airplanes as ambulances for the military. By 1913 the French were pushing for the Geneva Convention to be extended to provide protection for air ambulances (although their efforts were met with scorn at first). French medical officer Gautier famously said that airplanes would "revolutionize war surgery if [they] could be adapted as a means of transport for the wounded."[20-23]

It was in 1915, during World War I, that the first successful aeromedical evacuation occurred. During the Serbian retreat from the Albanian mountains, French Captain Dangelzer and Lieutenant Paulhan evacuated wounded men from Mitrovica to Valona by airplane. Although this spurred more interest in airplane use for patient transport, it was 1917 by the time modifications were made to a Dorand AR II aircraft to make space in the fuselage specifically for patient stretchers. In 1918 two of these modified planes were used to evacuate patients from the Battle of Flanders. These initial successes demonstrated the viability of air medical evacuation.[20-23]

During the International Conference of the Red Cross in 1923, attendees debated the role and use of air ambulances. The result of these debates led to a supplement to the Geneva Convention that provided protection of air medical units from belligerent action. Medical aircraft were prohibited from carrying any armament or photographic equipment, they could not fly over (or even approach) the battle lines, and all air medical units had to have the Red Cross insignia prominently displayed.[20-23]

The French continued to expand on the use of air medical evacuation following World War I. During the smaller conflicts in Morocco and Syria after World War I, they used airplanes to evacuate the wounded. By 1925 the French had established the Medical Air Transport Service. This service not only introduced the concept of flying the wounded, but it also introduced flying surgeons and doctors to the patients. This concept was not as successful because of safety and logistical concerns, and the focus of the Medical Air Transport Service remained on evacuating the wounded back to the medical facilities. By 1929 the French had 43 aircraft assigned to the Medical Air Transport Service.[20-23]

Other countries were far behind the French efforts and mostly relied on an informal system of volunteers. The British used a system of volunteer aviators operating under the British Red Cross Society. The US Army was modifying de Havilland airplanes to accommodate two patients and a physician. In 1926 the United States made its first successful air medical evacuations in Nicaragua. Other European countries were cautiously following the French and/or British examples in a limited fashion.[24-27]

In 1928 the first civilian air medical airplane service was established in Australia. The Australian Inland Mission sought to provide medical services to people in remote areas of the Australian Outback. Initially they provided clinics or hospitals in remote communities. As they struggled to provide medical personnel for these locations, Lieutenant Clifford Peel suggested using airplanes to fly physicians out to these isolated locations. From that suggestion, the Australian Inland Mission Air Medical Service was finally created in 1928 when enough funds were raised – 10 years after Lieutenant Peel's suggestion.[24-27]

The Australian Inland Air Medical Service completed 50 flights in its first year, relying on fundraising and donations for financial support. By 1932 their service had become so successful and popular that there was a push for a network of "flying doctors" across Australia. In 1934 the Australian Aerial Medical Service was formed and created sections across the continent with coverage areas. In 1942 the service was renamed the Flying Doctor Service, and in 1955 the appellation Royal was added.[24-27]

Today the Royal Flying Doctor Service of Australia operates 66 aircraft in 23 locations. They provide transport of healthcare personnel to remote locations, transport of patients from remote locations, telehealth services, education, and consultation for remote healthcare providers. The service is still run as a not-for-profit organization and relies on community support for funding.[24-27]

The first civilian air ambulances in the United Kingdom started in 1933 with the evacuation of a patient from the Isle of Islay in Scotland. Eventually the UK Department of Health for Scotland sponsored the development of air ambulances for Scotland (which continues to this day as the Scottish Ambulance Service Air Wing). In 1934 the first civilian air ambulance service was established in Africa by French nurse and pilot Marie Marvingt, and by 1957 a group of surgeons would establish the Flying Doctors in Africa. Austin Airways started operating in Canada in 1934, becoming the first North American private air ambulance. Swiss Air-Rescue (Rega) was established in 1952, and it not only flies patients in Switzerland but also retrieves Swiss citizens from anywhere in the world.[26]

From its beginnings in wartime, the airplane has played a significant role in patient transport. It has continued to be an important part of the healthcare system, especially in rural or underserved areas of the world. It has also become a valuable asset in transporting patients to specialty care facilities or repatriating injured or sick citizens back to their home country.

Patient Transport by Helicopter

Leonardo da Vinci was likely the first person to conceive an idea for what could be considered a helicopter. His "aerial screw" design dates back to 1493 and consisted of a platform with a helical screw driven by a rudimentary turning system powered by humans. Although his design was never created, and likely would not have flown as designed, it illustrates that the rotor wing/vertical flight concept has existed for a long time.[18–27]

Contrary to popular misconception, it was French engineer Paul Cornu that designed and built the first rotary wing (helicopter) aircraft to achieve flight. Like the Wright brothers, he was primarily a bicycle manufacturer that tinkered with aviation designs. In 1907 he successfully flew his twin-rotor helicopter for 30 seconds. Although his early work had limited success, it proved the concept of rotor wing flight.[18–27]

In 1909 Russian Engineer Igor Sikorsky returned from Paris (then the center of the aviation world) and began designing rotor wing aircraft. By 1910 Sikorsky had designed a helicopter capable of flight that also overcame the technical problems of controlling the aircraft in flight. By 1912 Sikorsky had designed helicopters able to carry passengers and even developed plans for airplanes with multiple engines. Sikorsky and his significant early contributions have cemented his name as the "father" of the helicopter.[18–27]

German engineer Henrich Focke built on Sikorsky's successful work. In 1936 he created the dual-rotor FA-61, which is generally considered to be the first practical and functional helicopter because it could fly at a speed of about 90 kilometers per hour (56 miles per hour) with a 230-kilometer (143-mile) range and ceiling limit of 3427 m (11,243 feet). The conflict in Europe (which would grow to become World War II) spurred Focke to iterate improvements. By 1940 the dual-rotor FA 223 Drache ("dragon") became the first helicopter to enter into mass production as World War II threw most of the world into conflict. Although few of the Drache were made, it could reach speeds and altitudes twice that of the FA-61 and carry a significant number of ordinances.[18–27]

Although Sikorsky was successful in Russia, he immigrated to the United States in 1919, where there was more opportunity and a chance to escape the economic turmoil of Europe. Sikorsky formed the Sikorsky Manufacturing Corporation in 1923. In 1929 he developed the first twin-engine airplane in America, the S-29. The financial success of the S-29 allowed Sikorsky to work on new helicopter designs, leading to the VS-300 design in 1940. The VS-300 used a single main rotor with an antitorque tail rotor, which is the most common configuration of helicopters today.[18–27]

Because of the helicopter's ability to get into smaller areas than airplanes, the US Army quickly realized the potential of Sikorsky's work. It commissioned Sikorsky to develop helicopters for military use, and they were initially used to position special military units in remote areas. In April 1944 the helicopter was first used to evacuate a patient; a US Army Sikorsky YR-4B transported a wounded British soldier from more than 100 miles behind Japanese lines in Burma.[5,12–27]

The military focus on helicopters until now was on their role either as combat aircraft or as troop transports. When the United States entered into the Korean War, the helicopter gained a new focus, casualty evacuation. Two weeks after the start of the conflict, Marine Corps pilots used their HMR-161 helicopters to evacuate patients. A special helicopter unit was soon formed with the express purpose of patient evacuation from the front lines to the Mobile Army Surgical Hospitals.[5,12–27]

This new unit used the smaller, and unarmed, Bell 47 helicopter that could transport two patients on external patient litters. During the Korean War, over 20,000 medical evacuations by helicopter took place. The combination of rapid transport by helicopter and nearby surgical hospitals greatly reduced the casualty rate, cementing the helicopter as a tool for rapid patient transport (see Fig. 1.2).[5,12–27]

In 1958 a California businessman named Bill Mathews decided to organize a civilian air medical service based on the successes of helicopters in Korea. Mathews lived in the small northern city of Etna, California, and partnered with the town physician, Granville Ashcroft, to transport patients. The helicopter was even used to transport medications for the town pharmacist during emergencies. This short-lived service was the first civilian helicopter medical operation in the United States. Meanwhile, REGA had conducted its first use of helicopter rescue in 1952 and fully embraced its use by 1959.[5,12–27]

During the Vietnam War, the care and transport of injured personnel continued to expand. During the conflict, over 200,000 injured were evacuated by helicopter to field hospitals and even further. A significant change in this conflict was the use of a much larger helicopter, the Bell UH-1 (often referred to as a Huey). The UH-1 could carry more patients and personnel inside the aircraft, allowing army medics to provide care during the transport. A more comprehensive system was developed, which allowed the injured to be evacuated to field hospitals while receiving care and then often transported to specialty care later by airplane or helicopter.[5,12–27]

During the 1960s Europeans as well as Americans had begun to embrace the use of helicopters for civilian medical transport. REGA was setting an example for helicopter use in Europe. They presented their rescue tools (the rescue line and horizontal net) and techniques for helicopters to attendees at their first helicopter symposium in 1966. REGA is believed to be the first civilian helicopter service to routinely use a hoist for rescue operations. When REGA began to exhaust its financial resources in the late 1960s, the Swiss government declined to fund it further. Instead, REGA offered a patronage system to the public: in exchange for a minimum donation, Swiss citizens received free emergency air transport. This system has fundamentally remained unchanged to this day and has been copied or modified by many other air medical services (Fig. 1.3).[5,12–27] As mentioned, the publication of *Accidental Death and Disability: The Neglected Disease of Modern Society* by the National Institutes of Health in 1966 had a profound effect on emergency medical services in the United States. This paper pushed for the Department of Transportation to set the national standards for ambulances and emergency medical technicians, which before this were largely unregulated. In addition to setting the standards for modern emergency medical services, this paper

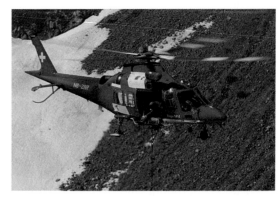

• **Figure 1.3 Swiss Air-Rescue.** (Courtesy REGA.)

provided an impetus for the growth of civilian air medical services based on the military model.[5,12–27]

In 1969 the US government implemented two programs to study the effect of medical helicopters on mortality and morbidity rates: Coordinated Accident Rescue Endeavor, State of Mississippi (Project CARESOM), and the Military Assistance to Safety and Traffic (MAST) in Texas. CARESOM used purchased helicopters located and staffed at three geographically different hospitals, whereas MAST used military helicopters and personnel to augment civilian emergency medical services. Both programs were successful at demonstrating the need for civilian air medical services.[5,12–27]

Meanwhile, the state of Maryland received a grant to purchase Bell Jet Ranger model helicopters. Maryland purchased four of them and strategically placed them throughout the state for quick response to emergency calls. The helicopters were staffed with a paramedic that was also trained as a law enforcement agent. When the helicopter was not being used for patient transport, it could be (and often was) used for law enforcement activity. The Maryland State Police Aviation Command still functions in this manner today, albeit with much larger aircraft than the Bell Jet Ranger.[5,12–27]

In Europe, Germany began operating its first civilian medical helicopter in 1970. Christoph 1, named after St. Christopher, was a resounding success. By 2015 Germany had over 75 medical helicopters with a combination of government and nonprofit programs. England was slower to develop its air medical services, outside of the Scottish Ambulance Service Air Wing, and air medical services funded by charities did not take root until 1980.[5,12–27]

In 1972 the first hospital-based helicopter medical program was established at Loma Linda Medical Center in California, but financial difficulties ended the program after 6 months. In that same year, St. Anthony's Hospital in Denver started its Flight for Life program with an Alouette III helicopter. Flight for Life is still in operation today, making it the longest-running hospital-based flight program in the United States (Fig. 1.4).[5,12–27]

The National Highway and Transportation Safety Administration (NHTSA) released a study in 1972 on helicopter use in emergency medical services and transport. NHTSA stated that the use of helicopters was of limited use in urban settings, and a follow-up study in 1981 suggested that air ambulances were not equipped to handle critically ill or injured patients. The criticism led the Federal Aviation Administration to demand better equipment and specially trained crews for air ambulances, and many individual states started to set requirements for air ambulances.[5,7,12,28–31]

In the 1980s hospital-based helicopter air medical programs opened at a rapid pace in the United States. By the late 1980s over 150 programs were in operation, and that number continued to rise. By 2003 the number of air medical helicopters had increased to 540, and by 2015 the number had nearly doubled from 2003. Europe and the rest of the world have seen similar growth in air medical programs, but not at the same pace as the United States.[5,7,12,28–31]

In the Gulf War of 1990 the US military underwent a significant shift in its medical response system. Before the collapse of the Soviet Union, the military focus on casualty evacuation had centered on conflict as part of smaller isolated incidents or a larger conflict in the European continent. By 1991 US personnel were stationed in the Middle East, and the Air Force Medical Service was the only substantial medical presence.[4,6,11,27–30] In 45 days the Air Force had deployed 15 hospitals, and before the offensive operation Desert Storm, the Air Force and Army were prepared to evacuate 3600 patients per day from the front line to hospitals by helicopter and 1000 to 2000 per day from these hospitals back to military hospitals in Europe or America. Although the casualty rate never came close to these estimates, it showed the preparation and commitment to air medical evacuation by the military.[5,7,12,28–31]

In 1994 there was a marked change in battlefield trauma care standards. The US special operations forces community began to develop and embrace the doctrine that would become tactical combat casualty care. This doctrine and approach focused on preventing battlefield deaths by focusing on the quick stabilization of immediate life-threatening injuries and delaying treatment for injuries that were not immediately life-threatening. The doctrine also emphasized the use of "damage control" treatment by using tourniquets and hemostatic agents instead of more complicated or time-consuming treatments.[5,7,12,28–32]

The combined US military operations in the Middle East precipitated by the events of 9/11 built on lessons learned regarding medical evacuation in previous conflicts. The military medical doctrine continued to focus on rapid and aggressive care and transport to definitive surgical care. Helicopters were still used for rapid evacuation of injured personnel to nearby surgical care, followed by later evacuation via airplane to hospitals in Europe or America for long-term treatment. This system, along with new practices and treatments, significantly reduced mortality among injured personnel. Lessons learned by medical personnel have slowly disseminated into civilian medicine, including air medical programs.[5,7,12,28–32]

Air Medical Program Models

Although air ambulance programs outside the United States have mostly remained nonprofit/charity or governmental programs, the United States has several different models of operation. Today there are four basic models of air medical programs in the United States. The oldest is the so-called "traditional model," in which hospitals or another healthcare agency contracts a third-party operator to provide aircraft, pilots, and maintenance while providing

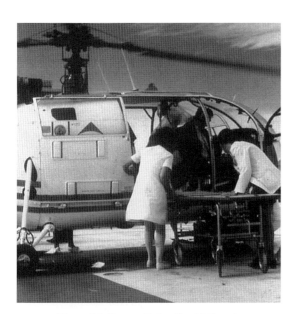

• **Figure 1.4** Nurses Unloading Helicopter.

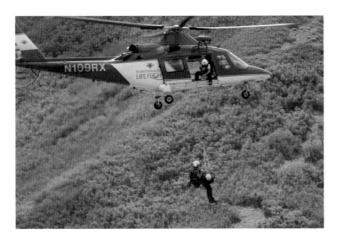

• **Figure 1.5** Intermountain Life Flight Hoist Rescue Operation. (Photo courtesy Intermountain Life Flight.)

medical personnel and management themselves. These programs have declined recently as other air medical program models have emerged and hospitals look to cut costs (Fig. 1.5).[5,7,12,28–33]

Next is a "community-based model," in which a company manages the helicopters, personnel, and support separate from a specific local hospital/healthcare agency. This model can be organized as a for-profit agency or as a nonprofit agency, but the key to the model is that the company running the program is not a governmental agency. Generally, this model is very similar to a private ambulance service in which the company bears all the costs and seeks reimbursement for services from insurance, Medicaid/Medicare, or private payment.[5,7,12,28–33]

One of the newest models is the so-called "alternative delivery model" or "hybrid model," which is a mix of the traditional and community-based models. In this model, a partnership exists between a healthcare agency and a private company. The specifics can vary, but the partnership allows both the private company and the healthcare agency to contribute something to the program. Sometimes this partnership can also be between a private company and a governmental agency to provide air medical services to a specific region or underserved area.[5,7,12,28–31,33,34]

The third model of the helicopter EMS (HEMS) is the "government-operated" version, in which governments take direct responsibility for providing air ambulance operations in specific regions. This is the least common of the models in the United States; most of these programs operate as part of a law enforcement agency such as the Maryland State Police Aviation Command.[5,7,12,28–31]

Nursing in Critical Care Transport

Florence Nightingale is generally considered the founder of modern nursing practice. She was one of the first nurses to practice outside the confines of a hospital and was in charge of the Female Nursing Establishment of the English General Hospitals during the Crimean War. Her leadership helped reduce the mortality rate from 47% to less than 3%.[5,1,7,12,28–31]

In the United States Clara Barton became the symbol of nursing practice. She was committed to providing aid to all patients needing care, regardless of race, creed, or belief. She was an advocate of providing care to patients on the battlefield during the American Civil War, and in 1882 she founded the American Red Cross. Since Nightingale and Barton, nurses have been actively involved in the care of patients at the front lines of conflict and involved in their care during transport.[5,1,7,12,28–31]

The first flight nurse, and founder of flight nursing, was Marie Marvingt (1875–1963). She was a trained surgical nurse and licensed pilot and even designed an airplane that was capable of carrying a stretcher. Following World War I, she devoted herself to advocating for air medical evacuation. She gave thousands of seminars and conferences on the subject and established the first civilian air medical service in Africa in 1934. She also appeared in two documentaries on air ambulances, and in World War II she served as a surgical nurse. In 1955 at age 80, she earned a helicopter pilot license and even flew a supersonic fighter jet. Marie Marvingt remains the most decorated woman in the history of France, and her contribution to air medical transport and flight nursing cannot be overstated (Fig. 1.6).[5,1,7,12,28–31]

American Flight Nursing starts with the Emergency Flight Corps, formed in 1933 by Lauretta M. Schimmoler, who pressured the US military to open a flight nurse training program in 1942 at the 349th Air Evacuation Group. This training program was a 6-week course that included flight physiology and transport considerations for patients. To enter the program, a nurse had to apply and work for 6 months at an Army Air Force Hospital. Once a candidate was approved and completed the training program at the 349th Air Evacuation Group, a nurse could request the designation "Flight Nurse" from the Commanding General of the Army Air Force. This designation was highly prized because it represented the elite of the nursing corps (Fig. 1.7 and Boxes 1.1 and 1.2).[5,1,7,12,28–31]

During World War II 1.5 million patients had been flown with flight nurses in attendance. By the end of the war 217 nurses had died (or were missing) in the line of duty. Following World War II flight nurse training was conducted by the US Air Force (which had separated from the US Army). Flight nurses were used during the Vietnam and Korean Wars, although their role remained as care providers inside field hospitals or during the transport of a patient from a field hospital to definitive or long-term care.[1,5,7,12,28–31]

The first civilian air medical programs in the United States were hospital-based programs. As a result, they often used a nurse along with a physician as the care providers. The expansion and growth of air medical programs throughout the United States has led to the discipline of flight nursing becoming a specialty type of nursing outside the military. Flight nurses today are generally referred

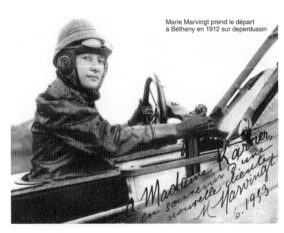

Marie Marvingt prend le départ á Bétheny en 1912 sur deperdussin

• **Figure 1.6** Marie Marvingt, Reims, 1912. (From Hargrave L. The pioneers: Aviation and aeromodeling–interdependent evolutions and histories. Marie Marvingt [1875–1963], Pioneer Aviatrix [monash.edu.au]. Accessed August 14, 2022.)

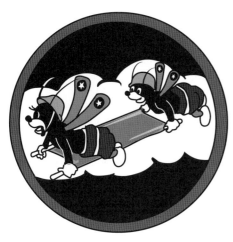

• **Figure 1.7 Bees Insignia.** Insignia of the US Army Air Force's School of Air Evacuation was a dark blue disk with two honeybees, whose bodies were or (gold) and sable (black) with argent (white) wings bearing stars, carrying a brown litter, all in front of an argent cloud. Blue and gold are the Air Corps colors. The honeybees, helmeted and wearing Red Cross armbands, are indicative of the industry displayed by the personnel of the organization. The litter is symbolic of evacuation of the sick and wounded, and the cloud is indicative of the area in which the mission is performed. The insignia was designed by Mrs. Don Rider of Buechel, Kentucky, who was greatly impressed by the work of the air evacuation personnel during the flood in Louisville in 1942.

• BOX 1.1 **"The Song of the Army Nurse Corps"**

We march along with faith undaunted beside our gallant fighting men;
Whenever they are sick or wounded, we nurse them back to health again;
As long as healing hands are wanted, you'll find the nurses of the Corps;
On ship, or plane, on transport train, at home or on a far off shore;
With loyal heart we do our part, for the Army and the Army Nurse Corps.

Copyright 1944 by MCA Music; Lou Singen, composer; Hy Zaret, lyrics.

• BOX 1.2 **Flight Nurses' Creed**

I will summon every resource to prevent the triumph of death over life.

I will stand guard over the medicines and equipment entrusted to my care and ensure their proper use.

I will be untiring in the performance of my duties, and I will remember that upon my disposition and spirit will in large measure depend the morale of my patients.

I will be faithful to my training and to the wisdom handed down to me by those who have gone before me.

I have taken a nurse's oath reverent in man's mind because of the spirit and work of its creator, Florence Nightingale. She, I remember, was called the "lady with the lamp."

It is now my privilege to lift this lamp of hope and faith and courage in my profession to heights not known by her in her time. Together with the help of the flight surgeons and surgical technicians, I can set the very skies ablaze with life and promise for the sick, injured and wounded who are my sacred charges.

...This I will do. I will not falter, in war or in peace.

David N.W. Grant
Major General, USA
Air Surgeon

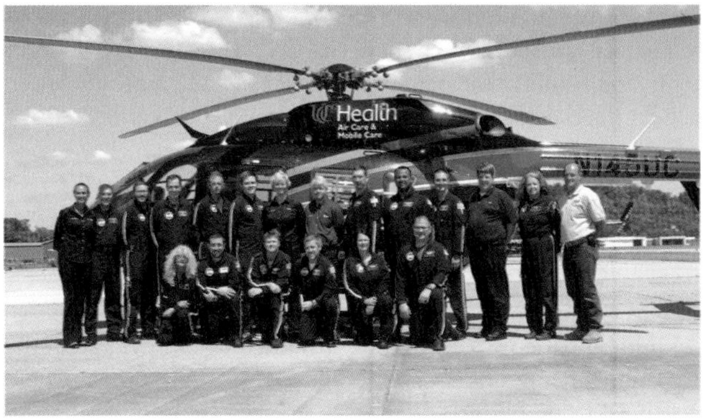

• **Figure 1.8** University Air Care Air Medical Transport Crew. (Photo courtesy University Hospital, Cincinnati, Ohio.)

to now as transport nurses. This includes both ground and air medical nurses providing care during the transport process.

In 1991 the Certified Flight Registered Nurse (CFRN) examination was created to reflect the role specialization of transport nurses. This exam was created by the Board of Certification for Emergency Nursing (BCEN).

In 2006, the BCEN created a certification exam for those nurses who primarily transported patients by ground. This exam is called the CTRN or the certified transport registered nurse.

Many critical care and air medical programs worldwide use nurses as part of the care team. Many transport teams primarily use nurses exclusively (Fig. 1.8).[1,5,7,12,23,28–31]

Paramedics in Critical Care Transport

The history of the paramedic can be traced back to early ambulance squads that provided aid during World War I. Although these squads provided little more than transportation of the injured, they did possess some basic first-aid training. In World War II, the military corpsman was a soldier trained to provide battlefield care to a wounded soldier. The corpsman evolved into the field medic, who could provide more advanced care and prepare a patient for helicopter evacuation. During the Vietnam War, the field medics were responsible for providing initial care and care for the injured soldier during the helicopter evacuation to a field hospital.[1–14]

As civilian ambulance services took root and spread, the focus began to shift to the training of the attendants and the care given during transport. By the 1960s ambulance attendants were generally trained and certified to some degree, but there was a noted disparity in the training requirements from country to country, and even within regions of the same country. In the United States the 1966 paper *Accidental Death and Disability: The Neglected Disease of Modern Society* along with President Lyndon Johnson's Committee on Highway Traffic Safety resulted in the standardization of emergency medical technicians and paramedic training programs by the Department of Transportation. The paramedic standards developed by the United States were the framework for paramedic programs throughout the world.[1–15]

In 1975 the paramedic profession gained official recognition as a healthcare occupation by the American Medical Association. As air medical programs began to emerge worldwide, many countries saw them as an extension of ambulance service and placed paramedics in them. In the United States paramedics were used as part of an air medical program as the number of programs grew and air medical helicopters began providing prehospital care and response.[32–35] The paramedic profession has grown and evolved as healthcare needs and the medical transport system have changed. The educational requirements and training for paramedics often include associate-level or bachelor-level degrees, and specialty disciplines and certifications for paramedics, such as the Certified Flight Paramedic (FP-C) and Critical Care Paramedic (CCP-C), are available.[36]

Most air and critical care transport medical programs worldwide use paramedics as part of the care team, and some countries and programs exclusively use paramedics. The roles of paramedics continue to expand to provide both prehospital and critical care for ill and injured patients. Community paramedicine provides community care to many underserved populations. Many programs are a part of EMS programs as well as supported by hospitals (https://www.ruralhealthinfo.org/topics/community-paramedicine).[32–35]

Recent Patient Transport History in the 20th and 21st Centuries

As the transport industry continues to grow and expand from its roots, several attempts have been made to describe what patient transport is, what impact it has, and how it might evolve.[37–44]

Several summits and surveys have been conducted and published within the transport environment that especially focus on air medical transport. The primary focus of these has been to identify where the field of patient transport is now and where it should be in the future. Table 1.1 provides a summary of a number of these events and publications including their focus and potential direction for transport safety, patient care, and research.

These issues continue to be important components related to patient transport, whether by air or ground. Associations have

developed that address specific parts of the transport industry. The following section contains information about the primary associations involved in patient transport.

Associations

The critical care and air medical industry is home to a multitude of member organizations that advocate for their members, profession, and the industry as a whole. Although this is not an exhaustive list, it covers some of the more significant associations that play a part in critical care or air medical transport.

Association of Air Medical Services

The American Society of Hospital-Based Emergency Air Medical Services, now known as the Association of Air Medical Services (AAMS), was established in 1980 as a nonprofit trade association.[38] Members of AAMS are the companies, associations, and related organizations that have a stake in critical care and medical transport. AAMS seeks to represent and advocate on behalf of their membership to enhance their ability to deliver quality, safe, and effective medical care and medical transportation for every patient in need. An example of AAMS advocacy includes Vision Zero, which focuses on safety in the transport environment, and publication of position papers that support the roles of transport programs in patient care.

Air and Surface Transport Nurses Association

The National Flight Nurses Association (NFNA), now known as the Air and Surface Transport Nurses Association (ASTNA), is a

TABLE 1.1	Industry Summits and Publications in the 20th and 21st Centuries	
Summit	**Focus**
1985 Safety Summit	Concern about escalating HEMS accidents focused on pilot fatigue. Recommended 12-hour shifts for pilots
2000 Safety Summit	Increase in number of HEMS accidents from 1988 to 2000. Development of AMSAC
1991 AAMS Air Medical Reimbursement Congress	Focused on coverage, reimbursement, billing, and cost-effectiveness
1996 AAMS Air Medical Transport Summit	What objective information existed that described patient transport and what needed to be identified and in what specific areas of transport including transport of specific patient populations such as neonatal and pediatric patients, economic advantage of helicopter transport, and airway management
2003 Air Medical Leadership Congress: Setting the Health Care Agenda for the Air Medical Community	Focused on safety, medical care, cost/benefit, and regulatory/compliance
A Blueprint for Critical Care Transport Research (2013)	"Go Zone" research ideas Safety Human factors Outcomes Utilization Financial Clinical care issues Education/training
AIRMED World Congress	Has been organized for over 30 years to address international issues related to defining the future of professional aeromedical services

AAMS, Association of Air Medical Services; *AMSAC,* Air Medical Safety Advisory Council; *HEMS,* helicopter emergency medical services.

membership association that advocates for nurses involved in patient transport.[38] The NFNA was founded in 1981 by a group of dedicated flight nurses. These nurses *developed* standards of practice including a safety committee that started the CONCERN Network, which is a communications system developed to relay critical incidents and processes from one program to another.

In addition, the Flight Nurse Advanced Trauma Course was an appointed committee that revised a course focused on advanced trauma care by flight nurses. This course originally was a part of the Advanced Trauma Course from the American College of Surgeons. It was known as the Flight Nurse Advanced Trauma Course (FNATC). The focus of the original course was to provide knowledge, competencies, and skills for injured patients including such skills as chest tube insertion and cricothyrotomy. The FNATC has evolved into the Transport Professional Advanced Trauma Course (TPATC). There is now also a Pediatric Advanced Transport Course. These courses are available online or in person (Air & Surface Transport Nurses Association [astna.org]).

In 1991 ASTNA partnered with the Board for Certified Emergency Nurses to develop both the CFRN and the Certified Registered Nurse (CTRN) certification examinations.

ASTNA is also responsible for the *Air and Surface Transport: Principles and Practice* text. This is a multidisciplinary, comprehensive text that addresses the principles and practice of patient transport. This text was the dream of a flight nurse named Carol Wickman and was brought to fruition by Genell Lee as the text *Flight Nursing Principles and Practice*, published in 1991. The fourth edition of the text *Air and Surface Transport Nursing: Principles and Practice* was awarded the *American Journal of Nursing* Book of the Year in 2011.

ASTNA is recognized worldwide as the professional organization for nurses practicing in the critical care transport industry.

International Association of Flight and Critical Care Paramedics

The National Flight Paramedic Association, now known as the International Association of Flight and Critical Care Paramedics (IAFCCP), was founded in 1984 and formally incorporated in 1986.[33,35] Although originally founded as a nonprofit association to represent the interests of flight paramedics, the association has expanded its depth and representation into critical care transport both in the air and on the ground. The IAFCCP is committed to providing education, representation, and advocating for the critical care and flight paramedic profession. Transport safety has remained a paramount concern for the association, and they have partnered with various other industry and governmental organizations in support of transport safety initiatives.

In 1998 founding association board member and past president Tim Hynes was killed in a tragic air medical crash in Utah. Tim's loss reaffirmed the association's commitment to averting future industry tragedies. In 2000 the association's Flight Paramedic of the Year Award was renamed the Tim Hynes Award and annually recognizes an association member for their outstanding contributions to leadership, education, and safety. In 2013 the IAFCCP facilitated the creation of a separate charity named the Tim Hynes Foundation. The foundation's goal is to create opportunities through career development, access to education, and programs to improve leadership abilities that will reinforce and advance medical transport safety. Currently, the foundation provides an annual scholarship to the Safety Management Training Academy.

The IAFCCP has furthered its dedication to transport safety through its continued support and membership with the industry's principal accrediting organization, the Commission on Accreditation of Medical Transport Systems (CAMTS). The IAFCCP was present at the first inaugural meeting of CAMTS in 1990 and has maintained steady representation on their board of directors to maintain a voice in developing and implementing industry standards that impact the role of critical care and flight paramedics. In 2016 the IAFCCP furthered its position as an international advocate for paramedic practice by serving as a founding member organization of the Commission on Accreditation of Medical Transport Systems–Europe (CAMTS-EU), which is based in Zurich, Switzerland.

In 2000 the IAFCCP undertook its most visible step in standardizing the practice of flight paramedicine with the introduction of the FP-C. To maintain the highest level of currency and applicability of the examination, the IAFCCP assisted in the creation of the Board for Critical Care Transport Paramedic Certification (BCCTPC) and turned over control of the examination process to this organization while maintaining representation on their Board of Directors. The BCCTPC subsequently expanded its examination offerings to include the CCP-C examination, which has become the first nationally accepted certification for critical care paramedics. Both the FP-C and CCP-C are currently recognized by CAMTS and have been embraced by the international transport community as well, with the first European offering of the FP-C examination occurring in Germany in 2009. The IAFCCP continues to directly support its membership through the examination process by providing a variety of examination preparatory courses, review texts, and discounts.

The IAFCCP continues to foster positive working relationships with other air medical and EMS industry organizations and has continued its pledge of advocacy by participating in several governmental meetings and lobbying activities. In 2010 the IAFCCP participated in the Federal Interagency Committee of EMS meeting; the 2011 EMS stakeholder's meeting in Washington, DC; and in the 2012 National Association of Emergency Medical Technicians, "EMS on the Hill Day." The association continues as a supporting organization of both the annual Air Medical Transport Conference and the Critical Care Transport Medicine Conference.

Founded in 1986, the *National Flight Paramedic Association* (NPFA) was originally created to advocate for paramedics that are involved in critical care transport by air. Over the years the association has grown to advocate for paramedics that operate in many nontraditional roles, and in 2022, its name was changed to the International College of Advanced Practice Paramedics (I-CAPP). "The I-CAPP provides advocacy, leadership development and educational opportunities for Advanced Practice Paramedics practicing in traditional and nontraditional roles and environments. We strive to strengthen and unite critical caregivers to enhance safe, efficient, and quality patient care worldwide."

Commission on Accreditation of Medical Transport Systems

CAMTS is an independent, nonprofit agency established in 1990 (as Commission for the Accreditation of Air Medical Service [CAAMS]) that audits and accredits fixed-wing and rotary-wing air medical transport services as well as ground interfacility transport services in the United States based on a set of industry-established criteria.[40]

The idea of CAMTS came from individuals in the transport environment who were concerned about the number of accidents and lack of standards in the air transport industry. Led by a flight nurse, Eileen Frazer, who is now the CAMTS Executive Director, representatives from all who are involved in patient transport established standards that encompass the education and training of personnel, the function and safety of transport vehicles, and medical care of ill and injured patients.

CAMTS first enacted its Accreditation Standards in 1991, which were developed by its member organizations as well as with extensive public comment and input. The criterion includes patient care standards, safety standards, and logistical and financial standards. The 12th edition of these standards will be published in 2023.

The CAMTS Accreditation Standards address issues related to patient care and safety for rotor wing, fixed wing, ground critical care, ALS, BLS, and Medical Escort Services. There is now CAMTS Global, which has accredited several transport services around the world. In recent years, accreditation has been made available for Special Operation Services (https://www.camts.org/standards/).

International Association of Medical Transport Communications Specialists

The International Association of Medical Transport Communications Specialists (IAMTCS), formerly known as the National Association of Air Communication Specialists (NAACS), was founded in 1989.[41] IAMTCS is a not-for-profit professional organization whose mission is to provide advocacy in medical patient logistics for operational control air and ground communications specialists. IAMTCS has helped create standards and training tools for communication specialists in critical care and air medical transport with the Certified Flight Communicator certification.

Air Medical Physician Association

The Air Medical Physician Association (AMPA) is an international organization committed to patient-focused, quality critical care transport medicine by promoting excellence in medical direction, research, education, safety, leadership, and collaboration.[42] AMPA published the *Principles and Direction of Air Medical Transport,* which is a comprehensive text that lays the foundation for transport medicine. The second edition of this text, published in 2015, provides additional information and tools to assist medical directors and transport team members in providing safe and competent care in the transport environment. AMPA is the largest worldwide professional organization of physicians dedicated to air medical and critical care ground transport.

National Emergency Medicine Service Pilots Association

The National EMS Pilots Association (NEMPSA) was founded in 1984.[43] NEMSPA is a professional organization dedicated to serving pilots involved in the air medical transport industry and to improving the quality and safety of those services. It has published position papers such as *Night Vision Goggles in Helicopter Emergency Medical Services, Sleep and Fatigue Management* and created online tools for Risk Assessment and Helipad Safety. NESMPA is recognized worldwide as the professional organization for pilots operating specifically in air medical transport.

Summary

Patient transport has been a part of patient care since patients required movement for definitive care, originating with the transport of patients from the battlefield to areas of safety.

Transport nursing originated through the work of nursing pioneers, such as Florence Nightingale, Clara Barton, Marie Marvingt, and Lauretta M. Schimmoler, whose theories and work became integral to patient care before and during transport. As the principles of flight and ground transport care were incorporated into civilian care, hospital-based transport programs were started and staffed by transport nurses.

Paramedics have been involved in patient transport since the beginning of the 20th century from their origins as battlefield care providers. Their role in critical care transport has continued to expand to critical care paramedics and flight paramedics.

In 1988 the US Department of Transportation published the Air Medical Crew National Standard Curriculum. This publication encompasses basic and advanced curriculum for the education and training of air medical transport teams. In 1990 the CAAMS, now known as CAMTS, began evaluating both helicopter and fixed-wing air medical transport services. Today, CAMTS is now evaluating ground and international transport programs.

The history of patient transport provides an understanding of where we in transport have come from and where we are going. We must be familiar with and take pride in our origins as we forge into the future. Combining the expertise of many professions provides optimum patient care during all modes and phases of the transport process.[44]

References

1. Corbett P, Wolfe AC. *A Legacy of Caring: Generations of Critical Transport.* Air and Surface Transport Nurses Association; 2018.
2. *History of Patient Transport.* 2016. https://aneskey.com/1-history-of-patient-transport/. Accessed June 27, 2023.
3. Barkley K. *The Ambulance.* Exposition Press; 1990.
4. Bell R. *The Ambulance: A History.* McFarland & Company; 2009.
5. Blumen I (Editor in Chief). *Principles and Direction in Air Medical Transport.* 2nd ed. Air Medical Physicians Association; 2015.
6. Dick W. Anglo-American vs. Franco-German emergency medical services system. *Prehosp Disaster Med.* 2003;18(1):29–35.
7. Donahue P. *Nursing: The Finest Art.* 2nd ed. Mosby; 1996.
8. Eisenberg M, Pantridge J, Cobb L, et al. The revolution and evolution of cardiac care. *Arch Intern Med.* 1996;12(26):1–15.
9. Browne B, Jacobs L, Pollack C. *Emergency Care and Transportation of the Sick and Injured.* 7th ed. Jones & Bartlett; 1999.
10. Gonsalves D. Historical background of emergency medical services in the United States. *Emerg Care Q.* 1988;4(3):77.
11. Haller J. *Battlefield Medicine: A History of the Military Ambulance From the Napoleonic Wars Through World War I.* Southern Illinois University Press; 1992.
12. Holleran RS. *Prehospital Nursing: A Collaborative Approach.* Mosby; 1994.
13. Link MM, Coleman HA. *Medical Support of the Army Air Forces in World War II.* Society for Military History; 1955.
14. McCall W. *The American Ambulance: 1900–2002.* Enthusiast Books; 2002.
15. Division of Medical Sciences, Committee on Trauma and Committee on Shock. *Accidental Death and Disability: The Neglected Disease of Modern Society.* National Academy of Sciences-National Research Council; 1966.
16. Porter R. *The Greatest Benefit to Mankind: A Medical History of Humanity.* Knopf; 1999.

17. Skandalakis P, et al. To afford the wounded speedy assistance: Dominique Jean Larrey and Napoleon. *World J Surg.* 2006;30(8): 1392–1399.
18. Carter G. The evolution of air transport systems: A pictorial review. *J Emerg Med.* 1986;6(6):499–504.
19. Helicopter EMS: Part I: A brief history. 2016. Accessed July 10, 2016. http://www.emsworld.com/article/10319182/helicopter-ems
20. McNab A. Air medical transport: "Hot air" and a French lesson. *J Air Med Trans.* 1992;11(8):15–16.
21. Ortiz J. The revolutionary flying ambulance of Napoleon's surgeon. *U.S. Army Med Dep J.* 1998;8:17–25.
22. WWII helicopter evacuation. 2016. Accessed July 9, 2016. http://olive-drab.com/od_medical_evac_helio_korea.php
23. Lam DM. Marie Marvingt and the development of aeromedical evacuation. *Aviat Space Environ Med.* 2003;74(8):863–868.
24. Royal Flying Doctor Service. Our history. 2016. Accessed July 9, 2016. https://www.flyingdoctor.org.au/about-the-rfds/history/
25. History of Queensland Ambulance Service. 2016. Accessed July 10, 2016. http://www.ambulance.qld.gov.au/about/
26. Rega History. 2016. Accessed July 9, 2016. https://en.wikipedia.org/wiki/Rega_(air_rescue)
27. State of Mississippi. *Extension of Project CARESOM: Final Report.* State Press; 1971.
28. Bader GB, Terhorst M, Heilman P, et al. Characteristics of flight nursing practice. *Air Med J.* 1995;14(4):214–218.
29. Grimes M, Mason J. Evolution of flight nursing and the National Flight Nurses Association. *Air Med J.* 1991;10(11):19–22.
30. Thomas F. The early years of flight nursing. *Hospital Aviation.* 1986;5(10):6–8.
31. Lee G. History of flight nursing. *J Emerg Nurs.* 1987;13(4):212.
32. Wheeler D, Poss W. Pediatric transport medicine. In: Wheeler D, Wong H, Shanley T, eds. *Resuscitation and Stabilization of the Critically Ill Child.* Springer-Verlag; 2009:125–136.
33. Kuehl A, ed. *Prehospital Systems and Medical Oversight.* 3rd ed. National Association of EMS Physicians; 2000.
34. Jaynes C, Werman H, White L. A blueprint for critical care transport research. *Air Med J.* 2013;32(1):30–35.
35. International Association of Flight and Critical Care Paramedics. 2016. Accessed July 9, 2016. http://www.iafccp.org/
36. International Board of Specialty Certification. 2016. Accessed August 6, 2016. http://www.ibscertifications.org/about/about-us
37. Thomas F, Robinson K, Judge T, et al. The 2003 Air Medical Leadership Congress: Findings and recommendations. *Air Med J.* 2004; 23(3):20–36.
38. Association of Air Medical Services. 2016. Accessed July 9, 2016. http://aams.org/
39. Air and Surface Transport Association. 2016. Accessed July 9, 2016. http://aams.org/
40. Commission on Accreditation of Medical Transport Systems (CAMTS). 2016. Accessed July 9, 2016. http://www.camts.org/
41. International Association of Medical Transport Communication Specialists. 2017. Accessed January 18, 2017. http://www.iamtcs.org
42. Air Medical Physicians Association. 2016. Accessed July 9, 2016. http://www.ampa.org/
43. National Association of EMS Pilots. 2016. Accessed July 9, 2016. http://www.nemspa.org/index.php
44. Mattera C, Hutton K, Allenstein T. No box of chocolates. *Air Med J.* 2001;20(5):4–5.

2

Members of the Transport Team and Preparation for Practice

JULIUS J. MCADAMS

Patient transport has become a widespread theme in the provision of care for many ill and injured patients, and interfacility and emergent patient transports have continued to increase in recent years.[1] In the out-of-hospital setting, transport may be required for significantly ill or injured patients who are unable to be stabilized in the prehospital setting. Transport may also be needed for patients that require treatment by specialty medical teams, technologies, or equipment that is not available at a referring facility. Critical care transport is a collaborative practice and process that requires coordination between clinical teams at the referring facility, the receiving facility, and the transport team. The scope and mission of the transport program, types of patients transported, and regulations of state nursing boards and emergency medical services (EMS) authorities contribute to transport team configurations. It is of utmost importance that the members of the transport team are able to provide the level of care needed by the patient and mission profile. The transport program must be able to safely and competently provide the level of care described in its mission statement and scope of care.

A team approach to patient transport is paramount. The goals of a transport team are to maintain or enhance the level of care from the referring facility or agency and render interventions as appropriate. This chapter will provide an overview of some of the members of the transport team along with the preparation needed to fulfill the responsibilities for those roles.

Transport Team Members (Air and Surface)

With advances in medical care came the need to maintain the care for increasingly complex cases that require a level of care equivalent to intensive care units (ICUs) at tertiary care hospitals during transport. The role of the transport professional has evolved over time to include individuals from all disciplines. Crew pairing may involve professionals with similar training and experience or differing skill sets and education. Both configurations have demonstrated benefits in consideration of the patient demographic, scope of practice, mode of transport, and accepted or recognized clinician practice. Although some general characteristics do exist among these professionals, the specific responsibilities and practice protocols depend on the mission profile of the type of service provided, the crew matrix, the type of vehicles used for transport, and state regulations.[2]

In 1998, the Emergency Nurses Association and the National Flight Nurses Association (now known as the Air and Surface Transport Nurses Association [ASTNA]) released a joint position paper that described the role of nursing in the prehospital environment.[3] This document denotes that nurses who practice in the prehospital care environment need to be appropriately educated to function successfully in that role. It further recommends that nurses who practice must be regulated by the state boards of nursing in the state(s) in which the transport nurse practices in place of EMS agencies governing nursing practice. The different training and expertise of nurses, paramedics, respiratory therapists (RTs), advanced practice providers such as nurse practitioners (NPs) and physician assistants (PAs), and physicians complements the transport team, providing focused care for patients requiring transport. The evolution to air rescue has required those professionals that routinely practice within the confines of the hospital to leave that setting and learn the nuances of providing care in the out-of-hospital arena. Simultaneously, specialized skills that were once reserved for the hospital setting have found their way into the paramedic scope of practice.[4,5]

ASTNA acknowledges that staffing with the most appropriate healthcare provider reduces the risk of poor patient outcomes. State boards of nursing, local EMS regulations, and even some national paramedic and physicians' associations have provided input into the practice of transport professionals. Clinical staffing models based on the level of care required by the patient during the transport have been routinely accepted within the transport industry; however, no consistent nexuses recognized beyond state and local regulations exist today.

The Commission on Accreditation of Medical Transport Services (CAMTS) is a nonprofit organization dedicated to improving the quality and safety of medical transport services. CAMTS accreditation standards address issues of patient care and safety in fixed and rotary-wing services, as well as ground interfacility services, providing critical care transports. Each standard is supported by measurable criteria that are used to benchmark a program's level of quality. The accreditation process is a voluntary evaluation of compliance with accreditation standards demonstrating the ability to deliver service of a specific quality.[6] Because of the level of accreditation standards set forth by CAMTS, achieving this accreditation is considered a prestigious accomplishment and is the standard used by many originations in the transport industry. CAMTS has defined team members based on the level of care required to fulfill the mission of the transport. Table 2.1[7] describes the different types of missions and clinical crew configurations based on the scope of care as defined by the CAMTS standard.

While transport team configurations may vary based on the scope of care dictated by patient needs, all team members must possess some level of training and education regarding the environment they will be operating in, and the equipment they will be utilizing. For example, team members must be familiar with aircraft and/or ground vehicle safety practices, proper use of radios or communication devices, emergency survival training, clinical equipment, and medications. Transport team staffing and education should be commensurate with the mission statement and scope of care of the medical transport service. The transport vehicle, by virtue of how it is staffed and medically equipped, becomes a patient care unit specific to the needs of the patient. The team that transports that patient must be appropriately educated and trained in patient management before, during, and after the transport process.[8–12]

The Transport Nurse

The RN has had a role in patient transport and the prehospital environment for numerous years. Discussion continues about what qualifications a nurse should have to practice in the transport environment. The ASTNA developed a position paper that addresses some of these issues. The preparation for patient care required to practice nursing, along with the appropriate experience and education, provides a sound foundation for practice in the prehospital and transport environments. However, that preparation rarely includes the skills needed to deliver patient care in the prehospital environment. ASTNA supports State Boards of Nursing or, in other countries, the equivalent regulatory bodies for the profession of nursing. It believes that services providing critical care transport are functional extensions of hospital emergency departments and critical care or specialty units and that staffing for these services should minimally consist of at least one professional transport nurse. ASTNA pursues recognition by state EMS agencies, or their equivalent, for the unique role of an RN to practice in the prehospital environment. The RN who practices

TABLE 2.1	Transport Team Definitions	
Mission	**Definition**

Basic life support (BLS)	Preface – appropriate AHJ applies
	1. Scope of Care
	   Capability to deliver prehospital basic life support care
	2. System
	   State-recognized agency or AHJ with a medical director who meets requirements listed below
	3. Clinical Crew
	   At a minimum, one crew member has EMT status (paramedic preferred) or equivalent national training
	   Vehicle operator is EVOC trained (or equivalent) and keeps training properly updated
	4. Medical Director
	   The medical director should be board certified in emergency medicine, but if he or she is not, it is strongly recommended that the medical director be board certified in family medicine, internal medicine, surgery, or pediatrics with demonstrated EMS education (e.g., NAEMSP medical director course) or 5 years of experience in emergency medicine
	5. Equipment
	   Oral/pharyngeal airway
	   Pulse oximeter
	   Automatic external defibrillator
	   Bag-valve mask
	   Glucometer
	   Adequate oxygen source
	   Hemorrhage control supplies/equipment (such as tourniquets, packing materials)
	   Depends on state/local or national requirements, or medical director requirements (e.g., autoinjector)
	6. Medications
	   EMT may assist patient in taking own medication
	   Depends on state/local or national requirements, or medical director requirements
	7. Interventions
	   Bag-valve mask ventilation and oxygenation
	   Selective spinal immobilization
	   Noninvasive vital sign measurement (e.g., blood pressure, pulse oximetry)
	   Control of bleeding (refer www.stopthebleedingfoundation.org)
	   Exposure (infection) control
	   Depends on state/local or national requirements, medical director requirements

Advanced life support (ALS)	Preface – appropriate AHJ applies – also includes all aspects of BLS
	1. Scope of Care
	   Capability to deliver prehospital advanced life support care
	2. Clinical Crew
	   A minimum of two medical personnel who are licensed/certified according to state and/or national requirements. The vehicle operator may be the second crew member for surface ALS if he/she is at minimum an EMT and is EVOC-trained (or equivalent) and his/her training is kept current.
	   One is a paramedic with National Registered Paramedic (NRP) or national equivalent preferred.

Continued

TABLE 2.1 Transport Team Definitions—cont'd

Mission	Definition
	3. Medical Director The medical director should be board certified in emergency medicine, but if he or she is not, it is strongly recommended that the medical director be board certified in family medicine, internal medicine, surgery, or pediatrics with demonstrated EMS education or 5 years of experience in emergency medicine. 4. Equipment – includes all equipment in BLS plus: Ventilation – ventilators and noninvasive ventilators (CPAP/bilevel positive airway pressure) with the capability to utilize blended gases Cardiac monitoring (e.g., ECG monitor with 12-lead capabilities, pacemaker, manual defibrillator) Noninvasive monitoring (e.g., waveform capnography, pulse oximetry) 5. Medications – include all medications in BLS plus: Resuscitative medications by national EMS education and practice standards. 6. Interventions – includes all interventions in BLS plus: Advanced airway management (endotracheal intubation, supraglottic airway) Needle thoracostomy Intraosseous placement Peripheral IV
Critical care	Preface – appropriate Authority Having Jurisdiction (AHJ) applies – also includes all aspects of BLS and ALS 1. Scope of Care Capability to deliver out-of-hospital care during the acute resuscitation phase before definitive care is provided (e.g., comparable to emergency department stabilizing care or an ICU transfer to more definitive care) 2. Clinical Crew A minimum of two medical personnel (who are licensed according to state and/or national requirements) who provide direct patient care plus a vehicle operator The primary care provider of the clinical crew may be a resident or staff physician, advanced practice nurse, registered nurse, physician assistant, or paramedic. The primary care provider must have 3 years of critical care experience. (Critical care experience is defined as no less than 4000 hours' experience in an ICU or an emergency department.) In addition, nurses, physician assistants, and paramedics clinicians in the primary care provider role must have prehire experience and/or education in the medications and interventions as defined in the program's scope of care and services listed below as well as IABP management (if part of scope of care), central line monitoring, left arterial wedge pressure monitoring, and ventilator management. Additionally, medical directors and clinical leadership must have direct responsibility to qualify the experience and competencies of applicants for a primary care provider role and set the minimums as they pertain to the autonomous care required for their specific scope of service. If crew member is a paramedic, 3 years (minimum of 4000 hours) of ALS experience is required. If crew member is a respiratory therapist, then 3 years (minimum of 4000 hours) of ED or ICU experience is required; ICU experience may be a combination of dealing with adult, pediatric, and/or neonatal patients (see section 03.05.01 3. Competencies for advanced certifications). 3. Medical Director Board-certified based on the program scope of care. Additional specialty and/or subspecialty physician liaison(s) as required 4. Equipment – includes all equipment in BLS and ALS plus: Ventilation – multimodality ventilators capable of invasive ventilation (pressure, volume, ventilator appropriate to all age groups transported) Invasive hemodynamic monitoring (e.g., transvenous pacemakers, central venous pressure, and arterial pressure) 5. Medications – includes all medications in BLS and ALS plus: Management of continuous infusions (e.g., vasopressors, antihypertensives, antidysrhythmics, bronchodilators, neuromuscular blockade, and sedation) 6. Interventions – includes all interventions in BLS and ALS plus: Medication-facilitated airway (including intubation) rapid sequence induction (medication facilitated) Surgical airway Ability to manage tube thoracostomy Ability to manage central line Blood product infusion management Continuous targeted temperature management (i.e., therapeutic hypothermia) Ability to perform decompressive thoracostomy (if in scope of care)

TABLE 2.1	Transport Team Definitions—cont'd
Mission	**Definition**
Specialty care	1. Scope of Care Capability to deliver out-of-hospital care at a specialty or subspecialty level during interfacility transport (e.g., comparable to that of a tertiary or quaternary such as an ICU, PICU, NICU, or tertiary perinatal center). Neonatal transport is defined as the ability to support the care of infants that continue to need mechanical thermoregulation and/or respiratory support. Respiratory support should include the capability to provide blended gases. Neonatal transport includes both preterm and term infants who require critical care or any infant under 5 kg. Specialty high-risk OB transports are defined as transports that include the use and interpretation of external fetal monitor, fetal Doppler, and tocolytics. The transporting of obstetrical patients to, and requiring care from, a subspecialty care (Level III) or regional perinatal healthcare center (Level IV) as defined by the American College of Obstetricians and Gynecologists (ACOG). A specialty care pediatric transport is defined as the ability to support an infant or child with life-threatening physiologic derangement, including respiratory, cardiac, and/or central nervous system, and meeting criteria for admission to a pediatric ICU. 2. Clinical Crew (as appropriate to the scope of care) 3. Medical Director Board-certified based on the program scope of care. Additional specialty and/or subspecialty physician liaison(s) as required by the scope of care 4. Equipment – includes all equipment in BLS, ALS, and critical care (as appropriate to the scope of care) Transcutaneous ventricular assist devices (e.g., LVAD, BiVAD, RVAD). Extracorporeal membrane oxygenation (ECMO) therapies and devices. Inhaled gases (e.g., nitric oxide, Heliox, aerosolized prostacyclin). Neonatal isolette with heart rate monitoring device and size-appropriate ventilator (with blender for adjustable oxygen delivery), thermoregulation control, and infusion devices (syringe pumps). Fetal Doppler/fetal heart rate monitoring device (if transporting high-risk obstetrics – HROB). For long-range transports, external cardiotocography monitoring device is required. 5. Medications – includes all interventions in BLS, ALS, and critical care (as appropriate to the scope of care) Maintenance of tertiary/quaternary critical care formulary (tocolytics for HROB) 6. Interventions include all interventions in BLS, ALS, and critical care (as appropriate to the scope of care) Ability to place central line (if in scope of care) Managing cardiac assist device Managing extracorporeal oxygenation device Ability to place endotracheal tube and maintain oxygenation and ventilation on a multimodality ventilator with capabilities for all age populations transported, including the capability to deliver inhaled specialty gases

in the out-of-hospital and transport environment must be properly prepared to deliver patient care safely and competently in this exceptional and challenging environment.

In 2015, ASTNA published a specific position paper that recommends the qualifications a transport nurse should have before being hired as a member of a transport team. These qualifications are summarized in Box 2.1.[8]

Additionally, CAMTS requires the Transport RN to have a current transport-specific nursing certification Certified Flight Registered Nurse (CFRN) or Certified Transport Registered Nurse (CTRN) pertinent to the scope of care and patient population (such as Certified in Neonatal Pediatric Transport (C-NPT) for teams that transport neonatal or pediatric patients).[7]

The CFRN and the CTRN were created through the work of ASTNA (formally known as the National Flight Nurses Association) and the Board of Certification for Emergency Nursing. A member of ASTNA is appointed to the board, and transport nurses are item writers for the examinations. ASTNA publishes the *Flight and Ground Transport Nursing and Paramedic Core Curriculum*, which contains the knowledge needed for transport nursing practice. ASTNA also publishes review manuals and has other materials available for review for preparation for both the CFRN and the CTRN examinations. More information about these resources can be found at http://astna.org/.

• BOX 2.1 Qualifications for Transport Nurses

- Registered nurse (with appropriate state/provincial licensure)
- Minimum 3 years' critical care or emergency department experience
- Specialty certification commensurate with previous experience (CEN, CCRN, CFRN, or CTRN within 2 years of hire)
- Basic cardiac life support or equivalent
- Age-specific ACLS and/or PALS, NRP, PEPP, and ENPC or equivalent
- TPATC, ATLS, or equivalent
- Objective assessment of the transport nurse applicant's qualifications for transport based on, but not limited to, the following characteristics:
  - Educational and experiential background
  - Technical and clinical competence
  - Leadership skills
  - Critical thinking skills
  - Proficient communication and interpersonal skills
  - Appreciation of public and community relations

ACLS, Advanced cardiac life support; *ATLS,* advanced trauma life support; *CCRN,* Critical Care Registered Nurse; *CEN,* certified emergency nurse; *CFRN,* Certified Flight Registered Nurse; *CTRN,* certified transport registered nurse; *ENPC,* Emergency Nursing Pediatric Course; *NRP,* Neonatal Resuscitation Program; *PALS,* pediatric advanced life support; *PEPP,* Pediatric Education for Prehospital Professionals; *TPATC,* Transport Professional Advanced Trauma Course.

The Advanced Practice Registered Nurse (APRN) has been a part of many transport teams for years, especially neonatal NP. As the role of the APRN has developed and grown, some services have included them, especially the acute care NP, who has been specifically educated to manage the critically ill or injured patient. However, as previously noted, transport teams need to be composed of the appropriate members based on their mission and scope of service.[12]

The Transport Paramedic

The International College of Advanced Practice Paramedics (I-CAPP; formally known as the International Association of Flight and Critical Care Paramedics) supports the utilization of paramedics in air medical and critical care transport environments.[13] The

certified flight paramedic (FP-C) examination and the certified critical care paramedic (CCP-C) certifications were developed to help clarify what preparation is necessary for an advanced role as a paramedic performing air medical and critical care ground transport, respectively. Box 2.2 provides a summary of the I-CAPP's recommendations for the qualifications for flight and critical care transport paramedics.[13–15]

Like the Transport RN, CAMTS requires the Transport Paramedic to have a current transport-specific board certification for the environment that they are operating in: FP-C for flight and CCP-C for ground critical care.[7]

To combat this ambiguity and the lack of a nationally recognized flight paramedic examination, the National Flight Paramedics Association (now known as the I-CAPP) introduced the FP-C examination. This examination was created on the premise that

---

• BOX 2.2   Qualifications for a Transport Paramedic

- Minimum of 3 years' experience or full-time employment as a paramedic in a busy advanced life support EMS system
- Education
- Primary: Successful completion of the paramedic National Standard Curriculum or equivalent
- Secondary: Successful completion of a critical care education program that meets or exceeds the educational objectives of this position statement, including didactic sessions, practical sessions, skill proficiency demonstration, and clinical rotations
- Tertiary: Continuing mentored didactic education, skill maintenance, and clinical opportunities that maintain the educational objectives of this position statement
- Certifications:
  - Advanced Cardiac Life Support (ACLS)
  - Transport Professional Advanced Trauma Course (TPATC), International Trauma Life Support (ITLS) Adult and Pediatric, Prehospital Trauma Life Support (PHTLS), or Advanced Trauma Life Support (ATLS)
  - Pediatric Advanced Life Support (PALS) or Advanced Pediatric Life Support (APLS)
  - Neonatal Resuscitation Program
  - Or an equivalent education in each of the previously mentioned areas
- Knowledge of the assessment for the critically ill or injured patient
- Advanced adult and pediatric airway management including, but not limited to, the following:
  - RSI intubation
  - Alternative and rescue airways
  - Surgical cricothyroidotomy
  - Continuous waveform capnography to monitor $ETCO_2$
  - Mechanical and noninvasive ventilation theory, troubleshooting, and competence
  - Chest tube thoracostomy management and insertion (if applicable)
  - Obtain and maintain peripheral venous, central venous (if applicable), and/or intraosseous access
  - Administration of blood and blood products
  - ECG monitoring and 12-lead ECG interpretation
  - Defibrillation; cardioversion; and transcutaneous and transvenous pacing monitoring, maintenance, and treatment
  - Circulatory management and support including invasive hemodynamic monitoring and IABP management (theory, transport considerations, troubleshooting, and operations, if applicable)
  - Intracranial pressure monitoring and management
  - Pharmacology included in the National Standard Curriculum augmented by knowledge of analgesics, antibiotics, antidysrhythmics, antiepileptics, paralytics, sedatives, and vasoactive medications
  - Laboratory value interpretation including arterial blood gas analysis
  - Targeted radiology study interpretation

- Patient management:
  - Acute respiratory emergencies
  - Cardiovascular emergencies
  - Hypertensive emergencies
  - Shock and multiorgan system failure
  - Infectious diseases
  - Neurologic emergencies including stroke and intracranial hemorrhage
  - Trauma
  - Spinal cord injury
  - Burn
  - Trauma in pregnancy
  - Pediatric trauma
  - Critical pediatric emergencies
  - Obstetric emergencies
  - Neonatal emergencies (if applicable)
  - Environmental emergencies
  - Poisoning/toxic exposure/hazardous material awareness
  - Bioterrorism
- Transport medicine:
  - Safety
  - Vehicle operations and emergency procedures
  - Critical care transport equipment
  - Patient/family factors
  - Human factors (including but not limited to AMRM or equivalent)
  - Evaluation of appropriateness for transport based on required level of care
  - Transport logistics
  - Critical care transport equipment (ventilator, IABP, neonatal isolette, etc.)
  - Patient packaging for safety and accessibility
  - Radio and communication technology
  - Transport physiology
  - Interaction and communication with medical oversight
  - Medical provider communication/transfer of care
  - Documentation
- Quality management: Understanding principles and best practice
- Certification examination: Successful completion of a critical care paramedic certification examination. Along with the FP-C, the I-CAPP and CAMTS recognizes the CCP-C as a valid certification examination for the critical care paramedic

AMRM, Air medical resource management; *CCP-C,* Critical Care Paramedic Certification Examination; *ECG,* electrocardiogram; *EMS,* Emergency Medical Service; *ETCO₂,* end-tidal carbon dioxide; *FP-C,* certified flight paramedic; *IABP,* intraaortic balloon pump; *IAFCCP,* International Association of Flight and Critical Care Paramedics; *RSI,* rapid sequence induction.

most flight paramedics function as critical care providers. Therefore, the certification process that defines the practice of the flight paramedic not only is based on an understanding of basic paramedic skills and flight physiology but also incorporates an understanding of critical care theory and practice.

Following the success of the FP-C examination, a separate board, the Board for Critical Care Transport Paramedic Certification (BCCTPC), was created to oversee the continued development of the FP-C examination and the eventual creation and implementation of a critical care ground transport–specific paramedic certification, the CCP-C. The focus of the CCP-C board certification is on the knowledge level of experienced paramedics who practice as a member of a critical care transport team. The examination is not meant to test entry-level knowledge. In January 2016, the BCCTPC moved to expand its role within specialty certifications, thus forming the International Board of Specialty Certification (IBSC), which currently oversees the FP-C and CCP-C examinations as well as a variety of other specialized transport and paramedic certifications.[16–18]

Respiratory Therapist

Although nurse-paramedic team configurations are the predominant dynamic, many transport teams include an RT as either a primary team member or an additional team member. Ventilatory management is an integral part of the management of critically ill and injured patients and, in many cases, includes the use of ventilatory equipment and assessment parameters that other members of the transport team do not consistently use. RTs typically work in hospitals, in which they perform assessments, diagnostics, intensive critical care procedures, and patient interventions for all patient populations, from the neonate to the geriatric.[19]

Respiratory care requires education in physics (gas laws), biology, pharmacology, chemistry, and microbiology. An RT possesses specific skill sets to perform multiple clinical interventions valued in the out-of-hospital critical care setting. For example, RTs are often trained in arterial line and chest tube insertion; intubation; surgical airways; medication administration (inhalation and parenteral); and management of high-technology medical equipment such as mechanical ventilation, intraaortic balloon pump, and pulmonary artery catheter monitoring.[19]

The American Association of Respiratory Care has a section for surface and air transport members that provides specific information about the roles of a transport RT. The therapist's role on the team must be well defined and, again, within the scope of practice in the geographic area in which he or she practices.[5] Like the other members of the transport them, the qualifications, education, and training for transport RTs are based on the scope and mission of the transport program for which they work. This training should include safety, survival, and operating within individual transport vehicles.[19]

Physicians

Physicians have been members of transport teams in some areas of the United States and the world since the inception of hospital-based helicopter programs.[20] Reasons cited for the use of a physician as a part of a transport team include medical/clinical judgment, technical skills, clinical experience, and the marketing value of having a physician on board.[20,21]

Physicians may contribute to the care provided by the team directly or indirectly: directly as a member of the critical care transport team and indirectly through the provision of medical direction or clinical oversight responsible for all aspects of care provided or as a liaison with other specialty care physicians. The level of expertise of transport physicians may range from that of a resident physician to that of an experienced board-certified physician specialist.

The transport environment can provide physicians with valuable training experience. The physician can bring medical expertise, possibly reduce medical legal issues, and provide important public relations in the prehospital environment.[12]

In programs in which physicians are not used as transport team members, control of medical direction of the transport team is often provided by assigning a physician responsible for the actions of the transport team. This medical control physician has the responsibility of overseeing that the correct team (e.g., adult, pediatric, neonatal), appropriate team configuration (e.g., RN/paramedic, paramedic/paramedic, RN/RN, RN/RT, specialty care team), correct equipment (e.g., ALS, BLS, specialized), and appropriate mode of transport (e.g., helicopter, fixed-wing, ground) are selected to meet the patient's transport medical needs and that appropriate medical backup is available to the transport team.

Physician Medical Director

The primary responsibility of the physician medical director is to provide administrative medical oversight and medical quality management and improvement over the transport program. Specifically, the physician medical director's role includes but is not limited to (1) helping develop, review, and approve medical protocols or guidelines; (2) providing oversight of medical crew member training; (3) providing oversight of medical control physicians; (4) providing quality improvement oversight for the medical care rendered by the transport service; (5) providing support for medical team members; and (6) assisting in the clarification and resolution of transport issues that may arise during the transport or from the referring or receiving agency.

The educational and experiential qualifications of an individual medical director are dictated by the mission profile of the relevant service. For patients who need specialty transports, medical direction may remain with the program medical director. Specialty-trained physicians (i.e., neonatologist, pediatric, adult critical care–trained) may be consulted, or the responsibility to provide medical control or oversight for specific cases may be delegated to that individual.[11,22]

The CAMTS standards provide educational and clinical recommendations for physicians involved in critical care transport. Moreover, Air Medical Physician Association (AMPA) offers robust resources for medical directors in their course Medical Director Core Curriculum and in the textbook *Principles and Direction of Air Medical Transport*.[11,23]

Identify Medical Protocols

For the transport service that does not routinely use physicians as transport team members, the medical director is responsible for identifying, reviewing, and approving medical protocols or guidelines that enable the transport team to initiate care treatments and procedures considered outside the routine practice of their individual disciplines. Although the transport medical director may not directly write these protocols, they are the physician that is ultimately responsible for the content and accuracy of these protocols. Team members, in conjunction with the medical director, develop and revise policies, protocols, or guidelines that guide medical care.

Ensure Adequate Training

The medical director is actively involved in the development of training that ensures that the transport team members can meet the expected level of medical care related to the transport environment. Prospective training occurs through introduction courses to emergency and critical care transport. Such training includes altitude physiology, transport medical care, and advanced procedures (i.e., difficult airway management, chest tube insertion, arterial line insertion, central line insertion, management, etc.). In addition to the initial training, the medical director is actively involved in continuous training and updating of the transport team members regarding new innovations in patient care. The use of items identified in quality improvement retrospective reviews of transport care via transport run report/patient chart review provides feedback for reinforcing or modifying care delivered by the transport team members.

Oversight of Medical Control Physicians

One role of the medical director is to ensure that physicians who provide medical control are educated about the mission and capabilities of the transport service. Clinical discrepancy between medical control and medical flight team members can arise. Under these circumstances, the medical director clarifies the recommended standard of practice for the transport service to both parties. Likewise, control physicians can determine whether additional training may be necessary for selected team members. Contacting the medical director regarding these training issues ensures that proper steps can be taken by the medical director to improve the quality of clinical care.

During transport, the control physician serves as the sounding board and provides medical support to the transport team members. This support may be done before transport so that the physician can provide the transport team members with information regarding the patient's status and with possible diagnostic or therapeutic suggestions. This support can also be provided during the transport, when the transport team recognizes that additional medical input may be beneficial in diagnosing or providing care to the patient.

After the transport, the transport team may discuss the possible diagnostic and therapeutic options related to the patient's condition with the control physician. Such interactions are beneficial because the transport team members gain additional insight and the medical director is able to recognize any need for additional transport team training.

Continuous Quality Improvement

One of the most important roles of the medical director is to provide quality improvement of the medical care provided by the medical team. Carrubba noted[11] that the medical director is specifically responsible for the following:
- Empowerment of flight crew members to identify quality improvement issues and to develop appropriate strategies to study these issues
- Recognition of pertinent quality assurance/continuous quality improvement (CQI) expertise both within and outside the program
- Internal collaboration with institutional quality management coordinators to link the air medical quality management plan to the organizational quality management program
- Contribution of time, knowledge, and action to all aspects of quality management in the program

- Vigorous support for the acquisition of necessary resources and executive-level commitment to all quality management activities

Communication Specialists

Communication is the first step in the transport process. The National Association of Air Medical Communication Specialists has developed a description of the role of the communication specialist in the transport process. In addition, operational control is an integral component of communications and the transport process, which ensures that the operator who holds the aircraft-operating certificate issued by the Federal Aviation Administration (FAA) is fully aware and involved in each movement of the aircraft throughout the transport. More components of the role of the communication specialist, particularly specific functions, are discussed in Chapter 7.

The communication specialist is responsible for obtaining patient information; initiating the operational control process for the transport; tracking the transport (air or ground); and notifying appropriate personnel before, during, and after the transport process. The transport team must always remember that the communication specialist is the "voice" of the transport team and should be treated as a team member and included in decision-making and stress management.

Pilots

Clinical team and pilot interactions play a critical role in the performance of air medical teams. Team-level and organizational factors may enhance or impede the ability of well-trained individuals to work together effectively and efficiently. Each team member's position must be clearly stated and defined, which establishes structure and determines the flow of communication.

The National EMS Pilots Association is dedicated to pilots involved in patient transport and focused on improving the quality and safety of air medical transport.

Pilot-in-Command Qualifications

The FAA mandates that the pilot-in-command (PIC) is responsible for the safety of the aircraft, crew, and passengers, as stated in the Federal Aviation Regulations, Part 91. The pilot is accountable for nonmedical aspects of the flight and has final authority in all flight-related issues. CAMTS outlines the PIC qualifications for both rotorcraft-helicopter and fixed-wing aircraft.[24,25]

The PIC must help maintain a balanced, predictable environment while responding to changing situations. This responsibility implies that shifts of balance occur and that each crew member should understand that they have the responsibility to participate fully and professionally in every flight.

The PIC must establish clear leadership and command authority and appropriately apply the use of authority based on the current situation. He or she will ensure the safety of the flight through strict adherence to the Federal Aviation Regulations as well as the general operations manual of the employer, which may be an air operator company rather than the transport program itself. The pilot must command respect but, at the same time, create an atmosphere conducive to crew participation.

Transport team members assist in flight-related duties as outlined by the individual program or vendor's policies or general operations manual and as reinforced by the PIC. Flight team members offer assistance in a variety of flight duties. Some of their contributions include air or ground traffic sightings, hazard and obstacle sightings, obstacle avoidance procedures (landing zones), cargo (medical equipment) securing, passenger briefing, radio monitoring, and minor participation in the computation of weight and balance requirements.

When time and safety permit, the pilot may also assist the flight team by helping load and unload patients. In addition, the pilot can transport needed medical equipment to the flight team and relay medical information to the receiving hospital.

To optimize program safety, an expectation of safety must override all other considerations. The adage "all to go, one for no" reflects the expectation that any member of the transport team can turn down a flight for safety concerns, and a program's safety environment must support such decision-making. Although an administrative request for justification is reasonable, unjust consequences toward pilots or other transport team members should not exist for turn-downs/flight aborts. Team members should feel safe to prioritize decision-making on the basis of established safety practices, program minimums, and previous flight experience.

The bond between established team members and the air medical staff could become quite strong. The eight goals for a successful relationship between the pilot and transport team members are as follows:
1. Communicate positively.
2. Direct assistance as needed.
3. Announce decisions clearly.
4. Offer assistance.
5. Acknowledge the actions of others.
6. Be specific.
7. Know and understand the team's aviation roles and responsibilities.
8. Be vigilant in understanding the interaction between the team members, the machine, and the environment.

Emergency Vehicle Operators

Drivers of the ground units or mobile ICU are often referred to as emergency vehicle operators (EVOs). The EVO is an active team member but is primarily responsible for the safe operations of the vehicle at all times. The individual must be trained, licensed, and qualified to practice safely and professionally within the unit. He or she must demonstrate proficiency in the mechanical operations of the vehicle, routine vehicle maintenance, emergency vehicle operation as regulated by state and local authorities, proper use of the communication equipment, operation of the patient care equipment, knowledge of the supplies, and possess driving adeptness in varying weather and familiarity with the service area. The EVO may participate in the loading and unloading of the patient and be an active transport team member when the vehicle is not in motion.

Program Manager

In most critical care transport programs, the program manager or director is responsible for coordinating the administrative activities of the transport service. The program director may be an RN, physician, pilot, paramedic, or nonclinical administrator. CAMTS provides some recommendations for the role of a program manager.

The major responsibilities of the program director include formulating administrative policies, directing CQI activities, managing vehicle contracts, negotiating medical equipment purchases or leases, navigating vendor relationships, maintaining the communications system, preparing and monitoring components of the budget, participating in strategic planning and marketing, serving as a resource for problem-solving, and serving as a community liaison.

The Association of Air Medical Services offers a Medical Transport Leadership Institute (MTLI) that has a mission to enhance the management of medical transportation services. This 2-year program offers courses in human resource management, leadership and administration, financial operations, program development, and asset management.[26] Program directors, medical crew supervisors, operators, lead pilots, and other leadership personnel in critical care transport are provided with a framework to strengthen or develop their leadership and administrative skills. A graduate-level program is also offered, which expands on foundational concepts, providing further opportunity for interactive dialog and problem-solving. Networking with proven transport industry leaders is a daily occurrence at all levels and provides excellent opportunity for participants to realistically hone their acquired skills.

Each critical care transport program dictates the role of the program director. The transport team must know and understand the director's role in the program and the program's organizational chart and how the transport team functions in the program.

Other Members of the Transport Program

Depending on the structure of the transport program, there may be many different types of leadership positions. These may include Chief Flight Nurse or Paramedic, Safety Officer, Clinical Team Lead, Business Manager, Medical Manager, Performance Improvement Officer, or Education Program Manager. Each of these positions should come with defined job descriptions and recommended qualifications. The addition of transport team members will depend on the size of the program operations or the type of model that a particular program uses.

Preparation for Practice

Critical care patient transport requires skilled and experienced personnel to meet the needs of complex cases in a challenging environment. It also necessitates clinical competency, critical thinking skills, and flexibility. Both ASTNA and I-CAPP have developed position papers that address some of the issues identified with the nurse practicing outside of the hospital and paramedic practice at the critical care level, beyond the routine care provided by EMS paramedics. The customary hospital-specific orientation or prehospital training does not include the knowledge and skills needed to deliver patient care in the critical care transport environment.[3,22,27]

The education, clinical proficiency, and knowledge needed to provide this care before, during, and after the transport must be diverse and comprehensive. The expertise of the healthcare professional should include established tenure within the area of expertise and age-specific life-support and advanced trauma training. The healthcare professional should also demonstrate a merit of knowledge specific to the scope of care with the successful completion of industry-specific advanced certifications.[7]

The CAMTS standards provide an outline for the initial training program requirements for each of the mission types (air or surface/ground) for transport programs.[6] These requirements provide a strong framework on which a program's initial orientation and continuing education are built. A summary of these requirements is found in Box 2.3.[7,14]

• BOX 2.3 Commission on Accreditation of Medical Transport Systems Initial Training Program Requirements

Didactic Component

- Advanced airway management
- Anatomy, physiology, and assessment for adult, pediatric, and neonatal patients as included in the program's scope of care and patient population
- Burn emergencies (thermal, chemical, and electrical)
- Cardiac emergencies and advanced cardiac critical care
- Environmental emergencies
- Equipment education specific to the equipment used by the program
- GI and abdominal emergencies
- Infectious and communicable diseases
- High-risk obstetric emergencies
- Mechanical ventilation and respiratory physiology for adult, pediatric, and neonatal patients specific to the equipment used by program
- Metabolic endocrine emergencies
- Multisystem trauma
- Neonatal emergencies (respiratory distress, surgical, cardiac)
- Neurological emergencies
- Pediatric medical emergencies
- Pediatric trauma
- Pharmacology
- Respiratory emergencies
- Sepsis
- Shock
- Toxicology

Clinical Component (on Basis of the Program's Scope of Care)

- Critical care (adult, pediatric, and neonatal)
- Emergency care (adult, pediatric, and neonatal)
- Invasive procedures on mannequin equivalent for practicing of invasive procedures
- Neonatal intensive care
- Obstetrics
- Pediatric critical care
- Prehospital care
- Tracheal intubations (and alternative airway management)

Transport-Specific Topics

- Altitude physiology/stressors of flight (RW/FW)
- Disaster and triage
- EMS radio communications
- Highway scene safety management (RW/S)
- Infection/exposure control and prevention in transport environment
- Medical patient transport considerations (assessment/treatment/stabilization/preparation/handling)
- Oxygen quality controls include: hazard awareness, knowledge of how to read cylinder levels, basic understanding of Compressed Gas Association (CGA) connections, knowledge of how to safely transport liquid oxygen cylinders (if utilized), and knowledge of cylinder durations as per local and national regulations (e.g., FDA Section 211.25(a) and NFPA 53M)
- Scene management/rescue/extrication
- State EMS rules and regulations rules regarding surface and air transport
- Transport vehicle orientation/safety and in-transport procedures/general vehicle safety including all types of vehicles the team may be exposed to, including depressurization procedures for fixed wing (as appropriate)

General Quality, Safety, and Compliance Topics

- Compliance issues and regulations
- Human factors – Crew Resource Management (CRM) and/or Air Medical Resource Management (AMRM)
- "Just culture" or equivalent education (strongly encouraged)
- Quality management – didactic education that supports the medical
- Transport service's mission statement and scope of care
- Examples of evidence to exceed compliance: TEAMSTEPPS and LEAN are examples of processes that provide teamwork, root cause analysis, and problem-solving
- Risk management training (strongly encouraged)
- Safety
- Sleep deprivation, sleep inertia, circadian rhythms, and recognizing signs of fatigue
- Stress recognition and management/resilience

A comprehensive orientation can be provided in numerous ways. With the use of adult learning principles, an educational program can be designed that uses self-directed learning packets, traditional lectures with discussion, or case scenario teaching.[9–11]

In addition to the didactic information, a practical component of skills training is needed. This training should include various inpatient and prehospital care clinical experiences and an invasive skills laboratory.[7,10,11]

After the initial education and training is complete, the new transport team member should complete an internship or preceptorship, which provides further role definition, recognition of the need for additional education or training, and an opportunity to "put into practice" all the previous learning. Although evaluation is an ongoing process, a final evaluation during the orientation process assists new transport team members in assessing their experience and the need for any further education.

Adult Learning Principles

Incorporation of adult learning principles and the use of various teaching methods should be included in a comprehensive orientation program. Adult learning today is influenced by generational differences, technology advancements, and differing learning styles. These should be considered in the development of any

orientation or educational program for new team members. Adult learning also requires various educational techniques including but not limited to traditional lecture with discussion, case presentation/scenario-based teaching, internet-based learning, multimedia applications, simulation training, and self-directed learning packages.[28–30] In addition to the didactic component, transport clinicians require additional skills with a practical clinical component. These skills should include various prehospital care and inpatient clinical experiences in addition to simulation training with tools such as synthetic models and mannequins or computer simulations.[28–31]

With the advancement of technology, simulation training has become a popular and common method of providing orientation, ongoing clinical skills, and exposure to uncommon clinical problems. The development of accreditation options for simulation training centers has helped to develop and elevate the quality and standards with the use of simulation. Many transport programs are no longer part of a hospital system, so finding clinical environments for education and practice has become limited,[28] and thus far, there is minimal literature describing the ideal way to orient transport team members to the critical care transport environment.[31,32] However, simulation-based training can be standardized based most appropriately on the scope and mission of the transport service.

As described previously, after the initial education and training is complete, standard practice is for a new transport team member to participate in a period of preceptorship or internship. Because of the variety of adult learning styles in today's education world and the knowledge that adult learners progress at different paces, emphasis and due consideration are needed in the evaluation of progress through the period of preceptorship. The duration of orientation and preceptorship for new team members should vary according to the needs of the transport program and the individual member. Many transport teams have reported that the most helpful resources they found for the development of new transport members were case reviews, additional time in the mode of transportation they were to use with a preceptor, and experiences with task trainers and mannequins.[31]

Competency-Based Education

Competency-based learning is a method of education that allows for flexibility and builds on previous knowledge. Competency-based instruction provides an opportunity for regular feedback and assessment of competency at the end of the various stages of the program, which provides positive response for progression through to the next stage and the ability to assess competency development as the transport nurse learns. An example is advanced airway management skills. The plan is an outline of requirements for competency in advanced airway skills. The orientation member then initiates the plan. An assessment of the member's ability to perform advanced airway management is done, and the plan is then modified. Evaluation is continuous.

ASTNA has developed a list of the minimal competencies that are recommended for nurses who practice in the transport environment.[8,33] A summary of these competencies is found in Box 2.4.

In addition, Johnson[29] has also developed a competency-based manual that provides several references and outlines for the orientation of transport personnel.

Each transport program, on the basis of the program's mission and scope of practice, has a standard of technical competencies and skills necessary for clinical practice. During the orientation period, new staff members are required to demonstrate competence in the specified requisites for progression to independent practice. Once demonstrated, these skills are built on by the novice practitioner and provide a continuing checklist for the experienced provider for continuing professional development. Additional individual skill sets, or a blend of technical, interpersonal, and critical thinking as identified in a specific job description, need to be measurably shown by the end of the orientation program. These objectives may also form the basis for an annual performance development review or personal evaluations within the transport program. Feedback regarding performance from a variety of sources, including peer reviews, self-reflection, and posttransport debriefings, provides honest evaluation and is often powerful motivation for self-development.

ASTNA recommends that clinical competencies be evaluated with use of written examinations, simulated practice/skills laboratories, transport preceptor/mentor supervised skills practiced during actual transports, case presentations, and oral examinations conducted by peers and the medical director. Staff meetings offer excellent opportunities to teach both new and experienced transport personnel using case studies from actual transports.

Coaching, mentoring, and clinical supervision programs should be available to new transport team members. Mentors fulfill a different role than that of the preceptor. They help new nurses in a role to deepen their knowledge and develop professionally, whereas clinical supervision allows the practitioner to share clinical, organizational, developmental, and emotional experiences with another professional to enhance knowledge and skills.

Continuing Professional Development

Continuing professional development has a fixed portion of training determined by standards, regulations, and the transport program, including skills/technical training, occupational health and safety, and local and state requirements. Additional sources of continuing education may include current textbooks related to transport medicine, professional journals, online discussion forums, and continuing education courses.

• BOX 2.4   Air and Surface Transport Nurses Association – Recommended Competencies for Transport Nurses

Advanced patient assessments skills to include anatomy, pathophysiology, assessment, and treatment for the age group and patients that are transported by the program (e.g., neonatal, pediatric, adult, geriatric):
- Acute and chronic respiratory disease
- Cardiovascular abnormalities
- Surgical problems
- Infectious diseases
- Musculoskeletal abnormalities
- Neurologic and spinal cord emergencies
- Gastrointestinal emergencies
- Genitourinary disorders
- Integumentary disruption
- Hematologic disorders
- Metabolic/endocrine disorders
- Genetic/disorders of dysmorphology
- Disorders of the head, eyes, ears, nose, and throat
- Trauma
- Environmental and toxicologic emergencies
- Adult and child maltreatment

- Airway management (basic and advanced)
- Vascular access
- Medication administration
- Intraaortic balloon pump management
- Ventricular assist device management
- Needle decompression
- Chest tube insertion
- Pericardiocentesis
- Pacing devices
- Immobilization skills
- 12-Lead electrocardiographic interpretation
- Arrhythmia analysis and treatment
- Invasive monitoring
- Fetal heart monitoring
- Radiographic interpretation
- Interpretation and treatment of clinical laboratory data
- Thermoregulation
- Psychological/bereavement support and crisis intervention
- Transport equipment management

• BOX 2.5   Commission on Accreditation of Medical Transport Systems Continuing Education/Staff Development

Didactic

- Human factors – Crew Resource Management (CRM) and/or Air Medical Resource Management (AMRM)
- Infection exposure control
- "Just culture" or equivalent education – strongly encouraged
- Safety and risk management training on an annual basis (strongly encouraged)
- Sleep deprivation, sleep inertia, circadian rhythms, and recognizing signs of fatigue
- State EMS rules and regulations regarding surface and air transport
- Stress recognition and management/resilience

Clinical/Laboratory

- Critical care (adult, pediatric, and neonatal)
- Emergency/trauma care
- Invasive procedures laboratories
- Labor and delivery
- Prehospital experience
- Skills maintenance program documented to comply with the number of skills required in a set period according to the policy of the medical transport service (e.g., endotracheal intubations, chest drains)

- Clinical competency maintained by currency in the following or equivalent as appropriate for position description, mission statement, and scope of care:
  - BLS: Documented evidence of current BLS certification according to the AHA
  - ACLS: Documented evidence of current ACLS according to the AHA
  - ATLS: According to the American College of Surgeons, ATLS audit, ATLS for Nurse or TPATC
  - PALS or APLS according to the AHA and ACEP, or equivalent education
  - NRP: Documented evidence of current NRP according to the AHA or American Academy of Pediatrics
  - Current transport-specific nursing certification (CTRN or CFRN) are required for nurses who have been employed for more than 2 years
  - Current paramedic certifications (FP-C or CCP-C) required for paramedics who conduct critical care transports and have been employed for more than 2 years

ACEP, American College of Emergency Physicians; *ACLS,* advanced cardiac life support; *AHA,* American Heart Association; *APLS,* advanced pediatric life support; *ATLS,* advanced trauma life support; *BLS,* basic life support; *CCRN,* Critical Care Registered Nurse; *CEN,* Certified Emergency Nurse; *CFRN,* Certified Flight Registered Nurse; *CTRN,* Certified Transport Registered Nurse; *EMS,* Emergency Medical Service; *NRP,* Neonatal Resuscitation Program; *PALS,* pediatric advanced life support; *TPATC,* Transport Professional Advanced Trauma Course.

Commission on Accreditation of Medical Transport Systems Recommendations

CAMTS outlines specific components of transport education and skills that should be reviewed annually (Box 2.5).[7]

In addition to these requirements, transport team members have a further responsibility to identify their own educational needs aside from any regulatory or accreditation standard requirements. As discussed previously, adult learners need a variety of experiences to learn and remain competent. Team members must maintain and continue to gain knowledge to meet patient needs and carry on the growth of the profession of transport nursing. This continuing education is an important part of the development and maintenance of expert practice in the field of transport medicine.

Clinical Decision-Making

Clinical decision-making or clinical judgment is a process in which the clinician identifies, prioritizes, establishes plans, and evaluates data, which leads to the formation of a judgment to provide patient care.[34,35] In transport medicine, complex clinical decisions are made on a daily basis, in collaboration (Fig. 2.1) with transport team members. In dealing with increasing patient complexity and technological advancement, transport clinicians must rely on sound decision-making skills to deliver up-to-date, evidenced-based care and help facilitate positive patient outcomes.

Reflective Practice

The use of reflective practice (application of learning experiences and current evidenced-based knowledge) in clinical decision-making enhances patient care delivery. A higher level of learning is achieved by applying learned material to current situations. This application of reflective practice associated with learning from experience is an important strategy for health professionals who

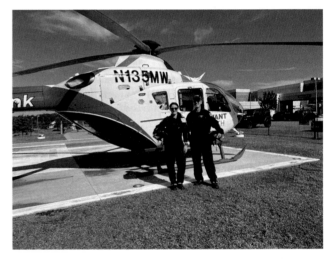

• Figure 2.1 Transport Nurse and Paramedic. (Courtesy Novant Health AirLink.)

engage in continual learning.[36] The act of reflection is seen as a way of promoting the development of autonomous, qualified, and self-directed health professionals.

Engagement in reflective practice is associated with improvement in the quality of care, stimulation of personal and professional growth, and closing of the gap between theory and practice. If clinicians are not thinking autonomously on a regular basis, they risk losing competence in their decision-making abilities.[36]

Summary

For effective patient transport, multiple resources are necessary. The mission of the transport service is to design the transport team and define the roles of all disciplines involved. Transport professionals require experience, advanced skills, and continuing education so that the transport team is able to function autonomously and in collaboration with all others who may be involved in the transport process. Patient care and management during transport occur in diverse multidimensional situations. The development of a sound orientation and strong preceptorship training program, in conjunction with continuing values-based professional development, provides the transport professional with the skills and ability to care for patients in diverse and sometimes difficult situations.

References

1. NHTSA. *Guide for Interfacility Patient Transfer*. 2006. https://www.nhtsa.gov/people/injury/ems/interfacility/index.htm
2. Kupas F, Wang H. Critical care paramedics – a missing component for safe interfacility transport in the United States. *Ann Emerg Med*. 2014;64(1):17–18.
3. Air & Surface Transport Nurses Association (ASTNA). Role of the Registered Nurse in the Out-of-Hospital Environment. ASTNA; 2015.
4. Sjolin H, Lindstrom V, Rinsted C, Kurland L. What an ambulance nurse needs to know: A content analysis of curricula in the specialist nursing programme in prehospital emergency care. *Int Emerg Nurs*. 2015;23:127–132.
5. Treadwell D, Arndt K, Werth R. Standards for Critical Care and Specialty Transport. Air and Surface Transport Nurses Association; 2015.
6. Camts.org. 2022. ABOUT US – CAMTS. [online]. Accessed August 1, 2022. https://www.camts.org/about/
7. Commission on Accreditation of Medical Transport Systems. Accreditation Standards. 12th ed. Commission on Accreditation of Medical Transport Systems; 2022.
8. Air & Surface Transport Nurses Association (ASTNA). *Qualifications, Orientation, Competencies, and Continuing Education for Transport Nurses*. ASTNA; 2015.
9. Air & Surface Transport Nurses Association (ASTNA). *Staffing of Critical Care Transport Services*. ASTNA; 2015.
10. Bader GB, Terhorts M, Heilman P, et al. Characteristics of flight nursing practice. *Air Med J*. 1995;14(4):214–218.
11. Carrubba C. Role of the medical director in air medical transport. In: Blumen I, ed. *Principles and Direction of Air Medical Transport. Advancing Air & Ground Critical Care Transport Medicine*. 2nd ed. Air Medical Physicians Association; 2015:90.
12. Stocking J. Crew configuration. In: Blumen I, ed. *Principles and Direction of Air Medical Transport. Advancing Air & Ground Critical Care Transport Medicine*. 2nd ed. Air Medical Physicians Association; 2015:50–56.
13. International Association of Flight and Critical Care Paramedics. Preparatory Outline for FP-C and CCP-C Exams. Accessed August 1, 2022. http://www.iafccp.org/?page=ExamPrep
14. International Association of Flight and Critical Care Paramedics. FAQs About Critical Care and Flight Paramedicine. Accessed August 1, 2022. http://www.iafccp.org/?page=CareerFAQ
15. Gryniuk J. The role of the certified flight paramedic as a critical care provider and the required education. *Prehosp Emerg Care*. 2001;5(3):290–292.
16. International Board of Specialty Certification. About Us. Accessed August 1, 2022. https://www.ibscertifications.org/about/about-us
17. International Board of Specialty Certification. Exam Preparation, FP-C. Accessed August 1, 2022. https://www.ibscertifications.org/resource/pdf/FP-C%20EXAM%20OUTLINE.pdf
18. International Board of Specialty Certification. Exam Preparation, CCP-C. Accessed August 1, 2022. https://www.ibscertifications.org/resource/pdf/CCP-C%20EXAM%20OUTLINE.pdf
19. American Association for Respiratory Care. 2016. http://www.aarc.org/?s=Air+Transport+Section
20. Stone K. The air medical crew: Is a flight physician necessary. *J Air Med Transp*. 1991;10(11):7–10.
21. Taylor C, Jan S, Curtis K, et al. The cost-effectiveness of physician staffed Helicopter Emergency Medical Service (HEMS) transport to a major trauma centre in NSW, Australia. *Injury*. 2012;43(11):1843–1849.
22. Carrubba C. Role of the medical director in air medical transport. In: Blumen I, ed. Principles and Direction of Air Medical Transport. Air Medical Physicians Association; 2015:89–96.
23. Air Medical Physician Association (AMPA). Medical Direction & Medical Control of Air Medical Services. AMPA; 2012.
24. Federal Aviation Administration. Pilot in command. 1997. Accessed August 1, 2022. http://www.faa.gov/about/initiatives/cabin_safety/regs/legal/media/pic_responsibility_fa_duty_rest.pdf
25. 14 CFR part 91—general operating and flight rules (FAR part 91). https://www.ecfr.gov/current/title-14/chapter-I/subchapter-F/part-91. Accessed June 22, 2023.
26. Raynovich W, Hums J, Stuhlmiller D, Bramble J, Kasha T, Galt K. Critical care transportation by paramedics: A cross-sectional survey. *Air Med J*. 2013;32:280–282.
27. International Association of Flight & Critical Care Paramedics (IAFCCP). Critical Care Paramedic Position Statement. IAFCCP; 2009.
28. Grisham L, Vickers V, Biffar D, et al. Case study feasibility of air transport simulation training: A case series. *Air Med J*. 2016;35(5):308–313.
29. Johnson J. *Competency Based Orientation and Continuing Education for Critical Care Transport*. Air and Surface Transport Nurses Association; 2007.
30. Knapp B. Competency: An essential component of caring in nursing. *Nurs Admin Q*. 2004;28(4):285–287.
31. Alfes C, Steiner S, Rutherford-Hemming T. Challenges and resources for new critical care transport crewmembers: A descriptive exploratory study. *Air Med J*. 2016;35(4):212–215.
32. Alfes M, Steiner S, Manacci C. Critical care transport training: New strides in simulating the austere environment. *Air Med J*. 2015;34(4):186–187.
33. Treadwell D, Santiago JP. *Standards for Critical Care Specialty Transport*. ASTNA; 2019.
34. Pugh D. A Phenomenologic study of flight nurses' clinical decision-making in emergency situations. *Air Med J*. 2012;21(2):29–36.
35. Miller M, Babcock D. *Critical Thinking Applied to Nursing*. Mosby; 1996.
36. Goudreau J, Pepin J, Larua C, et al. A competency-based approach to nurses' continuing education for clinical reasoning and leadership through reflective practice in a care situation. *Nurse Educ Pract*. 2015;15(6):572–578.

3

Aviation for Medical Personnel

JACOB A. MILLER

COMPETENCIES

1. Apply aviation principles to medical practice, recognizing the limitations that the environment, aircraft, and medical configuration may have on transport considerations.
2. Make an informed decision about whether to accept a flight based on current, forecast, and trending weather patterns.
3. Maintain situational awareness of the aircraft during instrument conditions.

Both the medicine and aviation industry are considered high-reliability organizations, where meticulous care must be taken during complex, high-hazard operations to prevent serious, potentially catastrophic incidents from occurring.[1] Although critical care transport (CCT) medical providers are primarily responsible for providing direct patient care, knowledge of basic aviation and aeronautical concepts can increase the crew's overall situational awareness and enhance operational safety. This chapter will review some of the concepts necessary for a working understanding of aviation and operational safety. Practical application of these topics to flight physiology, patient safety, and CCT crew safety will be discussed in later chapters.

Introduction to Aviation Terminology

Most CCT medical crewmembers are intimately familiar with the "jargon" of medical care. We can easily make sense of a protocol necessitating ASA for a STEMI, or to hold NTG for an SBP <90. What may be less familiar to the novice CCT medical provider is the language of aviation. Indeed, aviation has its own set of unique terms and abbreviations that rival that of the medical field. While it is impractical to provide a comprehensive list of aviation terms in this text, one resource for aviation terminology may be the Pilot/Controller Glossary that can be found in the Publications section at www.faa.gov/air_traffic/publications/.

Time

Just like in medicine, aviation uses 24-hour clock time. However, because the nature of air travel easily allows flights to cross several time zones, aviation commonly uses *Zulu*, or Coordinated Universal Time (UTC). In civilian terms, UTC is the same as Greenwich Mean Time (GMT) and needs to be converted to your local time zone and account for any additional variance from observed Daylight Savings Time. See Table 3.1 for US time zones relative to UTC.

TABLE 3.1	Time Zone Conversion From Zulu (UTC)	
Time Zone	**Conversion**	**Example at 22:00 Zulu**
Atlantic Standard Time	UTC − 4:00	18:00
Eastern Standard Time	UTC − 5:00	17:00
Eastern Daylight Time	UTC − 4:00	18:00
Central Standard Time	UTC − 6:00	16:00
Central Daylight Time	UTC − 5:00	17:00
Mountain Standard Time	UTC − 7:00	15:00
Mountain Daylight Time	UTC − 6:00	16:00
Pacific Standard Time	UTC − 8:00	14:00
Pacific Daylight Time	UTC − 7:00	15:00
Alaska Standard Time	UTC − 9:00	13:00
Alaska Daylight Time	UTC − 8:00	14:00
Hawaii–Aleutian Standard Time	UTC − 10:00	12:00

UTC, Coordinated Universal Time.

Altitude

Altitude within the United States is measured in feet. With few exceptions, most altitudes are expressed relative to mean sea level (MSL). One common exception is cloud reporting, which is reported in feet above ground level (AGL) at the reporting location. See Fig. 3.1 for an example of these different altitudes.

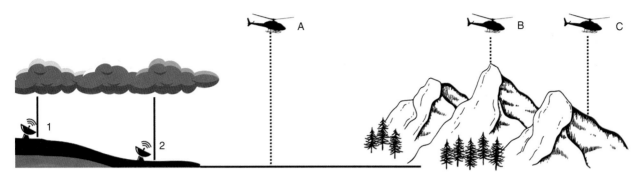

• **Figure 3.1** Altitudes Above Ground Level and Relative to Mean Sea Level. The helicopter is flying at a constant 10,000-feet altitude above mean sea level (MSL). At location **A,** the aircraft is both 10,000 feet MSL *and* 10,000 feet above ground level (AGL). At location **B,** the aircraft is only 2000 feet AGL (although the altimeter will still read 10,000 feet MSL). At location **C,** the aircraft is now 4000 feet AGL (although the altimeter will still read 10,000 feet MSL). Cloud cover, on the other hand, is reported in feet AGL at the observation location. Observation stations 1 and 2 are situated at different elevations. Observation station 1 would report the cloud ceiling at 2000 feet, but observation station 2 (at a lower elevation) would report the same cloud ceiling at 3000 feet.

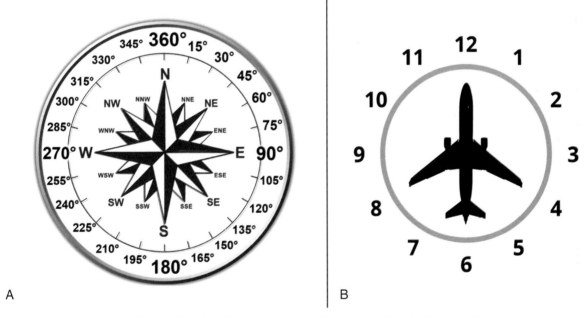

A   B

• **Figure 3.2** Relative Directions for Navigation and Hazard Reporting. **A.** Compass directions with degrees for cardinal directions. **B.** Clock position to describe objects relative to the aircraft.

Relative Directions

Directions provided for *navigation* purposes are described using compass degrees (Fig. 3.2A), where 360° is direct north, 90° is east, 180° is south, and 270° is west. This direction, relative to the current location of the aircraft, is sometimes referred to as the "bearing." In some rotor-wing flight programs, the aircraft may depart for a scene flight with a preliminary distance and bearing prior to receiving or entering exact GPS coordinates for the designated landing zone.

Airport runways are also numbered using this concept but omit the final digit in the compass heading. For example, Runway 9 faces directly east (90°); the opposite direction on the same runway would be labeled Runway 27 because it faces directly west (270°).

Directions provided to communicate locations *relative to the aircraft* are provided using a clock description (Fig. 3.2B), where the nose of the aircraft is 12:00, the right side of the aircraft (when looking forward) is 3:00, the tail is 6:00, and the left side of the aircraft (when looking forward) is 9:00. Clock positions are always relative to the aircraft nose, regardless of the navigational direction an aircraft is facing.

Airport Patterns

In addition to understanding runway headings, it is also beneficial to understand the terminology associated with airport patterns. The National Traffic Safety Board (NTSB) identifies failure to see and avoid other aircraft as a significant contributing factor to midair collisions.[2] Understanding airport patterns, and monitoring air-to-air communications during flight, can enhance situational awareness for medical crew and help identify traffic hazards during flight.

There are different ways to enter a traffic pattern, and that is beyond the scope of this chapter, but the following terminology can help identify where to look relative to the runway or airfield[2,3]:

- The *centerline* of a runway is a straight line that extends out from the long axis of the runway on the runway heading in either direction.
- An *upwind* leg describes movement parallel to, and in the same direction as, the referenced runway.
- A *crosswind* leg is perpendicular to the runway at the departure end.
- The *downwind* leg refers to movement parallel to, and *opposite*, the direction of the referenced runway.
- The *base* leg is also perpendicular to the runway but on the approach end (i.e., prior to landing).
- The *final approach* is at the approach end of the referenced runway along the centerline.

Pilots may additionally call out directional modifiers (i.e., right or left) with the traffic pattern; these directions indicate the turns the pilot must make to continue the pattern. Thus, a *left downwind* means the aircraft is flying on the *left* side of the indicated runway and must make left-hand turns to enter the base leg and final approach. Fig. 3.3 shows a graphical depiction of each of these terms.

Distance and Speed

Distance can be measured using statute miles (SM) or nautical miles (NM), depending on context. A statute mile is the "mile" we're most familiar with in the civilian world: 5280 feet. A nautical mile is slightly longer (approximately 6076 feet), and 1 NM is equal to about 1.15 SM. Speed, on the other hand, is almost universally measured in nautical miles per hour, or "knots" (abbreviated kt). The concept of speed is identical regardless of unit: distance over time. Thus, if miles per hour (mph) represents the number of (statute) miles traveled in 1 hour, knots represent the number of nautical miles traveled in 1 hour. For this reason, the conversion factor between distance and speed is identical: 1 NM ≈ 1.15 SM, so 1 kt ≈ 1.15 mph.

Aviation Fundamentals

Aircraft pilots are required to possess an in-depth knowledge of aircraft performance and aerodynamics to safely perform their duties. This section will provide a brief overview of some fundamental aspects of aviation that may be pertinent for the CCT medical provider to consider.

Physics of Aviation

There are several principles from physics that govern aviation and explain how aircraft can overcome the force of gravity. Some foundational principles will be discussed in this section; those interested in additional information can visit the National Aeronautics and Space Administration (NASA) Beginner's Guide to Aerodynamics at https://www1.grc.nasa.gov/beginners-guide-to-aeronautics/learn-about-aerodynamics/.

An aircraft is subject to a combination of forces at any given time. Recall Newton's first law of motion: An object at rest will remain at rest, and an object in motion will remain in uniform motion in a straight line, unless compelled to change that state by the sum of outside forces. Practically speaking, this means that forward motion in any plane can only occur if the forward force is sufficient to overcome the opposing force. Thus, as is demonstrated in Fig. 3.4, the aircraft must be able to generate sufficient lift to overcome the weight of gravity in order to get off the ground, and it must be able to generate sufficient thrust to overcome drag in order to maintain forward motion. This is true at the basic level for both fixed-wing and rotor-wing aircraft, although the way those forces are generated differs.[1,4,5]

Newton's second law of motion, which states, "*Force is equal to the change in momentum per change in time; at a constant mass, force*

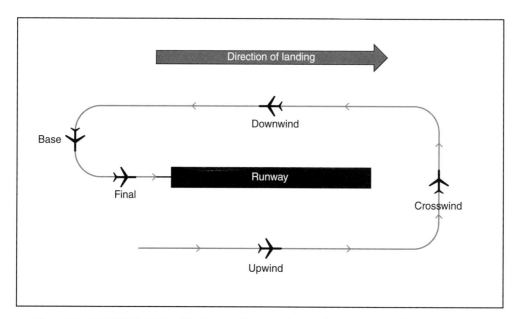

• **Figure 3.3** Airfield Traffic Pattern Terminology. Example of a standard left-hand traffic pattern. This is a "left" traffic pattern because the aircraft must make left-hand turns as it flies the pattern.

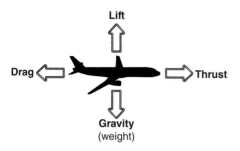

• **Figure 3.4** Forces Acting on an Aircraft. A general overview of forces affecting aircraft motion. In general, lift opposes gravity and thrust opposes drag.

equals mass times acceleration," describes the relationship between these forces and the mass of an object. Rearranged, this law maintains that for any given force, the acceleration will be inversely proportional to the mass of the object. A heavier object requires additional force to achieve the same acceleration.[1,4]

The last of Newton's laws to discuss, the third law of motion, states the following: *For every action, there is an equal and opposite reaction.* In a helicopter, the downward propulsion of air through the rotor disk generates an opposing force used to create both lift and forward thrust when the rotor disk is rotated slightly forward; this thrust can be applied in different directions by manipulating the rotor disk. In a fixed-wing aircraft, the air pushed backward through a propeller, or the exhaust ejected from a jet engine, works to provide a forward thrust for a fixed-wing aircraft. Lift, however, is better explained using Bernoulli's principle: *When the velocity of a fluid increases, its pressure decreases.* As an airfoil, like an airplane wing, passes through fluid (air), the fluid particles traveling over the top of the airfoil have a higher velocity than those traveling over the bottom (Fig. 3.5). This generates a lower relative pressure over the airfoil than below it. This pressure differential leads to lift.[1,4,5]

Factors Affecting Aerodynamics

One important concept to understand about the physics of aviation is that the forces acting on the aircraft in flight arise primarily from the fluid through which it is traveling, namely, air. Aircraft performance is, therefore, dependent on variations in that fluid or variations in the aircraft itself.

Environmental Factors

The principles of aviation physics mentioned previously are calculated assuming standard atmosphere conditions (temperature of 15°C [59°F] and sea-level pressure of 760 mm Hg [29.92 in Hg]).

As those environmental factors change, there is a resulting change in the air density. Air density describes the number of gaseous air molecules per volume of air – as air density increases, the air molecules are spaced closer together; as air density decreases, the molecules are spaced further apart. Generally speaking, lower air density results in decreased aircraft performance:

• Aircraft engines take in less air, leading to reduced power.
• Fewer air molecules traverse and interact with airfoils, causing a reduction in lift.
• Propellers and helicopter rotors also interact with fewer air molecules, making thrust and, for rotorcraft, lift inefficient.

Because lift must be sufficient to counteract the force of gravity (Fig. 3.4), operating in less-dense environments places limitations on the amount of weight the aircraft is able to safely carry, especially for helicopters and smaller fixed-wing aircraft, or the effective service ceiling for the aircraft.[1–5]

Temperature, barometric pressure, and, to a lesser extent, humidity all affect the air density and, therefore, aircraft performance. Although physiologic applications of gas laws will be discussed in greater detail in the flight physiology chapter, now is a good time to introduce the *ideal gas law*[6]:

$$pV = NkT$$

where p is absolute pressure, V is volume, N is the number of gas molecules, T is temperature, and k is simply a constant necessary to balance the equation (in this case, the Boltzmann constant). Because our use of the ideal gas law concerns the density of a constant number of air molecules, N remains a constant value. From this information, we can derive other gas laws and their application to aircraft performance (Fig. 3.6).[6]

Temperature (Charles's Law)

Charles's law states that temperature and volume are proportional at constant pressure; thus, as the temperature of a gas increases, the volume (or space) the gas occupies also increases.[6] The same number of molecules over a larger area means there is a lower air density. Thus, from an aerodynamic perspective, increased temperature leads to decreased air density and degraded aircraft performance. The opposite is true, then, with lower temperatures: as the temperature falls, air density increases, and aircraft performance improves.[1–5] Outside air temperature decreases at a standard lapse rate of 2°C for each 1000 feet altitude increase.

Pressure (Boyle's Law)

Boyle's law states that the volume of a gas is inversely proportional to pressure at a constant temperature; thus, with the fall in pressure

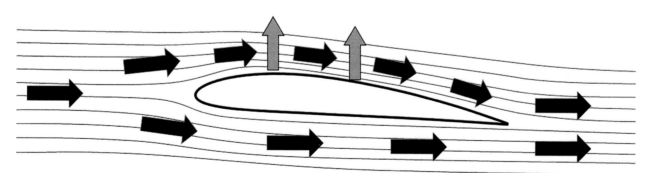

• **Figure 3.5** Airfoil Function. Air traveling over the top of the airfoil moves faster than air traveling below (*dark arrows*). This leads to a relatively lower pressure above the airfoil and higher pressure below, resulting in a lift force (*light arrows*).

The Ideal Gas Law:

$$pV = NkT$$

Because the number of molecules and the Boltzmann constant are constant values, we can simplify to:

$$pV \propto T$$

From here we can set up an equation to see how the different variables affect each other:

$$\frac{p_1 V_1}{T_1} = \frac{p_2 V_2}{T_2}$$

Finally, from here we can derive other relevant gas laws:

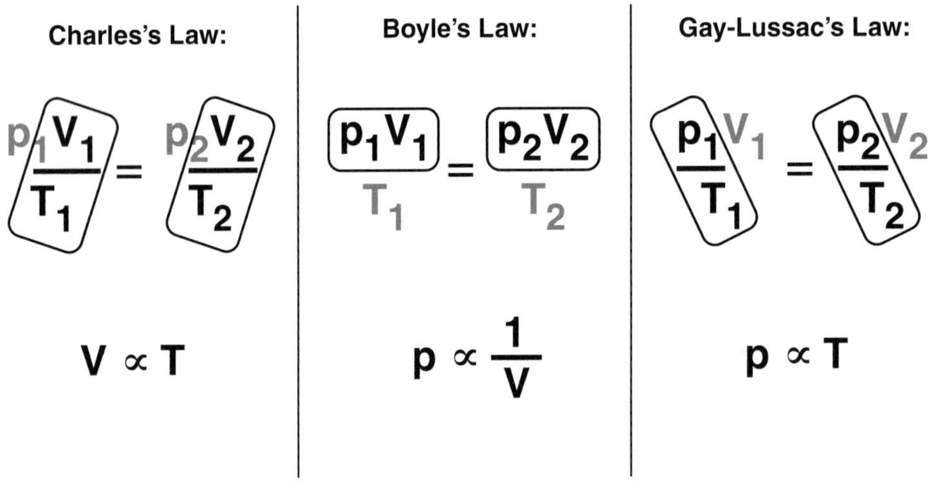

Charles's Law:	Boyle's Law:	Gay-Lussac's Law:
$$\frac{p_1 V_1}{T_1} = \frac{p_2 V_2}{T_2}$$	$$\frac{p_1 V_1}{T_1} = \frac{p_2 V_2}{T_2}$$	$$\frac{p_1 V_1}{T_1} = \frac{p_2 V_2}{T_2}$$
$$V \propto T$$	$$p \propto \frac{1}{V}$$	$$p \propto T$$

• **Figure 3.6** Gas Law Derivation. *k*, Boltzmann constant; *N*, number of molecules; *p*, absolute pressure; *T*, temperature; *V*, volume; α, proportional to.

incurred with increasing altitude, the volume of gas expands. This means that lower barometric pressure also results in a lower air density.[6] CCT medical personnel familiar with flight physiology will remember that as altitude increases, temperature and pressure *both* decrease – and these have opposing effects on air density. Generally speaking, however, the fall in pressure with increasing altitude outweighs the fall in temperature, so the net effect is a lower air density.[4] As this applies to CCT, aircraft performance is decreased when operating at higher altitudes, including geographic locations situated at high elevations.

Density Altitude

The term *density altitude* is used to describe the altitude above sea level at which a given air density would be found *in the standard atmosphere*. It is used most commonly to correct for nonstandard temperature variations. As noted before, air density has significant effects on aircraft and engine performance, especially for aircraft commonly used for air medical operations. Regardless of its true altitude above sea level, an aircraft's performance will mimic an aircraft

operating at an altitude equal to the density altitude. As an example, an aircraft is departing a runway at sea level. The density altitude is reported to be 2500 feet. Therefore, the pilot must consider that the aircraft will perform as though it were departing from a runway at 2500 feet above sea level, *not* from its actual location at sea level.[1–5]

Aircraft Weight

The lift generated by the aircraft must be able to overcome the force of gravity, which, for practical purposes, represents the weight of the aircraft (Fig. 3.4). In addition to the environmental factors just identified that affect the lift of the aircraft, CCT medical personnel must also be aware of aircraft considerations, the most controllable of which is total aircraft weight. As the weight of the aircraft increases, the aircraft must be able to generate sufficient lift to become airborne and remain aloft. Conversely, as environmental factors limit the performance of the aircraft and affect the lift that can be generated, there may be limitations on the amount of fuel, medical equipment, personnel, or patient weight that can be accommodated.[4,5]

Operating at Altitude

As altitude increases, air pressure and density both decrease. The decrease in air density means that fewer molecules of air occupy the same volume. Importantly, atmospheric air contains the oxygen necessary for cellular respiration and physiologic function. At higher altitudes, then, the same volume of air inhaled into one's lungs (i.e., tidal volume) contains fewer oxygen molecules to diffuse into the pulmonary circulation and can quickly lead to hypoxia. Respiratory physiology generally considers the *pressure* of various gases, not necessarily their *density*, although both concepts are closely related. Dalton's law of partial pressures states that the partial, or fractional, pressure of any gas is equal regardless of the total pressure.[6] Therefore, oxygen always comprises 21% of the atmospheric air regardless of the barometric pressure. This means that at sea level at standard pressure (760 mm Hg), oxygen has a pressure of around 159 mm Hg. At an altitude of 10,000 feet MSL (standard barometric pressure, 523 mm Hg), oxygen pressure is reduced to about 109 mm Hg. For this reason, Federal Aviation Regulations (FARs) require supplemental oxygen to be available for pilots and crew for flights above 12,500 feet MSL and must be available for all occupants on flights above 14,000 feet MSL.[7]

To combat the lower oxygen available at altitude, most fixed-wing aircraft that regularly fly above 12,500 feet MSL have a system to pressurize the air within the cabin. These systems are designed so that at maximum cruising altitude, the pressure inside the cabin is equivalent to the ambient pressure at 8000 feet MSL.[4] CCT medical crew should take into consideration the patient's current physiologic state and oxygen demands. It may be possible to request a cabin pressure closer to sea level to facilitate oxygenation for critically ill patients, but this requires advanced planning and should be communicated with the pilot as early as the potential need is identified (e.g., during preflight planning prior to initial departure). In all cases, if cabin pressure is lost at altitude, supplemental oxygen must be quickly applied by crew and passengers to prevent incapacitation from hypoxia.

Aviation Regulations

In the United States, aviation is governed by the Federal Aviation Administration (FAA), and the regulations thereof are published in Title 14 of the Code of Federal Regulations (CFR). The portions of the CFR that apply to aviation are commonly referred to as the FARs. These regulations pertain to air traffic control, airports, pilot and crew requirements, visual and instrument flight rules, and aircraft operations. CCT medical providers regularly participating in international flights from the United States should also be familiar with the regulations of the respective international country. Likewise, CCT members based or practicing in another country should be familiar with the local aviation regulations.

Federal Aviation Regulations

Foundationally, 14 CFR Part 91 sets the floor for regulations and broadly addresses general aviation operations and flight rules for all aircraft flying in US airspace. 14 CFR Part 121 applies to scheduled domestic flights; although this Part does not typically apply to air ambulance operations, medical escort flights may occur on Part 121 flights aboard commercial airlines. 14 CFR Part 135 provides more specific rules for unscheduled, on-demand aircraft operations, including air ambulance operations. The Part 135 regulations are often more strict than Part 91 regulations. Most civilian air medical services, whether fixed-wing ambulance or helicopter air ambulance (HAA), are regulated under Part 135 of the FARs because of the nature of transporting passengers or persons for compensation.[3,7-10] Because there is not one blanket regulation that universally addresses every leg of every air ambulance flight, it is important for the CCT clinician to understand the operations of their specific organization and the regulations under which each flight leg is operated.

Helicopter Air Ambulance Regulations

In 2014, the FAA expanded 14 CFR Part 135 to outline specific requirements for HAA equipment, operations, and training requirements in response to several recommendations from the National Transportation Safety Board (NTSB).[8,11,12] Among the requirements of the HAA Part 135 regulations are the following:

- Aircraft conducting HAA operations must be equipped with an approved helicopter terrain awareness and warning system (HTAWS) and flight data monitoring system.
- Specific weather minimums for Part 135 HAA operations are defined (see Table 3.2).
- Certificate holders with 10 or more HAA aircraft must have an operational control center staffed with qualified personnel and able to communicate with each aircraft.
- CCT medical personnel must receive either 8 hours of FAA-approved training every 24 calendar months *or* must receive a preflight briefing prior to each HAA flight. The briefing requirements are listed in Box 3.1.

TABLE 3.2 Part 135 VFR Weather Minimums for Helicopter Air Ambulance (14 CFR 135.609)

	Day Operations		Night Operations		Night Operations With HTAWS or NVIS	
	Ceiling (ft)	Visibility (SM)	Ceiling (ft)	Visibility (SM)	Ceiling (ft)	Visibility (SM)
Nonmountainous local flying areas	800	2	1000	3	800	3
Nonmountainous nonlocal flying areas	800	3	1000	5	1000	3
Mountainous local flying areas	800	3	1500	3	1000	3
Mountainous nonlocal flying areas	1000	3	1500	5	1000	5

ft, feet; *HTAWS*, Helicopter Terrain Awareness and Warning System; *NVIS*, Night Vision Imaging System; *SM*, statue miles.
Local flying area may be defined by the individual program in a manner approved by the FAA, not to exceed 50 nautical miles from a base; *Mountainous* regions are specifically defined in 14 CFR Part 95.

Medical crew members must be briefed on the following prior to each flight:
- Passenger briefing requirements prescribed in §135.117
  - Prohibition against smoking
  - Use of safety belts, including instructions on securing and removing
  - Required seat position for takeoff and landing
  - Location and operation of exit doors
  - Location of safety/survival equipment
  - Location and operation of fire extinguishers
  - As applicable:
    - For overwater flights: ditching procedures and location/use of flotation equipment
    - For flights above 12,000 feet MSL: normal and emergency use of oxygen (by crew members)
- Physiologic aspects of flight
- Patient loading and unloading
- Safety in and around the helicopter
- In-flight emergency procedures
- Emergency landing procedures
- Emergency evacuation procedures
- Efficient and safe communications with the pilot
- Operational differences between day and night operations
  The briefing for medical personnel may be omitted if **all** medical personnel have received FAA-approved medical personnel training, including 4 hours of ground training *and* 4 hours in/around the aircraft on all of the above topics, within the preceding 24 months.

MSL, Mean sea level.

Visual vs. Instrument Rules

There are two broad categories of flight operations: those operating under *visual flight rules* (VFRs) and those operating under *instrument flight rules* (IFRs). Flights conducted under VFRs require the pilot to be able to maintain visual separation from obstacles and other air traffic, and the prevailing conditions must meet the weather minimums defined in the FARs. The weather conditions necessary for VFR flight are generically classified as *visual meteorologic conditions* (VMCs) and are further described in the next section. By default, weather conditions that fall below VMC minimums are referred to as *instrument meteorologic conditions* (IMCs).[3,7–9]

Although IFR operations may allow for flights to be conducted in IMC weather, there are numerous logistical considerations that may make these operations impractical, especially for helicopter operations. Flights conducted under IFR require specific procedures, pilot rating, and pilot currency on use of the aircraft instruments. Landing in IMC requires using specific airports or helipads with an FAA-approved instrument approach. A flight plan must be filed with air traffic control (ATC) prior to entering IMC, and that flight plan must include the identification of a contingency plan and alternate landing area in the event the weather conditions deteriorate at the intended landing area, along with assurance that the aircraft maintains sufficient fuel to reach the alternate landing area. An IFR-rated pilot and aircraft may opt to fly under an IFR flight plan even in VMC weather, but a VFR-only pilot or aircraft cannot knowingly fly into IMC weather.[3,7–9]

A condition known as *inadvertent instrument meteorologic conditions* (IIMC) occurs when a flight operated under VFR suddenly encounters degraded weather and visual reference is lost. This can result in sudden disorientation and may have catastrophic results if the crew does not immediately recognize and accept that they have entered IIMC, the pilot is unfamiliar with IFR operations, and/or the crew and pilot do not take immediate actions necessary to safely recover and operate the aircraft. For this reason, VFR flight into IIMC is considered an emergency condition.

Weather Minimums

The FARs define explicit minimum ceiling and visibility requirements that must be in effect for an aircraft to operate within consistent safety standards. The technical definition and determination of *ceiling* and *visibility* are described later in this chapter, but generally, the ceiling describes the height of the overhead cloud cover and visibility describes the visible forward distance from the aircraft. Weather minimums differ between flights conducted under VFR and those conducted under IFR; the minimums also differ for flights conducted under Part 91 regulations and those conducted under Part 135.[3,7–9] In addition to the Part 135 regulations for HAA VFR operations outlined in Table 3.2,[8] Part 135.207 also requires visible ground (or, at night, ground light) reference to be maintained during helicopter flights conducted under VFR.[9] Lastly, it should also be noted that an individual fight program may set its own minimums *exceeding* those prescribed by the FARs.

Weight and Balance Considerations

Weight and balance requirements are important for helicopter and fixed-wing aircraft as specified in the airplane or rotorcraft flight manual. The manual contains aircraft performance data regarding maximum certified gross weights, center-of-gravity limits, and runway lengths that fixed-wing aircraft use for takeoff. In accordance with Part 91 regulations, the pilot must ensure that the aircraft is always loaded within weight and balance limits.[7] The gross weight of the aircraft is predetermined by the aircraft flight manual, which must account for the weight of the aircraft, fuel, pilot, CCT medical personnel, and usual equipment. The weight of any additional equipment or persons (e.g., the patient and any extra medical crew or patient family members) must be added during appropriate legs of flight, so the CCT medical personnel should attempt to obtain and relay this information to the pilot as soon as practical. The pilot has final authority for weight limitations and may decide that family members or other persons may not accompany the patient. In addition, the pilot may decide to decrease fuel loads, rearrange the seating of passengers, unload unnecessary equipment, leave behind unnecessary passengers or medical personnel, or depart from an airport with a longer runway to accommodate changes in the aircraft's weight and balance.[3]

A second important aspect of weight and balance is that aircraft should be loaded within the center-of-gravity range or limitations, also specified in the aircraft flight manual. Once the maximal weight has been determined, the weight *distribution*, or where the weight is placed in an aircraft, is critical for aerodynamic performance and safety while the aircraft is in flight. The weight must be properly distributed about the center of gravity, both fore and aft as well as laterally, per the manufacturer's flight manual.[3]

Aircraft Maintenance Regulations

The FARs prescribe generic maintenance intervals for every aircraft operated in the United States.[13] In addition to those intervals noted in the FAR, different airframes may have specific maintenance intervals prescribed by the manufacturer. These may include routine inspections, preventative items, or replacement of certain parts at the end of their service life. Maintenance regimens may be based on actual flight time (e.g., a "50-hour inspection" would occur after the aircraft has accumulated 50, 100, 150, etc., hours of flight) or based on calendar days (e.g., an "annual inspection" that must occur once every 12 months regardless of flight time). For these reasons, it might be necessary to remove an aircraft from duty, perhaps mid-shift, if it becomes due for one or more scheduled inspections or maintenance periods.

In addition to understanding *when* maintenance may occur, it is also important for medical personnel to understand *who* is qualified to perform maintenance on the aircraft. Which items must be performed by a qualified mechanic may be prescribed in the FARs, the aircraft manufacturer's documentation, or an individual program's operations manual; in general, however, an FAA-qualified mechanic must perform major maintenance items. Most maintenance items must also be documented in the aircraft logbook. Unlike ground ambulances or your personal vehicle, the amount of troubleshooting that the medical crew, or pilot, can perform may be incredibly limited. It is therefore always prudent to check with a pilot or mechanic before performing any alterations or modifications to the aircraft or when attempting to troubleshoot any aircraft or cabin malfunction that arises during transport.

Minimum Equipment List

Under the FARs, all instruments and equipment on an aircraft must be functional prior to each flight. However, an air carrier may adopt the FAA's master minimum equipment list (MMEL) for their airframe or develop their own minimum equipment list (MEL), to provide an allowance for flying with inoperative equipment that is determined to be nonessential for safety of flight. The MMEL is specific to each airframe and identifies critical instruments and equipment that must be operational for safe flight. Because this master list applies to all airframes and does not account for operational nuance, most air carriers develop their own, more restrictive, MEL. Colloquially in air medical transport, when a specific item is said to be "MEL'd" on an aircraft, it means the item is inoperative, but, based on the air carrier's approved MEL, the aircraft may still operate without that piece of equipment functioning. In some cases, inoperative equipment may restrict the ability to perform certain flights. For example, an MEL might list an inoperative autopilot system as permissible for VFR flights but might prohibit the aircraft from operating under IFR conditions until that system is repaired.[4,7,9]

Medevac Status

The term "medevac" is used to identify an aircraft requiring priority handling in the ATC system for those missions of an urgent medical nature. This may include response to an emergent patient (e.g., a primary scene response or time-sensitive interfacility transfer) or when a patient is on board and their condition warrants expeditious handling. Medevac status affords the aircraft priority handling with taking off, landing, or routing through congested airspace, but importantly, priority handling remains at the discretion of the air traffic controller. Especially in congested metropolitan airspace or at busy international airports, declaring medevac status can provide significant time savings; however, the disruption to commercial and private aviation caused by expediting medevac traffic may be significant and lead to costly delays. Therefore, an air medical service must reserve medevac status for those times when it is absolutely necessary. Medevac status does not negate the need to comply with Transportation Security Administration reporting requirements.[3]

The National Transportation Safety Board and Federal Aviation Administration

Aviation incidents that occur within the United States are investigated by the NTSB. Based on investigative findings of aviation incidents and accidents, the NTSB publishes recommendations to enhance safe operations. Importantly, however, the NTSB recommendations are just that – recommendations; only the FAA may enact legislation to require changes in aviation operations or requirements. Although compliance with FAA regulations is mandatory, air medical services should consider reviewing and integrating NTSB recommendations into their daily operations when practical to mitigate identified safety hazards.

Notice to Air Missions

Notices to Air Missions (NOTAMs) are issued to provide pilots with information about temporary conditions that may affect the safety of flight. Preflight procedures should include reviewing NOTAMs available in the area of planned flight operations. NOTAMs may include information about airspace safety hazards (e.g., construction cranes or other obstructions near a landing area, unlit towers, etc.); runway, taxiway, or ramp restrictions at an airport; special communications situations; status of navigational aid or weather service availability; or other pertinent information.[3]

Temporary Flight Restrictions

Temporary flight restrictions (TFRs) are a form of NOTAM that is issued when necessary to restrict access to certain airspace. TFRs may be enacted for several reasons, including hazardous conditions, local or national security (e.g., mass gatherings), to protect an airspace for public safety operations (e.g., search and rescue operations or wildland firefighting), or other general warnings as deemed appropriate. Although legitimate medevac flights are often exempted from TFR restrictions, it is important to be aware of the specific details of the TFR and follow any necessary procedures prior to entering (e.g., even if exempted, it is often necessary to notify ATC of the need to enter the TFR area for medevac purposes).

Weather Considerations

A significant consideration for CCT medical crew is the basic understanding of weather conditions and their effect on aircraft operations. Adverse weather conditions are a major contributing factor to aviation accidents, second only to human error.[14–16]

Weather Reporting Sources

It is important that only official weather sources be utilized to obtain weather information. Within the United States, official weather reports and forecasts can be obtained through the National Oceanic and Atmospheric Administration (NOAA) and National Weather Service (NWS) and found on the Aviation Weather Service (AWS) website at aviationweather.gov.[3,4] The following weather report types can be located on the AWS website and are useful for CCT medical crew to understand:

- Meteorological Aerodrome Reports (METARs): METARs provide the most current observed conditions at a reporting location. METAR information is most commonly obtained by an Automated Surface Observing System (ASOS) or Automated Weather Observing System (AWOS) with or without additional manual

KTRI 062353Z 31008G20KT 3SM RA SCT023 BKN031 OVC070 22/18 A3028
(1)   (2)   (3)   (4)   (5)   (6)   (7)   (8)

• **Figure 3.7** An Example METAR Report. Components of a METAR include the following:
(1) Station identification *KTRI, or Bristol/Tri-Cities Airport, Tennessee*
(2) Date (first 2 digits) and time (next 4 digits) the METAR was issued *6th day of month at 23:53 Zulu*
(3) Wind direction (first 3 digits) and speed (next 2 digits); "G" indicates wind gusts *Wind from 310° (northwest) at 8 knots, with wind gusts up to 20 knots*
(4) Visibility *3 statute miles*
(5) Current weather (if applicable); "+" indicates "heavy," "–" indicates "light" *rain*
(6) Current cloud cover, in hundreds of feet *Scattered layer at 2300 feet, broken layer at 3100 feet, and overcast at 7000 feet*
(7) Temperature and dewpoint, in degrees Celsius *Temperature 22°C, dewpoint 18°C*
(8) Altimeter (barometric pressure), in inches of mercury *30.28 in Hg*

human augmentation. METAR information at an ASOS/AWOS station is also available by phone or may be accessed during flight as part of the Automatic Terminal Information Service (ATIS) radio frequency at each airport with a reporting station. METARs are only valid for one hour and updated hourly at approximately 55 minutes past the hour, but may be updated more frequently if necessary. Fig. 3.7 shows an example of METAR. Table 3.3 provides a list of common abbreviations used to report weather conditions in a METAR, although many METAR sources, including the AWS website, provide an option to receive a "decoded" METAR in plain English.

• **Terminal Aerodrome Forecast (TAF):** These represent short-term (up to 24–30 hours) forecasts for prevailing conditions near select airports. TAFs are issued by the NWS Weather Forecast Office.

• **Significant Meteorological Information (SIGMET):** SIGMETs are issued to advise pilots of weather that may be hazardous to all aircraft. SIGMETs are valid for up to 4 hours but may be updated or re-issued if conditions persist. **Convective SIGMETs** indicate conditions favorable to the development of severe thunderstorms, which may result in high winds, hail, tornadoes, severe turbulence, severe icing, and/or low-level wind shear.

• **Airmen's Meteorological Information (AIRMET):** An AIRMET describes weather conditions that may be significant but are less severe than those requiring SIGMET issuance. AIRMETs may contain information about prevailing IMC conditions, mountain obscuration, turbulence, strong surface winds, or icing levels.

• **Pilot Reports (PIREP):** Reports issued by pilots during flight, which may include information about cloud cover, current weather conditions, icing or turbulence severity, or other pertinent conditions.

• **Weather Cameras:** Official weather cameras are a newer initiative spearheaded by the FAA, allowing pilots to observe real-time

TABLE 3.3 Common Abbreviations Used in METAR and TAF Weather Reporting

Qualifiers (used prior to a weather phenomenon to qualify it)

"+" = Heavy	"–" = Light	"VC" = Vicinity (5–10 miles from station)

Descriptors (used prior to a weather phenomenon to describe it)

BC = Patches	BL = Blowing	DR = Drifting	FZ = Freezing
MI = Shallow	PR = Partial	SH = Showers	TS = Thunderstorm

Weather Phenomena

Precipitation

DZ = Drizzle	GR = Hail	GS = Small hail	IC = Ice crystals
PL = Ice pellets	RA = Rain	SG = Snow grains	SN = Snow
UP = Unknown			

Obscuration

BR = Mist (>⅝ SM)	DU = Dust	FG = Fog (<⅝ SM)	FU = Smoke
HZ = Haze	PY = Spray	SA = Sand	VA = Volcanic ash

Other

DS = Dust storm	FC = Funnel cloud	SQ = Squall	SS = Sandstorm
+FC = Tornado or waterspout			

Examples: RA indicates rain, −RA indicates light rain, VCRA indicates rain in the vicinity but not directly over the reporting station, and +TSRA indicates heavy rain and thunderstorms.

weather at covered locations. These cameras are used heavily across Alaska, Hawaii, and Canada and are starting to be implemented in the continental United States. FAA weather cameras can be located at weathercams.faa.gov.

Ceiling and Visibility

Proper flight planning requires the knowledge of current and forecasted ceiling and visibility, especially when flights are planned to be conducted under VFR only. As noted previously, VFR flights require minimum ceiling and visibility thresholds, such as those listed for HAA operations in Table 3.2.[8] Ceiling and visibility are automated and obtained from ASOS/AWOS stations. These stations break the horizon circle into eight segments and use this information to determine cloud cover and prevailing visibility distance.[3,4]

The METAR and TAF will report actual and forecast cloud layers, respectively, but do not use the term "ceiling." There are five possibilities for cloud cover, as reported by ASOS/AWOS stations, based on the number of horizon segments in which clouds are detected:
- SKC (sky clear): no observed cloud in any of the 8 horizon segments
- FEW (few clouds): clouds are detected in 1 or 2 of the 8 segments
- SCT (scattered): clouds are detected in 3 or 4 of the 8 segments
- BKN (broken): clouds are detected in 5 to 7 of the 8 segments
- OVC (overcast): clouds are detected in all of the 8 segments

As defined in the FARs, a "ceiling" refers to the height, AGL, of the lowest cloud layer reported as BKN or OVC or the lowest level of some other obscuration (e.g., smoke, volcanic ash, etc.).[3,4] The ceiling for the METAR shown in Fig. 3.7 would be 3100 feet, even though there is a lower layer of scattered clouds at 2300 feet.

There are a few important points to understand about ceiling reporting: First, FEW and SCT cloud layers are not usually considered a ceiling but may still pose a hazard for visual flight operations and should be taken into consideration during flight planning. Some programs may opt to consider these layers part of the "ceiling" to enhance their safety of flight, especially during night operations. Second, the reported cloud cover is that which is observed *above ground level* and *at the reporting location*. If a flight is operating in a region with variable terrain, the actual cloud cover relative to the ground at any given location may be higher or lower than that reported at the nearest weather observation station (Fig. 3.1).

Cumulonimbus (CB) and towering cumulus (TCU) clouds deserve special attention. CB clouds are reported on both METARs and TAFs when applicable, whereas TCU clouds are only reported on METAR data; the cloud type is listed after the level representing its base. For example, OVC020CB indicates CB cloud formation with a solid (overcast) base at 2000 feet AGL. TCU clouds are often a precursor to CB clouds and indicate atmospheric instability. They are frequently accompanied by turbulent air in and around the cloud formation. CB clouds contain a large amount of moisture and are associated with significantly hazardous weather, including thunderstorms, lightning, hail, wind shear, and potentially even tornadoes.[4]

The term "visibility" refers to the greatest horizontal distance one can observe with the naked eye. Visibility is determined by identifying whether specific objects, situated at a known distance from the observation station, are visible under current atmospheric conditions. The prevailing visibility reported in a METAR must be present for at least one-half (4/8) of the horizon circle, but it does not necessarily have to be contiguous.[3,4] This again poses important considerations for flight planning. Although prevailing visibility may be reported at, or just above, VMC minimums, there may be areas of degraded visibility below those minimums.

As FAA weather cameras become more widely adopted, this will enable aircrews to have real-time observations of the conditions at covered locations. Most weather cameras have an annotated clear-day visual reference accompanying each camera angle, identifying various static reference points (e.g., buildings, towers, or vegetation) at known distances on the horizon to help determine visibility.

Ambient Temperature and Dewpoint

Temperature is another important consideration for air medical transport for two primary reasons: First, as temperature increases, air density typically decreases, leading to degraded aircraft performance at higher temperatures. For example, HAA flights may not be able to accommodate additional passengers in the hot summer months because of their loss of lift in the higher temperatures. Second, the relationship between temperature and dewpoint can be useful in determining relative humidity. The dewpoint is the temperature at which the air will become fully saturated with water vapor and moisture is likely to condense out of the air. As these two values converge, the risk of fog, clouds, or precipitation increases.[4]

Ambient temperature also plays into logistical considerations during flight planning. Consider the amount of time the aircraft will spend on the ground, because air conditioning or heating cannot be left on for more than a few minutes during this time unless the aircraft is kept running or an auxiliary power unit is used. Unfortunately, auxiliary power units may not be available at smaller airports, remote helipads, or improvised landing zones where most rotor- or fixed-wing transports originate.

Another temperature consideration is evident at higher altitudes, at which point the ambient temperature decreases. As the altitude increases, temperature decreases. The fuselage circumference of most air medical fixed-wing aircraft tends to be relatively small, and insulation of the walls is such that the walls and floor feel cool. The cumulative effect of these factors is often a cooler environment in a fixed-wing aircraft.

A third temperature consideration is encountered when descending into tropical or humid climates. On descent, windows may become fogged and other types of condensation may occur inside the aircraft.

Wind

Wind speed and direction is useful for takeoff/landing and en route calculations. Because air is needed to move over the airfoil of an aircraft wing to generate lift, at lower speeds and altitudes (i.e., takeoff and landing), travel *into* the wind during these phases of flight improves aircraft performance. Takeoff into a headwind reduces the required groundspeed (and, therefore, runway distance) necessary to achieve takeoff. Conversely, takeoff with a tailwind can significantly increase the necessary groundspeed (and, therefore, runway distance) necessary to achieve takeoff and may prevent the aircraft from achieving lift prior to the end of the runway in severe circumstances.[2,4,5] The effect of head- and tailwinds can be observed with winds at any angle relative to the aircraft but have more of an effect the stronger they are and the closer they are to the nose or tail of the aircraft, respectively.

Once aloft, however, wind speed and direction can be used to determine the relative groundspeed of the aircraft and provide for an estimated travel time to reach a destination. In general, the aircraft groundspeed is the airspeed of the aircraft (as indicated on the aircraft's airspeed indicator) *plus* any direct tailwind, or *minus* any direct headwind. As an example, an aircraft flying with a 100 kt airspeed in the absence of any winds will also show a groundspeed of 100 kt. That same aircraft flying into a 20 kt headwind will have a groundspeed of 80 kt (100 kt airspeed – 20 kt headwind) and will therefore take a longer time to cover the same distance.[4]

METARs and TAFs report both wind speed and direction. The first three digits of a wind report are the distance *from which the wind is coming*, using the magnetic compass (Fig. 3.2A). The second two digits are the wind speed in knots. Thus, wind reported as "09005" on a METAR indicates a 5 kt wind coming *from 90°*, or from the *east* moving *west*. Thus, if the aircraft is traveling directly east (a bearing of 090°), this would be a 5 kt headwind. If the aircraft were traveling directly west (a bearing of 270°), this would instead be a 5 kt tailwind.[3,4]

In addition to obtaining current wind information from METAR and ATIS reports, wind cones (commonly referred to as windsocks) are required to be present at each FAA-certified airport or heliport.[17,18] Wind cones indicate relative wind speed, with higher wind speeds causing the cone to be more fully extended. FAA specifications require wind cones to be fully extended at wind speeds of 15 kt, and the wind cone must be able to indicate wind direction with winds of at least 3 kt.[17] Contrary to popular belief, there are no requirements that (a) the wind cone be striped or (b) the individual segments tell a specific wind speed (e.g., a wind cone that is half extended does not necessarily indicate a wind speed of 7.5 kt).

Wind Gusts

Another concept to understand is the effect of wind *gusts*. Wind gusts reflect sudden changes in the wind speed over a short period of time. This can lead to turbulent air and may be unpleasant for crew and patients alike, especially patients not used to air travel and turbulence. In general, the larger the spread between the prevailing wind speed and the peak gust, the more likely the aircraft is to experience turbulence.[4] Wind gusts are designated in METARs and TAFs with the letter "G" and the peak gust speed following the prevailing wind direction and speed. For example, 09005G15 indicates a prevailing wind of 5 kt from the east with gusts up to 15 kt.

Wind Shear

Wind shear is a sudden, significant change in the speed and/or direction of wind over a small area. Wind shear can occur at any altitude but is particularly concerning when it occurs at low levels due to the aircraft's proximity to the ground. As a result of the sudden change in wind, the aircraft may experience sudden updrafts, downdrafts, or horizontal movements. At low altitudes, this may lead to a rapid gain or loss of altitude and in severe situations may cause unintended collision with obstacles or terrain. Wind shear is most commonly encountered near frontal activity, in areas of convection or thunderstorms, during temperature inversions (where there is an area of temperature *increase* with increasing altitude), or near-surface obstructions.[4,19]

Weather Trends

In a similar manner to how CCT medical personnel can trend a patient's vital signs to predict clinical deterioration and anticipate the need for further interventions, one can trend weather observations over time to predict the possibility of degraded conditions prior to accepting a flight request. The AWS website (aviationweather.gov) can provide both current and recent METAR reports for requested reporting stations. Rapidly falling barometric pressure ("altimeter" pressure on the METAR) may indicate the approach of inclement weather and potentially severe thunderstorm activity. A narrow temperature/dewpoint margin trending toward convergence, especially when coupled with light or no surface winds to disperse the water vapor, makes sudden fog formation and degraded visibility a distinct possibility.[4] In addition to trending METAR readings, comparing current METAR observations with TAF predictions can help understand how reliable future weather predictions may be. For example, if the TAF is predicting deteriorating weather in the next several hours, but METAR observations indicate current conditions are already below the forecast values, it's likely that the weather will deteriorate more rapidly and/or more significantly than what is currently forecast.

Overview of Aircraft Instruments

The most common HAA crew configuration involves two medical providers with a single pilot, even for programs operating IFR aircraft.[20,21] Thus, it is not uncommon for a CCT medical provider to be seated in the cockpit of the aircraft for flight legs without a patient on board, especially for rotor wing operations. Although many newer airframes are transitioning to a "glass cockpit" with advanced digital instruments and electronic flight displays, analog instruments (or digital representations of familiar analog faces) remain a prevalent feature in the cockpit of most air medical aircraft. Understanding basic information provided on these instruments may help improve situational awareness for the CCT medical crew and may aid in assisting a single pilot during planned IFR flights or during inadvertent flight into IIMC. The same information is usually available on electronic flight displays, but the nuance of each model is beyond the scope of this text.

The Pitot-Static System

All aircraft are equipped with a pitot-static system that is used to obtain critical information about airspeed and air pressure used to provide data to the airspeed indicator, vertical speed indicator, and altimeter. The static pressure, or actual ambient barometric pressure, is obtained through small holes located in an area of the aircraft likely to experience undisturbed air. The pitot tube captures the total pressure, including both static and dynamic pressure, as the aircraft moves through the air. The airspeed indicator bases its readings off of the dynamic reading (i.e., the pitot input minus the static input), whereas the altimeter and the vertical speed indicator use only static input.[2,4,5] As an important word of safety, aircraft pitot tubes are often heated to prevent moisture or ice from entering the tube, and these will remain hot for a period of time after landing and shutting down the aircraft. Care should be taken to avoid contacting the pitot tubes when operating in close proximity to the aircraft.

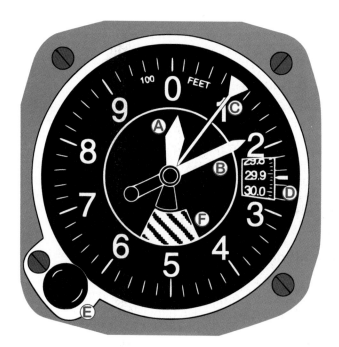

• **Figure 3.8** Altimeter. Although altimeter models may differ considerably, common features on many altimeters include: **(A)** a short, fat dial for thousands of feet; **(B)** a longer dial for hundreds of feet; **(C)** a longer, narrow dial for tens of thousands of feet; **(D)** a display of the current altimeter pressure setting; **(E)** a knob to set the altimeter pressure; and **(F)** a "cross-hatch flag" that displays at altitudes below 10,000 feet. In this example, the altimeter is calibrated to 29.92 in Hg pressure and is displaying an altitude of around 10,180 feet.

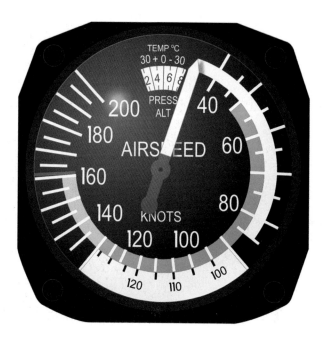

• **Figure 3.9** Airspeed Indicator. The airspeed indicator shows the *indicated airspeed*. Different aircraft will have different ranges for acceptable airspeeds. The maximum airspeed, or V_{NE}, of this aircraft, indicated by the *red line*, is around 162 knots indicated airspeed (KIAS).

Altimeter (Altitude Indicator)

The altimeter (Fig. 3.8) provides the altitude of the aircraft above a given pressure altitude; in aviation, the altimeter is set to the sea level pressure, so altitude is expressed relative to mean sea level (MSL). Although *standard* sea level pressure is 760 mm Hg, or 29.92 in Hg, changes in atmospheric conditions lead to varying *actual* sea level pressures. Thus, it is necessary to calibrate the altimeter to the local sea-level barometric pressure. This pressure is provided on the METAR as the "altimeter" and is usually provided by ATC controllers upon first contact with the tower. Failure to calibrate the altimeter to account for the local barometric pressure can lead to an inaccurate altitude display. If the altimeter setting is *higher* than the actual sea-level barometric pressure, the aircraft's true altitude will be *lower* than that displayed, and vice versa. It is worth reiterating that the altimeter displays altitude relative to MSL, not altitude above the ground. It is critical that the pilot know the elevation and topography of the local area to ensure that the aircraft remain free of terrain.[4]

Radio Altimeter

Unlike a pressure altimeter, a radio (or radar) altimeter uses radio-frequency signals to determine the aircraft's altitude above the ground. Because the signal is sent from and received by the aircraft directly, this allows for precise altitudes even with changing terrain.

Airspeed Indicator

The airspeed indicator (Fig. 3.9) displays the indicated airspeed (IAS) of the aircraft as measured using the pitot-static system. The

IAS does not account for head- or tailwinds and may therefore not reflect the actual groundspeed of the aircraft (true airspeed [TAS], which does account for windspeeds, is usually available on newer digital instruments). The abbreviation KIAS is used to note speeds in *knots of indicated airspeed*, referencing the speeds obtained from the airspeed indicator.[4]

The airspeed indicator has standard markings (Fig. 3.9), although the range of values for the different markings are unique to the specifications of a given airframe. The green arc represents normal operating airspeeds. The yellow arc indicates a cautionary range and should generally only be entered in smooth air, and even then, it should be done with extreme caution. The red line on the airspeed indicator reflects the "never-exceed speed" (V_{NE}) of the aircraft. Some rotor-wing aircraft may also have a blue line representing the maximum allowable airspeed for autorotation. White arcs may also be present on fixed-wing airspeed indicators representing permissible speed ranges with flap use.[2,4,5]

Vertical Speed Indicator

The vertical speed indicator (Fig. 3.10), also called the vertical velocity indicator, displays the rate of the aircraft's climb or descent in feet per minute. A reading of zero indicates level flight. An upward movement of the needle indicates that the aircraft is on a climb. A downward movement of the needle indicates that the aircraft is descending. In purely analog systems, the needle may take a few seconds to stabilize on the actual rate of climb or descent.[4]

Attitude Indicator (Artificial Horizon)

The attitude indicator (Fig. 3.11), sometimes called the "artificial horizon," depicts the *attitude* of the aircraft relative to the true horizon. The attitude indicator provides simultaneous information about pitch (upward or downward direction of the aircraft nose) and bank (side-to-side rolling of aircraft). This can be a

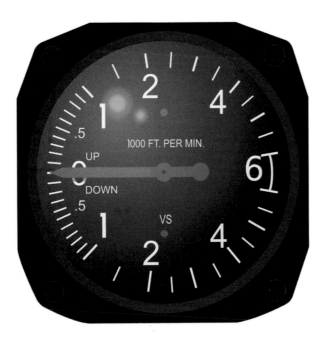

• **Figure 3.10** Vertical Speed Indicator. Vertical speed indicator showing thousands of feet per minute. An upward movement indicates climb, and a downward speed indicates descent.

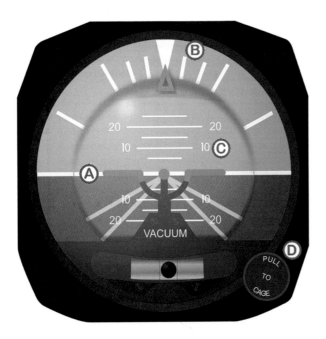

• **Figure 3.11** Attitude Indicator. The attitude indicator displays a representation of the aircraft "wings" relative to the horizon, where *blue* indicates the sky and *brown* indicates terrain **(A)**. During a turn, or banking event, the wings on the attitude indicator will display a turn relative to the horizon. The degree of banking, or bank angle, is identified at the top of the attitude indicator **(B)**. When the aircraft is pitching upward, the center dot between the two wings will be above the horizon (into the *blue area*); the degree, or angle, of upward pitch is noted with the horizontal bars **(C)**. Similarly, during a downward pitch, the center dot between the wings will move below the horizon into the *brown area*. "Caging" the attitude indicator **(D)** essentially locks the attitude indicator; it should be uncaged prior to flight.

critical resource for detecting, and correcting, the actual aircraft attitude during sudden loss of visual reference that may occur with IIMC flight.[4]

Other Gauges

A myriad of other gauges exists in the cockpit of rotor- and fixed-wing aircraft, providing information on other aspects of aircraft performance. These gauges may include temperature and pressure of various components of the engines and transmissions, torque, rotor speed (for rotor-wing aircraft), flap settings (for fixed-wing), and a variety of other information necessary for safe operation of the aircraft. Gauges monitoring critical aspects of aircraft performance are often accompanied by warning lights when conditions exceed predetermined thresholds.

Air Medical Resource Management

The concept of air medical resource management (AMRM), an extension of the crew resource management (CRM) used across general aviation, is designed to enhance situational awareness and improve communication and teamwork among all personnel involved in the flight.[22] The information contained in this chapter presents only a high-level overview of each topic but is written to enhance the awareness of pertinent aspects of aviation for the CCT medical team. It is hoped that this information can facilitate appropriate discussion between CCT medical team and their aviation counterparts prior to, during, and when debriefing an air medical flight. Although the pilot in command maintains ultimate authority and responsibility for the safe operation of the aircraft, AMRM principles empower any member of the transport team to speak up or ask questions as they arise, especially if there is a concern regarding the safety of the flight.

Summary

This chapter provided only a brief overview of some concepts felt to be beneficial to novice flight medical providers. Because each airframe can have nuanced differences, it is helpful for each air medical provider to review the specific instrumentation, limitations, and safety features of the aircraft in which they will be operating. For additional reading, the FAA publications referenced in this chapter may be freely accessed at the FAA's website.

References

1. Torenbeek E, Wittenberg H. *Flight Physics: Essentials of Aeronautical Disciplines and Technology, With Historical Notes.* Springer; 2009.
2. Federal Aviation Administration. *Airplane Flying Handbook.* FAA; 2021. Publication FAA-H-8083-3C.
3. Federal Aviation Administration. FAR/AIM 2022: *Federal Aviation Regulations and Aeronautical Information Manual.* Aviation Supplies & Academics; 2021.
4. Federal Aviation Administration. *Pilot's Handbook of Aeronautical Knowledge.* FAA; 2016. Publication FAA-H-8083-25B.
5. Federal Aviation Administration. *Helicopter Flying Handbook.* FAA; 2019. Publication FAA-H-8083-21B.
6. Pisano A. *Physics for Anesthesiologists and Intensivists: From Daily Life to Clinical Practice.* 2nd ed. Springer; 2021.
7. General operating and flight rules. 2018; 14 C.F.R. § 91.
8. Helicopter air ambulance equipment, operations, and training requirements. 2014; 14 C.F.R. § 135.601.

9. Operating requirements: Commuter and on demand operations and rules governing persons on board such aircraft. 2018; 14 C.F.R. § 135.

10. Operating requirements: Domestic, flag, and supplemental operations. 2018; 14 C.F.R. § 121.

11. Helicopter air ambulance operations. 2015; Advisory Circular 135-14B.

12. Helicopter air ambulance, commercial helicopter, and part 91 helicopter operations. 2014; 79 Fed. Reg. 9,931.

13. Maintenance, preventive maintenance, rebuilding, and alteration. 2021; 14 C.F.R. § 43.

14. Fultz AJ, Ashley WS. Fatal weather-related general aviation accidents in the United States. *Phys Geogr*. 2016;37(5):291–312. doi:10.1080/02723646.2016.1211854

15. Hon HH, Wojda TR, Barry N, et al. Injury and fatality risks in aeromedical transport: focus on prevention. *J Surg Res*. 2016;204(2):297–303. doi:10.1016/j.jss.2016.05.003

16. Greenhaw R, Jamali M. *Medical Helicopter Accident Review: Causes and Contributing Factors*. FAA; 2021. Publication DOT/FAA/AM-21/19.

17. Heliport design. 2012; Advisory Circular 150/5390-2C.

18. Certification of airports. 2004; 14 C.F.R. § 139.

19. Federal Aviation Administration. *Wind Shear*. FAA; 2008. Publication FAA-P-8740-40.

20. Rasmussen K, Sollid SJM. The HEMS medical crew survey. *Scand J Trauma Resusc Emerg Med*. 2015;23(Suppl 2):A28. doi:10.1186/1757-7241-23-S2-A28

21. Coons J, Zalar C. 2015 Air medical safety survey. *Air Med J*. 2016;35(3):120–125. doi:10.1016/j.amj.2016.03.003

22. Mains R. Air medical resource management: our last line of defense. *Air Med J*. 2015;34(2):78–81. doi:10.1016/j.amj.2014.10.008

4

Military Patient Transport

JEFFREY MALER

COMPETENCIES

1. Describe the military en route patient care transport system.
2. Describe the military roles of care and their respective capabilities.
3. Describe the difference between CASEVAC and MEDEVAC in the military transport environment.
4. Identify military patient transport platforms.
5. Identify the military medical training for transport personnel.
6. Describe the activation of patient transport in both the intra and intertheater environments.
7. Recognize special military transport situations and teams.

Introduction

The US Military Health System is a dynamic organization comprising the Army, Air Force, Navy, and the Defense Health Agency (DHA) medical assets. The system is responsible for the care and treatment of the combat-injured as well as the health promotion and medical readiness of the entire military force and their families. The system spreads across the entire trauma continuum, from prehospital injury prevention to trauma treatment and recovery. Essentially the military health system is a state-of-the-art trauma system with integrated services across the globe. Similar to civilian healthcare and hospital systems, the military health system strives to be a high-reliability organization. Although not required, military medical treatment facilities (MTFs) are accredited by The Joint Commission. Understanding the entire military health system is critical to understanding the unique transport environment and en route modalities the military utilizes.

The recent establishment of the DHA aligned the Department of Defense's medical assets under one organization. While each service component's medical command remains responsible for the medical warfighting function, DHA provides sustainment and health promotion for service members, retirees, and family members. DHA created a system of Healthcare Markets to manage military hospitals and clinics, similar to many civilian healthcare networks. In 2018, military MTFs began the conversion to DHA markets. The markets create a global network of military and civilian healthcare systems to provide standardized care to all beneficiaries.

While the primary mission of the military healthcare system is the treatment of the combat-injured and the medical readiness of the military force, the military plays a significant role in support of humanitarian and civil support missions. For example, the Army MEDEVAC and Navy Search and Rescue (SAR) teams complete high-risk missions in remote or austere locations throughout the United States. The Army National Guard, Army Reserve and Active Duty MEDEVAC teams are frequently called to rescue stranded climbers in the mountains of Colorado or the tundra of Alaska, while the Navy frequently rescues stranded hikers in the mountains of California.

Within the US military, the Air Force, Army, and Navy each have their own independent service surgeon generals and operating doctrines. While each service is accountable for its primary area of responsibility, today's operating environment necessitates a joint operating battle space with multiservice integration. The military focuses on interoperability in the multidomain operating environment. The healthcare delivery model follows the same principle. In addition, coalition partners, host nation military, and other government agencies' resources are frequently embedded and integrated into healthcare operations. Joint Operations present a unique challenge to the military healthcare system and require creative solutions. The interdependent Air Force, Army, and Navy medical transport capabilities must be interoperable and interchangeable in the looming threat of large-scale combat operations (Fig. 4.1).

Roles of Care

Understanding the different roles of care provided by the US military and its separate services helps understand each service's unique transport considerations. Military roles refer to the capability of care. Roles are in sequential order of a patient's movement through the military medical system.[1] In the military system, the lower the role, the less medical capability available, unlike the civilian system established by the American College of Surgeons trauma levels. The purpose of the graduating roles is for service members to be evaluated, treated, and released at the lowest level possible. Patients are transported to the next level of care as needed for definitive or specialty care with the goal of returning

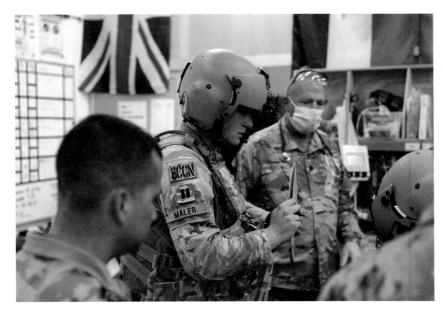

• **Figure 4.1** US Army En Route Critical Care Nurse (ECCN), a Flight Nurse, Receives Patient Report at a Role 2. (Courtesy Jeffrey Maler.)

the patient to duty. All military roles of care are highly mobile and modular; each role is able to move with the maneuver unit it supports. As warfighters advance on the battlefield, the medical support follows. US military doctrine follows the North Atlantic Treaty Organization (NATO) definition of roles of care. The similarities between the United States and NATO doctrine result in an interchangeable medical force with a shared understanding of the care provided at each level. Throughout the Afghanistan and Iraq wars, NATO partners worked side by side with US medical assets and all levels of care.

In the current operating environment, it is not uncommon for a patient to be transported directly from the Point of Injury (POI) to a Role 2 or a Role 1 to a Role 3. However, with the inevitability of large-scale combat operations, the roles of care will play a larger part in the treatment and movement of patients.

Point of Injury

Similar to "scene calls" in the civilian environment, POI is a term used for treatment performed at the location of the injury, for example, the location of a firefight or ambush. The treatment provided on the scene is first completed by the casualty, a nonmedical provider, or a basic medical provider. The focus of care provided at the POI is rapid assessment, stabilization, and transport to higher roles of care. The treatment provided at POI and subsequent care is in accordance with the Tactical Combat Casualty Care (TCCC) Guidelines.

TCCC was created by the Joint Trauma Services (JTS) to replace the legacy "Self-Aid Buddy Care." TCCC is designed for all service members to treat the preventable causes of death on the battlefield. The most common preventable causes of death, as identified by JTS, include massive hemorrhage, airway compromise, and tension pneumothorax. Of the 4596 casualties from 2001 to 2011, 24.3% of those deaths were deemed potentially survivable.[2] Most of those battlefield deaths were caused by massive hemorrhage. Standardizing the curriculum, training, and learning outcomes guarantees that every service member, regardless of service component, is capable of

treating the most common battlefield injuries. The TCCC curriculum follows a four-tiered provider approach, advancing skills and knowledge with each tier. All the tiers follow the same MARCH algorithm and contain three phases: Care Under Fire (CUF), Tactical Field Care (TFC), and Tactical Evacuation Care (TACEVAC). Each phase contains different treatment goals and outcomes to address the casualty and mission needs during that phase (Fig. 4.2).

The first phase of TCCC is CUF. During this phase, the primary goal is to suppress the enemy, get the casualty to cover, and prevent further injuries or casualties. The only treatment recommended in this phase is moving the casualty to cover and safety and stop life-threatening extremal hemorrhage. External hemorrhage control is best accomplished by a Committee on Tactical Combat Casualty Care (CoTCCC)–approved tourniquet. Tourniquets placed during CUF are applied following the "high and tight" method, placed proximal to the injury and over the uniform.

TFC begins when fire superiority is gained, the scene is made safe, and a perimeter is established. Attempting care before establishing a safe scene places the casualty and rescuer at risk of harm. TFC begins with the triage and identification of the number of patients. Care is provided following the MARCH algorithm for the identification and treatment of life-threatening injuries (Table 4.1). Treatments during this phase may include the application of tourniquets, the establishment of a surgical airway, needle chest decompression, chest seal application, IV or IO access, administration of blood products, hypothermia management, and the treatment of pain. Documentation of the interventions and treatments is paramount in the continuum of care. Care during all phases of TCCC is documented on the TCCC Card (DA 1380). The TCCC Card follows the MIST (Mechanism, Injuries, Symptoms, and Treatments) format to hand over patient care safely.

The Tactical Evacuation Care phase begins during the TFC phase with submitting a 9-line MEDEVAC or patient movement request. In the civilian world transport can be within minutes; on the battlefield, it can be hours to days depending on severity. Providers at all levels must be prepared to treat and hold patients until evacuation arrives. Once the transport modality arrives,

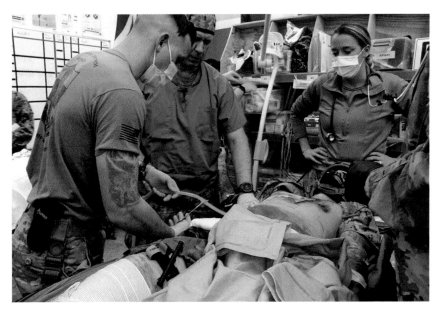

• **Figure 4.2** US Navy Expeditionary Medical Unit (EMU) Role 2 Surgical Team Provides Interventions on a Simulated Casualty. (Courtesy Jeffrey Maler.)

TABLE 4.1	TCCC March Algorithm

TCCC March Algorithm
M – Massive hemorrhage
A – Airway
R – Respiratory
C – Circulation
H – Hypothermia/head injury
P – Pain
A – Antibiotics
W – Wounds
S – Splints

whether CASEVAC or MEDEVAC, the TFC transitions to Tactical Evacuation Care. TACEVAC guidelines mirror the care provided under the TFC phase with the addition of advanced procedures and by appropriate providers. The only significant variation between TFC and Tactical Evacuation Care is the initiation of cardiopulmonary resuscitation (CPR). Casualties with extensive torso trauma or polytrauma who lose pulse or respirations during care under TFC should be treated with bilateral needle decompressions for the possible treatment of tension pneumothorax. If unsuccessful in the TFC setting, a provider should not initiate CPR as it will be unsuccessful and resource exhausting. During TACEVAC, however, a provider may initiate CPR after bilateral needle chest decompression if the casualty does not have any apparent fatal wounds and will arrive at a surgical facility within a short duration of time.[3]

The ground medic is the first medical provider a casualty will see on the battlefield. Organic ground medics, embedded in the operational unit, support nearly all maneuver units in the military.

Whether an Army Combat Medic, Air Force Medic, or Navy Corpsman, these ground medics are the first medical asset on the battlefield responsible for trauma care and stabilization. Furthermore, when not engaged with trauma care, these same medics are responsible for routine and preventative medical care. As part of the DHA transition, all enlisted medical personnel train at the same basic medical level at Fort Sam Houston at METC. All Army Combat Medics, Air Force Medics, and Navy Corpsmen are instructed and trained to the civilian level of EMT-B with extensive additional trauma training. While the Army and Air Force medics are required to obtain and maintain a National Registry EMT certification, it is only an option for selected Navy Corpsmen.

The US Army Combat Medic/Healthcare Specialists, commonly known by their MOS "68-Whisky," are trained at the Medical Center of Excellence (MEDCoE) at Fort Sam Houston, Texas. The 16-week advanced individual training (AIT) encompasses the National Registry of Emergency Medical Technicians (NREMT) curriculum and trauma education. The training 68W receives exceeds the standards of the NREMT EMT level. Within the next few years, initial entry Army medics will graduate with the AEMT, a move that best aligns with the skill set already taught and expected of the combat medic. Additionally, advanced skills in prolonged field care and blood transfusions are revolutionizing the combat medic of tomorrow. Upon completion of AIT, combat medics are sent to the units for continued on-the-job training. Combat medics must complete annual refresher training and biannual recertification by NREMT. Combat medics are assigned to medical companies of brigade combat teams (BCTs) to enable the treatment and transport of maneuver unit's casualties. Outside of maneuver units, combat medics are employed by medical battalions and brigades as resources to support the treatment and movement of casualties on the battlefield. Stateside medics can be found working in clinics, hospitals, or maneuver units supporting the medical readiness of the Army force.

The US Air Force Medic undergoes a 14-week initial training at Fort Sam Houston. The Air Force program with the Army completes the basic NREMT curriculum followed by service-specific tasks and skills. Air Force medics complete biannual NREMT refresher training at the unit and maintain an NREMT certification. The Air Force is the only service component that runs its own robust Emergency Medical Services; basic medics and paramedics respond to 911 emergencies on bases throughout the world. Air Force medics attend advanced courses to specialize in aerospace medicine, aeromedical evacuation (AE), operational medicine, or other specialties. A unique specialty in the Air Force is the Independent Duty Medical Technician (IDMT). IDMTs are forward-utilized or deployed medics with advanced training to operate pseudoindependently. These medics have an expanded scope of care with the ability to assess, diagnose, and treat basic diseases and medical complaints. In collaboration with a physician and a standardized formulary, IDMTs prescribe basic medication. IDMTs work in geographically remote units or with special operations forces that are not supported by larger medical assets.

Navy Hospital Corpsmen complete initial 14-week medical training (A-School) at Fort Sam Houston, Texas. Corpsmen complete the basic NREMT curriculum but are not required to be certified by NREMT. Upon completion, Corpsmen are assigned to Naval clinics, hospitals, and ships throughout the world. All Corpsmen are required to maintain the Hospital Corpsmen Skill Basic qualification. Corpsmen in specialty roles including respiratory therapy, laboratory technician, or pharmacy technician complete additional training (C-School). Specialty Corpsmen obtain certification and licensure in their respective specialty while maintaining basic skills qualification. Independent Duty Corpsman (IDC), similar to USAF IDMTs, complete advanced training to work as an advanced provider. IDCs support special missions and units in austere or remote environments. IDCs are most notably utilized on submarines and small ships where no other medical officer is available. Independent Duty Corpsmen are the peak of Navy Medicine. The Marine Corps, lacking its own organic medical assets, utilizes a Naval Corpsman and medical officers to service its Marines. Corpsmen assigned to Marine Corps maneuver units, as Fleet Marine Force Corpsman, acquire additional training to prepare to deploy with the Marines.

Role 1 (Emergent Care)

Military Role 1 is the unit level of medical care and is responsible for the immediate treatment and lifesaving interventions for medical and trauma ailments. Role 1 in large-scale operations becomes the staging location for casualties awaiting evacuation to higher echelons of care. Across the service components, a Role 1 is manned by a provider, either a physician or a physician's assistant, and several medics. In the combat environment, Role 1 provides initial and advanced TCCC and when available provides sick call and preventative medicine operations. When staffed by a provider, a Role 1 may provide basic invasive and medical interventions, including intubation, chest tube placement, and central line access.

Battalion Aid Station serves as the Role 1 asset. An aid station is staffed by a provider, and 2 to 4 medics, including a senior medic. The Army Role 1 is highly mobile; it is required to move with its maneuver unit to provide immediate medical services. The Navy and Marine Battalion Aid Stations are operated by a provider, numerous Corpsmen, and litter bearers. Both Aid Stations provide disease and nonbattle injury routine and emergency care to the maneuver units they support (Fig. 4.3).

Role 2 (Forward Resuscitative Care)

Military Role 2 provides advanced trauma management and emergency medical treatment, including the continuation of resuscitation initiated at the POI or Role 1. A Role 2 is focused on providing emergency and stabilization treatment rather than definitive care. Role 2s are limited in capabilities and are resource dependent. Without medical resupply and patient transport, Role 2s become limited to 72 hours of operation and limited patient hold capability. In addition to emergency surgical treatment, the Role 2 level of care includes full spectrum of services including integrated behavioral health, preventative medicine, dental, physical therapy, patient hold, laboratory services, and medical logistics. The military medical logistics chain is responsible for supplying medical

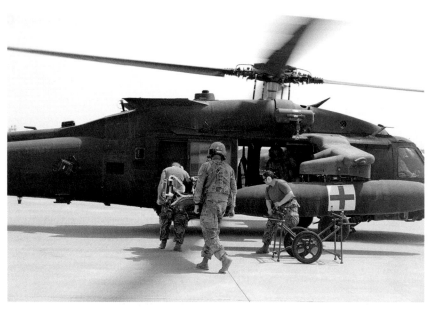

• **Figure 4.3** US Navy Expeditionary Medical Unit (Role 2) Members Load a Patient onto a US Army MEDEVAC HH-60M Helicopter for Transport to a Field Hospital (Role 3). Interoperability between services is vital in the care of casualties. (Courtesy Jeffrey Maler.)

equipment, medications, and blood products to units around the world in an expedited fashion.

Forward Resuscitation Surgical Detachments (FRSDs) provide the Army Role 2 surgical service. An FRSD can serve as a standalone asset or integrate with a collocated medical company to increase capabilities. The primary mission of an FRSD is to provide far-forward damage control resuscitation and damage control surgery to stabilize patients for further medical evacuation to the next higher role of medical care. An FRSD is made up of two identical elements comprising 10 personnel: an Emergency Physician, a General Surgeon, an Orthopedic Surgeon, an Anesthesia provider, a trauma nurse, a critical care nurse, a licensed practical nurse, a surgical tech, a combat medic, and administrative personnel. When combined, an FRSD provides emergency treatment, triage, and surgical intervention for 30 patients over 72 hours without resupply. A full FRSD can manage eight postoperative patients for 6 hours after surgery. During split operations, each 10-person element can manage 12 patients for 72 hours and hold 4 postoperative patients for 6 hours.[4] The modular design and organization of the elements allow for rapid deployment and movement with the maneuver elements to place surgical capabilities as far forward to the POI as possible. Full Role 2 services are provided by the Army's Medical Company Area Support (MCAS) and the Brigade Support Medical Company (BSMC). These units provide 8 out of 10 medical functions including medical treatment, evacuation, logistics, command and control, dental services, laboratory services, preventative medicine, and combat and operational stress control. The BSMC only lacks definitive hospitalization and veterinary services. Each Brigade Combat Team (BCT), which is the Army's maneuver element, contains one BSMC. Medical Brigades support larger maneuver element operations with supplemental MCAS units. The Army Role 2 is critical in treating and evacuating patients on and off the battlefield.[5]

Air Force Role 2 surgical services are provided by Ground Surgical Teams (GSTs). The GST is comprised of a surgeon, anesthesiologist, health service administrator, emergency physician, critical care nurse, and surgical services tech. The team provides damage control surgery, resuscitation, and emergency care for injured or critically ill patients in an austere environment. A GST is able to stabilize and prepare casualties for evacuation to high levels of care. The team can perform up to 10 surgical interventions and postoperative holding for up to 3 patients for 12 hours without resupply.[6] A GST can serve as a standalone entity or augment other medical assets for additional surgical capability. An Air Force GST, similar to an Army forward surgical detachment, depends on medical resupply and patient evacuation. The Air Force has additional Role 2 capabilities with the Expeditionary Medical Support (EMEDS) Health Response Team (HRT) and the EMEDS+10. The EMEDS HRT is the first increment of the EMEDS capability.[7] EMEDS is a modular medical support package that can build up to 25 patient beds. The smaller HRT provides surgical stabilization and patient hold for four patients for up to 24 hours. Within 24 hours of notification, the team can deploy and establish emergency room capabilities within 2 hours of arrival, with complete surgical services within 6 hours. The HRT contains surgical, dental, critical care, flight medicine, and radiological services. As the mission expands, the EMEDS system can continue to grow to the EMEDS+10 (additional 6 beds to HRT) or the EMEDS+25 (additional 15 beds to EMEDS+10). With the EMEDS+10 expansion, additional clinical services such as critical care, pediatrics, and OB/GYN can be attached.

The Navy provides the Marine Corps health support and management by assigning Sailors to organic Marine Corps units. The Marine Corps Role 2 is comprised of a Forward Resuscitative Surgery System (FRSS) and Shock Trauma Platoons (STPs), Surgical Company (SC), and Casualty Receiving and Treatment Ships (CRTSs), all staffed by Naval personnel. STPs are designed to bridge the gap between POI care and forward surgical care. STPs provide direct medical support to Marine Expeditionary Forces. As augments to Battalion Aid Stations, they can provide additional triage and pre/postoperative management. An STP directly supports FRSS by expanding the triage and patient hold capacity with 10 additional beds. The FRSS is the smallest unit that provides surgical care to Marine Corps casualties. The FRSS provides the full spectrum of trauma care, focusing on resuscitation and damage control surgery.[8] Similar to the Army FRSD and Air Force GST, the FRSS is limited in supplies and capacity; it can only hold a total of five patients for no more than 4 hours. While an FRSS can be a standalone asset, it is best served in cooperation with an STP or Battalion Aid Station (Fig. 4.4).

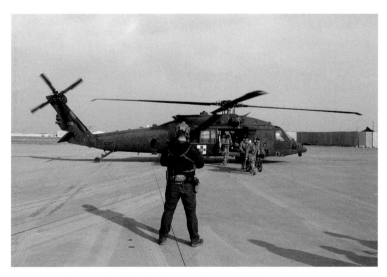

• **Figure 4.4** US Navy Personnel off load a Casualty from a US Army MEDEVAC HH-60M Helicopter. (Courtesy Jeffrey Maler.)

Casualty Receiving and Treatment Ships (CRTS) are large-deck amphibious ships augmented by Fleet Surgical Teams (FSTs) for the treatment and transport of casualties in the forward naval environment. An Amphibious Assault Ship can have up to 4 operating rooms, 15 intensive care beds, and 45 intermediate care beds when fully augmented with an FST and HSAP. In order to increase surgical support for the surface fleet, FSTs supplement medical assets on CRTS and other Amphibious Ready Groups assets. The team comprises 16 personnel: a chief surgeon, general surgeon, CRNA, internal medicine or emergency medicine physician, OR nurse, ICU nurse, respiratory therapist, medical admin officer, two OR techs, two lab techs, two general duty Corpsman, one radiology tech, and a senior enlisted advisor. There are currently nine FSTs worldwide. Much like the Army FRSD, the FST lacks prolonged patient hold capabilities and depends on patient evacuation and resupply Table 4.2.

After emergent stabilization and initial resuscitation, casualties are packaged for transport to the next role of care, an Army Field Hospital (FH), an Air Force EMEDS, or a Navy Fleet Hospital.

Role 3 (Theater Hospitalization)

Definitive theater level of care is provided at a Role 3 facility. A theater Role 3 provides care equivalent to stateside ACS Level 2 trauma centers, including initial resuscitation, stabilization, postoperative care, inpatient critical care, and outpatient care. Additional surgical and medical capabilities are contained at Role 3 that may not be available at a Role 2 asset, including CT capabilities, vascular surgery, OMFS, neurosurgery, urology, thoracic surgery, dental, critical care intensivists, psychiatric services, and logistical support. A major differentiating factor between Role 2 and Role 3 is the ability to provide hospitalization or the clinical and support services required to hold a patient for an extended period of time. Role 3 care is directed at providing care to return patients to duty or stabilization for transport.

The US Army Medical Command recently realigned Role 3 services from a Combat Support Hospital (CSH) to modular Hospital Centers (HCs) with corresponding Field Hospitals (FH). The change from CSH to FH allows Role 3 assets to be adapted for future operating environments. An HC is the command-and-control element for brigade-level medical assets and can doctrinally control up to two FHs. At maximum, an HC can support up to 240 beds when configured with FH and supporting augmentation detachments.[9]

Each FH is organically comprised of 32 beds, including ER, OR, ICU, and ICW capabilities. An FH is the smallest Army hospital element that retains the clinical capabilities of a Role 3 and is the cornerstone of deployed hospitalization. Augmentation detachments can expand the FH's patient hold and medical capabilities. A surgical detachment adds 24 critical care beds and thoracic, urology, and OMFS surgical capabilities. A medical augmentation detachment adds an additional 32 beds (12 ICU/20 ICW beds). An intermediate care ward provides 60 additional ICW beds with the appropriate nursing and support staff. HC and FH can add or subtract augmentation detachments as the military operation develops. The modular system is designed to place the appropriate medical assets in the appropriate locations to optimize combat casualty care and survival. Modularity enhances the mobility of the HC and FH, enabling medical assets to remain forward on the battlefield.[10]

The Air Force Role 3 builds upon the structure of the Role 2 EMEDS asset. The EMEDS + 25 and the Air Force Theater Level Hospital are designated military Role 3 assets. The third iteration of the EMEDS system, the EMEDS + 25, provides additional capabilities above that of the EMEDS + 10 to include an additional 15-bed capacity. The EMEDS + 25 provides expanded comprehensive care, including rehabilitation. Air Force Theater Hospital (AFTH) is the culmination of the Air Force expeditionary medical system. The AFTH provides dedicated in-theater and en route support with up to 12 critical care beds, 46 medical/surgical beds, and 6 operating room tables. The AFTH builds upon the EMEDS + 25 system with additional capabilities, including CT, optometry, ophthalmology, OMFS, vascular surgery, and urology. An AFTH can provide definitive care and treatment while patients await transport to stateside medical facilities.[7]

The US Navy provides theater-level hospitalization with Expeditionary Medical Facilities (EMFs) and its two hospital ships, the USNS Mercy and the USNS Comfort. The Navy hospital ship is a floating medical treatment center with 12 operating rooms, 88 intensive care beds, 400 intermediate care beds, and 500 minimal care beds. When fully staffed, these ships can provide care equivalent to a stateside Level 2 trauma center with over 1000 medical personnel onboard. Historically the USNS Comfort and USNS Mercy have provided care around the globe, supporting humanitarian and disaster relief missions on top of their combat mission.[11] The Navy, similar to the Army FH or the AFTH, deploys a 150-bed EMF with each maritime ship squadron. When fully established, the EMF contains 2 operating rooms, 20 intensive care beds, and 130 acute care beds. Similar to the Army FH, the EMF is modular and can be adapted from 10 to 150 beds to meet operational needs.

The Role 3 facility is designed for the treatment and evaluation of patients with the goal of returning the service member to duty. If patients are unable to return to combat duty, they are transported to their home unit or to one of the Role 4 hospitals for continued care and rehabilitation (Fig. 4.5).

Role 4 (Definitive Care)

Role 4 medical facilities are considered the final stop in the military medical system. These facilities focus on definitive medical and surgical treatment, rehabilitation, and convalescent care.

TABLE 4.2 US Navy Afloat Capabilities			
Type of Ship	OR Beds	ICU Beds	WARD Beds
Hospital ship	12	100	900
Aircraft carrier (Nimitz class)	1	3	48
Aircraft carrier (Ford class)	1	3	32
Amphibious assault ship (with FST)	1	3	12
Amphibous assault ship (with FST and HSAP)	4	15	45
Amphibious transport dock (LPD)	1	N/A	24
Landing ship (LSD)	N/A	N/A	8
Submarine tender	2	N/A	12

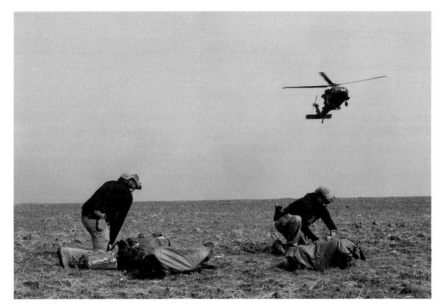

• **Figure 4.5** US Military Members Prepare Casualties at a Point of Injury (POI) Landing Zone for Patient Evacuation by US Army MEDEVAC Personnel. (Courtesy Jeffrey Maler.)

Stateside facilities include comprehensive rehabilitation centers designed to return service members to the best quality of life after a traumatic injury.

There are permanent Role 4 facilities stateside (CONUS) and overseas (OCONUS). Landstuhl Regional Medical Center (LRMC) in Germany and Tripler Army Medical Center (TAMC) are Role 4 facilities capable of providing comprehensive care and serve as gateways to stateside evacuation. Critical Care patients unable to make the long journeys from Southwest Asia or the Pacific to the continental United States stop at one of these facilities. These facilities provide additional medical support prior to continued evacuation. LRMC and TAMC provide surgical stabilization, revisions, and continued definitive care while the casualty waits for follow on transport. LRMC served as a staging location for patients returning from the Iraq and Afghanistan wars over the past 20 years. Casualties transported from the OCONUS Role 4 travel to either Bethesda Walter Reed National Medical Center in DC or Brooke Army Medical Center (BAMC) in Texas. Both Bethesda and BAMC provide all services necessary for the definite treatment of medical and surgical patients. These facilities additionally have collocated Centers for the Intrepid for rehabilitation. The Centers for the Intrepid are pioneering rehabilitative centers dedicated to providing a full spectrum of care to return service members to the highest level of physical, psychological, and emotional function. Additionally, once stateside, service members can receive follow-on and specialty care within Veterans Affairs and civilian hospitals closer to home.

Patient Movement

Patient movement involves the regulated and unregulated movement of casualties via CASEVAC, MEDEVAC, or AE from POI through the successive roles of care within and out of the theater. Patient movement is a collaborative effort of the entire military medical system. For example, it is not unusual for a wounded Marine to be treated initially by another Marine, followed by a Navy corpsman, an Army surgeon, and an Air Force flight nurse (FN), all during transport through Roles 1 to 4.

CASEVAC vs. MEDEVAC

CASEVAC, or casualty evacuation, is defined as any unregulated patient movement in a nonstandard vehicle. This transport may or may not include en route care provided by a layperson or a medical provider. CASEVAC tends to be a vehicle of opportunity, for example, a truck or a nondedicated helicopter. The decision to CASEVAC a casualty takes into count time, scene safety, and the medical transport platform used in the operational environment. Typically, CASEVAC is completed by a maneuver unit from a POI to a Role 1 or Role 2 asset. However, CASEVAC may be a means of getting a casualty to a location where medical evacuation can accrue, such as an ambulance exchange point or MEDEVAC landing zone. CASEVAC is the primary means of evacuation for Naval and Marine Corps assets lacking dedicated medical evacuation platforms (Fig. 4.6).[12]

MEDEVAC is defined as regulated patient movement on a dedicated medical transport asset with en route care provided. Unlike CASEVAC, which utilizes combatant assets, MEDEVAC is protected under the Geneva Convention and the Laws of War when properly marked and employed. With the Geneva Convention, MEDEVAC assets are considered noncombatants on the battlefield and are not supposed to be armed beyond personal protection. The US Army provides the only air and ground dedicated MEDEVAC assets, including the ground ambulance company and air ambulance company. This differentiation is essential as CASEVAC may routinely happen from POI to Role 1 or Role 2, while MEDEVAC, or transport by dedicated medical assets, transports patients to higher echelons of care.[13]

Intratheater vs. Intertheater Transport and Activation

Understanding the difference between intratheater and intertheater transportation is vital in determining which type of patient movement is required and how the transport is activated. Intratheater is the movement of patients within the theater of operations.

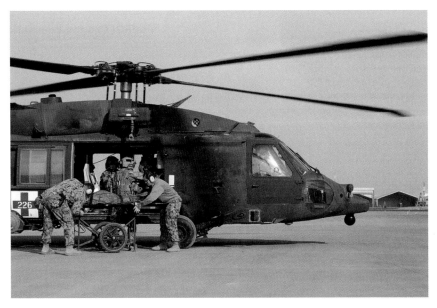

• **Figure 4.6** US Navy Role 2 Members Download a Patient from a US Army MEDEVAC HH-60M Helicopter. (Courtesy Jeffrey Maler.)

An example of intratheater movement is a patient moved from the Navy Role 2 Team in Erbil, Iraq, to the Army Role 3 Hospital in Baghdad, Iraq. Intratheater transport can be accomplished by CASEVAC, ground MEDEVAC, air MEDEVAC, or AE. Intertheater patient movement is the transport of patients from one theater of operation to another. An example of intertheater patient movement is a patient moved from the Army Role 3 hospital in Baghdad, Iraq, to LRMC (Role 4) in Germany. The Air Force AE system exclusively completes intertheater patient transport.

Intratheater Patient Movement Requests

A traditional "911" call is not used in a combat zone, but the ability to initiate MEDEVAC capabilities on the scene is just a call away. The MEDEVAC 9-line request is utilized to start the MEDEVAC process for both scene calls and urgent or critical role-to-role transfers. The 9-line MEDEVAC request is standardized across the military, including NATO and government agency partners (Table 4.3). The request passes through maneuver units' command and control elements to the Patient Movement Center (PMC). The PMC works with both the Army and Air Force air liaisons to determine which transportation modality is most expeditious and appropriate for the transport. Within 15 minutes of an urgent 9-line approval, an Army MEDEVAC helicopter can launch to the POI or request role of care. Intratheater movement between roles of care will also utilize a Patient Movement Request (PMR) to the PMC. A PMR gives a quick synopsis of the casualty's demographics, injuries, and treatments requiring transport. The PMR is similar to civilian facility transfers and requires a physician-to-physician handover if operationally capable. When fixed-wing transport is required, a PMR rather than a 9-line request is utilized to activate Air Force assets to move the patient throughout the roles of care. A PMR is validated by the theater flight surgeon, who allocates the appropriate resource for AE with the Patient Movement Requirements Center.

Intertheater Patient Movement Request

Intertheater AE is accomplished in the same way as intratheater AE. The sending physician completes and submits a PMR to the theater Patient Evacuation Center (PEC). The theater PEC coordinates with Theater Patient Movement Requirements Center (TPMRC) and AE Control Team (AECT) to allocate the appropriate aircraft and AE to move the patient. The AE categories of evacuation precedence differ from those utilized by the 9-line MEDEVAC process. An urgent patient must move immediately to save life, limb, or eyesight or prevent serious illness complications. Priority patients require prompt medical care that must move within 24 hours. Finally, routine patients should move within 72 hours on routine or scheduled flights.[11]

Types of Patient Movement

Ground MEDEVAC

The US Army has the largest intratheater medical ground evacuation capacity for collecting, treating, and transporting casualties. Numerous medical ground transport platforms exist in the Army inventory. These platforms are large dedicated field ambulance vehicles operated by two basic medics with typical basic life support medical supplies and equipment, similar to that found in a civilian ambulance. Patients from POIs or from Roles 1 to 2s are transported via ground on tactical vehicles such as the armored HMMWV (M996), Stryker Medical Evacuation Vehicle (M1133), Armored Personnel Carrier Ambulance (M113A3), MRAP (mine-resistant ambush protected vehicle), or a Front-Line-Ambulance ("FLA" M997).[13] In the modern combat environment, patients are transported in the heavily armored ground ambulance (HAGA) rather than the soft-skinned FLA traditionally associated with Army ambulance companies. Army ground ambulances are controlled by ground ambulance company, ambulance platoon of area support medical company, evacuation platoon of BSMC, and ambulance squads of BCTs. Each ambulance platoon contains eight ambulance teams made up of an ambulance aide, vehicle commander, and ambulance driver. Each Ground Ambulance Medical Company contains two platoons of 12 ambulances. The style of the ambulance is dependent on the maneuver unit's capability the ambulance company supports.

TABLE 4.3	9-Line MEDEVAC Request
Line 1	Location of pickup site (grid)
Line 2	Radio, frequency, call sign, and suffix
Line 3	Number of patients by precedence A – Urgent B – Urgent surgical C – Priority D – Routine E – Convenience
Line 4	Special equipment A – None B – Hoist C – Extraction equipment D – Ventilator E – Other
Line 5	Number of patients by type L – Litter A – Ambulatory
Line 6	Security of pickup site N – No enemy in the area P – Possible enemy in the area E – Enemy in the area X – Enemy in the area (armed escort required)
Line 7	Method of marking pickup site A – Panels B – Pyrotechnic signal C – Smoke D – None E – Other
Line 8	Patient nationality status A – US military B – US civilian C – Non-US military D – Non-US civilian E – Enemy prisoner of war
Line 9	CBRN contamination (wartime) C – Chemical B – Biological R – Radiological N – Nuclear

TABLE 4.4	Medical Ground Evacuation Platform Capacity		
Type	Litter	Ambulatory	Provider
M996 HMMWV	2	3	1
M997 HMMWV (FLA)	4	8	1
HAGA	4	4	1
STRYKER	4	4	1
Ambulance Bus (Ambus)	20	44	2

For example, a medical company supporting an Armored Brigade Combat Team (ABCT) will utilize an M113A3-tracked ambulance. A medical support company supporting a Stryker BCT will utilize a Stryker Medical Evacuation Vehicle. Each ambulance style is designed to carry four litter patients or up to eight ambulatory patients.[14] Patients are loaded into the ambulance, starting from least critical to most critical. Loading the most critical last allows that patient to be removed first and the first patient into the higher echelon of care (Table 4.4).

In the noncombat zone, the US Air Force maintains a fleet of civilian-styled ambulances responsible for base and flight line response worldwide. The Air Force has the most extensive organic stateside EMS system among all the service components. Most of these ambulances are staffed to the civilian equivalent with an Air Force EMT and Paramedic that provides real-world emergency response. The Air Force does not provide routine ground transport in the combat environment.

Rotary Wing Transport

MEDEVAC is traditionally associated with the Army Air Ambulance Companies, known as DUSTOFF. The Army utilizes HH-60M/L/A Blackhawk aircraft for the transport of casualties throughout the world, both in noncombat and combat operations. The HH-60M model of the Blackhawk is a highly modified aircraft specifically designed for patient transport. The HH-60, with a prefix meaning Hospital Helicopter, is designed for patient care with the newest models including oxygen generating systems, power outlets, built-in suction, and automatic litter pans adjustable for loading and transport. All MEDEVAC aircraft are equipped with a 300-feet hoist. Both ambulatory and litter patients are extracted via hoist out of locations where a helicopter may not be able to land. Flight medics train on hoist operations utilizing the SKED litter, rescue seat, and jungle penetrator. MEDEVAC units have hoisted patients off the side of mountains or other difficult situations in Iraq and Afghanistan but also stateside in Colorado or Washington. Per Army doctrine, the newest model, the HH-60M, is capable of transporting up to six litter patients, eight ambulatory patients, or a combination of both. Each MEDEVAC company contains 15 aircraft across 5 Forward Support Medical Platoons (FSMPs).[14] In combat, FSMPs are collocated with maneuver units to create concentric circles of MEDEVAC coverage. Complete coverage of the combat environment ensures MEDEVAC's ability throughout the area of responsibility (Fig. 4.7).

MEDEVAC helicopters, previously staffed with basic EMT combat medics, are today staffed by Critical Care Flight Paramedics. Advancing the certification of flight paramedics to Critical Care Flight Paramedics ensures the same level of care equivalent to civilian helicopter-based emergency medical service. Service members are now provided the same level of care as, if not better than, civilian trauma patients in the United States. Flight medics are assisted in MEDEVAC operations by aircraft crew chiefs. Crew chiefs primarily focused on aircraft operations are trained in basic medical tasks and skills. In the combat environment, DUSTOFF teams are augmented with En Route Critical Nurses (ECCNs), aka Flight Nurses or ECCNs. ECCNs provide a critical operational capability performing advanced critical care transport for patients across various casualty transport platforms that may include air, ground, ship, or other platforms of opportunity. These nurses provide additional clinical expertise and capabilities to the MEDEVAC mission. While the primary mission of ECCNs is the critical care transfer from roles of care, ECCNs have been instrumental in assisting with POI care.

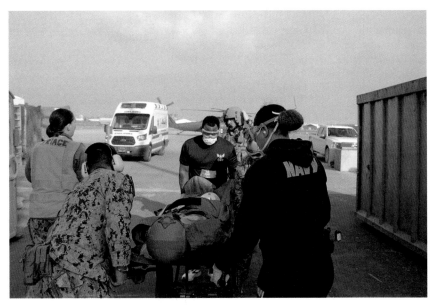

• **Figure 4.7** US Navy Personnel Triage a Casualty Arriving from a US Army MEDEVAC Helicopter for Treatment at a Role 2. (Courtesy Jeffrey Maler.)

In order to become an Army Flight Medic, a combat medic must have a minimum of 1 year of experience before applying to the Critical Care Flight Paramedic Program. The program is broken down into three phases: the paramedic, critical care, and aircrew member. After the 18-month pipeline, critical care flight paramedics are prepared for MEDEVAC duty. The training gained during the CCFP pipeline prepares flight medics to manage critical and routine medical and trauma patients. Critical Care Flight Paramedics are required to maintain an NREMT Paramedic level certification and are highly recommended to maintain the IBSC's Critical Care Flight Paramedic certification.

In 2004 the US Army initiated the JECC to give a more formal orientation to transport nursing. This course is now a triservice course coordinated by the Army School of Aviation Medicine at Fort Rucker, Alabama. Enroute Critical Care Nurses (ECCNs) are Army ICU- and ER-trained nurses with a minimum of 1 year of critical care or emergency nursing experience. The Joint En Route Care Course (JECC), also called the "flight nurse course," is open to Army nurses, paramedics, flight surgeons, physician assistants, Air Force Nurses, Navy nurses, and Corpsmen. JECC is required for both Army ECCNs, Naval En Route Care Nurses, and Naval Flight Nurses. The course includes extensive didactic education focusing on transport trauma management, flight physiology, water survival, combat survival, crew resource management, and effective communication. High-fidelity practical exercises challenge students' ability to transport critically ill patients in the rotary-wing environment (Table 4.5).

Navy/Marine Corps En Route Care

The Navy and Marine Corps lack dedicated air MEDEVAC assets and utilize aircraft of opportunity instead. Medical assets found in Aircraft Carrier Strike Groups and Marine Expeditionary Forces provide CASEVAC support on any Navy or Marine Corps utility platform, including rotary-wing, fixed-wing, and small transport ships. Aircraft include SH-60 Sea Hawk, CV-22 Osprey, CH-46 Sea Knights, and CH-53 Sea Stallions.

TABLE 4.5	Air Casualty Evacuation Platform Capacity		
Type	Litter	Ambulatory	Provider
HH-60L/M (MEDEVAC)	6	8	1
UH-60 (CASEVAC)	3	8	1
CH-47 Chinook	24	31	2
UH-72 Lakota	2	4	1
UH-1Y Huey	6	10	1
CH-46 Sea King	15	22	2
CH-53 Super Stallion	24	37	2
CV-22 Osprey	12	24	2

The Marine Corps En Route Care System (ERCS) provides essential follow-on care for FRSS, STP, and Surgical Companies. ERCS can provide medical care for two critically injured/ill, but stabilized, patients for 2 hours during flight.[15] ERCS is flexible and can integrate with various modes of transportation, rotary-wing/fixed-wing aircraft, and sea transport platforms. The En Route Care Team (ERCT) is comprised of a critical care nurse and a flight Corpsman. Both members of the ERCT must attend the Army JECC; additionally, Corpsmen attend the Flight Medic course at the Naval Aerospace Medicine Institute. The Flight Medic Course trains Corpsmen to conduct SAR, CSAR, air ambulance, CASEVAC, and MEDEVAC missions. Training includes basic and advanced trauma life support, emergency care, and critical care transport on rotary- or fixed-wing assets.[16]

Naval Aviation Search and Rescue (SAR) units provide both afloat and land base SAR support. Whether on land or at sea, these units provide SAR capabilities to all military branches. At the request of local authorities, Navy SAR can support rescue operations outside the Navy area of responsibility. Civilian support in the past included natural disaster response, stranded climber rescue, or difficult technical rescue. An SAR team may include a Naval Search and Rescue Medical Technician (SMT) and a Rescue Swimmer. Naval Rescue Swimmers train primarily in rescue operations but may be trained to the NREMT Basic EMT level. Navy SMTs are minimally trained to the EMT Basic level, with an increasing requirement for Paramedic training. SAR Medical Technicians provide emergency medical treatment in support of SAR and CASEVAC missions for the Navy and Marine Corps. Additionally, SMTs provide en route CASEVAC support for patient movement from ship to higher echelons of care.

Fixed Wing

Fixed-wing transport is completed by the Air Force AE system. This mission uses fixed-wing resources to evacuate casualties under the care of qualified AE crew members, both intratheater and intertheater. The Air Force can deploy assets at a moment's notice around the world in order to receive and transport casualties. Crews are prestaged around the world to facilitate rapid movement. AE crew are trained and qualified to transport casualties on almost the entire Air Force inventory, but most commonly on the C-130 for intratheater and the C-17 or KC-135 for intertheater. Aircraft and mission dependent, the AE crew is able to transport patients on C21s, which are civilian Learjet 35s converted for military use. Other opportune fixed-wing aircraft can be utilized if available. AE crews are specially trained to perform in-flight medical care and are experts in aircraft configuration.

The AE crew, comprised of FNs and AE technicians (AETs), provides the en route medical care necessary to provide safe patient transport. The number of crew members depends on the length of flight, patient acuity, number of patients, and aircraft type. An urgent or priority intratheater mission can be accomplished in a short time period with a minimal crew of an FN and two AETs. Crews for extended flights from Southwest Asia to Landstuhl, for example, require two FNs and three AETs. For missions with extended crew duty days (24 hours), the standard crew will be augmented with another FN and AET. The AE environment is dynamic, and each crew member must maintain clinical expertise, accountability, knowledge, and skill to manage patients in flight.[17]

Both FNs and Aeromedical Technicians are trained at the Air Force School of Aerospace Medicine at Wright Patterson AFB, Ohio. The school's En Route Care Training Department provides initial, advanced, and continuing en route care and education for nurses, physicians, medical technicians, and respiratory therapists across the Department of Defense (DoD). The department maintains high-fidelity simulators and KC-135, C-130, C-17, KC-46, and UH-60 fuselages to provide enhanced training in realistic delivery environments.[17] Originally developed in the 1940s, the 3-week initial FN/AET course covers communication, logistics, safety, air operations, patient considerations, the stresses of flight, altitude physiology, altitude-related illnesses, and the effects of altitude on other diagnoses. The course extensively covers the aircraft and equipment used in the AE system, the logistics of patient movement items, and the maintenance of the equipment. The AE crew train to rapidly construct the AE litter stands and transport equipment in the aircraft before patient arrival. As aircrew members, FN and AETs undergo an additional 2-week survival course that covers combat survival, evasion, and water survival (Table 4.6).

TABLE 4.6	USAF Aeromedical Evacuation Platform Capacity		
Type	Litter	Ambulatory	Provider
C-130 (Intratheater)	74	92	2 flight nurses 3 AE techs
C-17 (Intertheater)	36	31	2 flight nurses 3 AE techs
KC-135	15	33	2 flight nurses 3 AE techs
KC-10	8	24	2 flight nurses 3 AE techs
C-12	1	8	1 flight nurse 1 AE tech
C-21	1	5	1 flight nurse 1 AE tech

Reflects the maximum number of all litter or all ambulatory patient loads; a combination of litter and ambulatory patients decreases capacity.

En Route Critical Care

Critical care transport is accomplished by specialized augmentation teams called a CCATT (critical care air transport team). CCATTs assist in the patient movement mission to supplement en route care capabilities by providing an advanced level of care to critically ill patients. A CCATT team indeed provides an intensive care unit (ICU) capability in the sky for the military patient movement system.[18] The team can transport up to three critical care patients or up to six stabilized patients. A CCATT team consists of a physician (emergency, critical care, anesthesia, or pulmonology), critical care nurse (emergency or critical care trained), and respiratory therapist (cardiopulmonary technician). Members are experienced in the care of critically ill or injured patients with multisystem trauma, head injuries, shock, burns, respiratory failure, multiorgan failure, and other life-threatening complications. As an augmentation team, CCATT requires an AE crew in order to conduct patient transport. The AE crew provides all logistical and aircraft support. Historically, CCATTs have typically been embedded in AE units. In future operations, there may be situations where CCATTs deploy outside the traditional AE force to provide critical care support in the en route care continuum.[19]

Members of the CCATT team have a minimum of 1 year of emergency or critical care experience prior to attending the CCATT Initial Course at Wright Patterson AFB, Ohio. The initial course covers CCATT operations, capabilities, and aircraft familiarization. Following the initial course, students attend the CCATT Advance Course at the University of Cincinnati Medical Center in Ohio. In the advanced course, students are placed in trauma ICUs to refine clinical skills while also participating in high-fidelity simulations taking care of complex polytrauma patients. Once complete, CCATT-trained nurses, physicians, and techs are prepared for the CCATT mission. CCATT members are not considered part of the aircrew and therefore do not attend the survival course that AE crew members attend.

Subspecialty Teams

Numerous subspecialty CCATTs include a neonatal and pediatric team, heart and lung team, and special operation team.

Neonatal intensive care teams are located throughout the military medical system and are responsible for the safe transport of NICU patients to higher roles of care. The NICU team transports neonatal military dependents from smaller military treatment facilities (MTFs) to larger MTFs with robust NICUs. The NICU team is comprised of a NICU provider, including Neonatal Nurse Practitioners, a NICU-trained nurse, and a respiratory therapist.

Heart and Lung Team

The most advanced CCATT team is the Heart and Lung team, also known as the ECMO team. The team, supplemented with an additional ECMO primer, is able to respond worldwide to initiate heart and lung protective ECMO and transport the patients back to BAMC. The Heart and Lung team was crucial during the Iraq and Afghanistan wars in transporting casualties in acute respiratory distress or other acute lung injuries. In the recent COVID-19 epidemic, the ECMO team transported critically ill COVID-19 patients to BAMC for specialized care. These teams initiated ECMO at local hospitals and transported the patients via ground or air to BAMC.

TCCET

Tactical Critical Care Evacuation Team (TCCET) provides damage control resuscitation and critical care support in the perioperative phase of care across the spectrum of unregulated to regulated portions of the evacuation process. The team provides critical care stabilization in uncertain or hostile environments. The three-person teams are comprised of an emergency medicine or critical care physician, a certified nurse anesthetist, and an emergency department nurse or intensive care/critical care nurse. The TCCET-E is an enhanced five-person team specializing in emergency trauma care with an in-flight surgical capability to transport and treat patients with acute, life-threatening injuries. TTCET/E transport on opportune modes of transport, typically with special operations forces.[20]

SOCCET

The Air Force Special Operations Critical Care Evacuation Team (SOCCET) is a special operations command organic asset ready for forward deployment to transport critically ill special forces operators. Unlike traditional CCATT teams, they are not limited by the AE system and routinely utilize transport of opportunity, whether ground, air, or sea, to transport the casualty to higher roles of care.[21]

US Army Burn Flight Team

The DoD's only verified burn center is part of the Army Institute for Surgical Research at BAMC. The USAISR Burn Center provides specialty care for burn and burn-like injuries to civilians and military beneficiaries worldwide. The Institute for Surgical Research provides advanced resuscitation and rehabilitation care while conducting research to optimize combat casualty care in the future. As the only verified Burn Center, it provides 24-hour consultation for the entire DoD. A medic on the ground in Southwest Asia or a Physician in LRMC can call the burn center's hotline and receive immediate critical care recommendations. When that call is initiated, it also activates the DoD's only Burn Flight Team.

The USAISR Burn Flight team is an additional augmentation team to the Air Force CCATT and AE crew specializing in burn resuscitation and treatment. Since 1951, the US Army Burn Flight Team has provided worldwide assessment, treatment, and AE of casualties sustaining thermal injuries related to combat and non-combat-related events. The team, comprised of Army burn specialized nurses, respiratory therapists, and physicians, complete the Air Force CCATT training and work full-time in the Burn ICU. The team is ready for worldwide deployment within hours of notification and is available anytime, anywhere.[22]

The Air Force AE system is supported by an extensive ground organization responsible for staging and preparing patients for AE (Fig. 4.8). The En Route Patient Staging System (ERPSS) provides dedicated support to the AE mission by supplying rapid patient staging, patient hold, and ground transportation

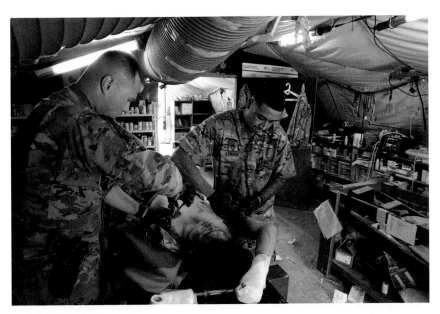

• **Figure 4.8** Army Medical Personnel Treat a Simulated Casualty in an Aid Station (Role 1) in a Combat Environment. (Courtesy Jeffrey Maler.)

between medical facilities and fixed-wing AE aircraft. The modular ERPSS concept can support operations ranging from 10 to 250 beds for patients to be held from 6 to 72 hours while awaiting AE. ERPSS most commonly supports ground transportation between aircraft and medical centers with the iconic Ambu-bus. The ambulance bus transports up to 20 litter patients or 44 ambulatory patients and medical crew. The coordination by ERPSS between medical and AE elements ensures that patients are prepared for flights.[11]

Special Operations Teams

The unique mission of special operations forces requires unique and innovative solutions to forward medical care and patient evacuation. Special operation forces maintain organic and inorganic medical assets, including regulated and unregulated patient movement. Each service component's special operation force contains specific medical assets. The Navy Seals and Marine Special Operations Command is supported by Special Operations Independent Duty Corpsman (SOIDC) and Naval Special Warfare Team Medics trained for the unique water, dive, and amphibious mission. The Army's Ranger and Special Forces groups are supported by advanced medics and Special Operations Medical Sergeants (18D). The Air Force special operations command is supported by Pararescue Jumpers (PJs), the DoD's Combat SAR element. Nearly all SOF medics attend the Special Operations Combat Medic (SOCM) course at the JFK Special Operations Warfare School Center and School. The medics train to the civilian Paramedic level with additional training in Prolonged Field Care, Advanced Surgical Interventions, and Advanced Tactical Medicine. Special operations teams are additionally supported by specialized en route care providers and forward resuscitation teams.

Pararescue Jumpers (PJ) – The US Air Force Special Operations Command's Pararescue Jumpers are responsible for Combat Search and Rescue (CSAR) and Personnel Recovery for all service components. As a combatant unit, PJs are responsible for direct support of Special Operation's mission while providing firepower support. The PJ team is comprised of advanced paramedic-trained PJs, Combat Rescue Officers (CROs), and special operations aircrew members who fly specially modified HH-60G aircraft.[21] Unlike the Army's MEDEVAC aircraft, these aircraft are armed and are not protected by the Geneva Convention. The en route care provided by PJ is considered CASEVAC care. The Jolly's HH-60Gs are capable of inflight refueling, hoist, and low-visibility operations. PJ's hoist capabilities allow the rescue of downed aircrew members no matter the terrain or environment. While primarily utilized in combat for SAR downed aircrew members and special operation teams, stateside and abroad, PJs support humanitarian and SAR missions. In recent years PJs have supported the rescue and transport of victims of natural disasters, most notably hurricanes in the southern United States.

160th Soar Flight Medic/Flight Surgeon Team – The Army Special Operations Command's aviation element, 160th Special Operations Aviation Regiment (160th SOAR), provides helicopter aviation support to special operations forces. The aviation support includes CASEVAC operations with and without medical personnel. The unit has Flight Paramedics and Flight Surgeons that support special operations missions providing unregulated en route medical support. The 160th flight medics attend the SOCM course at the Joint Special Operations Medical Training Center and obtain a civilian Critical Care Flight Paramedic certification. The medics provide tactical operational medical support and sustainment support to aviators, including preventive and occupational medicine.

Joint Medical Augmentation Unit (JMAU) – The Joint Medical Augmentation Unit is a specialized surgical team comprised of an ER Physician, a General Surgeon, a Certified Registered Nurse Anesthetist (CRNA), and a Special Operations Medic. This team may be further augmented by an Ortho Surgeon or other specialized provider. These teams directly support Special Operations missions by providing the most advanced care as close to the POI as possible. The JMAU team is able to provide surgical support in any structure or vehicle, even while in flight on the 160th's highly modified MH-47 Chinook. The mobile team carries all their equipment and supplies.[20]

Joint Trauma Service

The DoD's JTS is the center of collaboration for improving trauma readiness and outcomes through evidence-driven performance improvement. The JTS supports performance improvement projects, publishes trauma education and training, regulates the DoD's Trauma Registry, publishes Clinical Practice Guidelines (CPGs), and facilitates medical readiness. As the authority on military combat casualty care, the Joint Trauma System coordinates the Committees on TCCC, En Route Care, and Surgical Care. Publications and training created by JTS support the United States, partner nations, and civilian trauma casualty care.

For further information or to explore the DoD's JTS's Clinical Practice Guidelines, including the *Critical Care Flight Paramedic Standard Medical Operating Guidelines (SMOG)*, visit the JTS's website at https://jts.health.mil.

Summary

Military medical systems are utilized for a wide spectrum of operations, including humanitarian relief, disaster response, homeland security, small-scale contingencies, and major theater war.

The military medical system is planned, deployed, and constructed from the ground up to support military action or humanitarian relief. The medical system must be able to support this action anytime and anywhere in the world. Within the military medical system, the Air Force, Army, and Navy work to combine different military medical transport platforms that move patients rapidly from the POI to definitive care. Soldiers, marines, airmen, and sailors know that if they are ever injured, even in the most remote location, they will be rapidly triaged, treated, and transported to the highest level of medical care necessary. The interdependence of the Air Force, Army, and Navy patient transport system is supported by highly skilled and trained transport medical personnel. By providing joint interoperable and interchangeable platforms, military en route care and patient transport saves lives. Many lessons learned in military medicine during combat operations have been applied to and now benefit medicine in the civilian sector (Fig. 4.9).

The views expressed in this chapter are that of the author taken from published articles and the Department of Defense and service component doctrine. It is not an official policy or position of the Department of Defense, the US Army, or the US Government.

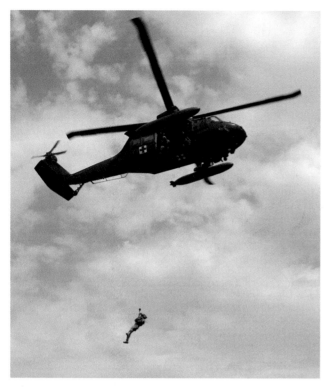

• **Figure 4.9** A MEDEVAC HH-60L Demonstrates Hoist Capabilities by Hoisting the Flight Medic from the Ground into the Helicopter. The hoist allows the MEDEVAC team to extract patients in a variety of situations including when the helicopter cannot land due to terrain. (Courtesy Jeffrey Maler.)

References

1. Borden Institute. *Emergency War Surgery.* Chapter 2, Roles of medical care (United States). 2013. Accessed May 9, 2017. https://medcoeckapwstorprd01.blob.core.usgovcloudapi.net/pfw-images/dbimages/Ch%202.pdf

2. Eastridge BJ, Mabry RL, Seguin P, et al. Death on the battlefield (2001–2011): implications for the future of combat casualty care. *J Trauma Acute Care Surg.* 2012;73(6 Suppl 5):S431–S437. https://www.east.org/content/documents/MilitaryResources/b/TCCC%20Eastridge%20Death%20on%20the%20Battlefield%20J%20Trauma%202012.pdf

3. Joint Trauma Service Committee on Tactical Combat Casualty Care. *Tactical Combat Casualty Care Guidelines.* 2021. Accessed July 4, 2022. https://deployedmedicine.com/market/31/content/40

4. Department of the Army. *The Medical Detachment, Forward Resuscitative and Surgical.* 2020. ATP 4-02.25. Accessed July 21, 2022. https://armypubs.army.mil/productmaps/pubforms/details.aspxPUB_ID=1021369

5. Department of the Army. *Army Health System Doctrine Smart Book.* 2021. Accessed July 21, 2022. https://milsuite.gov

6. Department of the Air Force. *Tactical Doctrine: Ground Surgical Team (GST).* 2018. AFTTP 3-42.77. Accessed July 21, 2022. https://static.e-publishing.af.mil/production/1/af_sg/publication/afttp3-42.77/afttp3-42.77.pdf

7. Department of the Air Force. *Tactical Doctrine: Expeditionary Medical Support (EMEDS) and Air Force Theater Hospital (AFTH).* 2014. AFTTP 3-42.71. Accessed July 21, 2022. https://static.e-publishing.af.mil/production/1/af_sg/publication/afttp3-42.71/afttp3-42.71.pdf

8. Office of the Joint Chiefs of Staff. *Joint Publication 4-02: Joint Health Services.* 2018. JP 4-02. Accessed July 4, 2022. https://www.jcs.mil/Portals/36/Documents/Doctrine/pubs/jp4_02ch1.pdf

9. Department of the Army. *Field Manual: Army Health Systems.* 2020. FM 4-02. Accessed July 21, 2022. https://armypubs.army.mil/epubs/DR_pubs/DR_a/ARN31133-FM_4-02-000-WEB-1.pdf

10. Department of the Army. *Army Techniques Publication: Theater Hospitalization.* 2020. ATP 4-02.10. Accessed July 21, 2022. https://armypubs.army.mil/epubs/DR_pubs/DR_a/ARN30125-ATP_4-02.10-000-WEB-1.pdf

11. Lemay Center for Doctrine. *Air Force Doctrine Publication (AFDP) 4-02 Health Services.* 2019. AFDP 4-02. Accessed July 21, 2022. https://www.doctrine.af.mil/Portals/61/documents/AFDP_4-02/4-02-AFDP-Health-Services.pdf

12. Department of the Army. *Army Techniques Publication: Casualty Evacuation.* 2021. ATP 4-02.13. Accessed July 21, 2022. https://armypubs.army.mil/epubs/DR_pubs/DR_a/ARN32888-ATP_4-02.13-000-WEB-1.pdf

13. Department of the Army. *Army Techniques Publication: Army Health System Support Planning.* 2020. ATP 4-02.55. Accessed July 15, 2022. https://armypubs.army.mil/epubs/DR_pubs/DR_a/pdf/web/ARN21532_ATP_4-02x55_FINAL_WEB.pdf

14. Department of the Army. *Army Techniques Publication: Medical Evacuation.* 2019. ATP 4-02.2. Accessed July 18, 2022. https://armypubs.army.mil/epubs/DR_pubs/DR_a/pdf/web/ARN17834_ATP%204-02x2%20FINAL%20WEB.pdf

15. Marine Corps. *Health Service Support Field Reference Guide.* 2018. MCRP 3-40A.5. Accessed July 10, 2022. https://www.marines.mil/Portals/1/Publications/MCRP%203-40A.5.pdf?ver=2017-03-29-090106-597

16. Department of the Navy. *Patient Movement.* 2013. NTTP 4-02.2M. Accessed August 14, 2022. https://www.marines.mil/News/Publications/MCPEL/Electronic-Library-Display/Article/1739363/mcrp-3-40a7-formerly-mcrp-4-111g/

17. Department of the Air Force. *Tactical Doctrine: Aeromedical Evacuation.* 2019. AFTTP 3-42.5. Accessed July 21, 2022. https://static.e-publishing.af.mil/production/1/af_a3/publication/afttp3-42.5/afttp3-42.5.pdf

18. Air Force Medical Service. *AFMS Capability: Critical Care Air Transport Team.* 2022. Accessed July 17, 2022. https://www.airforcemedicine.af.mil/Platforms/AFMS-Capability-Critical-Care-Air-Transport-Team

19. Department of the Air Force. *Tactical Doctrine: Critical Care Air Transport Team (CCATT).* 2015. AFTTP 3-42.51. Accessed July 21, 2022. https://static.e-publishing.af.mil/production/1/af_sg/publication/afttp3-42.51/afttp3-42.51.pdf

20. Baker J, Northern M, Frament, C, et al. Austere resuscitative and surgical care in support of forward military operations – Joint trauma system position paper. Mil Med. January–February 2021; 186(1–2):12–17. doi: 10.1093/milmed/usaa358

21. Department of the Air Force. *Tactical Doctrine: USAF Medical Support for Special Operations Forces.* 2017 AFTTP 3-42.6. Accessed July 21, 2022. https://static.e-publishing.af.mil/production/1/af_sg/publication/afttp3-42.6/afttp3-42.6.pdf

22. USAISR. *Deployed Resources: Burn Flight Team.* Accessed July 15, 2022. https://usaisr.health.mil/index.cfm/burn_center/deployed

5

Transport Physiology

CHARLES F. SWEARINGEN

COMPETENCIES

1. Understand pertinent gas laws and their effects in the transport environment for optimal patient management.
2. Provide interventions to prevent the adverse effects of barometric pressure changes during patient transport.
3. Identify specific management of stresses that may occur during transport.

Patient transport requires an understanding of the physiologic stressors that may occur in this environment. Understanding the concepts of transport physiology is crucial because they are the basis for the special skills used in transporting patients within the air medical environment via fixed-wing or rotor-wing (RW) aircraft. This chapter specifically discusses gas laws and physiologic stressors related to transport, in addition to their potentially negative effects on patients and transport teams.

Gas Laws

In the air medical environment, transport personnel must possess in-depth knowledge of altitude physiology and its effects, since patients transported via aircraft will experience these physiologic changes. Because of this, it is incredibly important that we understand and anticipate those changes for optimal patient care. Altitude physiology is based upon the ideal gas law concept that $PV = nRT$, where the relationships among temperature (T), pressure (P), volume (V), ideal gas constant (R), and mass of gases (n) interact. Imagine you are at a beach. There is a column of gas from the top of your head to outer space. That column has a weight to it and exerts its weight as pressure. The higher you go into the atmosphere, the column of gas on top of you becomes smaller, and subsequently, less pressure is exerted upon you.

We have evolved, or were divinely created depending upon your perspective, to live within a certain pressure range. Too much pressure and our tissues will be crushed. Too little and the gasses dissolved in our body fluids will leave their compartments. This affects physiology since we rely on dissolved gasses in our tissues to behave appropriately. When gasses misbehave, physiology is affected, and the results can range from discomfort to death.

While you may never think of the ideal gas law during patient care, an understanding of its foundation in all gas laws and its applications are incredibly important. To best understand how the gas laws grossly function relative to patient management, the factors that influence gas behavior need to be defined. As previously mentioned, the four basic variables that affect gas volumetric relationships are temperature, pressure, volume, and the relative mass of a gas, or the number of molecules of the gas. These variables (T, P, V, and n) are defined as follows[1-11]:

1. *Temperature (T)* indicates the level of energy a gas sample possesses and is related to the movement of the molecules of a substance. The faster they move, the more temperature they possess. It can be measured using three common scales: Kelvin (K), Celsius (°C), or Fahrenheit (°F).
2. *Pressure (P),* defined as absolute or total exerted pressure, is conventionally expressed in atmospheres (atm) or torr (1 torr = 1/760 atm), or as a given column of mercury in millimeters (mm Hg) or of water balancing the pressure in centimeters (cm H_2O).
3. *Volume (V)* is expressed in cubic units, such as cubic meters (m^3), cubic centimeters (cm^3), or in liters (L).
4. *Relative mass* of a gas or the number of molecules (n) or ions is expressed in gram molecules (the molecular weight of the substance in grams).

Gas laws govern the body's physiologic response to barometric pressure changes by these four variables. When the transport team is caring for the patient during air transport, these changes become particularly important on ascent and descent.

Boyle's Law

Boyle's law, which originated from experiments conducted by Robert Boyle in 1662, states that at a constant temperature, the volume of gas is inversely proportional to its pressure. This law applies to all gases and may be expressed as follows:

$$P_1 \times V_1 = P_2 \times V_2 \text{ or } P_1/P_2 = V_2/V_1$$

where V_1 is initial volume, V_2 is final volume, P_1 is initial pressure, and P_2 is final pressure.

An example of Boyle's Law is how the gas in a balloon expands as the balloon ascends. This occurs because there is less pressure exerted on the balloon as it ascends higher into the atmosphere, thus allowing the volume of gas in the balloon to expand. Ultimately, the higher someone ascends into the atmosphere, the less pressure they experience, and therefore gases are allowed to expand.

The effects of this law can be seen in several clinical situations. As an unpressurized aircraft ascends, patients can exhibit pneumothorax expansion, rupture of air from endotracheal tube (ETT) cuffs (or other air-filled bladders), and gastric distention – all because Boyle's law allows gas expansion with increasing altitude. If gas expansion is ever a concern during air medical transport, consider requesting the pilot to fly at the lowest, safest altitude. It is important to always be aware of the effects of Boyle's law on patients.[1-11]

Dalton's Law (Law of Partial Pressure)

Dalton was a chemist who in 1803 observed that the total pressure of a mixture of gasses is equal to the sum of the partial pressures of each gas in the mixture. Dalton's law is expressed using the following formula:

$$P = P_1 + P_2 + P_3 + \dots P_n$$

P is the total pressure of the gas mixture, and P_1, P_2, and P_3 ... P_n are partial pressures of each gas in the mixture.

The partial pressure of each gas in the mixture is derived from the following equation[12]:

$$P_1 = F_1 \times P$$

where P_1 is the partial pressure of gas 1, F_1 is the fractional concentration of gas 1 in the mixture, and P is the total pressure of the gas mixture.[1-11]

In other words, the pressure a gas mixture exerts (like the atmosphere, for example) is due to the fraction of each individual gas multiplied by the barometric pressure. Thus, each individual gas present in a mixture exerts a partial pressure that when summed equals the total pressure of the mixture of gases.[1-11]

A mathematic illustration of Dalton's law is shown in the following example, in which the partial pressure of oxygen (PO_2) at sea level is calculated:

$$PO_2 = 20.95 \ (21\%) \times 760 \text{ mm Hg} = 159.6$$

Since the atmosphere is made up of mostly oxygen and nitrogen, calculating the partial pressure of nitrogen and adding it to the partial PO_2 will total close to the weight of the atmosphere, or about 760 mmHg.

$$PN_2 = 78.03 \ (78\%) \times 760 \text{ mm Hg} = 592.8$$

$$PN_2 \ (592.8 \text{ mm Hg}) + PO_2 \ (159.6 \text{ mm Hg}) = 752.4,$$
which is not far from 760 mm Hg.

Barometric pressure, or atmospheric pressure, is the pressure exerted against an object or a person by the atmosphere (Table 5.1). At sea level, this pressure is 15 psi, or alternatively measured as 760 mm Hg or 760 torr. Increased altitude results in decreased barometric

TABLE 5.1 Summary of the Stages of Hypoxia

Gas Law	Action	Practical Application
Boyle's law	↑ Altitude = ↓ Pressure = ↑ Volume	With higher altitudes, gases expand: pneumothoraces get bigger, ETT cuffs can expand and rupture, free air in the stomach can expand and prevent adequate ventilation
Dalton's law	Total pressure = $P_1 + P_2 + P_3 \dots P_n$	As altitude increases, the partial pressure decreases; therefore, supplemental O_2 is needed at higher and higher altitudes
Charles' law	↑ Temperature = ↑ Volume	As the air heats up, it expands and therefore is less dense; colder air is therefore more dense; this allows a wing to create more lift; thus the aircraft can pick up heavier patients or cargo
Gay-Lussac's law	↓ Pressure = ↓ Temperature	At higher altitudes, pressure will decrease and thus will be cooler; clinicians and patients may need more warmth and oxygen tank pressures may change between takeoff and at altitude (colder temperatures shrink gases)
Henry's law	↑ Pressure = ↑ Gas solubility	At depth, a diver is subjected to incredibly high pressures, which pushes nitrogen molecules very close together; this increases the solubility of nitrogen and should the diver come up too fast, this nitrogen will quickly come out of solution and cause decompression sickness
Graham's law	↑ Diffusion = ↓ Molecular weight	Lower-molecular-weight molecules have higher diffusion rates
Fick's law	↑ Partial pressure = ↑ Oxygenation ↑ Surface area ↓ Thickness	By adding FiO_2 and PEEP, partial pressure and surface area will be increased, and the thickness of the alveolar capillary membrane will decrease

ETT, Endotracheal tube; *PEEP*, positive end expiratory pressure.

pressure. Barometric pressure multiplied by the concentration percent of a gas is equal to the partial pressure of the gas[1-11]:

barometric pressure $\times$ gas concentration = gas partial pressure

760 mm Hg $\times$ 21% O_2 = 159.6 mm Hg PO_2[a]

Dalton's law can be utilized to calculate the FiO_2 needs during flight and at the destination. Because there are fewer oxygen molecules per volume at altitude than at sea level, additional oxygen may be needed to maintain an appropriate oxygen saturation (SpO_2). Consider a patient on a ventilator with an FiO_2 of 0.7 (or 70% oxygen delivery). If this patient was transported from sea level to a destination at altitude, then at the destination they would need more FiO_2. To calculate this, we use a version of Dalton's law. Here is the equation:

[(Pressure at Sending Facility)(FiO_2 at Sending Facility)/ (Pressure at Destination)] = Needed FiO_2 at Destination

For any flight legs, the "Destination" terms can be swapped for "Altitude."

To obtain the data needed for the equation, the flight clinician needs to look up the barometric pressure at the destination. Additionally, the flight leg in a pressurized cabin can be calculated by asking the pilot what they will pressurize the cabin to during flight. The result of the equation is the new FiO_2 that should maintain the patient's current SpO_2 – assuming there are no medical or traumatic changes that would cause a decrease in SpO_2.

Charles' Law

An additional development in the early formulation of the laws of ideal gases came from the French physicist Jacques Charles who concluded, "When pressure is constant, the volume of a gas is very nearly proportional to its absolute temperature." This law is expressed as[1-11]:

$$V_1/V_2 = T_1/T_2 \text{ or } V_1/T_1 = V_2/T_2$$

where V_1 is initial volume, V_2 is final volume, T_1 is initial absolute temperature, and T_2 is final absolute temperature.

Thus, the volume is directly proportional to the temperature when expressed on an absolute scale with all other factors constant (P and n are constant).[13] Consequently, if a mass of gas is kept under a constant pressure as the absolute temperature of the

---

[a]Note: Oxygen concentration remains at 21%, regardless of altitude. However, oxygen availability decreases with altitude because the oxygen molecules are farther apart, which could potentially result in hypoxia. This is a difficult concept to understand when you are first studying flight physiology. While on a beach, you take a breath ($\sim$500 mL), and you pull in 100 air molecules (21% O_2, 78% N_2, and some trace elements). This means you pull in 21 oxygen molecules at sea level. You actually pull in about 25 sextillion (25 with 21 zeros behind it), but let us consider only 100 for the purposes of the example. If you ascend to 10,000 feet, then one breath (still $\sim$500 mL) has 70 air molecules (14.7 O_2 molecules and 54.6 N_2 molecules). At 30,000 feet, one breath (still $\sim$500 mL) only contains 25 air molecules (5.25 O_2 molecules and 19.5 N_2 molecules). If you ascend to 50,000 feet and take a breath (again still $\sim$500 mL), it only contains 3 air molecules (0.63 O_2 molecules and 2.34 N_2 molecules). As you ascend, the percentage of oxygen stays the same, but since there is less atmospheric pressure, the molecules are allowed to get further apart. This means that at altitude, you are physically bringing in less oxygen molecules than you do at sea level despite inhaling the same volume of air.

gas is increased or decreased, the volume increases or decreases accordingly.[1-11]

Charles' law describes how aircraft, especially RW aircraft, are affected by atmospheric temperatures. In colder months, the air is denser because gases contract as temperature decreases. The contracting of gases in cold temperatures illustrates a decreasing volume with higher density. An aircraft's wing can produce greater lift in cold temperatures; therefore, the transport team may be able to transport a bariatric patient in an aircraft in the winter that it could not pick up in the summer. This law affects aircraft but has little effect on human physiology because humans normally maintain a constant temperature, not to mention that the heat needed to expand our physiologic gases would damage our tissue irreparably.[1-11]

Gay-Lussac's Law

Gay-Lussac's law relates pressure and temperature and is expressed as:

$$P_1/T_1 = P_2/T_2 \text{ where V and n are constant.}$$

Thus, the pressure of a gas, when volume is constant, is directly proportional to the absolute temperature for a constant amount of gas.[1-11] As the transport team ascends into the atmosphere, it is subjected to less pressure; therefore, as altitude increases, pressure and temperature decrease. Ultimately, as passengers and equipment travel higher in an unpressurized aircraft, they will experience colder temperatures. This means the passengers may need warmer clothes at altitude and oxygen tanks may reflect lower pressures than what was measured before takeoff. An astute flight clinician should be prepared for the oxygen tank pressures to lower slightly at altitude and then return to pressures close to what they were at takeoff.[1-11]

Henry's Law

Henry's law deals with the solubility of gases in liquids. The law states: "The quantity of gas dissolved in 1 cm[9] (1 mL) of a liquid is proportional to the partial pressure of the gas in contact with the liquid." The absolute amount of any gas dissolved in liquid under conditions of equilibrium is dependent on the solubility of the gas in the liquid, the temperature, and the partial pressure of the gas.[9] A simpler conception of Henry's law is that the weight of a gas dissolved in a liquid is directly proportional to the solubility of the gas within the liquid.[1-11]

Ultimately, gases can be forced to dissolve into a solution (like body fluids); as the pressure surrounding the fluid rises, more gas is dissolved into the fluid. This means that as high pressure is removed, the gas will tend to come out of the solution. This can be illustrated by a soda can being opened. Before opening, the contents of the can have been pressurized, allowing the carbon dioxide (CO_2) to be dissolved into the soda. Once the can is opened, the pressure in the can equalizes to the atmospheric pressure (which is much less than when the can was pressurized), and the gas violently escapes.

Another example of this phenomenon is the adage that blood will boil in space should an astronaut take off their helmet during a spacewalk. Boiling is the heating of a substance to a temperature where it becomes vapor. Technically, blood does not boil in space, but vapor, or gas, does leave solution. All of our body fluids have gases dissolved into them (such as oxygen, CO_2, and nitrogen). The pressure of our atmosphere pushes these molecules closer together and allows them to dissolve easily into our body fluids. So if an astronaut took off their helmet in space, where there is no atmospheric pressure, the gas molecules in their body fluid would move further apart, thereby reducing the solubility in their body fluids and allowing the gases to escape their body fluids and enter space. To prevent this from happening, we need space suits that allow us to apply pressure around our bodies similar to atmospheric pressures. This in turn pushes the gas molecules closer together, thus maintaining their physiologic solubility and preventing them from leaving our body fluids.

Clinically, Henry's law applies to scuba divers via the same mechanism as it applies to astronauts: lower barometric pressures reduce the solubility of physiologic gases which therefore exit their body fluids. When a scuba diver ascends too rapidly from a deep dive, they are exposed to exponentially lower barometric pressures, allowing nitrogen bubbles to form in the blood and causing decompression sickness. To manage these patients, one treatment modality is a hyperbaric chamber. Placing a patient in a hyperbaric chamber allows medical staff to increase the pressure surrounding the patient to levels that push gas molecules very close together and subsequently increase the gases' solubility. This forces those gases back into solution (back into body fluids), thus eliminating the problem of the trapped gas. This treatment modality can also be used for air embolisms. Consider a patient who experiences a large air embolism. By exposing them to hyperbaric therapy, the air embolism may be dramatically reduced and eliminated, thus weaponizing Henry's law as a therapeutic intervention.

Graham's Law (Law of Gaseous Diffusion)

Graham's law states that the rate of diffusion of a gas through a liquid medium (such as the membranes throughout the body) is directly related to the solubility of the gas and inversely proportional to the square root of its density or gram molecular weight.[9] In other words, Graham's law simply states that substances with lower molecular weights will dissolve faster through a membrane and that gases with higher solubility stay in liquids longer.[b] This does not have a direct impact on patient care or equipment management but is discussed to offer a thorough review of the gas laws.

Fick's Law

Fick's law, another diffusion law, states that the diffusion rate of a gas is proportional to the difference in partial pressure and the surface area of the membrane and is inversely proportional to the thickness of the membranes. This law directly relates to oxygenation with respect to ventilator management. By increasing the FiO_2, the partial PO_2 delivered to the patient is increased, resulting in an increased SpO_2. In a disease process like emphysema, the alveolar walls are destroyed. Subsequently the surface area of the alveoli shrinks and oxygenation decreases. In a disease process like congestive heart failure with pulmonary edema, there is an increase in the thickness of the alveolar capillary membranes, which results in decreased oxygenation. Therefore, to increase oxygenation in patients on a mechanical ventilator, increase the FiO_2 (partial pressure) and positive end expiratory pressure to ultimately increase the alveolar surface area and thins the alveolar capillary membranes.[1-11]

---

[b]Note: Carbon dioxide is more soluble than oxygen.

Stresses of Transport

Multiple stresses that may be caused by air medical transport have been identified. According to the US Air Force,[3] which has done the most research about stresses related to flight, stresses of flight include:
Stressors of flight (altitude based):
- Hypoxia
- Hyperventilation
- Barometric pressure
- Gastrointestinal (GI) changes
- Thermal changes
- Humidity
- Cabin pressurization

Stressors of flight (non-altitude based):
- Noise
- Vibration
- Fatigue
- Gravitational forces
- Aircraft motion
- Spatial disorientation
- Flicker vertigo
- Fuel vapors

Hypoxia

Within the air medical environment, different types of hypoxia are found. An understanding of the terms *hypoxia*, *hypoxemia*, and *hypercapnia* is essential to establish a foundation of knowledge about the effects of decreased partial PO_2.

Hypoxia is a general term that describes the state of oxygen deficiency in the tissues. It refers to a decrease in tissue oxygen or an oxygen supply inadequate to meet tissue needs.[1-5,10,11,13,14] Hypoxia disrupts the intracellular oxidative process and impairs cellular function.[10,11]

Many factors may interfere with a blood cell's ability to carry oxygen to the body. Anemia, altitude, alcohol, medications, carbon monoxide poisoning, and heavy smoking can all decrease the blood's ability to absorb and transport oxygen.

Hypoxemia refers to a decrease in arterial blood oxygen tension (PaO_2). A normal PaO_2 does not guarantee adequate tissue oxygenation; conversely, a low PaO_2 may not indicate tissue hypoxia and may be clinically acceptable.[1-5,10,11,13,14]

Hypercapnia refers to an increased amount of carbon dioxide in the blood.[10,15,16]

Causes

Hypoxia has multiple causes: (1) deficiency of alveolar oxygen, (2) reduction of oxygen-carrying capacity of the blood, (3) reduction of blood flow to the tissues, and (4) tissue poisoning.

Characteristics

The onset of hypoxia may be gradual or insidious. An example of insidious onset of hypoxia is that of intellectual impairment, demonstrated by slowed thinking, faulty memory of events, lessened immediate recall, delayed reaction time, and a tendency to fixate.

Early Signs and Symptoms

The individual symptoms of hypoxia can be identified in subjects under safe and controlled conditions in an altitude chamber. Once recognized, these symptoms do not vary dramatically in similar time exposures or among subjects. Hypoxia can be classified by objective signs (those perceived by an observer) or subjective symptoms (those

TABLE 5.2	Signs and Symptoms of Hypoxia
Objective Signs	**Subjective Symptoms**
Confusion	Confusion
Tachycardia	Headache
Tachypnea	Stupor
Seizures	Insomnia
Dyspnea	Change in judgment or personality
Hypertension	
Bradycardia	Dizziness
Arrhythmias	Blurred vision
Restlessness	Tunnel vision
Slouching	Hot and cold flashes
Unconsciousness	Tingling
Hypotension (late)	Numbness
Cyanosis (late)	Nausea
Euphoria	Euphoria
Belligerence	Anger

perceived by the subject).[17] Signs and symptoms that appear on both lists in Table 5.2 may be seen by observers and recognized by the hypoxic subject when they occur.[10,15–17]

Cyanosis has been determined to be an unreliable sign of hypoxia because the oxygen saturation must be less than 75% in persons with normal hemoglobin levels before it is detectable.[10,15–17]

Four Stages of Hypoxia

The distinct four stages of hypoxia need to be considered when examining their effects on human pathophysiology. These four stages are divided by altitude. The first stage is the *indifferent stage.* The physiologic zone for this stage starts at sea level and extends to 10,000 feet. In this stage the body reacts to the lessened availability of oxygen in the air with a slight increase in heart rate and ventilation. Night-vision deterioration occurs at 5000 feet. The second stage is the *compensatory stage,* which occurs from 10,000 to 15,000 feet. In this stage, the body attempts to protect itself against hypoxia. Increases in blood pressure, heart rate, and depth and rate of respiration occur. Additionally, efficiency and performance of tasks that require mental alertness become impaired. The third stage is the *disturbance stage,* which occurs between 15,000 and 20,000 feet. This stage is characterized by dizziness, sleepiness, tunnel vision, and cyanosis. Thinking becomes slowed, and muscle coordination decreases. The *critical stage* is the fourth stage of hypoxia. This stage occurs between 20,000 and 30,000 feet and features marked mental confusion and incapacitation followed by unconsciousness, usually within a few minutes.[11] Table 5.1 contains a summary of the hypoxia stages and their effects on humans.

Types of Hypoxia

Based on the physiologic effects elicited on the body, hypoxia can be divided into four different types: hypoxic hypoxia, hypemic hypoxia, stagnant hypoxia, and histotoxic hypoxia.

Hypoxic hypoxia is a deficiency in alveolar oxygen exchange. A reduction in PO_2 in inspired air or the effective gas exchange area of the lung may cause oxygen deficiency. The result is an inadequate oxygen supply to the arterial blood, which in turn decreases the amount of oxygen available to the tissues.[10] Decreased barometric pressure at high altitudes causes a reduction in the alveolar partial pressure of oxygen (PaO_2). The blood oxygen saturation, which is ~98% at sea level, is reduced to ~87% at 10,000 feet and ~60% at 22,000 feet. This reduction in the amount of oxygen in the blood decreases the availability of oxygen to the tissues and causes an impairment of body functions.[10] Hypoxic hypoxia is also referred to as altitude hypoxia because its primary cause is exposure to low barometric pressure. Hypoxic hypoxia interferes with gas exchange in two phases of respiration: ventilation and diffusion. During the ventilation phase, a reduction in PaO_2 may occur. Specific causes include breathing air at reduced barometric pressure, strangulation/respiratory arrest/laryngospasm, severe asthma, breath holding, hypoventilation, breathing gas mixtures with insufficient PO_2, and malfunctioning oxygen equipment at altitude. Causes of reduction in the gas exchange area include pneumonia, drowning, atelectasis, emphysema (chronic obstructive pulmonary disease), pneumothorax, pulmonary embolism, congenital heart defects, and physiologic shunting. Some causes of diffusion barriers are pneumonia and drowning.[9,11]

Hypemic hypoxia is a reduction in the oxygen-carrying capacity of the blood. If the number of red blood cells per unit volume of blood is reduced, as from various types of anemia or from a loss of blood volume, the oxygen-carrying capacity and thus the oxygen content of the blood are reduced.[9] Even with normal ventilation and diffusion, cellular hypoxia can occur if the rate of oxygen delivery does not satisfy metabolic requirements due to poor saturation of oxygen in red blood cells.[1–5,10,13,14] Hypemic hypoxia interferes with the transportation phase of respiration and causes a reduction in oxygen-carrying capacity. Specific causes of hypemic hypoxia include anemia, hemorrhage, hemoglobin abnormalities, use of drugs (e.g., sulfanilamides, nitrites), and intake of chemicals (e.g., cyanide, carbon monoxide).[1–5,10,13,14] Carbon monoxide is significant to air medical crews because it is present in the exhaust fumes of both conventional and jet-engine aircraft. It is also present in cigarette smoke and any fire or smoke inhalation situations. Carbon monoxide binds with hemoglobin 200 times more readily than does oxygen and displaces oxygen to form carboxyhemoglobin.[1–5,9,13,14]

Stagnant hypoxia occurs when conditions result in reduced total cardiac output, pooling of the blood within certain regions of the body, decreased blood flow to the tissues, or restriction of blood flow.[9] Stagnant hypoxia interferes with the transportation phase of respiration by reducing systemic blood flow. Specific causes include heart failure, shock, continuous positive pressure ventilation, acceleration (g-forces), and pulmonary embolism. A reduction in regional or local blood flow may be caused by extremes of environmental temperatures, postural changes (prolonged sitting, bed rest, or weightlessness), tourniquets (restrictive clothing, straps), hyperventilation, embolism by clots or gas bubbles, and cerebral vascular accidents.[1–5,9,13,14]

Histotoxic hypoxia (tissue poisoning) occurs when metabolic disorders or poisoning of the cytochrome oxidase enzyme system results in a cell's inability to use molecular oxygen.[1–5,9,13,14] Histotoxic hypoxia interferes with the utilization phase of respiration because of metabolic poisoning or dysfunction. Since every cell of the body needs oxygen and glucose to engage in metabolism, without oxygen, normal metabolism cannot occur. Poisons such as carbon monoxide, cyanide, and alcohol all prevent oxygen from cellularly uniting with glucose, and anaerobic metabolism is allowed to occur.[1–5,9,13,14] It is important to mention that carbon monoxide poisoning can cause both hypemic and histotoxic hypoxia, but it has a greater effect on hypemic hypoxia.[1–11]

Effective Performance Time and Time of Useful Consciousness

These two terms are frequently used synonymously relative to what happens when crew members are exposed to low-oxygen environments. *Effective performance time* (EPT) denotes the amount of time an individual can perform useful flying duties in an environment of inadequate oxygen.[7,11] *Time of useful consciousness* (TUC) refers to the elapsed time from the point of exposure to an oxygen-deficient environment to the point at which deliberate function is lost.[5,7,8,11] These concepts were originally developed independently from military aviation studies which targeted the responses pilots had to lower oxygen concentrations. EPT focused on slow, steady withdrawal of oxygen, while TUC focused on rapid decompression. In 2015, the FAA printed an advisory circular where the value of slow vs. rapid changes in altitude experience was highlighted. This circular acknowledged TUC and EPT as synonymous and added a third time column for "Following Rapid Decompression." Additionally, it mentioned that the provided times are averages, and each individual may experience high altitude effects differently based on multiple extraneous variables, such as fitness, alcohol consumption, comorbidities, and others.[18]

With the loss of performance in flight, an individual is no longer capable of taking the proper corrective or protective action.[5,7,8,11] Thus, for air medical personnel the emphasis is on prevention. In addition to altitude, factors that influence EPT/TUC are rate of ascent and an individual's physical fitness, physical activity, temperature, tolerance, and self-imposed stresses, such as smoking, intake of alcohol and medication, and fatigue.[10] Another factor that dramatically reduces both EPT/TUC is rapid decompression, which occurs when a quick loss of cabin pressure occurs in a pressurized aircraft at high altitudes. On decompression at altitudes above 10,058 m (33,000 feet), an immediate reversal of oxygen flow in the alveoli takes place, which is caused by a higher PO_2 within the pulmonary capillaries. This event depletes the blood's oxygen reserve and reduces the EPT at rest by up to 50%. Exercise also reduces the EPT/TUC considerably.[5,7,8,11] Table 5.3 presents altitude and EPT/TUC.

Treatment

The general treatment for hypoxia is administration of 100% oxygen. The type of hypoxia needs to be determined so that specific treatment can be administered accordingly. The following are required steps for transport team members:

1. **Administer supplemental oxygen under pressure.** Provision of adequate supplemental oxygen is the prime consideration in the treatment of hypoxia. Consideration must be given to the altitude and the cause of the oxygen deficiency. Equipment malfunction or altitude exposure above 12,192 m (40,000 feet) cannot be corrected without the addition of positive pressure.[c]

The physiologic requirements for breathing are as follows:

Normal	Positive Pressure
Inspiration – active	Inspiration – passive
Expiration – passive	Expiration – active

The proper method of positive pressure breathing is:

Inhale slowly → Pause → Exhale forcibly → Pause

2. **Monitor breathing.** After a hypoxic episode, the resulting hyperventilation must be controlled to achieve complete recovery. A breathing rate of 12 to 16 breaths per minute or slightly lower aids recovery.
3. **Monitor equipment.** The most frequently reported causes of hypoxia are lack of oxygen discipline and equipment malfunction. A conscientious preflight check of equipment and frequent in-flight monitoring reduce this hazard. Inspection of oxygen equipment when hypoxia is suspected may detect its cause. Ground-transport team members must also conduct the same careful inspection of their equipment before and after transport to prevent any problems with their oxygen-delivery system during transport. Correction of a malfunction should bring immediate relief to the hypoxic condition. If treatment for hypoxia does not remedy the situation, oxygen contamination should be suspected. Use of an alternative oxygen source, such as the emergency oxygen cylinder or portable assembly, should be considered. Descent should be initiated as soon as possible, and the contents of the oxygen system should be analyzed.
4. **Descend.** Increasing the ambient oxygen pressure by descending to lower altitudes, particularly below 3048 m (10,000 feet), is also beneficial. Descent to a lower altitude compensates for malfunctioning oxygen equipment that may have caused the hypoxia.[10,15,16]

The primary treatment of hypoxia for any patient being transported is prevention. The transport team must remember that the patient's condition is already compromised and that stresses related to transport increase the risk of patient hypoxia unless the transport team continuously monitors the patient and accurately anticipates the oxygen needs of the patient during transport.

Hyperventilation

Hyperventilation at altitude is an important consideration for air medical personnel and for the air medical patient. Hyperventilation is of concern because it produces changes in cellular respiration. Although the causes are unrelated, the symptoms of hyperventilation and hypoxia are similar and often result in confusion and inappropriate corrective procedures. Despite increased knowledge and training and improved life-support

TABLE 5.3	Average Time of Useful Consciousness for Nonpressurized Aircraft	
Altitude (in feet)	**Time**
18,000 and lower	30 minutes
25,000	3–5 minutes
30,000	90 seconds
35,000	30–60 seconds
40,000 and higher	15 seconds or less

---

[c]Positive pressure breathing is the opposite of normal breathing.

equipment, both hypoxia and hyperventilation are hazards in flying and diving operations.[10,17] *Hyperventilation* is an abnormal increase in the rate and depth of breathing that upsets the chemical balance of the blood[10,11,15,16]; it is commonly caused by psychological stress (e.g., fear, anxiety, apprehensiveness, and anger) and environmental stress (e.g., hypoxia, pressure breathing, vibration, and heat). Certain drugs, such as salicylates and female sex hormones, also cause or enhance hyperventilation, and any condition that creates metabolic acidosis results in hyperventilation at high altitudes.[10,11,15,16]

Treatment

At high altitudes, hyperventilation and hypoxia are treated in the same way because of similarities in the signs and symptoms. The following steps describe the treatment:
1. Administer 100% oxygen.
2. Begin positive pressure breathing, which is the same as supplemental oxygen under pressure.
3. Regulate breathing and watch for hyperventilation.
4. Check equipment.
5. Descend.

The treatment for hyperventilation in the air medical patient is the administration of oxygen. If treatment is successful, the amount of oxygen in the blood increases. Oxygen transfers from air to blood 20 times slower than carbon dioxide, and carbon dioxide transfers 20 times faster from blood to air than oxygen, which explains why the amount of carbon dioxide in the blood is directly associated with ventilation. When a patient is hyperventilating from anxiety, the act of putting a mask on the face to administer oxygen probably heightens the anxiety and increases tidal volume. Primarily, tidal volume must be reduced.[17] More favorable responses can be obtained by talking to patients to distract them, identifying the hyperventilation causes, and suggesting specific exercises to reduce respiratory rate. Several helpful exercises are listed as follows:
1. The patient should count to 10 slowly while exhaling.
2. The patient should inhale and exhale only 10 times per minute.
3. Using a watch with a second hand, the patient should set a respiratory rate between 10 and 12 breaths per minute.
4. The air medical team member can provide counterpressure by suggesting isometric or active-passive exercises[6] that cause the patient to hold their breath and reduce the respiratory rate.

Barometric Pressure Changes

Boyle's law states that at a constant temperature, the volume of a gas is inversely proportional to the pressure. On ascent, gases expand; on descent, gases contract. Therefore, trapped or partially trapped gases within certain body cavities (e.g., the GI tract, lungs, skull, middle ear, sinuses, and teeth) expand in direct proportion to the decrease in pressure.[2,5,8,10,11,15,17,19]

Middle Ear

The *middle ear cavity* is an air-filled space connected to the nasopharynx by the eustachian tube. The eustachian tube has a slit-like orifice at the throat end that allows air to vent outward more easily than inward. During ascent, air in the middle ear cavity expands and then normally vents into the throat through the eustachian tube when a pressure differential of approximately 15 mm Hg has been reached. A mild fullness is usually detected but disappears as equalization occurs. This constitutes the *passive process*.[4,5] On descent, however, a different situation exists. The eustachian tube remains closed unless actively opened by muscle action or high positive pressure in the nasopharynx. If the eustachian tube opens, any existing pressure differential is immediately equalized. If the tube does not open regularly during descent, a pressure differential may develop. If this pressure differential reaches 80 to 90 mm Hg, the small muscles of the soft palate cannot overcome it, and either reascent or a maneuver that is not physiologic is necessary to open the tube.[10,11,15,16,20] On descent, equalization of pressure in the middle ear can be accomplished by performing the Valsalva maneuver, yawning, swallowing, or moving the lower jaw and via topical administration of vasoconstrictors or use of a bag-valve mask. These procedures are examples of the *active process*. Please note that gum chewing is not recommended as a method of pressure equalization because it causes swallowing of air and then subsequent gastric distention and discomfort.

Barotitis Media

Barotitis media, frequently referred to as an ear block, results from failure of the middle ear cavity to ventilate when going from low to high atmospheric pressure (i.e., on descent).[10,11,15,16] Pressure in the middle ear becomes increasingly negative, and a partial vacuum is created. As the pressure differential increases, the tympanic membrane is depressed inward and becomes inflamed, and petechial hemorrhages develop. Blood and tissue fluids are drawn into the middle ear cavity, and if equalization with ambient pressure still does not take place, perforation of the tympanic membrane may occur. Severe pain, tinnitus, and possible vertigo and nausea can accompany acute barotitis media.[10,11,15,16] Priority is placed on patient briefing before flight and adequate instructions for air medical crews. The ears should be equalized on descent with the methods previously described. Patients who are sleeping should be awakened before descent so that they can also equalize their ears in a normal manner.

Patients with viral or bacterial upper respiratory tract infections must be closely monitored during both ascent and descent for swollen eustachian tubes, which interferes with normal equalization procedures.[10,11,15,16] Air medical crew members with upper respiratory tract infections should not fly.

If patients have ear pain during ascent, which rarely occurs, air medical personnel should not have them execute a Valsalva maneuver because that would only aggravate the problem; instead, personnel should have them swallow or move their jaw muscles or administer a mild vasoconstrictor.[3]

If an ear block occurs, mild vasoconstrictors should be administered early, and the aircraft should reascend to a higher altitude until symptoms lessen or the patient's ear block clears. A patient's nose should be sprayed with a decongestant solution to attain maximal shrinkage of the mucosa. Additional ear block interventions include the use of the Politzer bag or a source of compressed air. For the Politzer bag method, the olive tip is placed in one nostril, the nose is compressed between the air medical crew member's fingers, and the patient is then instructed to say "kick, kick, kick" while the bag is squeezed, increasing the pressure in the nasopharyngeal cavity to the point at which the eustachian tube is opened and the middle ear space ventilated.[3]

In review, the treatment is as follows:
1. Patient performs Valsalva maneuver.
2. Crew member administers vasoconstrictor spray.
3. Crew member administers Politzer bag or bag-valve-mask.
4. Aircraft reascends.

Delayed Ear Block

A delayed ear block, which occurs after the flight is terminated, results from breathing 100% oxygen during flight. As the ears equalize during descent, 100% oxygen is forced into the middle ear cavity.[3,10] In addition, the absorption of oxygen by the middle ear and mastoid mucosa contributes to the relatively negative pressure in those cavities. The patient may be symptom free immediately after flight, but if the oxygen in the middle ear is not replaced with air, the surrounding tissues absorb it, thereby creating a negative pressure within the cavity. Delayed barotitis media occurs when oxygen absorption is the primary factor in the development of a pressure differential.[3,10,19] This condition causes a tightness or "stopped-up" sensation in the ears and slight to possibly severe pain. To prevent delayed ear problems, the patient should perform the Valsalva maneuver periodically after the flight.[3] However, if a flight is completed in the late-evening hours or during the night and the individual retires a short time later, a significant pressure differential may develop during sleep because of the combined effects of oxygen absorption and infrequent swallowing.[20] Patients who are maintained on 100% oxygen during flight are especially susceptible to this problem.[10,11,15,16]

Flight crew members who continue to have ear pain after flight can treat it with decongestants and analgesics. If symptoms persist, flying at high altitudes should be avoided until the symptoms subside. If the team member has had a ruptured tympanic membrane, several days to weeks may be needed before it heals, and they should not fly until cleared.[1]

Barosinusitis (Sinus Block)

The sinuses usually present a little problem when subjected to changes in barometric pressure. Because a free flow of air exists between the sinus cavities and the exterior, the sinuses automatically equalize with ambient pressure when the air in them expands or contracts.[1]

Barosinusitis is an acute or chronic inflammation of one or more of the paranasal sinuses produced by the development of a pressure difference, usually negative, between the air in the sinus cavity and that of the surrounding atmosphere.[2,20] Common causes of barosinusitis are viral and bacterial upper respiratory tract infections. Patients with such problems should be closely monitored during ascent and descent.[2,20] The symptoms of barosinusitis are usually proportional to its severity and may vary from a mild feeling of fullness in or around the involved sinus to excruciating pain. Pain can develop suddenly and be incapacitating.[2,20] Another symptom is possible persistent local tenderness. The immediate treatments for barosinusitis are to reascend until the pressure within the sinus equals the cabin pressure, administer vasoconstrictors to reduce swelling, and descend as gradually as possible to afford every opportunity for pressure equalization.[2,20]

Barodontalgia

Barodontalgia, or aerodontalgia, is a toothache that is caused by exposure to changing barometric pressures during actual or simulated flight.[2,20] The precise cause of barodontalgia has not been determined; however, exposure to reduced atmospheric pressure is obviously a significant factor. This exposure is evidently a precipitating factor, with disease of the pulp the primary cause. Pressure changes do not elicit pain in teeth with normal pulps, regardless of whether a tooth is intact, carious, or restored.[2,20]

Some pathologic conditions may cause no symptoms at ground level but be adversely affected by a change in barometric pressure. Barodontalgia commonly occurs during ascent, with descent bringing relief.[4] Moderate to severe pain that usually develops during ascent and is well localized generally indicates direct barodontalgia. The patient or crew member is frequently able to identify the involved tooth. This condition can usually be prevented by high-quality dental care with an emphasis on slow, careful treatment of cavities and the routine use of a cavity varnish. Indirect barodontalgia is a dull, poorly defined pain that involves the posterior maxillary teeth and develops during descent.[10] If patients have tooth pain during descent, especially involving the upper posterior teeth, they may have barosinusitis and should be treated accordingly.[2,20]

A crew member who undergoes dental treatment involving deep restorations should be restricted from flying for 48 to 72 hours after treatment to allow time for the dental pulp to stabilize.[2,20]

Gastrointestinal Changes

Gas contained within body cavities is saturated with water vapor, the partial pressure of which is related to body temperature. In determining the mechanical effect of gas expansion, one must account for the noncompressibility of water vapor, which causes wet gases to expand faster than dry gases.[2,20] The stomach and intestines normally contain a variable amount of gas at a pressure that is equivalent to the surrounding barometric pressure. On ascending to high altitudes, however, the gases in the GI tract expand. Unless the gases are expelled by belching or the passing of flatus, they may produce pain and discomfort, make breathing more difficult, and possibly lead to hyperventilation or syncope.[2,20] Severe pain may cause a vasovagal reaction that consists of hypotension, tachycardia, and fainting. Abdominal massage and physical activity may promote the passage of gas. If this treatment is unsuccessful, a descent should be initiated to an altitude at which comfort is achieved.[20] Because the possibility of decompression does exist, however, certain precautionary measures should be taken to reduce the chances of GI gas-expansion difficulties. Such measures include avoiding hasty and heavy meals before flight, such as gas-forming foods; carbonated beverages; and foods that are not easily digested.[2,11,20] Normally, the average GI tract has approximately 1 L of gas present at any one time.

One useful example is a pediatric patient with abdominal distention. Gas expansion in the abdominal cavity, if untreated, can increase to such a volume that it raises the diaphragm. With diaphragmatic crowding, lung volume and expansion are decreased. If this distention is large enough, the great blood vessels in the area are compressed, which alters the blood supply to vital organs.[2,10,11]

Patients with an ileus (bowel obstruction) or recent abdominal surgery should have a gastric tube placed before transport. The gastric tube should not be clamped but should be vented for ambient air or low intermittent suction during transport. After abdominal surgery, pockets of air may remain in the abdominal cavity. For this reason, general recommendations are that patients should not be transported by air until 24 to 48 hours after the surgery. Patients who have undergone colostomy should be advised to carry extra bags because of more frequent bowel movements that result from gas expansion.[9–11,15,16] Colostomy bags should be emptied and properly vented before air medical transport. Penetrating wounds allow ambient air to travel along the wound tract. According to Boyle's law, penetrating wounds to the eyes, neck, thorax, abdomen, and lower extremities can cause the introduction of emboli, in addition to irreparable damage to nerves and surrounding tissues.

Thermal Changes

An increase in altitude results in a decrease in ambient temperature. Consequently, cabin temperature fluctuates considerably depending on the temperature outside the aircraft.[3] The ratio of altitude to temperature is fairly constant from sea level to approximately 35,000 feet. Temperature decreases by 1°C for every 100 m (330 feet) increase in altitude. From flight level (FL) 350 to FL 990, the temperature fluctuates from ±3°C to 5°C. The temperature remains relatively isothermic at approximately –50°C from FL 350 to FL 990.[2,10]

Vibrational forces and temperature alterations can yield both antagonistic and synergistic physiological effects on the human body. The body's primary response to heat exposure is vasodilation and activation of cooling mechanisms. Exposure to whole-body vibration appears to interfere with the normal human cooling responses in a hot environment by reducing blood flow and decreasing perspiration.[6] Exposure to cold and vibration stimulate vasoconstriction and decreased perspiration.[2]

Turbulence can be produced by high and low temperature changes in the air. Turbulence increases stress during flight by promoting fatigue and increasing one's susceptibility to motion sickness and disorientation.

The transport team must also keep in mind that some medications can also interfere with the maintenance of a constant body temperature. Sedatives, analgesics, some psychoactive agents, and neuromuscular blocking agents are only a few examples of medications that can place the patient at risk for problems with body temperature regulation.

Both hyperthermia and hypothermia increase the body's oxygen requirement. Hyperthermia increases the metabolic rate, and hypothermia increases energy needs because of shivering; thereby, both conditions increase the body's oxygen consumption.[3] Air medical crews can facilitate maintenance of adequate body temperature with blankets, warm clothing, and warm liquids.[6] An additional way to facilitate thermoregulatory control is with a first-aid thermal blanket, which is sometimes called a space blanket.

Decreased Humidity

Humidity is the concentration of water vapor in the air; as air cools, it loses its ability to hold moisture. Because temperature is inversely proportional to altitude, an increase in altitude produces a decrease in temperature and, therefore, a decrease in the amount of humidity. The fresh-air supply is drawn into the aircraft cabin from a very dry atmosphere.[3] Before takeoff, small amounts of moisture are present in the cabin air from clothing and other items on board that retain moisture, in addition to expired air from crew members, patients, and other passengers. As the aircraft altitude increases, the air exhausted overboard carries away trapped moisture. Eventually, all the original moisture is lost. The only moisture that remains is supplied by crew members, patients, other passengers on board, and the fresh-air system.[2,4,6] For example, on a typical flight of a military jet aircraft known as a C-141 Starlifter, which is a high-speed, high-altitude, long-range aircraft used for troops, cargo, and air medical transport, less than 5% relative humidity remains after 2 hours of flight time. The military jet's relative humidity then decreases to less than 1% after 4 hours.[2,4,6,10] Propeller-type aircraft are not as dry inside because they do not fly as high; the lowest relative humidity levels reached on typical propeller aircraft flights range from 10% to 25%.[8] Patients and air crew members may become significantly dehydrated because of the decreased humidity at high altitudes. The ventilation systems on aircraft draw off what little moisture there is and contribute further to the decrease in the percentage of humidity. For a healthy person, low humidity results in nothing more than chapped lips, scratchy or slightly sore throat, and hoarseness. Steps that the medical crew member can take to minimize problems caused by decreased humidity include mouth care, use of lip balm, and adequate fluid intake. Patients who receive in-flight oxygen therapy are twice as susceptible to dehydration because oxygen itself is a drying agent. Humidified oxygen should be used on extended patient transports. The transport team must be certain that when humidifiers are used, they are changed often to prevent contamination.

Patients who are unconscious or unable to close their eyelids must be provided with eye care. The administration of artificial tears and the taping shut of lids prevent corneal drying. Before transport, patients with compromised conditions predisposed by age, diet, or preexisting medical or surgical complications need special consideration with respect to decreased humidity.

Transport team members should also maintain adequate fluid intake to prevent dehydration. Water or other appropriate liquids need to be available during both air and ground transport.[21]

Noise

Sound is any undulatory motion in an elastic medium (gaseous, liquid, or solid) that is capable of producing the sensation of hearing. Normally, the medium is air.[12,21] *Sound waves* are variations in air pressure above and below the ambient pressure.[12,21] Sound is described in terms of its intensity, spectrum, and time history. The *intensity* of a sound wave is the magnitude by which the pressure varies above and below the ambient level. It is measured with a logarithmic scale that expresses the ratio of sound pressure to a reference pressure in decibels (dB), which are the units used to describe levels of acoustic pressure, power, and intensity.[21] The *spectrum* of a sound represents the qualities present distributed across frequency. The frequency of periodic motion (e.g., sound and vibrations) is the number of complete cycles of motion that take place within a unit of time, usually 1 second. The international standard unit of frequency is the hertz (Hz), which is 1 cycle per second.[12] *Pressure–time histories* describe variations in the sound pressure of a signal as a function of time. The frequency content is not quantified in pressure–time histories of signals, so analytic techniques must be applied to the signal in order to obtain frequency or spectrum characteristics.[9,21]

Theoretically, sound waves in open air spread spherically in all directions from an ideal source. Because of this spherical dispersion, the sound pressure is reduced to half its original value as the distance is doubled, which is a 6 dB reduction in sound pressure level.[9,21] Hence, several factors are involved in the creation of sound. In relation to the definition of sound, it is usually easier to think of sound as comprising of intensity, which is commonly thought of as loudness, in decibels; frequency, in cycles per second and pitch; and duration.

Thus noise, which is dependent on sound, can be more easily defined. *Noise* may be defined subjectively as a sound that is unpleasant, distracting, unwarranted, or in some other way undesirable.[9,21] The human hearing mechanism has a wide range and is fairly tolerant, but at times in an aircraft, this tolerance is exceeded and may lead to the following potential effects:

- Communications in the form of speech and other auditory signals inside the aircraft, air-to-air, or air-to-ground may be degraded.

- The sense of hearing may be temporarily or permanently damaged.
- Noise, acting as a stress, may interfere with patient care and safe transport.
- Noise may induce varying levels of fatigue.[9,21]

The A-level of a decibel (dBA) is a unit of noise measurement that correlates most closely with the way a human ear accommodates sound or noise. The dBA is a single measurement that incorporates both amplitude and the selective frequency response features that most closely parallel those of the human ear. When ambient noise levels exceed 80 to 85 dBA, a person must usually shout to be heard.[9,21] Essentially, unprotected exposure to noise can produce one or more of the following three undesirable auditory effects: interference with effective communication, temporary threshold shifts (auditory fatigue), or permanent threshold shifts (sensorineural hearing loss).[9,21] Auditory fatigue incurred by noise is frequently accompanied by a feeling of "fullness," or high-pitched ringing, buzzing, or a roaring sound in the ears (tinnitus). Tinnitus usually subsides within a few minutes after cessation of the noise exposure; however, for some individuals, the tinnitus may continue for several hours.[3] Most of the truly significant forms of undesirable response to acoustic noise, such as nausea, disorientation, and excessive general fatigue, are associated with only very intense noise, which air medical personnel rarely encounter during normal airlift operations.[9,21] Other hazards of exposure are loss of appetite and interest, diaphoresis, salivation, nausea or vomiting, headache, fatigue, and general discomfort.

Noise in the transport environment also impairs the ability of the transport team to perform patient assessments before and during transport. Aircraft noise, sirens, and traffic and crowd noise can interfere with the evaluation of breath sounds, with auscultation of blood pressure, or even when obtaining patient information. Propeller aircraft noise is a loud tonal noise from piston or turbo propeller engines in the cabin. A beating noise may occur when the tonal noises from two propellers are at similar levels but differ slightly in frequency. Rotorcraft cabin noises can come from impulsive, periodic, and broadband noises from rotors and structures such as the gearbox. The noise from a helicopter contains both high-level and low-frequency noise. Jet aircraft also produce high-frequency-level noise that increases with liftoff and climbing out until cruising altitude is reached.[9–12,15–17,21]

Transport team members need to rely on monitoring devices to measure patient blood pressure and monitor oxygen saturation, ETT placement, and overall perfusion. Visible signs of distress or discomfort, such as increased respiratory rate, changes in skin color, and grimacing, may provide additional information about a patient's condition and comfort in a noisy transport environment.

Table 5.4 provides an example of the numbers of decibels that result from certain sources. Whenever the noise cannot be controlled at a desirable level, ear protection devices that attenuate the noise on its way from the surrounding air to the tympanic membrane must be worn, whether in an aircraft or ground transport vehicle. Ear protection devices include helmets, earplugs, and earmuffs. Because effectiveness can vary considerably depending on the device's basic performance and personal fit, all transport team personnel should be carefully instructed regarding its quality and size selection and techniques for use.[10] Earplugs are inert devices, and headsets and earmuffs are occluding devices. Earplugs must fit tightly to offer the maximum allowable attenuation; the only requirement for using airtight earplugs during flight operations is that they be removed before descent. Pressure

TABLE 5.4	Decibels and Source
Decibels	Source
60	Normal conversation at 1 m
80	Garbage disposal
88	Propeller aircraft flyover at 1000 feet
90	Noisy factory / Cockpit of light aircraft
103	Jet flyover at 1000 feet
117	Jet on runway in preparation for takeoff
110–130	Construction site during pile driving

changes that result from decreased altitude tend to pull the plugs inward toward the tympanic membrane.[3] Transport team members should have their hearing evaluated on a yearly basis.

The Commission on Accreditation of Medical Transport Systems (CAMTS)[13] requires that all RW personnel wear helmets during patient transport operations. This requirement should help decrease the risk of hearing damage related to RW transport and improve team member communications during transport.[13]

A patient's hearing, particularly that of an unconscious patient, needs to be protected during transport; therefore, a headset or earmuffs should be placed on all patients.

Vibration

Vibration is the motion of objects relative to a reference position (usually the object at rest) and is described relative to its effect on humans in terms of frequency, intensity (amplitude), direction (regarding anatomic axes of the human body), and duration of exposure.[3,9–12,15–17,21] Most vehicles contain two principal sources of vibration: the first originates within the vehicle, specifically from the power source, and the second comes from the environment, which encompasses the terrain over which the land vehicle travels, the turbulence of the air through which the aircraft flies, or the status of the sea in which the ship sails.[2,9,10] Thus, both air and ground vehicles cause vibration.

Helicopter vibration occurs with broadly similar intensity in all three axes of motion. Large differences in the amplitudes of specific harmonics in different modes of flight may exist, but the overall amplitude of vibration tends to increase with airspeed and with the loading of the aircraft. Vibration is usually worse during transition to the hover position.[3,9–12,15–17,21]

In fixed-wing aircraft, any vibration from the power source is usually at a higher frequency than in helicopters. The main source of vibration encountered in fixed-wing aircraft is the atmospheric turbulence through which the aircraft flies. Consequently, the most severe vibration usually occurs during storm-cloud penetration or during high-speed low-level flight. The response of the aircraft to atmospheric turbulence is determined by the aerodynamic loading on the wings. An aircraft with a large wing area relative to its weight undergoes greater amplitude low-frequency excursions from level flight because of turbulence.[2,9–12,15–17,21]

Resonant frequencies of body structures produce a more pronounced effect than do nonresonant frequencies.[9] Vibration between 1 and 12 Hz has been firmly established to cause performance decrement in the cockpit. For example, low-frequency vibration can induce motion sickness, fatigue, shortness of breath, and abdominal and chest pain.[9] Research has established that a human's sensitivity to external vibration is highest between 0.5 and 20 Hz because the human system absorbs most of the vibratory energy applied within this range, with maximal amplification between 5 and 11 Hz. The most physiologically harmful frequencies lay between 0.1 and 40 Hz.[9]

When the human body is in direct contact with a source of vibration, mechanical energy is transferred and some of this energy becomes degraded into heat within tissues that have dampening properties. The response to whole-body vibration is an increase in muscle activity to maintain posture and possibly to reduce the resonant amplification of body structures. This response is reflected in an increased metabolic rate and a redistribution of blood flow with peripheral vasoconstriction. The increased metabolic rate during vibrations is comparable to gentle exercise. Respiration is also increased to achieve greater carbon dioxide (CO_2) elimination.[2–4,9,10,13] Disturbances in dynamic visual acuity, speech, and fine-muscle coordination result from vibration exposure.[2–4,9,10,13] The effects of vibration on the body can be reduced by attention to the source of vibration, modification of the transmission pathway, or alteration of the dynamic properties of the body.[2–4,9,10,13] Pain from injuries, such as fractures or disease states, can be increased, which then causes the need for additional analgesia and sedation.

Vibrations can also interfere with transport equipment, such as cardiac and blood pressure monitor readings. Additionally, sensors, electrodes, leads, ETTs, and intravenous lines may become disconnected or dislodged. These devices may be difficult to replace during transport. The equipment should be secured in the transport vehicle in a manner least conducive to vibrations.[2–4,9,10,13]

Aircraft manufacturers have eliminated severe vibrations by improving designs and materials; however, some vibrations still occur as a result of engine operation, flap and landing gear extension and retraction, and general aircraft movement. To minimize reactions to vibrations in either air or ground transport vehicles, transport crew members should properly secure patients, encourage and assist them with position changes, and provide adequate padding and skin care.[2–4,9,10,13]

Fatigue

Many operational stressors of transport may induce fatigue to some degree. Fatigue is an inherent stress of transport duties. Erratic schedules, hypoxic environments, noise and vibration, and imperfect environmental systems eventually take their toll; therefore, in transport, fatigue is always a potential threat to safety.[9–12,15–17,21]

Fatigue is the end product of all the physiologic and psychological stressors of flight associated with exposure to altitude.[9–12,15–17,21] Fatigue can also result from self-imposed stressors regardless of the type of transport. Box 5.1 shows self-imposed stresses that can have disastrous results.

Gravitational Force

In terms of practical application for civilian air medical transports, the effects of gravitational force (g-force) are limited and, in most cases, negligible. For an examination of g-force as a stress of flight, an understanding of speed, velocity, acceleration, and mass is helpful to clarify the concepts of exerted forces.

• BOX 5.1 **Factors That Affect Tolerance: DEATH**

Factors that affect tolerance to the stresses of flight can be summarized using the acronym DEATH.

D = Drugs. Use of over-the-counter drugs and antihistamines, misuse of prescription drugs, and use of stimulants such as caffeine can cause insomnia, tremors, indigestion, and nervousness.

E = Exhaustion (fatigue). Exhaustion can lead to judgment errors, limited response, falling asleep on the job, narrowed attention, and change in circadian rhythm.

A = Alcohol. Use of alcohol can cause histotoxic hypoxia, affect the efficiency of cells to use oxygen, interfere with metabolic activity, and result in a hangover.

T = Tobacco. Along with exposure of the body to nicotine, tar, and carcinogens, smoking of two packs of cigarettes per day results in 8% to 10% of the body's hemoglobin being saturated with carbon monoxide.

H = Hypoglycemia (diet). Poor dietary intake can cause nausea, judgment errors, headache, and dizziness.

Speed is the rate of movement of a body regardless of the direction of travel. *Velocity* is the rate (magnitude) of change of distance and direction of travel of an object and is, therefore, a vector quantity. The velocity of a body changes if its speed or direction of travel changes. It is expressed as the rate of change of distance in a specified direction. *Acceleration* is the rate of change of velocity of an object, and like velocity, it is a vector quantity.[5]

Weight is the force exerted by the mass of an accelerating body.[3,5] *Mass* is a measure of the inertia of an object (e.g., its resistance to acceleration).[3,5] Newton's three laws of motion define the relationship between motion and force[3,5]:

1. **Newton's First Law of Motion.** Unless it is acted on by a force, a body at rest will remain at rest and a body in motion will move at a constant speed in a straight line.
2. **Newton's Second Law of Motion.** When a force is applied to a body, the body accelerates, and the acceleration is directly proportional to the force applied and inversely proportional to the mass of the body.
3. **Newton's Third Law of Motion.** For every action, there is an equal and opposite reaction.

Two types of acceleration must be considered: linear and radial. *Linear acceleration* is produced by a change of speed without a change in direction. In conventional aviation, prolonged linear accelerations seldom reach a magnitude that could produce significant changes in human performance because most aircraft do not exert sufficient thrust to produce extended changes in linear velocity. However, significant linear accelerations that last 2 to 4 seconds are produced during catapult-assisted takeoffs, during arrested landings, and when reheat is engaged in certain high-performance aircraft. Large prolonged linear accelerations occur during the launching of spacecraft and during slowing on reentry into the Earth's atmosphere. *Radial acceleration* is produced by a change of direction without a change of speed. Such accelerations occur when the line of flight is changed. Aircraft maneuvers are, by far, the most common source of prolonged acceleration in flight. Accelerations on the order of 6 to 9 *g* or more can be maintained for many seconds by circular flight in agile military aircraft.[3,5]

When the main interest is the effect of acceleration on humans, the direction in which an acceleration or inertial force acts is described using a three-axis coordinate system (X, Y, and Z), in which the vertical (Z) axis is parallel to the long axis of the body.

Considerable confusion can result if a clear distinction is not made between the applied acceleration and the resultant inertial force because these, by definition, always act in diametrically opposite directions.[3,5]

Aircraft Motion

Because space is three-dimensional, linear motions in space are described with reference to three linear axes, and angular motions are described with three angular axes. In aviation, customary terms are the longitudinal (fore-aft), lateral (right-left), and vertical (up-down) linear axes, which are used to describe the roll, pitch, and yaw angular axes, respectively.[3,5]

Linear Axes	Angular Axes
Longitudinal axis (fore-aft)	Axis of roll
Lateral axis (right-left)	Axis of pitch
Vertical axis (up-down)	Axis of yaw

The relationship of this three-axis system with its action on humans is illustrated in Table 5.5.

Long-Duration Positive Acceleration

The crews of agile aircraft are frequently exposed to sustained positive accelerations ($+g_z$) with changes in the direction of flight, either in turns or in recovery from dives. Exposure to positive acceleration usually causes deterioration of vision before any disturbance of consciousness. For example, exposure to $+4.5 \, g_z$ typically produces complete loss of vision, or "blackout," but hearing and mental activity remain unaffected. Exposure to a positive acceleration stress that is slightly greater than that required to produce blackout results in unconsciousness. At moderate levels of acceleration (5–6 g), blackout precedes loss of consciousness; however, at higher accelerations, unconsciousness occurs before any visual symptoms occur.[3,5]

Long-Duration Negative Acceleration

Flight conditions that cause negative accelerations ($-g_z$) are outside loops and spins, in addition to simple inverted flight and recovery from such maneuvers. Tolerance for negative acceleration is much lower than that for positive acceleration, and the symptoms produced by even $-2 \, g_z$ are unpleasant and alarming. Furthermore, low levels of negative acceleration produce serious decrements in performance.[1,2,3,5,14,19]

Long-Duration Transverse Acceleration

Accelerations of long duration acting at right angles to the long axis of the body ($+g_x$) rarely occur in present-day conventional flight. They are usually confined to catapult launches, rocket-assisted and jet-assisted takeoffs, and carrier landings, although forces more than $-2 \, g_x$ may build up during flat spins. However, the forces in these maneuvers are small relative to human tolerance and do not cause problems.[1,2,5,14,19]

The definitions of the g force effects given here are applicable to high-performance aircraft, mostly fighter types, and emergency situations. The longitudinal axis is most important in air medical transports. However, the effects of g-forces are usually encountered only with forces greater than 1.5 g.

Cabin Pressurization

The pressure environment that surrounds the Earth can be divided into four zones: physiologic, physiologically deficient, space-equivalent, and space. These zones are characterized according to their physiologic effects as follows:

Physiologic zone: From sea level to altitudes up to 10,000 feet.
Physiologically deficient zone: Altitudes from 10,000 to 50,000 feet.
Space-equivalent zone: Altitudes from 50,000 to 250,000 feet.
Space: Altitudes beyond 250,000 feet.

In the physiologic zone, humans are well adapted. Although middle ear or sinus problems may be experienced during ascent or descent in this zone, most physiologic problems occur outside this zone and when proper protective equipment is not used. In the physiologically deficient zone, protective oxygen equipment is mandatory because of the decrease in barometric pressure, which can result in oxygen deficiency and subsequent altitude hypoxia.[8–12,15–19,21] Additional problems may result from trapped and

TABLE 5.5 Three-Axis Coordinate System for Describing Action on Humans Regarding Direction of Acceleration and Inertial Forces

Direction of Acceleration	Direction of Resultant Inertial Forces	Physiologic and Vernacular Descriptors	Standard Terminology
Headward	Head to foot	Positive g Eyeballs down	$+g_z$
Footward	Foot to head	Negative g Eyeballs up	$-g_z$
Forward	Chest to back	Transverse A-P-G Supine g Eyeballs in	$+g_x$
Backward	Back to chest	Transverse P-A-G Prone g Eyeballs out	$-g_x$
To the right	Right to left	Left lateral g Eyeballs left	$+g_y$
To the left	Left to right	Right lateral g Eyeballs right	$-g_y$

evolved gases. Travel in the space-equivalent and space zones requires either a sealed cabin or a full-pressure suit.

Generally, the most effective way to prevent physiologic problems is to provide an aircraft pressurization system so that the occupants of the aircraft are never exposed to pressures outside the physiologic zone. In cases in which ascent above the physiologic zone is necessary, protective oxygen equipment must be provided.[8–12,15–19,21] Aircraft pressurization consists of increased barometric pressure within crew and passenger compartments, which reduces the cabin altitude, creating near-the-Earth atmospheric conditions within the aircraft.[19] Commercial passenger aircraft normally pressurize to the equivalent of 5000 to 8000 feet, with the aircraft ascending a bit over 40,000 feet (FL 400).[8,12,15,17] The conventional method, used in virtually all current aircraft, is to draw air from outside the aircraft, compress it, and deliver it into the cabin. The desired pressure is maintained within the cabin with control of the compressed gas flow out of the cabin and into the atmosphere. The continuous flow of air ventilates the compartment; in most aircraft, this flow of air also controls the thermal environment within the cabin.[19]

The difference between the absolute pressure within an aircraft and that of the atmosphere immediately outside an aircraft is called the *cabin differential pressure*. Differential pressure is frequently controlled so that it varies with aircraft altitude. The two principal aircraft pressurization systems, isobaric and isobaric-differential, are described as follows[5]:

Isobaric system: Isobaric control maintains a constant cabin pressure while the ambient barometric pressure decreases. Many military and civilian aircraft are equipped with isobaric pressurization systems. This pressurization increases the comfort and mobility of the passengers, negates the necessity for the routine use of oxygen equipment, and minimizes fatigue.

Isobaric-differential system: Tactical military aircraft are not equipped with isobaric pressurization systems because the added weight severely limits their range and the large pressure differential increases the danger of rapid decompression during combat situations. Instead, these aircraft are equipped with an isobaric-differential cabin pressurization system. The isobaric function controls cabin pressure until a preset pressure differential is reached. With continued ascent, the preset differential is maintained. Thus, the apparent cabin altitude progressively increases as the aircraft ascends.

In air medical transport, cabin pressurization is especially important. Not only does it protect the occupants from the physiologic hazards of altitude, but it also provides more effective control of cabin temperature and ventilation, promotes greater mobility and comfort, and reduces fatigue. Cabin pressurization does not eliminate all problems, however. Cabin pressure can be lost as a result of structural failure, such as a window or a door blowing out, or through a mechanical malfunction of pressurization equipment.[4]

Decompression

A loss of cabin pressure is referred to as *decompression*. Aircraft decompression can be slow and gradual, over a period of several minutes, or it can be sudden, within a matter of seconds.[4,10] The risk of injury from decompression increases in proportion to the ratio of the area of the defect to the volume of the cabin and to the ratio of cabin pressure before and immediately after the decompression.[6,9] The following factors control the rate of decompression[15,16]:

- Volume of the pressurized cabin: The larger the cabin, the slower the rate of decompression if all other factors are constant.

- Size of the opening: The larger the opening, the faster the rate of decompression. The most important factor is the ratio between the volume of the cabin and the cross-sectional area of the opening.
- Pressure differential: The initial pressure gradient between the initial cabin pressure and the initial ambient pressure directly influences the rate and severity of decompression. The greater the differential, the more severe the decompression.
- Pressure ratio: Time is directly related to the pressure ratio between the cabin and ambient pressures. The greater the ratio, the longer the decompression.
- Flight pressure altitude: The altitude at which decompression occurs relates directly to the physiologic problems that occur after the incident.

Box 5.2 illustrates the physical characteristics of decompression.

The physiologic effects of rapid decompression are hypothermia, gas expansion, hypoxia, and decompression sickness. Hypoxia is by far the most important hazard of cabin decompression in aircraft flying at high altitudes.[15,16] The rapid reduction of ambient pressure produces a corresponding drop in the PO_2 and reduces the alveolar oxygen tension. A two- to threefold performance decrement occurs, regardless of altitude. The reduced tolerance for hypoxia after decompression is caused by (1) a reversal in the direction of oxygen flow in the lungs, (2) diminished respiratory activity at the time of decompression, and (3) decreased cardiac activity at the time of decompression.[15,16]

Crew members and passengers must protect themselves from the potential physiologic hazards caused by loss of cabin pressure. Because hypoxia is the most immediate hazard, all occupants must

---

• BOX 5.2 Physical Characteristics of Decompression

Slow Decompression
Onset is insidious and gradual and can occur without detection. Signs and symptoms are the same as for hypoxia. Decompression can be determined by checking the cabin altimeter.

Rapid Decompression
Onset is immediate, in 1 to 3 seconds, and is accompanied by noise, flying debris, and fog.

Noise
When two different air masses collide, a sound is heard that ranges from a swish to an explosion.

Flying Debris
On decompression, rapidly rushing air from a pressurized cabin causes the velocity of airflow through the cabin to increase rapidly as the air approaches the opening. Loose objects, such as maps, charts, and unsecured medical equipment, can be extracted through the orifice. Dust and dirt hamper vision for a short period of time.

Fog
During rapid decompression, both temperature and pressure suddenly decrease. This decrease reduces the capacity of air to contain water vapor and causes fog. The dissipation rate of fog is fairly rapid in fighter aircraft but considerably slower in larger multiplace aircraft.

Modified from Chase NB, Kreutzman RJ. Army aviation medicine. In: DeHart RL, ed. *Fundamentals of Aerospace Medicine.* Lea & Febiger; 1985; Heimbach RD, Sheffield PJ. Decompression sickness and pulmonary overpressure accidents. In DeHart RL, ed. *Fundamentals of Aerospace Medicine.* Lea & Febiger; 1985.

breathe 100% oxygen. Air medical personnel must first ensure that they are breathing 100% oxygen before attempting to assist their patients. Patients who already have oxygen deficiencies, such as patients with coronary disease, anemia, or pneumonia, must be closely monitored after decompression. After the prevention or correction of hypoxia, descent is made to an altitude below 10,000 feet, if possible.[3,9–12,15–17,21]

Decompression Sickness

The first human case of decompression sickness was reported in 1841 by M. Triger, a French mining engineer who noticed symptoms of pain and muscle cramps in coal miners who had been working in an air-pressurized mine shaft.[12,15–17] Because tunnel workers were first to have the syndrome now known as decompression sickness, early terminology describing this disorder was related to the mining occupation, hence the names *caisson disease* and *compressed-air illness.*[2,5,15,16]

A distinct difference is found between compressed-air illness and *subatmospheric decompression sickness,* although they share the same colloquial nomenclature for the common manifestations. Classically, the main manifestations are limb pain (the bends), respiratory disturbances (the chokes), skin irritation (the creeps), various disturbances of the central nervous system (the staggers), and cardiovascular collapse (syncope). These symptoms of subatmospheric decompression sickness virtually always subside or disappear during descent to ground level. Rarely, however, does recovery occur after recompression to ground level, and in some cases, the severity of the symptoms may increase, accompanied by a generalized deterioration in the individual's condition, which is known as *postdescent collapse.*[2,5,15,16]

Although the finer points of the pathologic processes that underlie some of the altitude decompression sickness manifestations remain unknown, the basic mechanism is supersaturation of the tissues with nitrogen.[9,12,15–17,21] Because the partial pressure of nitrogen in the inspired air falls with ascent to higher altitudes, nitrogen is carried by the blood from the tissues to the lungs, in which it exits the body in the expired gas. In addition, because the solubility of nitrogen in the blood is relatively low and some tissues contain large amounts of nitrogen, the rate of fall of the absolute pressure of the body tissues, which is associated with the ascent in altitude, is greater than the rate of fall of the partial pressure of nitrogen in the tissues. Therefore, these tissues become supersaturated with nitrogen. In certain circumstances, supersaturation gives rise to the formation of gas bubbles, primarily nitrogen, within tissues of the body. Gas exchange is the governing mechanism in the formation of gas bubbles, and these bubbles subsequently grow in size through the diffusion of nitrogen and other gases, such as oxygen and carbon dioxide, from surrounding tissue.

The driving pressure for gas bubble formation in a fluid is the difference between the partial pressure of the gas dissolved in the fluid and the absolute hydrostatic pressure.[12] Henry's law can be applied as follows: the amount of a gas that dissolves in a solution and remains in that solution is directly proportional to the pressure of the gas over the solution. Nitrogen is metabolically inert. At sea level, the amount of nitrogen dissolved in the body tissues and fluid is in equilibrium with the ambient pressure. At higher altitudes, nitrogen evolves in a manner similar to the formation of bubbles in a carbonated beverage when the bottle cap is removed. Decompression sickness is not usually encountered below a pressure altitude of FL 250.[4] The clinical manifestations of decompression sickness are shown in Box 5.3.[15,16]

• BOX 5.3 Clinical Manifestations of Decompression Sickness

Skin
Paresthesia (numbness or tingling sensation)
Mottled or diffuse rash of short duration
Itching
Cold or warm sensations

Joints
"Bends" pain (mild to severe) in muscles and joints, caused by nitrogen bubbles in the joint space
Pain is mild at onset, becomes deep and penetrating, and eventually becomes severe
Pain usually affects (in order) knee, shoulder, elbow, wrist or hand, and ankle or foot
Pain increases with motion

Lungs
"Chokes" (rare in both diving and aviation)
Deep sharp pain under sternum
Dry cough
Inability to take a normal breath
Attempted deep breath causes coughing (frequently paroxysmal)
Condition progresses to collapse if exposure to altitude is maintained
"False chokes" (caused by breathing cold, dry oxygen, which dries the throat and causes irritation and a nonproductive cough)

Brain
Visual disturbances
Headache
Spotty motor or sensory loss, or both
Unilateral paresthesia
Confusion
Paresis
Seizures

In a small number of cases, circulatory collapse or postdecompression collapse may occur. The clinical symptoms vary. Typically, the patient becomes anxious, develops a frontal headache, and feels sick. Facial pallor, coldness, and sweaty extremities may occur, and peripheral cyanosis almost always occurs. General or focal signs of neurologic involvement, such as weakness of the limbs, apraxia, scotomata, and convulsions, may occur. Arterial blood pressure is generally well maintained until late in the illness. Finally, in the worst cases, coma supervenes. Recovery can occur at any stage but is rare once coma has developed.[2,5,15,16]

In addition to supersaturation of the tissues with nitrogen, other factors that influence an individual's susceptibility to decompression sickness include the rate of ascent, altitude, time of exposure, reexposure to high altitude, body fat, age (if greater than 40 years), exercise before and after flight, presence of infection, and alcohol ingestion.[2,5,15,16]

The primary treatment of decompression sickness that arises at high altitudes is recompression to ground level as rapidly as possible. Breathing 100% oxygen also relieves the tissue hypoxia produced by the reduction of local blood flow. The actual management of a serious decompression sickness case depends on the geographic location and availability of a suitable hyperbaric chamber. Therefore, the preferred treatment, based on availability, is presented as follows[8,15,16,19]:

1. Immediate hyperbaric compression with or without intermittent oxygen breathing should be administered.

2. When there is not a hyperbaric chamber facility locally, air medical personnel should treat circulatory collapse and arrange for early transfer to a hyperbaric chamber facility that is within a reasonable time or distance (less than 6 hours of travel time) away. Surface transport is preferable; flight to a suitable chamber should be at an altitude below 1000 feet, if possible, and not higher than 3000 feet.
3. Air medical crew members should administer full supportive treatment for circulatory collapse if there is no possibility of transfer within a reasonable time to a hyperbaric chamber.

Due to the risk of decompression sickness, transport team members should not fly for at least 12 hours after diving.

Additional Stresses of Transport

Spatial Disorientation

Spatial disorientation is described as an individual's inaccurate perception of position, attitude, and motion in relation to the center of the Earth.[1] When persons experience spatial disorientation, they cannot correctly interpret or process the information they are given by their senses. Spatial disorientation primarily occurs during air transport.

During flight, the following three systems are involved in maintenance of equilibrium: visual, vestibular, and proprioceptive. These systems combine to allow the appropriate interpretation of input. However, the visual system plays the most important role.

Spatial disorientation can cause the following visual illusions[1,5]:
- Cloud formations being confused with the horizon or ground.
- Water or desert appearing to be farther away than it is.
- During night flights, the perception is that another aircraft is moving away when it is actually getting closer.

These visual illusions can cause significant motion sickness, which may render pilots or transport team members incapable of performing their duties or providing patient care. Spatial disorientation can also lead to misinterpretation of a landing area and result in a crash.

To prevent spatial disorientation, transport team members should use proper scanning techniques, never stare at lights, get adequate rest and nutrition, and provide conscious patients with a tactile reference during transport.

Flicker Vertigo

Flicker vertigo can occur when transport team members and patients are exposed to lights that flicker at a rate of 4 to 20 cycles per second.[1,5,10] It can cause nausea and vomiting. In severe cases, it can cause seizures and unconsciousness. Flicker vertigo commonly occurs when sunlight flickers through the rotor blades of a helicopter or an airplane propeller. It has also been triggered by light from rotating beacons against an overcast sky.

Transport team members or patients with a history of seizures are at risk for flicker vertigo. Wearing a hat with a bill and sunglasses can prevent flicker vertigo. Adequate rest and stress management may also decrease the risk.

Fuel Vapors

Both ground and air transport can expose transport crew members and patients to fuel vapors. Jet fuel, diesel fuel, and gasoline are a few examples of what may be used in transport vehicles. Exposure to fuel vapors can cause altered mental status, nausea, and eye inflammation.[1,5,10]

Fuel vapors may be an indication of a problem in the transport vehicle and, when detected, should be immediately reported by the transport team. Adequate ventilation can help decrease the effects of exposure.[1,5,10]

Summary

To become an effective healthcare provider in the transport environment, each transport team member must be thoroughly familiar with the effects of the stresses of transport on the human body. Implementation of correct interventions is an essential responsibility of each team member to minimize the effects of the stresses of transport upon themselves and their patients.

CASE STUDY

Transport Physiology 1

A 54-year-old man with a history of COVID-related pneumonia is being transported via FW aircraft for a higher level of care at a tertiary facility. His vital signs are: blood pressure 112/78 mm Hg, pulse rate 98 beats per minute (bpm; sinus tachycardia), respiratory rate (intubation on transport ventilator) 20 breaths per minute, and rectal temperature 38°C.

The patient has been prepared for transport in a PC 12. You recall the pilot mentioned he will be pressuring the cabin to 5500 feet. You will be taking off from sea level and landing at a location at 4000 feet elevation. Current ventilator settings include an FiO_2 of 0.8 and PEEP of 4 cm H_2O. Additionally, their SpO_2 has been 94% to 95%. The transport nurse uses Dalton's law to calculate the needed change in FiO_2 during flight as well as the FiO_2 needed at the destination.

After the patient is loaded into the PC 12, the flight nurse changes the FiO_2 to 0.97. Throughout the flight, the patient is monitored for any changes or needs. Upon landing at the destination airport, the flight nurse changes the FiO_2 to 0.93. The patient is then transported to the receiving facility.

Discussion
This situation describes patient management using Dalton's law. With the FiO_2 on the ventilator set to 0.8, it is important to consider the needed FiO_2 with

altitude applied. The higher the altitude, the more oxygen is needed. This calculation can be accomplished using this formula:

$$[(Pressure\ at\ sending\ facility)(FiO_2\ at\ sending\ facility)/(Pressure\ at\ destination)] = Needed\ FiO_2\ at\ destination$$

For the flight leg, the "Destination" terms can be swapped for "Altitude." In this case study, the flight nurse calculated an FiO_2 change from 0.8 to 0.97 at altitude/in flight (barometric pressure of 630 torr). This was achieved via the following calculation: $[(760\ torr)(0.8)/(630\ torr)] = 0.965$, or about 97%. This change will help maintain the patient's SpO_2 between 94% and 95%, which was the range experienced at the sending facility. Similarly, at the destination airport, which has a barometric pressure of 653.6 torr, the flight nurse changed the FiO_2 from 0.97 in flight to 0.93. This was calculated via the following: $[(630\ torr)(0.97)/(653.6\ torr)] = 0.934$, or about 93%.

CASE STUDY

Transport Physiology 2

A 9-month-old infant was involved in a one-car MVC with frontal impact. Upon impact the infant was secured in a car seat. His vital signs are 82/58 mm Hg, pulse rate 162 bpm (sinus tachycardia), respiratory rate 70 breaths per minute, oxygen saturation 88%, and rectal temperature 97°F. The patient appears very fatigued and is exhibiting see-saw respirations.

You and your partner decide to intubate the patient. The intubation is performed without incident. You package the patient for transport and prepare to transition the patient to the aircraft. An isolette is used to transport the infant. Just prior to departing the small county ER, the patient is on the mechanical ventilator and monitoring devices, and the patient seems to be stabilized. Upon departure, the patient's blood pressure is 91/61 mm Hg, pulse rate 154 bpm, and oxygen saturation 96%.

The pilot launches the rotor-wing aircraft and it reaches cruising altitude. Within minutes, the patient's blood pressure drops to an undetectable value, the carotid pulse weakens, and the oxygen saturation drops to 76%. The tracheal tube is confirmed to have correct placement between the vocal cords.

An isotonic crystalloid fluid bolus is administered. The FiO_2 is increased on the ventilator to 1.0. The patient's vitals do not correct with these treatments. Your partner makes a comment about how high up the aircraft is. You question the pilot as to your altitude and he replies that you are at 9500 feet.

You request the pilot to descend to the lowest safest altitude and needle decompress the chest with an 18-gauge IV catheter into the 4th intercostal space at the anterior axillary line. This results in an immediate return of stable vital signs.

Discussion

The patient developed a tension pneumothorax. The initial impact of the MVC caused a very small, undetectable pneumothorax. When the pilot ascended to 9500 feet, the lower pressure at this altitude allowed the pneumothorax to develop into a tension pneumothorax, as predicted by Boyle's law. A critical care transport team needs to be proactive in protecting their patients from the dangers of high flying. This was an actual patient transported in 2007.

References

1. Blumen I, Callejas S. Air transport physiology: a reference for air medical personnel. In: Blumen I, Lemkin DL, eds. *Principles and Direction of Air Medical Transport*. Medical Physicians Association; 2006.
2. Brashers V. Structure and function of the pulmonary system. In: McCance K, Huether S, eds. *Pathophysiology: The Biologic Basis for Disease in Adults and Children*. 7th ed. Elsevier; 2014: 1225–1247.
3. Department of the Air Force. *Aeromedical Evacuation*. US Air Force Pamphlet No 10-1403; 2011.
4. Egan F, Spearman CB, Sheldon RL. Gases, the atmosphere and the gas laws. In: Scanlon CL, Spearman CB, Sheldon RI, eds. *Egan's Fundamentals of Respiratory Therapy*. 4th ed. Mosby; 1982.
5. Hawkins H. The aircraft cabin and its human payload. In: Orlady HW, ed. *Human Factors in Aviation*. 2nd ed. Avebury Technical; 1993.
6. Kenefick W, Cheuvront SN, Castellani JW, et al. Thermal stress. In: Davis J, Johnson R, Stepanek J, eds. *Fundamentals of Aerospace Medicine*. 4th ed. Wolters Kluwer; 2008.
7. Martin TE. Clinical aspects of aeromedical transport. *Curr Anaesth Crit Care*. 2003;14(3):131–140.
8. Polikoff LE, Giuliano JS. Up, up and away: aeromedical transport physiology. *Clin Pediatr Emerg Med*. 2013;14(3):222–230.
9. Thibeault S. *Transport Professional Advanced Trauma Course Manual*. 6th ed. Air and Surface Transport Nurses Association; 2015.
10. Woodward GA, ed. *Guidelines for Air and Ground Transport of Neonatal and Pediatric Patients*. American Academy of Pediatrics; 2007.
11. Clark Y, Stocking J, Johnson J. *Flight and Ground Transport Nursing Core Curriculum*. Air and Surface Transport Nurses Association; 2007.
12. Rood GM. Noise and communication. In: Ernsting J, King P, eds. *Aviation Medicine*. 2nd ed. Butterworth; 1988.
13. Commission on Accreditation of Medical Transport Systems (CAMTS). *Accreditation Standards*. 10th ed. Author; 2015.
14. Banks RD, Brinkley JW, Allnutt R, et al. Human response to acceleration. In: Davis J, Johnson R, Stepanek J, eds. *Fundamentals of Aerospace Medicine*. 4th ed. Wolters Kluwer/Lippincott Williams & Wilkins; 2008.
15. Van Hoesen K, Bird N. Diving medicine. In: Auerbach P, ed. *Wilderness Medicine*. 6th ed. Elsevier Mosby; 2012:1520–1549.
16. Van Hoesen K, Bird N. Diving medicine. In: Auerbach P, ed. *Wilderness Medicine*. 6th ed. Elsevier Mosby; 2012:1549–1562.
17. Stepanek J, Webb JT. Physiology of decompressive stress. In: Davis JR, Johnson R, Stepanek J, eds. *Fundamentals of Aerospace Medicine*. 4th ed. Wolters Kluwer/Lippincott Williams & Wilkins; 2008.
18. Federal Aviation Administration. Advisory Circular 61-107B; Change 1, Aircraft operations at altitudes above 25,000 feet mean sea level or Mach numbers greater than 0.75. September 9, 2015. https://www.faa.gov/documentLibrary/media/Advisory_Circular/AC_61-107B_CHG_1_FAA.pdf
19. Pickard JS, Gradwell DP. Respiratory physiology and protection against hypoxia. In: Davis JD, Johnson R, Stepanek J, eds. *Fundamentals of Aerospace Medicine*. 4th ed. Wolters Kluwer/Lippincott Williams & Wilkins; 2008.
20. Phelan JR. Otolaryngology in aerospace medicine. In: Davis J, Johnson R, Stepanek J, eds. *Fundamentals of Aerospace Medicine*. 4th ed. Wolters Kluwer/Lippincott Williams & Wilkins; 2008.
21. Smith D, Gooman JR, Grosveld FW. Vibration and acoustics. In: Davis JR, Johnson R, Stepanek J, eds. *Fundamentals of Aerospace Medicine*. 4th ed. Wolters Kluwer/Lippincott Williams & Wilkins; 2008.

6

Scene Operations and Safety

CASEY GREEN AND MARIN PETERSON

COMPETENCIES

1. Explain the purpose of the Incident Command System.
2. Perform an initial scene evaluation to identify safety hazards.
3. Identify potential hazardous materials and safety positioning.
4. Verbalize general procedures for the decontamination process.
5. Understand general extrication principles/hazards as they apply to scene safety.
6. Define actions to take (e.g., THREAT) in an active shooter scenario.

Critical care transport personnel frequently participate in on-scene patient care. They are often preceded to the scene by other rescue personnel who have already managed scene hazards, freed trapped victims, and begun patient care. Nevertheless, extrication and scene management are important concepts for the transport team to thoroughly understand and be prepared for. Although familiarity with extrication, scene management, and hazardous material management exercises are generally included in transport team training, only transport team members with the appropriate training and personnel protective equipment (PPE) should participate in extrication or hazard management. More complex technical rescues, including hazardous material response, trench collapse, confined space, and rope rescue situations, are "high-risk, low-frequency" events that require specially coordinated, equipped, trained, and competent rescue personnel.

Most often, the transport team will operate in an environment in which other personnel manage the scene, extrication, and specialty rescues, while maintaining high situational awareness and attention to their personal safety. The failure of proper awareness and the failure to exercise personal and team restraint can result in direct injury, exposure, or contamination to both rescuers and victims and may delay patient care and transport.

Incident Command System

The Incident Command System (ICS) is a management method designed to clarify command relationships at incidents, foster interagency cooperation, and offer maximum flexibility for achieving strategic goals. ICS uses standardized terminology which facilitates communication. It also allows transitions with only minimal adjustments – it is easily scalable in real time, both for expansion and contraction. Any incident that taxes the assets of the responding rescuers is considered a mass casualty incident (MCI), ranging from a three-patient motor vehicle crash in a resource-limited area

to an event with overwhelming geographic scope or number of casualties. The ICS is designed to work effectively across the spectrum from minor incidents to complex MCIs or geographically disparate events.[1,2]

One or more individuals must always have authority over the incident, known as the command function. This can be a single person, the Incident Commander, or it may be a group of people who exert a unified command. Once command is established, usually by the most senior person in the initial response team, there are clear rules for the transfer of command and for the chain of command. Another key feature of ICS is a modular organization, allowing subgroups of the response team to be deployed to address needs. This modular function allows expansion and contraction, which is the feature that preserves the span of control (no individual is accountable for more than 3–7 people) (Fig. 6.1).[1,2]

There are five functional areas for major incidents: command, operations, planning, logistics, and finance/administration. For most incidents, command and operations are in place and planning, logistics, and finance/administration often are not deployed, except on very large-scale, extended duration incidents. Field personnel will usually be involved under the Operations component, which consists of an Ops branch and may include a dedicated air operations branch. A staging area may also be assigned under Operations. Divisions and Groups are components that may be under the Branches, depending on the size of the incident, and may be responsible for search and rescue (SAR) or triage, for example.[1,2]

One essential feature of the ICS is that members report to their designated supervisor, who has a known location and assignment within the pyramid of the command structure. For the transport team, this requires identification of the appropriate supervisor, a clear report to that person, and following the given assignment. The transport team will report to the commander for operators, or some subpart of the Operations group. The team rarely reports directly to the Incident Commander.[1,2]

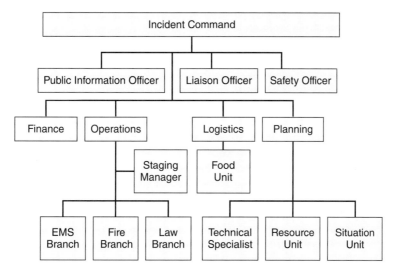

• **Figure 6.1** Sample incident command structure. (Modified from Sanders MJ, Lewis LM, Quick G, et al. *Mosby's Paramedic Textbook*. 3rd ed. Elsevier/Mosby; 2007.)

Scene Management

Prearrival/En Route Considerations

Scene evaluation begins when the communications center obtains information about potential problems and circumstances the rescuers may confront. The communication specialist should continue to seek information that could aid the rescuers throughout the incident, such as time of day, weather conditions, location, terrain, and number of victims, as well as information about fire, spilled fuel, toxic chemicals, overturned or entangled vehicles, and downed electrical lines. Before arrival, the communication center should relay contact information to on-scene providers. This information will be important for hazard communication, landing zone information for air operations, and postarrival deployment information. The transport team should discuss ingress and egress, hazards, and vehicle loading options prior to approaching the scene.

Approach to the Scene

Based on the scene size and characteristics, ambulances may be directed to a staging area and await further instructions, such as in a mass casualty scenario, or directly to the scene, such as in a small-sized, well-controlled scenario. At the scene, ambulances should generally park 100 feet from the scene, on the same side of the road, and allow enough room for traffic to pass. They should also be positioned uphill if there is a concern for hazardous materials. Law enforcement and other emergency response services should be present to secure the scene prior to the ambulance's arrival, although if the scene has not been secured, the ambulance may consider parking diagonally 50 feet in front of the scene to divert traffic further away and improve the safety of the scene. In addition, amber directional signals, rather than blinding and flashing lights, are preferred for traffic diversion.[3]

Proper placement of the helicopter for air medical transport is essential when approaching the scene. Landing zones should be secured by law enforcement or fire departments. The landing zone may be of sufficient distance from the incident that it requires a second traffic control zone to be established, in which case, the transport team should consider themselves as part of two separate

incidents with a need to operate safely in both and to plan the transit between scenes carefully.[1] If helicopters are left running at the scene, a tail guard must be in place. Personnel leaving and approaching the aircraft should do so within sight of the pilot, at a 3 o'clock or 9 o'clock approach (Fig. 6.2). When the aircraft is on a slope, always approach and depart downhill to maintain adequate distance from the rotor blades.

While approaching the scene, the transport team should complete a rapid assessment of the scene and surroundings. They should observe the terrain and attempt to understand the mechanism of injury and other hazards that may present themselves because of the accident (i.e., downed electrical lines, narrow bridges, or poor landscape access). This provides information to determine scene safety for everyone involved and if additional medical or ancillary services should be requested. For air operations, the opportunity to survey this information may be limited if the landing zone is located away from the accident. Information, such as wind direction and speed, is more easily gathered during daylight hours due to the decreased visibility at night, even with night vision goggles. Further landing zone requirements and operations are discussed in the operational safety and survival chapter 10.[3]

On-Scene Considerations

Once the vehicle has arrived, the transport team should wear reflective gear and the ambulance could use their scene floodlights for improved visibility and safety. The scene of a roadway incident must have an adequate traffic control zone in which responders can safely operate (Fig. 6.3). The traffic control zone, including roadways being used as landing zones or staging areas, should be blocked off with larger, well-lit emergency vehicles parked at an angle to deflect traffic away from the scene. Even with appropriate protective equipment, the risk of a secondary incident involving property damage or personal injury to responding personnel is real.[1,3] Factors associated with secondary incidents include the following:

- Lack of training
- Lack of situational awareness
- Failure to establish a sufficient traffic control zone for roadway incidents

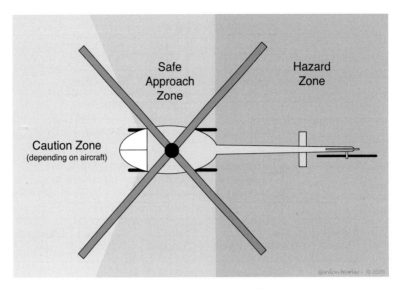

• **Figure 6.2** Landing zone safety.

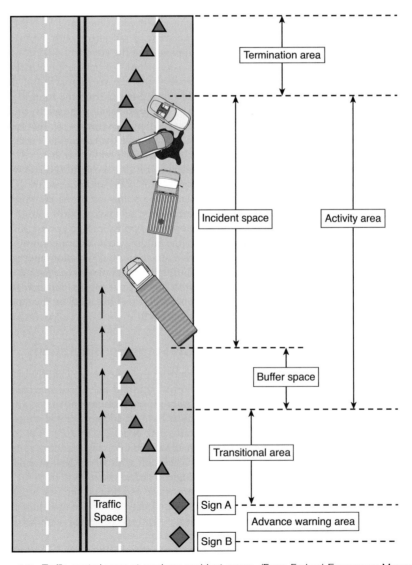

• **Figure 6.3** Traffic control zone at roadway accident scene. (From Federal Emergency Management Association publication. United States Fire Administration–Traffic Incident Management Systems. Publication FA-330, Fig. 3.5. https://www.usfa.fema.gov/downloads/pdf/publications/fa_330.pdf;2012.)

• BOX 6.1 Scene Management Guidelines

- Never compromise rescuers to aid victims.
- Evaluate the situation for potential safety hazards (e.g., traffic, utilities, gasoline, propane, fuel oil, water, sanitary systems, movement of vehicles, release of high-pressure systems).
- Report arrival to Incident Command and follow deployment instructions.
- Secure the accident scene and any traffic flow that may endanger rescuers.
- Wear personal protective equipment appropriate to the hazards on the scene (e.g., traffic vests, gloves, eye protection).
- Gain access to the patient only if trained and properly protected.
- Defer to specialty expertise for rescue and hazard management.

- Improper positioning of apparatus
- Inappropriate use of scene lighting
- Failure to use safety equipment[1]

It is important not to lose sight of equipment being used at the scene. Fire hoses, extrication tools, stabilization devices, and other equipment can occupy much of the ground around an accident. Awareness of the ground around your feet can prevent an injury. Lighting around the scene is important for all personnel involved in the extrication for safety and ease of work. Remember to defer to specialty expertise when necessary: the utility company should secure downed electrical lines, the fire department contains and controls hazardous materials, and scene security is usually provided by law enforcement personnel. Onlookers and the media should be kept well back from the operation (Box 6.1). If there ever is concern for personal safety due to traffic, violence, or nearby crowds, law enforcement should be immediately notified for assistance and transport personal may retreat to safety.[3]

Safety tactics that transport personal may utilize in an unsafe situation include the use of avoidance, retreat, concealment, and distraction. Avoidance is simply staying away from a potentially or known dangerous individual or environment. Tactical retreat is an immediate removal of oneself during a dangerous or violent situation. The mode and route of retreat should be the one that offers the least amount of exposure to the dangerous situation. Cover and concealment include the use of physical objects or structures as a means of protecting oneself and hiding oneself from danger, such as gunfire or a violent person. Distraction and evasive maneuvers can be used during retreat or when there are no other options. These maneuvers include blocking a door with furniture or throwing equipment toward an aggressor. These require the anticipation of the aggressor's movements and preplanning.[3]

Mass Casualty Triage

Triage is required when there is more than one victim present, but triage becomes more complicated in a mass casualty scenario when the number of victims can quickly deplete emergency medical resources. Sort, assess, lifesaving interventions, and treatment/transport (SALT) triage is a reputable method to categorize patients, prioritize patient care, and administer lifesaving care in an efficient manner.

S – Sort: This method begins with sorting the overall victim population for priority. This is done by asking the victims to walk to a designated area, which sorts out those that will be assessed last, or are labeled as third priority. Next, the victims should be asked to follow a command, such as wave. Those that successfully completed, the command will be second priority. Those that did not complete the command are those that require immediate attention.

A – Assess: In the priority group that requires immediate attention, brief lifesaving care will be provided to further assess their condition. This care includes controlling major hemorrhage, opening the airway without advanced airway devices, providing two rescue breaths if it is a child that requires ventilations, completing chest decompression, and/or administering auto-injector antidotes as needed.

L – Lifesaving interventions: Perform lifesaving interventions rapidly. Time should not be wasted by seeking additional equipment or supplies. Based on these interventions, the victims will be further categorized.

T – Treatment/transport: At this point, the victims should be categorized. Dead (black tag) is determined if the adult victim is not breathing after their airway has been opened or if the child victim is not breathing after the airway has been opened and two breaths were delivered. No further care is given to this category. Immediate (red tag) is the category that receives priority care, and their care is continued. To meet this category, the victim can have a "no" to having purposeful movements/follows commands, has a peripheral pulse, is not in respiratory distress, or has a controlled hemorrhage but the transport team member still believes that the victim is likely to survive with treatment. Expectant (gray, white, or blue tag) is the victim that can have a "no" to any of the previous questions but is not expected to survive even with treatment. This category of victim may receive treatment, but it will be after all the immediate victims have been cared for. Delayed (yellow tag) includes victims with serious injuries who can presumably tolerate a delay in their treatment. This category is determined if the patient has all of the following: a peripheral pulse, is not in respiratory distress, has their hemorrhage controlled, and can follow commands or make purposeful movements. Minimal (green tag) is the category of victim that has all the previously listed qualities and is ambulatory. These victims have the potential to help care for or transport other victims (see Fig. 6.4).[3]

Hazardous Materials Emergencies

The Department of Transportation (USDOT) defines hazardous material as any substance or material that could adversely affect the safety of the public, handlers, or carriers during transportation. Emergencies that involve hazardous materials occur in all areas of the United States, and transport teams are likely to be involved in the care of those who have been injured. The key for the transport team, and all responders, is to remain a safe distance away until the hazard is identified, to avoid entering the scene and risking danger to themselves, and to avoid contaminating themselves and their vehicles by ensuring that patients are decontaminated before entering the treatment area. When a hazardous material can be identified from an identification number or by its name, emergency service personnel may obtain advice regarding the emergency scenario from agencies that assist in the management of hazardous materials, such as the Chemical Transportation Emergency Center (CHEMTREC) or the US DOT.[2,4,5]

Not every transport vehicle or locality containing hazardous material is marked with a placard that identifies the specific material on board. More often, they have placards that identify only the category of material carried or a four-digit identification number (Fig. 6.5). The Emergency Response Guidebook (ERG), carried in all first response vehicles, provides the first responders with general information about hazardous materials. It focuses on the protection of the responders and the public and is meant to be used only during the initial response. The book is broken down

SALT mass casualty triage

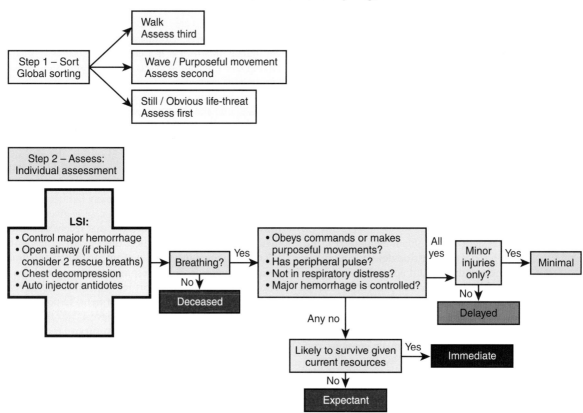

• **Figure 6.4** Sort, Assess, Lifesaving Interventions, and Treatment/Transport (SALT) mass casualty triage method. *LSI, Life-saving Interventions.* (From Sanders MJ, McKenna K, American Academy of Orthopaedic Surgeons. *Sanders' Paramedic Textbook.* 5th ed. Jones & Bartlett Learning; 2018.)

into six color-coded sections, each dealing with various aspects of a hazmat response. The ERG has been around since 1973 and is still widely used throughout the world.[2,4,5]

The National Fire Protection Agency developed a diamond sign to designate the distinct types and severity of hazards present on site. This diamond is made up of four different colored boxes, each representing a specific hazard class: blue for health hazard, red for flammability, yellow for reactivity, and white for special hazards. The special hazard box will also contain identification letters, such as AS (asphyxiant), W (water reactive), or O (oxidizing agent). The three colored boxes will have a number between 0 and 4, representing the increasing level of risk in the specific category.[2,4,5]

The shape of a transport vehicle or container can also provide some basic information. Rail and road transport units may have certain identifying characteristics. All pressure vessels will have rounded ends. High-pressure vessels will have fittings only at the top of the rounded vessel, whereas lower-pressure containers may have fittings elsewhere. Flammable products will be in containers with an oval cross-sectional shape and fittings on the bottom of the tank. Compressed gas transport trailers have multiple smaller rounded tanks stacked together, whereas a trailer containing corrosives will usually have a large black ring around the center of the trailer.[2,4,5] Transport teams responding to the scene of hazardous material emergencies follow these general guidelines[2,4,5]:

• Park the ambulance or land the aircraft uphill, upwind, and far enough away from the scene to prevent rotor wash from spreading hazardous materials. Pilots should avoid flying over the top of hazardous materials areas.

• Keep out of low areas in which heavier-than-air vapors can accumulate.

• Hazardous Material crews will establish "hot," "warm," and "cold" zones of operation. Transport teams should always stage in the Cold Zone to prevent the risk of personal injury or contamination of the vehicle. Only hazardous material responders trained to the technician or operations levels should operate in the Warm Zone, and only those trained to technician level should work in the Hot Zone (Fig. 6.6).[2]

• Rescuers should wear PPE that is appropriate for the situation, including respiratory and splash protection, as dictated by the nature of the hazardous material. EMS uniforms and flight suits are classified as Level D protection, the lowest level of protection possible.

• If there is a fire, some corrosive materials react violently with water. Defer to the personnel managing the scene before attempting to extinguish flames.

• Stay away from the ends of tank vehicles.

• Cool down uninvolved containers exposed to heat.

Radioactive Material Emergencies

Radioactive material emergencies are one variant of hazardous material emergencies. The degree of hazard varies depending on the type and quantity of the radioactive material, and individual risk varies with time of exposure, distance from the source, and attenuation or shielding. Exposure can come from inhalation, ingestion, or skin absorption. Although some radioactive materials

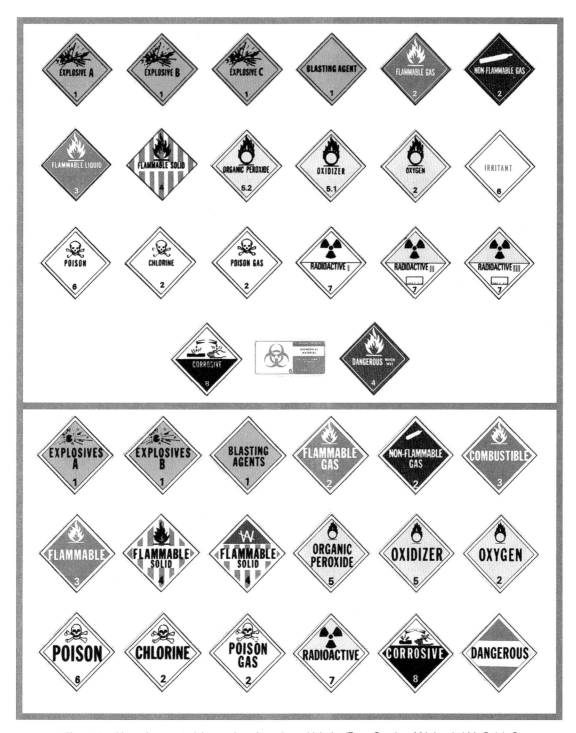

• **Figure 6.5** Hazardous materials warning placards and labels. (From Sanders MJ, Lewis LM, Quick G, et al. *Mosby's Paramedic Textbook.* 3rd ed. Elsevier/Mosby; 2007.)

may burn normally, they do not, as a class, ignite rapidly. Runoff from fire control or dilution activities can cause water pollution and potentially spread the contamination.[4,5]

Knowledge of the hazard is important. If only the yellow, black, and white "Radioactive Material" placards are visible on the carrier and the material being carried cannot otherwise be identified, people nonessential to the firefighting or rescue operation should be kept at least 150 feet upwind of the area; greater distances may be advised by the radiation authority (a division of the environmental protection agency). Persons and equipment exposed to the radioactive material must then be detained until the radiation authority arrives or other instructions are received.[4,5]

Decontamination

The decontamination corridor is called the Warm Zone and is located between the Hot and Cold Zones. This zone should be the only point of entry and exit to the Hot Zone. The following steps

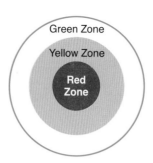

Red Zone—Hot (Contamination) Zone	Yellow Zone—Warm (Control) Zone	Green Zone—Cold (Safe) Zone
• Protective gear needed, highest potential for exposure • Number of personnel limited to those critical or necessary	• Surrounds contamination zone, decontamination takes place here • Prevents the spread of contamination • Protective gear needed • Emergency care and decontamination are performed	• Personnel sheds contaminated gear before entering, free from contamination • Normal care (triage, stabilization) and treatment here • Planning and staging area

• **Figure 6.6** Safety zones for hazardous materials incident.

have been recommended for use when a person needs decontamination after exposure to a hazardous material.

1. An entry point should be established for the "dirty" victims and rescuers to remove their clothing.
2. Surface decontamination should be performed with plenty of water unless the contaminant requires another decontaminant.
3. PPE should be removed and stored.
4. Other clothing may have to be removed, depending on the level of contamination.
5. Contaminated personnel and victims should be washed at least twice. Whenever possible, warm water with detergent should be used for decontamination.
6. Victims and personnel should be medically evaluated.
7. Injured individuals should be transported for definitive care.
8. The decontamination site must be cleaned up and contaminated materials disposed.
9. All equipment that has been used should be decontaminated and cleaned.
10. Contaminated clothing should never be taken home and cleaned or transported with the patient. Remember that clothing may be evidence.
11. Decontamination procedures must meet Occupational Safety and Health Administration requirements 29 CFR 1910.120.

The transport team needs to ensure that patients have undergone appropriate decontamination before being placed in any transport vehicle. Defer to expertise for determining appropriate decontamination. If the victim is not appropriately decontaminated, both the team and the transport vehicle can be contaminated. If the transport vehicle is contaminated, it needs to be taken out of service and decontaminated according to decontamination codes and guidelines.[4,5]

Transportation Emergency Scenes

Motor Vehicle Accidents and Extrication

Based on early estimates for 2021, the National Highway Traffic Safety Administration (NHTSA) reported that approximately 24,915 people died in motor vehicle traffic crashes, which is a 10.5% increase from 2020 and is the highest since 2005.[6] Responding to these increasingly fatal crashes are teams of rescue personnel. The makeup of these teams will vary according to the location, resources, and emergency preparedness model. Rescue teams should be trained on a regular basis to maintain proficiency with their equipment and the required skills along with the understanding of current technical rescue practices.[7]

Transport teams should not participate in rescue or operate around rescue scenes without sufficient protective equipment that is appropriate to the scene. The transport team may enter a vehicle after donning protective equipment, if trained or directed by trained personnel, and if the scene and vehicle are stabilized and deemed safe. Flight suits and regular EMS uniforms are considered the lowest level of protective equipment. Entering a car in which a heavy rescue is about to take place requires the transport personnel to wear the same level of protective equipment as the other public safety personnel working on the rescue.[7]

Rescue teams will utilize disentanglement, the process of spreading, cutting, or removing portions of a vehicle from a victim, and extrication, the process of removing a victim (Fig. 6.7). This team typically uses a systematic process that involves the stabilization of the scene, followed by the vehicle, and then the victim.[7]

To stabilize the scene, at least two rescue personnel should complete simultaneous outer and inner surveys. These surveys consist of 360-degree inspections to ensure that all hazards and accident details are identified. See Box 6.2 for the components of the outer and inner surveys. If any immediate danger to life and health (IDLH) hazards are identified, then all personnel on scene must be ordered to freeze until the hazards have been mitigated or resolved. A company officer will take the lead in this inspection and in granting permission to advance in the plan of action. They will communicate the safety status through an agreed-upon method, such as air horns for audio communication or hand signals for visual communication. In addition, they will continue to monitor the scene safety throughout the extrication process and communicate with the rescue team accordingly for the ongoing safety of everyone involved.[7]

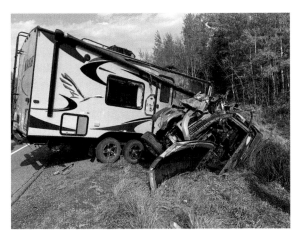

• **Figure 6.7** Trained rescue teams will utilize disentanglement and extrication techniques to remove victims from a motor vehicle accident.

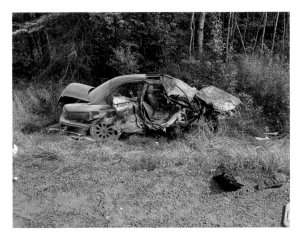

• **Figure 6.8** Once the scene and vehicle stability are deemed safe, extrication of the victim can be completed. This may require the use of hydraulic tools to obtain access points.

• BOX 6.2 Outer and Inner Scene Surveys at a Traffic Accident

Outer Survey (25–100 feet)
- Immediate danger to life and health (IDLH) hazards
- Potentially ejected victim(s)
- Walking wounded
- Additional vehicles
- Child car seats

Inner Survey (3–5 feet)
- IDLH hazards
- Type of vehicle (conventional, electric, hybrid)
- Status of the vehicle (Still running? In park or drive?)
- Number of victims
- Entrapment and its severity (minor, moderate, heavy)
- Obvious trauma to victim(s)
- Position and stability of vehicle
- Activation of airbags (deployed, live, and undeployed)
- Primary and secondary access plans, along with an emergency escape plan[7]

Any unanticipated vehicle movement is both unacceptable and unsafe for rescuers and occupants, so rescue teams must stabilize the vehicle before entry to prevent any potential movement. Vehicle stabilization methods include the placement of cribbing blocks underneath the vehicle, flattening tires, and attachment of stabilizing lines or struts. Continuous monitoring of the vehicle's stabilization should be done for ongoing safety assurance. Before proceeding with patient extrication, the rescue team should ensure that the vehicle's tires are chocked, the key/engine is turned off, the transmission is placed in park, and, whenever possible, the vehicle's battery is disconnected.[7]

Once the vehicle is stabilized, then the victim can be stabilized and extricated. When approaching a victim who is presumed to be entrapped, always remember to "try before you pry." Access to the victim may be gained by simply unlocking and opening any vehicle door that is undamaged or slightly damaged. The simplest solution is usually the fastest and safest for the rescuer. If the doors cannot be opened, then the windows may be broken to gain access. Broken glass is a hazard and should be managed appropriately. Breaking windows furthest away from the victim, announcing the plan to break a window prior to the breaking,

applying adhesive film to the window prior to breaking, utilizing appropriate PPE, and relocating broken glass to a safe area are all methods of mitigating the risks of broken glass.[7]

If more complex extrication is required, then the use of heavy extrication tools (hand-, electric-, and hydraulic-powered) should be used (Fig. 6.8). Depending upon how the stabilized car is positioned, extrication can be done through the vehicle's roof or doors. Hydraulic tools can be used to completely remove doors, remove the roof, or cut a U-shaped opening in the roof for access.

Occasionally, a victim's thorax becomes wedged between the forward-displaced seat and the rearward-displaced steering wheel or column, or a victim's feet and legs become trapped under the downward-displaced dashboard and the accelerator or brake pedal. A quick option to create more room between the victim, the seat, and the steering wheel is to manually slide the seat back (if it remains operational). Multiple rescuers should control the seat and the patient to avoid unnecessary movement and possible risk of further injury. Alternatively, hydraulic tools can displace the vehicle's dash and steering column off an entrapped victim in a dash roll technique or a dash lift technique. Another valuable extrication tool is the high-pressure air-lift bag. This tool, along with cribbing, can effectively lift a vehicle that is pinning a victim underneath. All rescue equipment should only be operated by trained personnel for the safety of the rescue team and victims.[7]

During extrication, rescue teams must be aware of potential hazards. Airbag systems, fuel runoff, and vehicles with alternative fuels can be dangerous to rescuers and entrapped victims during extrication unless extra caution is taken. Driver and front-passenger airbags are mandatory in all vehicles. Other airbag locations, such as side-impact, center, knee, seat cushion, rear set, and seat belt airbags, and their inflation cylinders vary and depend on the vehicle manufacturer. The inflation systems use a stored compressed-gas system, pyrotechnic propellant gas-generation system, or combination of both systems. These high-pressure systems work in milliseconds and tend to be located within cut zone areas, such as roof pillars or roof rales. Therefore, to avoid injury by accidentally deploying the airbag or triggering the inflators, it is recommended to recognize and identify these devices, disconnect the power supply, and ensure proper distance. Disconnecting the power may not fully prevent the airbag from deploying due to backup energy systems, so continue to ensure safe distancing throughout extrication. Additionally, attempting to disconnect

- Maintain proper procedures for disconnecting vehicle power and distancing from the airbags.
- Avoid placing personnel or objects in front of an undeployed airbag.
- Never try to contain the airbag by placing webbing or other containment equipment in front of the undeployed airbag.
- Inspection is critical! Expose the area prior to cutting, spreading, or pushing the vehicle structure to ensure no airbag components could potentially be damaged.
- Always consider the airbag's electronic control unit (ECU) when using tools around the center console and floorboards since every vehicle is designed differently.
- Always consider the side-impact airbags and sensors prior to using extraction tools on vehicle doors. Consider exposing the door hinges and cutting the hinges for a safer method.[7]

the inflator could accidentally trigger the airbag to deploy. The minimum recommended distance to maintain from driver-side airbags is 10 inches, passenger-side airbags is 20 to 25 inches, and side-impact airbags is 5 to 15 inches. Box 6.3 highlights considerations when completing extractions in vehicles with airbags.[7]

Vehicle fuel sources pose challenges and risks to rescue teams. Conventional vehicles use internal combustion engines that commonly burn petroleum-based fuels, such as gasoline or diesel. Fuel runoff can be dangerous if it encounters an ignition source, mixes with other chemicals at the scene, or leaks into the environment. Rescue teams can mitigate these risks by damming, diverting, diluting, or absorbing the fuel. Additionally, potential ignition sources should be kept away to avoid any potential exposure to fuel. Electric vehicles use a high-voltage electrical system with rechargeable batteries as a power source. The high-voltage wiring is contained in protective wrapping and/or within the framing. These vehicles have safety features that disable the electrical system when an accident, abnormally high temperature, or a leak or electrical disruption is detected. Depending upon the vehicle, it may take 5 to 30 minutes for the capacitor to fully discharge the voltage. The automatic disabling of the electrical system should not be assumed. To manually disable the voltage system, turn the key to the off position or take the smart key at least 20 feet away from the vehicle. Also, the vehicle's main fuse can be removed (and if the main fuse cannot be found, then remove all the fuses). Depending on the vehicle, the manufacturer may also recommend accessing the vehicle's service disconnects. Additionally, inspecting before cutting during the extrication process is crucial so battery packs and wiring can be avoided. Hybrid vehicles use a combination of petroleum-based fuel and electricity for power. The precautions for a hybrid vehicle are the same as the conventional and electric vehicles.[7]

Commercial Motor Vehicle Accidents

Commercial motor vehicles, such as commercial trucks and buses, pose unique challenges for the rescue team. Commercial trucks vary in cab configuration, size, and chassis design. Heavy-duty trucks can be over 33,000 pounds. Similarly, school buses or transit buses vary in cab configuration and size.[7]

The basic extrication process of these larger vehicles, compared to conventional vehicles, still requires the guarantee of a stabilized scene, vehicle, and then victim. Although additional caution must be used at the scene involving trucks and buses. Commercial

trucks may be carrying hazardous materials; therefore, anticipate and plan for this possibility and then utilize any placards or United Nations/North American Hazardous Materials Code identification numbers on the truck or available shipping papers regarding the cargo. Buses may have multiple passengers that have become victims with simple to severe injuries.[7]

The commercial vehicle may simply need to have the parking brake applied, engine turned off, and wheels chocked. Do not place anything under any portion of the vehicle until it is securely stabilized, especially since the air suspension system bellows may deflate without warning, in which case the body of some vehicles may drop suddenly to within inches of the roadway. If more advanced stabilization is required, a large 50/60-ton rotating tow unit with an articulating boom is the best equipment to use, but other feasible equipment includes struts, First Responder jacks with cribbing, and air-lift bags that can manage heavy equipment.[7]

Extrication from commercial vehicles requires the rescue team to enter a cab that is positioned higher and a structure that is heavier than the standard personal vehicle. Again, ensure that anyone entering the vehicle is wearing proper safety equipment. The rescue team should enter the commercial vehicle through the front door, if possible, but only after the vehicle is stabilized. If the rescuers cannot enter through the front door, they could attempt to enter the vehicle by removing the windshield, removing doors, or cutting through the roof. To extricate a pinned victim, the dash may be pushed out of the way.[7]

Specific to school buses, they have designated emergency exits which consist of a rear door or escape window, side windows, and roof hatches (Fig. 6.9A and B). Sidewalls can be removed for large extrication points by removing two adjacent windows. Obtaining roof access in a school bus may be challenging due to its heavier-gauged steel structure that is made of bowed trusses that run from the floors to across the roof and longitudinal stringers that run along the roof from the front to back. Similarly, the side walls are reinforced with steel rub (or guard) rails and crash rails that run the length of the bus to provide added crash protection for the passengers. If needed, bench seats from a bus can be quickly removed using a hydraulic spreader and cutter. Air-lift bags and cribbing can be utilized to lift a bus up for victims trapped underneath.[7]

Aircraft Accidents

Aircraft accidents can occur anywhere, have unique hazards, and require special precautions. All these accident scenes are under the jurisdiction of the National Transportation Safety Board (NTSB), an independent federal agency, and are treated like crime scenes to preserve the integrity of the scene and evidence for determining the probable cause of the accident. The Federal Aviation Administration (FAA) may be requested by the NTSB to assist in the investigation. Local law enforcement agencies are responsible for the initial scene safety and security. They will probably be responsible for the entire duration of scene security, but this will be determined by the NTSB or FAA once they arrive and throughout the investigation. The primary roles of local law enforcement, rescue teams, and first responders are to remove injured or trapped victims, protect the wreckage (i.e., evidence) from further damage, and protect the public from injury.[8]

Aircraft varieties include light sport models, experimental aircraft, certified airplanes, helicopters, and unmanned aircraft systems. Light sport aircraft include ultralights. They are generally flown for pleasure, use ballistic parachute systems, fit two or less individuals, utilize a small amount of fuel, and weigh less than

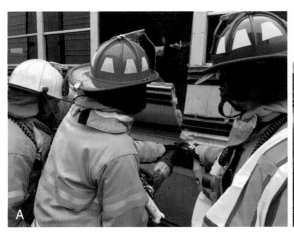
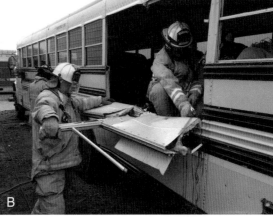

• **Figure 6.9** (A, B) School buses have designated emergency exits, although bus sidewalls can also be removed for larger extrication points.

1300 pounds. Experimental aircraft are also flown for pleasure but vary in size and design. Certified aircraft include small propeller-driven airplanes, single- or twin-engine planes, and small business jets. They are flown for pleasure or commercial operations, have more complex systems, and vary in size. Helicopters are primarily used for commercial operations. Unmanned aircraft systems are primarily used within the military and may contain weapons or lasers.[8]

In addition to knowing the typical characteristics of each type of aircraft, knowing the aircraft's mission can provide some insight into its potential hazards. Aircraft that complete agricultural applications will likely contain hazardous chemicals, such as pesticides. Law enforcement aircraft could potentially contain ammunition and weapons, and avalanche control aircraft may contain explosives. Emergency medical service aircraft will probably have oxygen tanks on board. Similarly, offshore aircraft may contain large nitrogen tanks for large emergency inflatable floatation bags. Lastly, prototype aircraft may have parachute systems or explosive escape hatches. Having this information can guide emergency planning and hazard mitigation.[8]

Aircraft hazards differ from motor vehicle hazards. Aviation fuel is volatile and may be still onboard or anywhere within the wreckage. Fuel is commonly stored within the wings but may also be in a fuselage tank. The engines will most likely be off by the time the rescue team arrives. If they happen to remain running, it is important to find a path that avoids the propellers, engine inlets, exhausts, and plane of rotation (which is the area perpendicular to the jet engine or propeller). The propellers should not be touched due to the risk of their movement causing kickback or even restarting of the engine. Another hazard includes the composite aircraft structure. The composite material is made from glass or carbon fibers with an epoxy resin. In an accident, this material creates a potential inhalation, instability, and penetration hazard. Fire burns away the epoxy resin which causes combustion products and fibers to become airborne. These can cause respiratory irritation, and some are even carcinogens. It is recommended to avoid these inhalation hazards by moving around from an upwind direction or utilizing a self-contained breathing apparatus (SCBA). This burned composite structure creates a secondary structure that can hold its form but cannot bear weight. Additionally, fracturing of the composite material can create shards that are capable of penetrating boots and loose fibers that can penetrate and irritate the skin. Due to these structural alterations, movement on and around the aircraft must be done

cautiously and minimum PPE should include a high-efficiency particulate air filter (HEPA) respirator and leather gloves. Newer aircraft have airbags that are located within seatbelts can be hazardous to the rescue team. They inflate up and outward from the individual and rapidly deflate to allow for emergency egress. The airbags can be identified by an unusually thick seatbelt. The associated inflator systems tend to be located below the seat and are pressurized to over 6000 psi. Therefore, extreme caution must be taken when cutting around the seat. Similarly, ballistic parachute systems may be present and are extremely dangerous hazardous features that include rockets to deploy parachutes. Rescue teams can identify these units from their physical appearance and warning placards. The parachute is in a pack with an attached rocket that is encased in aluminum and is the size of a 16-ounce can. Warning placards on the outside of the aircraft are required per federal regulations and label the panel in which the rocket is expelled from, which can be from a variety of different locations. This exit path must always be strictly avoided to mitigate harm to the rescue team, since even 1/4 to 1/2 inch movement of the actuation cable or heat can activate the parachute system. If extrication is required, the actuation cable in the aircraft cabin must be secured by ensuring the safety pin is in place and, if it is not, place a pin or zip tie within the safety pin hole. If the parachute is already deployed and inflated, do not enter the aircraft due to risk of aircraft movement and avoid the parachute along with suspension lines to avoid entrapment or entanglement. Attempt to deflate the parachute by dousing it with water or cutting the suspension lines. Once deflated, roll the parachute up and secure it or place a vehicle on it for security. Ultimately the ballistic parachute system's manufacturer should be notified to assist in its ultimate disengagement. Other aircraft hazards include components with stored energy, such as pneumatic systems, hydraulic systems, struts, wheels, fire extinguishers, and batteries.[8]

The FAA's recommended procedure for aircraft accidents:
1. Ensure that the NTSB and FAA are notified.
2. Establish a perimeter with only one entrance to allow for only authorized personnel (FAA, police, fire, EMS, medical examiner, investigation authority) and to minimize disruption of the scene.
   a. Multiple perimeters may be required if aircraft parts have departed the aircraft prior to the primary ground impact.
3. Cautiously approach the scene to avoid potential hazards, to search for occupants that may have been thrown from the aircraft, and to protect the scene and possible evidence. Approach upwind if possible.

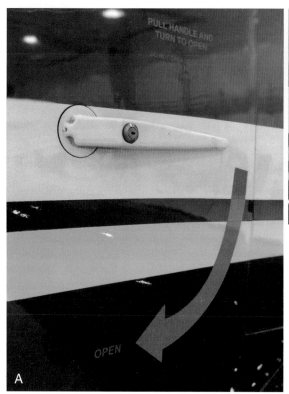
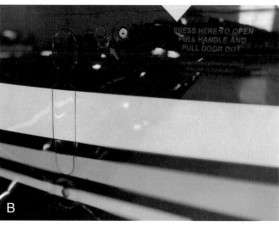

• **Figure 6.10 (A, B)** Aircraft doors and hatches utilize various opening mechanisms and should be labeled accordingly.

4. Don PPE. It is recommended to initially use an SCBA. As the scene and hazards are further assessed, then the PPE can be adjusted as needed.
5. Consider the stability of the aircraft. Take into account the surrounding landscape and the orientation of the aircraft wreckage.
6. Attempt to open doors and hatches to gain access first. Aircraft handles vary from automobiles. They tend to be flush and may pop out or require a panel to be pushed in for access to the handle (Fig. 6.10A and B).
   a. Main entry doors and emergency escape exits vary in design. Some doors require a two-hand approach – one hand presses a release button and the other hand turns the handle. Airstair doors have hinges at the bottom and require two hands to open and support the door for a controlled opening. Pressurized aircraft doors are a plug-type that push outward on the door frame and self-seal when the aircraft is pressurized.
   b. Emergency exits are often located over the wings. They usually have flush handles and are plug-type doors with no hinges (Fig. 6.11).
7. If first aid or rescue is not needed, then relocate to a safe distance and continue to maintain a secure perimeter.
8. If extrication is needed, different tools and techniques may be needed than for automobile extrication. Prior to cutting, inspect the area and know where you are cutting to avoid fuel lines, electrical lines, pressurized aircraft systems, and ballistic parachute systems.
   a. Aircraft windows are highly resilient and should be the last resort for extrication. The windows are designed to resist impact and hold cabin pressure loads.
   b. If the wreckage must be disturbed for extrication, photograph and document the area beforehand. This includes

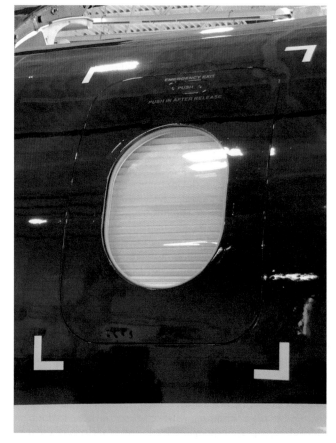

• **Figure 6.11** An example of a plug-type emergency exit that is located over the wing of an aircraft. Note that it has clear emergency markings and labeling.

switch and control positions, instrument and gauge readings, and the aircraft structure.

9. For accidents that require a mass casualty response, establish a second secured perimeter for the triage of victims.

10. Fatalities should be concealed from the media and bystanders for privacy. Prior to removing any fatalities, coordinate this with the NTSB to support the upcoming accident investigation. They also may recommend that a toxicology screen be completed before the coroner begins their embalming process.

11. When emergency vehicles are ready to depart the scene, they should back up from their current position to minimize disturbance to the scene.[8]

Railway Incidents

Railway transportation and incidents pose many challenges and dangers for emergency personnel. The main railway safety rule of thumb is to expect rail movement on any track, at any time, and in any direction. Trains, particularly freight trains, run all day and every day without a set schedule. It is important to note that trains always have the right of way, even over police, emergency vehicles, and pedestrians. This right of way includes the 25 feet area surrounding the area that extends from the center line of the tracks.[9]

In addition to the trains, railway systems include railroad tracks, road crossing equipment, and the surrounding land. All of this is privately owned. The US DOT only assists with the creation and enforcement of rail safety regulations. In the case of a railway incident, the initial and very important step is to contact the owner of the railroad track so their railway traffic can be immediately shut down and their emergency procedures initiated. Some railroad tracks are shared between multiple different organizations, therefore, do not assume that the organization listed on the train cars is the owner of the tracks. Also, if multiple tracks are present, they may have different owners and each owner will have to be notified to stop their rail traffic. For optimal safety, no emergency personnel should get within 25 feet of the railway incident until it is announced that all railway traffic has been definitely stopped. If it is unknown if the railway traffic has been stopped, flaggers can be used. Flaggers should be located two miles from the incident in both track directions. They will stand near the tracks (but not on the tracks) and use a brightly lit item, such as a light or flare, to wave horizontally, which is the universal sign for the train to stop.[9]

Freight trains can be over 1 mile in length with a series of freight cars that are pushed or pulled by one or more locomotives. Locomotives are the power unit of the train and can be located at either end of the train. Additional locomotives may be remotely controlled by the engineer in the lead locomotive. An average locomotive weighs approximately 200 tons (400,000 pounds) and a fully loaded freight train can reach up to 6000 tons. If a sudden stop is required, a freight train traveling at 55 miles per hour would require one mile or more to come to a complete rest.[9]

If an incident occurred near a railway system, contact the railroad track owner to notify them of the nearby emergency personnel presence and to potentially stop railway traffic. Due to this high-risk environment, never go around down crossing arms. Also, anyone near the tracks should understand that trains are generally closer and moving faster than they appear, and they may extend over 3 feet, or more, from the rail.[9]

Freight trains are generally run by a two-person crew. A conductor oversees the train and an engineer controls train movement. Additional crew, such as brakemen, inspectors, officials, or other railway employees from other trains, may also be present and would typically be in an extra locomotive. In case of a railway incident, the conductor should be immediately sought since they possess a consist, which are shipping documents of each train car's contents. This includes whether the contents are hazardous and if there are any special handling instructions. If the crew requires extrication, initially seek them out in the lead locomotive. The train seats do not have seat belts, therefore, look throughout the cab for a victim. Also check for the crew in the cab's bathroom and nose entry. Look along the tracks because the crew members may have jumped from the train prior to the incident. Additional train personnel may be located in the additional locomotives.[9]

Most freight trains are diesel-electric, and most passenger trains are electric power. Diesel-electric systems have large diesel engines that support an AC or DC generator which produces electricity for traction motors. The traction motors are mounted to each wheel set of a locomotive. Electric systems use electric traction motors that are supplied with high-voltage power from overhead catenary systems or electric third rails.[9]

Railway incidents may be challenging due to the potential scene length, various terrains and crossings, and potential hazards. In the case of a railway incident, it is beneficial to be aware of any railway tunnels or bridges that may be involved since these will hinder access to the scene or complicate the rescue. It is also important to be aware of high-risk areas within the incident vicinity, such as schools, hospitals, and waterways. If the train is transporting any hazardous materials, these high-risk areas may be negatively affected and may require risk mitigation at the incident scene or surrounding high-risk sites. Having existing knowledge of your local railway organization's contact information and commonly transported cargo will greatly assist in prompt incident planning. There are blue and white Emergency Notification System (ENS) signs that offer valuable railway emergency contact information present at every highway-rail grade crossing, which is the intersection of any road, street, or highway with railroad tracks (Fig. 6.12). The United States Federal Railroad Administration offers a website and mobile app that provide quick access to railway emergency information and contact numbers. When communicating with the railroad organization's dispatch center, use the track's mile marker, railway signal marker, or the US DOT rail grade crossing number as a reference for the incident's location. See Box 6.4 for railway incident recommendations.[9]

Emergency rescue in a railway incident poses many difficulties. Locomotives have a split-level design with crowded cabs. The lower portion includes a nose entrance, electronics bay, and bathroom. The electronics bay is a high-voltage area that houses the battery bus disconnect knife switch and fuse for the 74-volt DC electrical bus. This should be switched off, although caution must still be taken since some electrical systems could remain live. The upper portion includes the engineer's control stand (with the throttle, reverse, independent and automatic brakes, horn, bell, and sanding controls), the conductor's desk (with an emergency brake and communication equipment), and jump seats. Also within the cab is an electrical panel that houses an emergency fuel cut-off and engine stop button. Only shut down the locomotive if necessary due to the specific incident or for safety reasons since a running locomotive is required to maintain air pressure for its brakes. Also, if a train is shut down on uneven ground, it may begin to roll. To prevent this movement, the wheels can be choked, chained, or blocked. Manual hand brakes are located on the back of every locomotive. These should primarily be managed by any available train crew member but, if necessary, can be accessed by emergency personnel. There is a rotating manual hand

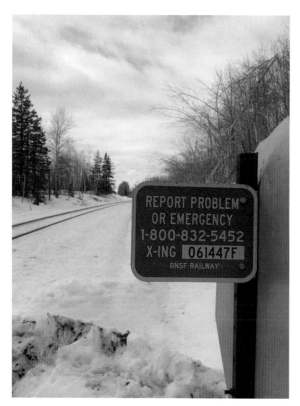

• **Figure 6.12** At every rail grade crossing, there should be a blue and white emergency notification system sign to provide emergency contact information.

•BOX 6.4   Railway Incident Recommendations

- Always contact the organization that owns the railroad tracks' dispatch, to report the incident and ensure that all railroad traffic has been stopped.
- Maintain constant situational awareness.
- Be vigilant about potential hazards.
- Never cross under train cars. Never walk between train cars unless there is a walking platform and all railway traffic has been stopped.
- Never stand between or next to train cars or sections of train cars.
- Never attempt to mount a moving train.
- Never approach a train until knowledge of what it is transporting and if it is hazardous. Ask for the train's consist.[9]

brake that uses a wheel turned clockwise to set the brake or a pump/level manual hand brake that uses a lever pumped up and down to set the brake. Overall, locomotive controls within the cab should be well marked and the primary component locations of a locomotive are generally standardized.[9]

Locomotives have narrow, heavy steal front and rear access doors. Additionally, they have a large windshield and sliding glass windows on each side of the cab that have heavy rubber gaskets and penetration-resistant glass (Fig. 6.13). Emergency entry or egress is best through the sliding windows due to their simple locks and sliding tracks, which allow for quick entry. The location is easily accessible in a tilted or overturned locomotive. They are also large enough for a backboard. The greatest drawback about using the sliding windows is their location. The cab of a locomotive is, on average, 15 feet high and these windows are near the top. Another potential egress is the windshield, which can also

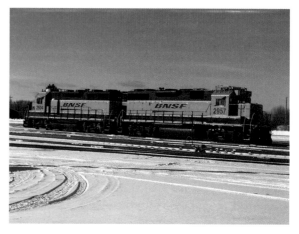

• **Figure 6.13** Locomotives are the power unit of the train. They pose many unique challenges for victim rescue and dangers for rescuers.

provide a quick entry. Glass can be broken using a Halligan tool or axe, or it can be cut through using a reciprocating saw. The doors, whether damaged or not, can be removed at the hinges using hydraulic tools or a reciprocating saw. The drawbacks to going through the doors are that the doors are heavy and narrow, this process is slower than the windows, and rigging may be required to remove the door. The roof can also be an extrication location. The roof is generally stable in an upright locomotive and can allow for a large opening. The drawback to roof extrication is the requirement for medium- to high-powered tools since a Halligan tool and chisel would be ineffective. Also, each locomotive model may have different challenges within this area, such as electrical wiring, internal framing and support structures, insulation, and so forth.[9]

On the outside of the locomotives, there are engine and fuel cut-off switches. In an emergency incident, these cut-off switches should be activated by pressing and holding on every locomotive present. It may take up to 1 minute, or more, for all of the fuel in the lines to burn off before the engine completely shuts down.[9]

Common railway hazards include[9]:

- Fuel: Locomotive fuel tanks can hold up to 6000 gallons of diesel fuel. This fuel is preheated before it is pressure injected into the engine, thereby causing a potential for diesel fumes to be present for combustion.
- Electrical: Locomotives must be treated like electrical substations. They can store up to 3000 volts in capacitors, which can be retained indefinitely, in the electrical room of the cab and in the rear section of the locomotive. Additionally, large lead batteries are present under the locomotive cab which are used for start-up and lights. These batteries can be accessed from external panels. Ensure that these batteries get disconnected since some locomotives are equipped with auto-start, and may automatically restart the engine unexpectedly. Electrical hazards also include electrical cabinets present at railroad crossings that hold electricity and batteries to run the crossing warning systems.
- Compressed air: Compressed air operates the train's brakes and horn. There are hoses with 80 to 110 psi between each train car and hoses with 140 psi between each train locomotive. These hoses should automatically uncouple if the cars accidentally separate. There are also tanks that hold large volumes of compressed air which require caution when operating around.
- Wreckage: Similar to other transportation scenes, the wreckage may be unstable and contain sharp edges that pose hazards.

Loaded train cars can weigh up to 286,000 pounds each, and the train wheels and their assemblies (trucks) can weigh up to 10 tons and are not permanently fixed to their frames. Also, empty train cars may contain hazardous material residue which can still pose as a safety hazard.

- Chemicals: Chemicals present on a train can include 400 to 500 gallons of lubrication oil, 50 gallons of sulfuric acid in batteries, and up to 6000 gallons of diesel fuel. The train cars may be transporting potentially hazardous chemicals, therefore, seek the train's consist for details regarding its cargo.
- Track and rails: Track rails may be slippery from the weather or spilled chemicals. The track ballast, the rocks that provide support underneath the tracks, may shift, be slippery, or contain jagged rocks. Track switches can be manually or remotely changed and may have associated gas or electric heaters. They may be a site for accidental hand or foot crush injuries or for gas or electricity risks.
- Tunnels or bridges: Never enter a tunnel or onto a bridge unless there is a guarantee that the railroad tracks are shut down. There is little clearance around the train and few escape zones at these locations. Also, tunnels may not have adequate ventilation, so consider an SCBA prior to entry.
- Railway yard: At railway yards, multiple tracks may be present along with multiple sections of connected cars. Within this environment, there may be poor visibility, a limited field of view, and distracting noise and activity. There may be humping of cars, which is the act of allowing a train car to roll independently down a hill and then is directed onto a selected track system. Material, such as banding or cabling, can overhang a moving train car, leading to harming nearby personnel. Mechanical failure may lead to the accidental uncoupling of a train car followed but unanticipated car movement.[9]

Industrial Emergency Scenes

Electrical Emergencies

Downed electrical lines or damaged electrical transformers can pose a great danger to rescue teams. At nighttime, streetlights or surrounding homes without power may be an indication of electrical involvement. A perimeter should be made around the electrical line or transformer by setting out traffic cones, lights, or barrier tape to keep rescue personnel and bystanders safe. The electrical utility company should be promptly contacted to discontinue the electricity and to provide assistance. While still energized, power lines can jump several feet, therefore, a safe distance must be maintained. For safety mitigation, never throw anything over the line, never attempt to move the line, and never assume that the power line is dead. Transformers may be suspended with overhead powerlines or located at ground level with underground electrical lines. Damage to these transformers may cause an open source of high voltage, toxic smoke and gas, an explosion with possible flying debris, or release of pressurized gas.[6]

If a victim is present around a downed electrical line, damaged transformer, or any other electrical environment, do not touch the person. A person actively receiving electricity may not be able to let go of the electrical source until it has been turned off and may pass the electrical current to the rescuer if touched. Never approach the victim on a metal platform or through water. A rescuer or victim that is present on a metal platform or object may receive an electrical shock that is equal to or worse than that of standing in water. Once the electricity has been turned off, the victim can be cautiously approached.[10,11]

Agricultural Emergencies

Agricultural environments have significant potential hazards, for agricultural workers and rescuers, that range from confined spaces to heavy machinery. Confined spaces have minimal entries and exist in addition to potentially poor ventilation that can support hazardous air conditions. Manure pits can create dangerous levels of hydrogen sulfide, methane, and carbon dioxide. Silos can create dangerous levels of nitrogen dioxide. In a confined area, these gases can result in a variety of physical complications from pulmonary irritation to asphyxiation. Rescue teams should immediately recognize these potentially life-threatening environments. Air quality should be tested, and a pressure-demand air-supplied respirator should be available. SCBA equipment could be utilized but may also be too bulky for some confined spaces. Additionally, the rescue team should be equipped with a harness and rope for rescuer safety. Radio communication should be maintained from within and outside of the confined space to ensure ongoing safe and efficient operations.[12,13]

Grain bin entrapment and suffocation may occur due to the movement of the loose grain (Fig. 6.14). This risk increases when the grain is being unloaded, especially from the bottom of the bin. This movement causes the victim to get pulled down into the grain. The victim inhales and swallows grain that subsequently inhibits oxygenation or the victim has chest wall restriction that inhibits respiration. Rescue teams must plan for safety in the bin before entering. They may initiate the bin's aeration fans to promote additional oxygen and ventilation. The next steps are to remove the

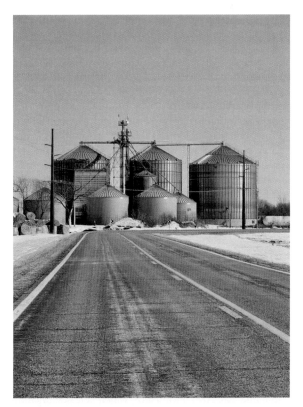

• **Figure 6.14** Agricultural environments are high-risk rescue scenes that pose many physical, electrical, and chemical threats, as seen in this photo.

grain in an orderly and rapid manner while gaining access to the patient. Safety should be continuously assessed for the well-being of the patient and the rescue team.[12]

Heavy machinery, such as tractors and farming implements, is another potential hazard for farmers and the rescue team. Tractor rollovers are the leading cause of farming fatalities. Farming implements, such as drivelines, augers, and power takeoffs (PTOs), tend to have powerful rotating parts that can quickly entangle clothing subsequently causing severe physical harm. Rescue teams require training and basic knowledge of farm equipment to safely extricate the victim and mitigate risks for their own safety.[12]

Additional agricultural hazards include industrial-strength fertilizers, pesticides, and herbicides. Rescuers should use appropriate PPE (e.g., eye protection, face mask, gloves, and protective clothing) to prevent chemical exposure throughout the rescue. The victim should be promptly removed from the hazardous environment. Contaminated clothing should be removed from the victim and appropriate decontamination procedures should be completed.[12]

Specific examples of common hazardous agricultural chemicals include anhydrous ammonia and organophosphates. Anhydrous ammonia is a highly dangerous, caustic nitrogen fertilizer that frequently causes respiratory, ophthalmic, and traumatic injuries. It is stored as a liquid through compression, but once it is released, it returns into a colorless gas, or potentially an opaque white gas cloud, with a pungent odor. If the anhydrous ammonia gas contacts the mucous membranes of an individual, the gas turns into a strong alkaline ammonium hydroxide solution. An individual who has been in contact with the anhydrous ammonia must be evacuated from the scene, have their contaminated clothing removed, and be washed down with cool water including thorough irrigation of their skin and eyes for at least 15 minutes. Respiratory distress symptoms can be treated with supplemental oxygen and bronchodilators as needed. Hospital admission for at least 24 hours of observation is recommended. Similarly, organophosphates are a group of hazardous chemicals that also pose a significant hazard to agricultural workers and rescuers. Organophosphates, and a similar group called carbamates, are acetylcholinesterase inhibitor insecticides. These chemicals are lipid soluble which allows prompt absorption into an individual's integumentary, respiratory, and gastrointestinal systems. Once into an individual's adipose, organophosphates and carbamates can cause a delayed or long-duration toxicity from acetylcholinesterase inactivation. Acetylcholinesterase inactivation causes excess acetylcholine at neuromuscular junctions leading to a collection of symptoms that can be presented with the mnemonic DUMBELS: defecation, urination, muscle weakness, bradycardia, bronchorrhea, bronchospasm, emesis, lacrimation, and salivation.[12] Seizures may also occur in severe cases. Like other exposures, this victim should be relocated to a safe location, have their clothing removed, and receive decontamination through the washing of their skin. Regarding medical treatment, carbamates tend to be shorter acting which allows them to be self-limiting and easily reversible with antidotal treatment. Organophosphates tend to be longer acting which makes them more resistant to antidotal treatment and potentially irreversible. The antidotal treatment for both insecticide classes is intravenous high-dose atropine boluses potentially followed by an atropine infusion. Specific to organophosphates, an additional antidote is pralidoxime (2-PAM, Protopam) which releases organophosphate and acetylcholinesterase binding. The victim of these insecticides require hospitalization for ongoing supportive and antidotal

treatment along with observation for rebound toxicity which may occur after several days post exposure.[12]

Trench Collapse

Regarding construction and industrial work, trenching and excavation are among the most dangerous operations. These workers and the responding emergency service personnel can be buried under tons of earth when unsupported trench walls collapse. Sheeting and shoring a trench are labor-intensive tasks but are absolutely necessary if a rescue operation is to be performed safely. Specifically, sheeting holds back loose debris and shoring prevents the unraveling or collapse of the trench wall. The steps to be followed in the case of a trench collapse are as follows[14]:

- Maintain a safe distance from the scene and determine who is in charge.
- Assess the immediate scene, including the estimated number of injured or presumed deceased, the possible location of the victims, and any possible hazards (water, electricity, sewage, natural gas, carbon monoxide, heavy equipment) within the trench. Determine whether the rescue team will operate in rescue mode or recovery mode; if the patient is obviously deceased, lives of rescuers should not be risked, and all operations should proceed slowly and methodically to prevent unnecessary harm or injury to rescuers.
- Plan for and utilize risk mitigation techniques, such as PPE, air supply systems for ventilation, trench lip protection, and escape ladders.
- Create a shoring plan that includes an assessment and evaluation of the trench and potential victims. Ensure that the trench lip is safe prior to beginning the shoring. Primary shoring provides rapid victim protection from further collapse. Secondary shoring ensures that the rescuers have a safe work area. Lastly, complete shoring expands and enhances all of the current shoring. Shoring typically utilizes struts, panels, wales (beams), and backfill.
- Complete hourly shoring performance assessment, which is a thorough physical inspection of the shoring.
- Once access to the trapped victims has been achieved, the rescuer should uncover each victim's head and chest immediately followed by emergency care measures. Once the victim is completely freed, they should be secured to an extrication device and removed from the trench.[14]

Wilderness Emergency Scenes

Wilderness Emergency Medical Services

Wilderness medicine includes the care of an individual within an environment that has set or dynamic geographic challenges that impair or direct the medical care or transport required (Fig. 6.15). These challenges directly affect the locating and treatment of the victim and the safety of the rescuers. Examples of wilderness medicine environments include geographically remote areas (e.g., deserts, mountains, caves, and oceans) and urban areas during a disaster. Wilderness medicine supports training and planning for theoretical events although the true response is generally spontaneous and improvised. The organized providers and systems that offer wilderness medicine are considered wilderness emergency medical services (WEMS) and include SAR teams, national or state park rangers, ski patrol organizations, and specialized law enforcement, fire department, or military teams. WEMS carry

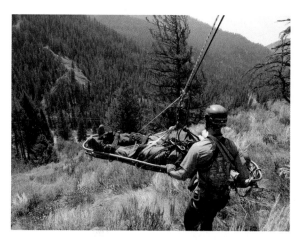

• **Figure 6.15** Air rescue in a mountainous environment. (Cooper DC, Smith W. Search and rescue. In: Auerbach PS, Cushing TA, Harris NS, eds. *Auerbauch's Wilderness Medicine*. 7th ed. Elsevier; 2017. Fig. 55.14 on p. 1234.)

supplies for their own personal survival in the wilderness setting along with enough medical supplies to adequately care for a potentially critically ill individual.[15]

Wilderness rescues include flat-terrain, low-angle, and high-angle rescues. Flat-terrain rescues include level ground that may be covered with large or small rock, loose soil, water, and various other ground textures and features that may create obstructions to safety move over. Low-angle rescue is a technique to be used on ground that is steep, but an individual can still walk it without the use of their hands. This rescue utilizes ropes to counteract gravity to assist walking and the carrying of a litter, thereby mitigating falls. Lastly, high-angle rescue is used for vertical terrain that hands and feet must be used to navigate, such as a slope greater than 60°, and is high risk for life-threatening falls. For this rescue, expert personnel use rope or aerial equipment along with rope and knot techniques for their own movement to the victim and for the hoisting or lowering the litter.[3]

Search and Rescue

SAR operations can be utilized within the natural wilderness to seek those that are lost or injured or within the urban environment to seek those that are missing after a natural disaster. SAR operations are mostly completed by the Civil Air Patrol, state police services, or local rescue agencies. Larger organizations, such as the US Air Force, US Coast Guard, and FAA, assist in coordinating and supporting SAR operations.[16]

There are five stages of SAR. Awareness is the first stage and is the notification of an actual incident. The second stage is the initial action stage. This stage requires the SAR team to assess their current information, attempt to obtain more information, and determine the severity of the emergency. The severity of the emergency is listed as one of three phases. The uncertainty phase concludes that there is doubt that an unsafe situation actually exists; the alert phase concludes that there is a potential and concern of an unsafe situation; and the distress phase concludes that there is most likely an immediate danger that requires immediate intervention. The third stage is the planning stage, which is essential for an accurately and effectively executed operation. Next is the fourth stage, which is the operations stage. This includes the finding, aiding, and rescuing of those in need. Last is the conclusion stage in which the operation was completed or determined to be not required.[16]

To locate the missing individual(s), initial information is gathered. The subsequent search can be indirect, which does not require an actual physical search, or direct, which has searchers physically searching an area. These searchers can incorporate dogs and/or human trackers that seek clues in the physical environment. Search principles include:
1. An urgent response.
2. Confine the suspected search area.
3. Search for clues.
4. Search at night, but only if the risks of the darkness can be mitigated.
5. Search with a plan and in an organized, systematic way.
6. Use a grid (high coverage) searching method as a last resort.[16]

Once the individual is found, the rescuers must gain access to them. This access can be simple, such as hiking down a trail, or complex, such as rappelling down a cliff ledge or during adverse weather. Once access is completed, the individual may require physical, medical, and emotional stabilization. Finally, transporting the patient out is arranged, which is usually done by foot or air.[16]

Whitewater Rescue

Whitewater, referring to moving water in a creek or river, offers an adventurous area to raft, kayak, or canoe. Personal flotation devices (PFDs) and helmets are the recommended safety equipment. Hazards stem from the size of the riverbed, volume of water in the river, gradient of the river, and hydrologic elements (e.g., waves, holes, and waterfalls).[17]

River hazards include eddies, hydraulics, undercuts, and waterfalls. Eddies form when water flows around an obstacle and causes the water to flow upstream leading to a higher level on the upstream side and lower level on the downstream side of the obstacle. The separation between the two currents is called the eddy line. This area gives the rescue boat a location to slow or stop their downstream descent and allows them to have a moment to survey the downstream area.[17]

Hydraulics are the most common hazard and are caused by water flowing over an obstacle. This water movement creates a depression and then vacuum force from the downstream water recirculating. This water tends to be very aerated and appears white and foamy. The force of this water hazard can overturn rafts and kayaks and can even trap them or people within the recirculating flow. During a rescue operation, these hazards must be identified. A preset rope should be placed below the hydraulic area to promote safe rescue from the site. If a person is entrapped within the recirculating water, the best exit is not to attempt immediate resurfacing, which causes re-entry into the circulation, but rather to stay submerged and allow downstream movement away from the recirculating water. Extra caution should be taken around low-head dams because they can form massive hydraulics with incredibly powerful recirculating power and since they stretch the length of the river, there is no escape route.[17]

Another hazard is an undercut. This is when a rock extends upstream above the water and not under the water. This causes the potential for an object or person to get pushed underneath the rock and become entrapped. This scenario can also occur when a swimmer goes to stand up or a person walks through the water and gets their foot wedged underneath an undercut rock or between rocks. If the current is fast, this person may lose their balance and could potentially drown in water that is less than three feet deep. Undercuts can be difficult to recognize and can be very dangerous.[17]

Lastly, waterfalls can pose as a hazard. It is possible for a person to fall in the water above a waterfall and ultimately be pushed over the waterfall, which may be of a great height, and onto rocks below. For safety, it is recommended that one should never cross moving water upstream of a waterfall and never climb up a waterfall.[17]

The safest way to maneuver through whitewater is from a boat rather than swimming, although boats in this moving water also have hazards. A boat can become wrapped around or pinned against an obstacle (broach). Also, a kayak or canoe can go over a drop and then become vertically lodged (vertical pin). In either of these hazardous positions, the water pressure can cause damage to the boat and entrap victims.[17]

If a rescuer falls into the water, the whitewater defensive swim position is to float on your back with toes pointed downstream. This position protects your head and neck, and it promotes keeping your toes out of the water which helps to prevent them from becoming pinned under or in an obstacle. Strainers are objects such as trees, fencing, or debris that are stuck between rocks or stick out from the shore. These objects become points of possible entrapment. If a strainer is observed and unavoidable, it is recommended to go head-first and on your stomach toward these obstacles. Once it is reached, then an attempt to climb up and over it should be made.[17]

Whitewater rescue utilizes throw ropes, carabiners and pulleys, webbing, Prusik loops, knives, and whistles. In most river rescue scenarios, throw bags are utilized. A throw bag contains between 15 and 21 m of braided polypropylene rope that has one end secured in the nylon bag along with a float. The unsecured end of the rope is held, and the bag is then thrown underhand to the victim. Prusik loops are functional loops of line that can help secure items, such as a trapped boat, or guide a rope's position. These items are vital for implementing a rescue strategy.[17]

Rescues can be made by using a wading technique. After scouting the river for potential hazards and mitigating any risks, the rescuer will face upstream and slowly wade into the water with a paddle for additional support and stability while walking. This method can also use a group of rescuers working together in the water to provide additional stability. A tagline rescue uses a rope that is stretched across the river downstream and is then moved upstream toward the victim. A floating tagline can use a PFD or throw bag to create floatation of the line, thereby allowing the victim to easily access the line and receive some floatation support (Fig. 6.16). A snag tag is a weighted line that can be walked upstream to a victim who has an entrapped body part (Fig. 6.17). Two throw bags can be weighed down with rocks and then serve as a method of weighing down the tagline to create the snag tag. These lines can help pull out entrapped body parts or body from entrapment. If a boat is caught on an obstacle, then ropes, pulleys, and Prusik loops can be used to create a vector pull or a Z-drag system. These systems are designed to amplify the amount of power available via pulleys to free the boat.[17]

Cave Rescue

A cave rescue is a complex environment that may present confined space, water, extreme temperature, height, and hazardous surface challenges. Additionally, navigating caves is a three-dimensional endeavor because the passages can go upward, downward, or sideways. This movement may require rappelling, crawling, climbing over a boulder, squeezing through a crack, and swimming through a dark, enclosed environment. Due to the

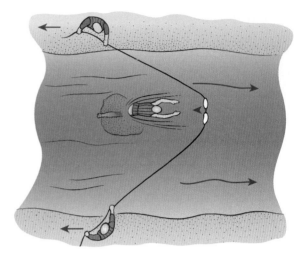

• **Figure 6.16** A floating tagline. (McGinnis HD. Whitewater medicine and rescue. In: Auerbach PS, Cushing TA, Harris NS, eds. *Auerbauch's Wilderness Medicine*. 7th ed. Elsevier; 2017. Fig. 62.19 on p. 1400.)

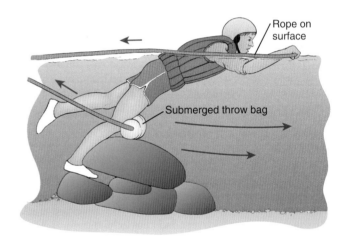

• **Figure 6.17** A submerged snag tag. (McGinnis HD. Whitewater medicine and rescue. In: Auerbach PS, Cushing TA, Harris NS, eds. *Auerbauch's Wilderness Medicine*. 7th ed. Elsevier; 2017. Fig. 62.21 on p. 1401.)

great dangers involved with a cave rescue, only trainer personnel should be involved.[13]

PPE for cave exploration and rescue includes protective suits made from a rubberized, vinyl-coated, or Cordura outer layer, a possible wet suit, mountaineering-style helmet, protective and warm gloves, and protective, lug-soled boots. Cave rescue requires the ability to read a cave map and have experience with cave navigation. The search process should be well planned and organized. During the search, clues will be sought, and a marking system should be used to mark passages that have already been searched. Once the victim is found, a litter may not be required or may not be feasible due to the narrow passages (Fig. 6.18). Other transfer devices such as a drag-sheet type litter (e.g., wraparound Sked Stretcher [SKED]) or a short board (e.g., Kendrick Extrication Device [KED] or Oregon Spine Splint II [OSS II]) may be feasible. Another route of extrication to consider is vertical. High-angle rescue is similar to above-ground techniques but is complicated by tight spaces, darkness, and lack of alternative routes. Ropes used for this rescue require low stretch and abrasion resistance, so static kernmantle ropes are usually used. Due to the cave layout, multiple different rigging locations may have to be set up for a successful vertical extrication.[13]

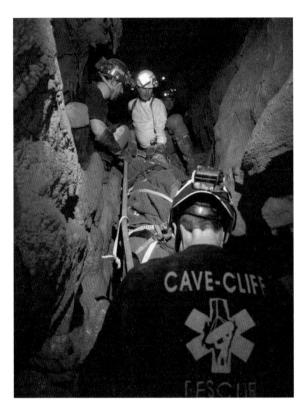

• **Figure 6.18** Victim securely strapped to a litter during a cave rescue. (McCurley L, Mortimer RB. Caving and cave rescue. In: Auerbach PS, Cushing TA, Harris NS, eds. *Auerbauch's Wilderness Medicine*. 7th ed. Elsevier; 2017. Courtesy Kris H. Green.)

Caves innately have hazards due to their extreme environments as previously discussed. These settings also have unique hazards secondary to their construction. Some caves have atmospheric hazards which include a potential for a lack of oxygen or build-up of toxic gases (e.g., carbon monoxide, carbon dioxide, methane, and hydrogen sulfide). These atmospheric hazards can be mitigated with the use of air monitors and SCBAs. Some caves are susceptible to flooding with or without any warning due to heavy rains and their natural design is to be water reservoirs or drainage systems. If a cave floods, the rescue may be delayed until the water naturally recedes. If a delay is not appropriate, the water can possibly be diverted through physical channels or damning. Pumping may be completed but the subsequent exhaust fumes of a fuel-driven engine, potential for electrocution of an electricity-driven engine, and risk of mechanical failure must be factored into the decision-making. The last resort, based on risks, is to have rescuers enter the flooded cave with scuba diving equipment. These rescuers should be cave-certified divers and have specialty equipment.[13]

Natural and Human-Made Disasters

Natural disasters are created "by biologic, geologic, seismic, hydrologic, or meteorologic processes"[18] which cause destructive phenomena, such as earthquakes, volcanic eruptions, severe storms, tornadoes, and floods. In contrast, human-made disasters are created through human attitudes, technology, and human–environment interactions. Examples of human-made disasters include transportation accidents, oil spills, and building collapses. Either type of disaster can cause complex emergency scenes that cover a large geographic area and pose a multitude of safety concerns. Safety hazards could

be unstable or collapsed structures, the presence of hazardous materials, adverse weather conditions, and dangerous environments. Rescuers must be trained to identify potential hazards within each disaster scenario, approach the scene in a safe manner, and utilize appropriate PPE to mitigate safety risks.[11,18]

Thunderstorms

During a thunderstorm, there is no safe place outside. Lightning should be considered a potential hazard and a safe shelter should be utilized. While outside, lightning can reach a rescuer or bystander through a direct strike, contact with a struck object, "splash" effect (or side flash) when the electrical current jumps from one object to another (object or person), or transfer from the ground. Safe shelters are primarily houses and substantially constructed buildings. If these are not available, then a fully enclosed, metal-roofed vehicle (e.g., car, bus, and ambulance) can be used as a safe shelter. Open-sided or small structures (e.g., golf, beach, or bus shelters) or tents do not offer lightning protection and may increase the risk of injury secondary to lightning.[19]

Law Enforcement–Related Situations

Law enforcement officials expect the cooperation of other emergency personnel regarding a police emergency. A cooperative relationship must exist to successfully mitigate a high-risk situation. Defer to law enforcement for scene safety and for control of a scene.

Active Shooter

Active shooter (AS) situations usually involve one or more suspects participating in a random or systematic shooting spree with the intent to harm or commit mass murder. These scenarios can easily fall into the category of an MCI. Law enforcement and EMS must focus on preparation to respond to these events with the intention of saving as many lives as possible.[20,21]

A group, convened by the American College of Surgeons and the Federal Bureau of Investigation in Hartford, Connecticut, developed a concept aimed at increasing survivability in an AS incident. Clinical evidence shows that the greatest cause of death in penetrating trauma is hemorrhage, therefore, the Hartford Consensus identifies hemorrhage control as the most important requirement in response to an AS/MCI. The consensus also outlines levels of threat in relation to the traditional hot/red, warm/yellow, and cold/green zones of safety, in which hot indicates an immediate or direct threat, warm indicates an indirect threat, and cold indicates no known threat. These zones and their associated level of threat guide the actions that should be taken. The Hartford Consensus uses the acronym THREAT to outline the critical actions required during an AS/MCI:

T – Threat suppression
H – Hemorrhage control
R/E – Rapid extrication to safety
A – Assessment by medical providers
T – Transport to definitive care

In the hot zone, the threat should try to be suppressed. Next, in the warm zone, hemorrhage control and extrication of victims should be attempted. Lastly, in the cold zone, victim assessment and transport should be completed.[3,21]

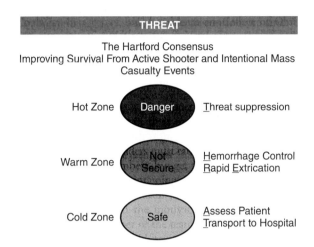

• **Figure 6.19** Response to active shooter/intentional mass casualty incidents. (Diagram of safety zones with level of danger and interventions recommended. From Schneidman D, Jacobs LM, Burns KJ. Strategies to enhance survival in active shooter and intentional mass casualty events: A compendium. *Bull Am Coll Surg.* 2015;100(1S):16–17.)

Other on-scene precautions in these situations include the following[21]:

- Cautious approach to the scene, lights/sirens off early, distance approach.
- Look out for secondary devices.
- Be prepared to withdraw to a safe area.
- Work in pairs.
- Responders must be easily identifiable.
- Advise hospitals early.
  See Fig. 6.19.

Evidence Preservation

Many investigations have been seriously hindered because emergency service personnel inadvertently disturbed or destroyed articles of evidence at a crime scene. Investigators look at everything; something that seems of little importance may be a valuable piece of evidence to law enforcement personnel. Anticipating if the scene is an actual or potential crime scene will direct the transport team's overall actions in order to preserve potential evidence. These actual or potential crime scenes may include violent acts, presence of drugs or drug manufacturing, obvious or reported suicides, obvious or reported accidents, and fires.[22]

Once scene safety is ensured, the transport team's priority is to provide medical care and secondly to protect the crime scene by creating minimal disruption to the surrounding environment. Unauthorized persons must be kept away from the scene. For authorized personnel, one entrance and exit should be utilized. Situational awareness must be maintained throughout the entire scene time. Blood or fluids on the ground and footsteps or other markings on the ground should be avoided to prevent contamination. The surrounding environment should not be touched unless it is vital for patient care. The transport team should also use gloves, not just for patient care, but to avoid leaving their fingerprints at the crime scene. If an item or the victim is moved, thorough and complete documentation of this must be made. If an item is removed from the scene, such as medication bottles, they should be placed in a brown paper bag and these actions should be documented. There is no reason the transport team should remove weapons or

shell casings from the scene. In cases of obvious victim death, minimal touching or moving of the body should be done.[3,22,23]

Special care is also required regarding the victim, which includes victims of physical and sexual assault. When the victim's clothing needs to be removed, never cut through knife or bullet holes, or through bloody or contaminated areas. Cut through intact, clean sections of clothing, then place the clothing into a paper bag. If the victim can independently remove their own clothing and it is medically necessary to remove the clothing prior to hospital arrival, they should remove it while standing on a sheet. This sheet may collect particulate evidence that falls off the clothing and should be included with the clothing as evidence. If the clothing is saturated with a fluid, place the clothing into a paper bag followed by a plastic bag. The victim's hands should be covered and sealed with paper bags to protect any evidence that may be present on their hands or underneath their nails. Additionally, avoid removing potential evidence from the victim's clothing or skin with medical solutions, such as skin antiseptics, unless required for medical care. All the packaged items should be labeled, sealed, and handed over to law enforcement.[3,22,23]

At vehicle crash scenes, items of significance to accident investigators are tire marks, runoff from radiators and crankcases, blood, broken glass, vehicle trim, motor parts, and even clods of dirt turned up by a vehicle's wheels. To assist police investigators, the transport team should keep their transport vehicles a safe distance away from the immediate scene as possible to not disrupt potential evidence, unless medical attention is emergent and the distance is not appropriate. Additionally, the transport team should rope off the crash site so physical evidence can be preserved in place and bystanders can be kept away. Photographs of the bottom of the victim's shoes can help in determining if breaking had been applied. Also, documenting if a seatbelt was used by the victim and was cut or unlatched by the victim or rescuers may help determine who was driving and offer additional valuable information for the investigation.[22]

Documentation should be thorough, fact based, and free from opinion. It should include quotes from the victim and details about the scene regarding the victim's presentation. The documentation should include specific details regarding the patient's physical condition, including specific injuries, and every intervention completed by the transport team. This documentation may be used in court, so be cognizant about the wording, such as avoiding the labeling of an "entrance" or "exit" wound; rather, simply label it as a wound with a thorough description.[3,22]

Weapons

A weapon, such as a knife or firearm, found at the scene must be left in the exact position in which it was discovered. Rescuers should assume the firearm is loaded and in operating order – even if it appears otherwise. Law enforcement should be called to manage the weapon. If the weapon must be moved for any reason before law enforcement arrives, that task should be delegated to a trustworthy person. Only one person should handle the weapon with gloves on until it can be turned over to the police officers. If a camera is available, a photograph can be taken of the weapon in place along with reference points, such as doors, windows, and furniture, to help investigators accurately identify the weapon's original placement. When moving a firearm, keep your fingers off the trigger and hammer, and point the barrel away from others. Never attempt to unload or manipulate the firearm. The number of live and expended rounds in a revolver, their position in the cylinder, and the status of the round under the hammer may be important to investigators.[3,22]

Explosive Materials Emergencies

There are four types of injuries seen with explosions: fragmentation, overpressure, impact, and head. Fragmentation injuries occur from fragments exploding and traveling at a high rate of speed that penetrate the body and do immeasurable damage. Overpressure injuries happen when a shock wave travels through the air and damages gas-containing organs in the body. Lungs are the most susceptible and can show a delayed effect as the damage starts to build. These patients will need to be monitored for the potential of an injury to progress. Impact injuries are a result of the body being thrown by the force of the explosion and striking an object on landing or injuries by objects landing on the patient. Head injuries may consist of open wounds or a closed head injury. Violent movement from falls and pressures can cause significant damage to the brain and other structures. Spinal injuries can be associated with trauma to the head and should be suspected.[24]

Intentional explosions are meant to cause massive damage and loss of life. Rescuers must watch out for any secondary devices that are present and intended for emergency responders. These devices may take the form of pipe bombs, backpacks, small packages, or a large vehicle or van. Larger communities have bomb disposal units that can clear an area. Structures around the blast must be watched for potential collapse issues. Full PPE is necessary because of the potential for widespread and large quantities of blood-borne pathogens. Explosions may also be intentionally contaminated with biological or radioactive materials.[24]

Summary

Although the transport team may not be directly involved in extrication or rescue activities, crew members should be prepared to help the rescue effort and not endanger themselves. The transport team should be aware of the unique safety challenges prior to, upon arrival, and at the scene, remaining vigilant during the entire response. Scene management of various incidents should be a training component for all transport teams. Transport teams can offer additional medical care and rapid transport to those injured in all types of incidents. Only transport teams that have had appropriate training, carry the correct equipment, and have experience performing rescues should be the rescuers. Without the proper equipment and training, the rescue crew may find themselves in need of rescue.

References

1. Federal Emergency Management Association publication. United States Fire Administration–Traffic Incident Management Systems. Publication FA-330, March 2012.
2. Sanders MJ. *Mosby's Paramedic Textbook*. 4th ed. Mosby; 2014.
3. Sanders MJ, McKenna K, American Academy of Orthopaedic Surgeons. *Sanders' Paramedic Textbook*. 5th ed. Jones & Bartlett Learning; 2018.
4. Occupational Safety and Health Administration. Hazardous Materials, 29 CFR 1910.120 (2022). Accessed August 1, 2022. http://www.ecfr.gov/cgi-bin/text-idx?SID=a0438214500657c98329 601f8fb58a02&mc=true&node=se29.5.1910_1120&rgn=div8
5. Welles WL, Wilburn RE, Ehrlich JK, et al. New York hazardous substance emergency events surveillance: Learning from hazardous substances releases to improve safety. *J Hazard Mater*. 2004;115:39–49.
6. National Highway Traffic Safety Administration. Newly Released Estimates Show Traffic Fatalities Reached a 16-Year High in 2021, 2022. Accessed July 19, 2022. https://www.nhtsa.gov/press-releases/early-estimate-2021-traffic-fatalities#:,:text=Preliminary%20 data%20reported%20by%20the,from%201.34%20fatalities%20 in%202020
7. Sweet D. *Vehicle Rescue and Extrication: Principles and Practice*. Revised 2nd ed. Jones & Bartlett Learning; 2022.
8. Federal Aviation Administration (U.S. Department of Transportation). First Responder Safety at a Small Aircraft or Helicopter Accident. Updated June 23, 2022. Accessed July 27, 2022. https://www.faa.gov/aircraft/gen_av/first_responders
9. Federal Railroad Administration (U.S. Department of Transportation). Law Enforcement/First Responders Resources. Updated April 15, 2022. Accessed July 28, 2022. https://railroads.dot.gov/highway-rail-crossing-and-trespasser-programs/first-responder
10. Berkeley Lab. Electrical Injury Emergency Response. Electrical Safety. Accessed August 2, 2022. https://electricalsafety.lbl.gov/electrical-safety/emergency-response/
11. Biddinger PD, Kemen KM. Natural disaster management. In: Auerbach PS, Cushing TA, Harris NS, eds. *Auerbauch's Wilderness Medicine*. 7th ed. Elsevier; 2017.
12. Brandenburg MA, Lafave M, Butterwick DJ. Ranch and rodeo medicine. In: Auerbach PS, ed. *Auerbauch's Wilderness Medicine*. 7th ed. Elsevier; 2017.
13. McCurley L, Mortimer RB. Caving and cave rescue. In: Auerbach PS, Cushing TA, Harris NS, eds. *Auerbauch's Wilderness Medicine*. 7th ed. Elsevier; 2017.
14. Zawlocki R, Dashner, C. *Trench Rescue: Principles and Practice to NFPA 1006 and 1670*. 4th ed. Jones & Bartlett Learning; 2022.
15. Hawkins SC, Millin MG, Smith W. Wilderness emergency medical services and response systems. In: Auerbach PS, Cushing TA, Harris NS, eds. *Auerbauch's Wilderness Medicine*. 7th ed. Elsevier; 2017.
16. Cooper DC, Smith W. Search and rescue. In: Auerbach PS, Cushing TA, Harris NS, eds. *Auerbauch's Wilderness Medicine*. 7th ed. Elsevier; 2017.
17. McGinnis HD. Whitewater medicine and rescue. In: Auerbach PS, Cushing TA, Harris NS, eds. *Auerbauch's Wilderness Medicine*. 7th ed. Elsevier; 2017.
18. Reed SB. Natural and human-made hazards: Disaster risk management issues. In: Auerbach PS, Cushing TA, Harris NS, eds. *Auerbauch's Wilderness Medicine*. 7th ed. Elsevier; 2017.
19. Cooper MA, Andrews CJ, Holle RL, Blumenthal R, Aldana NN. Lightning-related injuries and safety. In: Auerbach PS, Cushing TA, Harris NS, eds. *Auerbauch's Wilderness Medicine*. 7th ed. Elsevier; 2017.
20. Schneidman D, Jacobs LM, Burns KJ. Strategies to enhance survival in active shooter and intentional mass casualty events: A compendium. *Bull Am Coll Surg*. 2015;100(1S):16–17.
21. US Department of Homeland Security: FEMA. 2013. Fire/Emergency Medical Services Department Operational Considerations and Guide for Active Shooter and Mass Casualty Incidents. September 2013.
22. Price TG, O'Neill RM. EMS Crime Scene Responsibility. Updated September 26, 2022. In: *StatPearls* [Internet]. Treasure Island, FL: StatPearls Publishing; 2023. Available from: https://www.ncbi.nlm.nih.gov/books/NBK499999/
23. Sharma BR. Clinical forensic medicine-management of crime victims from trauma to trial. *J Clin Forensic Med*. 2003;10:267–273.
24. Polk JD. Response to blast injuries. *JEMS*. June 2012. Accessed March 12, 2017. https://www.jems.com/patient-care/trauma/response-blast-injuries/

7

Communications

JASON BOUTWELL, BRIAN FOSTER, AND ROBERT ANDREW HAMILTON III

COMPETENCIES

1. Demonstrate knowledge about communications systems and their use in patient transport.
2. Apply appropriate communication skills before, during, and after transport.
3. Demonstrate the use of appropriate communication equipment to provide safe and competent patient transport.

Communication is one of the most important skills and functions of everyday life. In the air medical industry, it encompasses more than the use of a radio or telephone; it is a total system, often an integrated system, that ensures the smooth operation of patient transports while supporting optimal patient care and transport team safety (Fig. 7.1). There is no one perfect communications system for all transport programs. Today's technology advances are happening so fast that staying informed on the latest advances including the advantages and disadvantages of various systems essential in today's Communications Center ecosystem.

All transport team members must have good communication skills and know-how to operate any equipment they may use for communication.[1] Communication equipment is influenced by the geographic location of the transport program, the primary response area, and the education and training of those who use the equipment.

All communication needs to be compliant with the Health Insurance Portability and Accountability Act of 1996 (HIPAA). Team members must remember that, like other forms of public communication, radio and verbal communications can be easily overheard and cause a breach of patient confidentiality.[1,2]

Because working in communications is a multifaceted role and applies to physical equipment as well as an intangible human action, this chapter will focus on the two aspects of communications: physical hardware and the human component of communicating.

Communication Centers

An integral part of the transport program, the communication center is often the first interaction a program will have with its customer: an intersecting hub for all electronic traffic communication and system-wide coordination efforts allowing the communication specialists (CSs) to bring together and provide a safe,

seamless, and effective transport for the crews and patients. There are many models of communication centers currently in existence. Some are single-service models such as police or fire only. Other models incorporate multiple programs such as fire dispatch and emergency medical services (EMS) into one integrated center. Flight dispatch centers often stand alone as an independent entity because of the intricacy and degree of commitment it takes to successfully coordinate just one air medical transport. The Commission on Accreditation of Medical Transport Systems (CAMTS) standards dictate that a CS must be assigned to receive and coordinate all requests for the medical transport service.[3] Federal Aviation Regulation 135.79 requires that the Part 135 certificate holder have procedures established for locating each flight for which a Federal Aviation Administration (FAA) flight plan is not filed.[4] CAMTS[3] lists the components that a communication center must contain (Box 7.1).

Communications Specialist

The complexities of organizing a communications system are unique with respect to its operation. Beyond dealing with electronic hardware and computer software, the program is faced with one of the most challenging of tasks – dealing with people.

Humans are both the strongest and the weakest points in a system. People represent a broad spectrum of personalities and opinions, especially while under the stress of a lifesaving situation; no two individuals are the same. A communications center, a CS, and good communication skills are mandatory to ensure a safe transport operation.

Roles and Responsibilities

The *CS* position is designated to coordinate requests for aircraft and ground responses. The title assigned to the person with the CS function varies from program to program. The only limitation

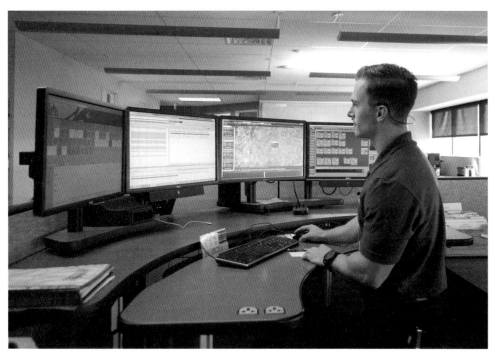

• **Figure 7.1** Communications Center. (Courtesy Clayton Smith.)

• BOX 7.1 Components of a Communication Center

At least one dedicated phone line.

A system for recording all incoming and outgoing telephone and radio transmissions, which should be stored for 90 days, with time recording and playback capabilities.

Capability to notify the transport team and online medical direction for a request and during transport.

Back-up emergency power when power outages occur.

A status board to follow transport vehicles and show who is on the transport teams, weather status, and so on.

Local aircraft service area maps and navigation charts.

Road maps available for ground transport.

Communication policy and procedures manual.

From Commission on Accreditation of Medical Transport Systems. *Accreditation Standards.* 10th ed. The Commission on Accreditation of Medical Transport Systems; 2015.

---

is that the FAA uses the term *dispatcher* to describe the person who decides whether an aircraft may legally accept a flight and take off. Unless this is the case in a program, another title should be used.

The CS is responsible for coordinating both the program and interagency communications pertaining to any phase of a transport, from a request to hospital admission. The role of the CS is to serve as a facilitator for the smooth integration of all the resources at the program's disposal, with the dual objectives of program safety and excellent patient care.

The CS must perform a variety of tasks including the following[5]:
• Listening intently
• Asking appropriate questions
• Accurately confirming what was said
• Anticipating the needs of the crew or patient (to be communicated to the crew)
• Reading maps (including using computer mapping software)
• Using spelling and professional grammar skills
• Using common and familiar medical, aviation, and EMS terms
• Setting, evaluating, and resetting priorities
• Providing customer service and good public relations

Candidate Selection

Applicants for CS positions should be screened as thoroughly as applicants for any of the other components of the transport team positions. Just as all persons who desire to be part of a transport team are not suited for the work, all persons who desire to be a CS may not be suited to the type of stress inherent in the job, even those employees that have been in similar fields.[6,7]

The decision about whom to hire as a CS must be determined by each individual program and the environment in which the CS role must function. Certain minimal educational requirements should be met in all cases, but some of the experience and background requirements should be driven by the expected functions of the CS. Many CSs specialize in "transfer-like" services for their hospital or program. Others may take emergent, nonemergent, and even scheduled transportation calls. When considering the development of a CS role and job description, consider the following:
1. Should the CS have medical field experience? If so, at what level and how much?
2. Should the CS have communications center experience? If so, what type of experience is acceptable, and how much experience is necessary?

Neither medical field experience nor communications center experience alone qualifies a person to be a CS.

CAMTS recommends that certifications, such as emergency medical technician, emergency medical dispatcher, and International Association of Medical Transport Communication Specialists (IAMTCS) Certified Flight Communications Course, be utilized as qualification requirements by transport programs.[3]

Training

Regardless of the background of the CS applicant, the person must be trained for the role that the communications specialist plays within the individual organization. The CAMTS standards that address communications state that the training of the designated communications specialist should be commensurate with the scope and responsibility of the Communications Center personnel. Box 7.2 contains a summary of the initial training. The IAMTCS has developed a specific course to train and educate the CS, and the components of this course are summarized in Box 7.3.

• BOX 7.2 **Summary of the Commission on Accreditation of Medical Transport Systems Initial Training of Communication Specialists**

1. Medical terminology and how to obtain patient information
2. Knowledge of emergency medical system, including roles and responsibilities of various levels of training
3. State and local regulations that govern the EMS systems in which the transport service operates
4. Familiarization with equipment used in the prehospital environment
5. Knowledge of Federal Aviation regulations and Federal Communications Commission regulations pertinent to medical transport services
6. General safety rules and emergency procedures pertinent to medical transportation and flight following procedures
7. Navigation techniques/terminology and flight following and map skills
8. Weather interpretation
9. Radio frequencies used in medical and ground EMS
10. Assistance with hazardous material response
11. Stress recognition and management
12. Customer services
13. Quality management
14. Air medical crew resource management
15. Computer literacy and software training
16. Post Accident Incident Plan
17. Sleep deprivation, sleep inertia, circadian rhythms, recognizing signs of fatigue
18. Landing zone safety, requirements, procedures, and coordination
19. Knowledge of local geography, facilities, and transport resources, as well as helicopter shopping and duplicate aircraft requests
20. Coordinator for long-range flights training

EMS, Emergency Medical Services.

• BOX 7.3 **Summary of the International Association of Medical Transport Certified Flight Communicator Training Course**

Post Accident Incident Plan
Flight following
Radio communications skills
Aviation weather
Aircraft emergencies
Medical terminology
Navigation and map usage
Customer service/public relations
Air medical crew resource management
Stress management
Federal Aviation Administration
Safety

Training must be an ongoing process to ensure currency and proficiency. During training, the CS should be given a variety of situations, be allowed to make decisions, and discuss why decisions were made. Just as many transport teams use their "most challenging transports" to teach others, the "most challenging communication situations" presented and discussed with new CSs may assist them in future work.

The CS should undergo periodic testing on all elements of the position. This person must be deeply familiar with the program, its capabilities, and its history and be able to use that information at a moment's notice with a high degree of accuracy. The communications center is often the first impression of the care a patient will receive from the rest of the team, so accuracy, confidence, and politeness are imperative in the delivery of the CS role to ensure that this first impression establishes a strong foundation that can be continued with the arrival of the transport team. The competencies within a communications center's scope and function are similar to that of their peers in aviation, maintenance, and clinical settings; they must be tested and improved upon on a continuous basis to maintain competence and expertise.

Communications Operations

Operations Control Centers

The FAA has mandated that any Helicopter Air Ambulance (HAA) certificate holder that operates 10 or more helicopters must have an Operations Control Center (OCC).[8] The OCC and communication center are often colocated due to the common use of radio, Internet, and other technological components.

Operational control (OC) requires the certificate holder to be responsible for all aspects of flight operations. The FAA recognized the challenge of ensuring the integrity of OC when different companies collaborate to provide joint services. As defined in Federal Aviation Regulation 1.1, OC is the authority to initiate, conduct, and terminate a flight. This authority lies ONLY with those individuals identified by the operator as having OC. The responsibility and authority of OC should never be in question, and the FAA provides guidance with Order 8900.1.[9]

Flight operations consist of crew member training; currency and certification; aircraft maintenance and airworthiness; "weather minimums, proper aircraft loading, center of gravity limitations, icing conditions, and fuel requirements"; and flight-locating requirements.

The roles and responsibilities of the OCC must not get confused with those of the CS or communication center. It is best practice to treat them as two separate entities, and communications with one department do not mean that the other will automatically relay that information, particularly concerning weather issues.

Selection and Training

Preferably, although not required, HAA Operations Control Specialists (OCSs) should be trained helicopter pilots and ideally highly experienced HAA pilots.

Each OCS must complete an 80-hour FAA-approved program to perform official duties. This is also an annual requirement for each OCS to maintain certification and may be reduced to 40 hours.

The program must include the following:
1. Aviation Weather
2. Navigation
3. Flight Monitoring

4. Air Traffic Control
5. Aviation Communication
6. Aircraft Systems
7. Aircraft Limitations and Performance
8. Aviation Policy and Regulation
9. Crew Resource Management
10. Local Flying Area Orientation

Roles and Responsibilities

While each certificate holder must describe the roles, responsibilities, and level of OC authority delegated to each OCS in their applicable operations manuals, at a minimum, the duties of an OCS include the following:

- Communications
  - Directly with the helicopter or relayed through the communications center.
- Weather Reporting
  - Using National Weather Service or FAA-approved weather sources.
- Monitoring Flight Progress
  - Ensuring deteriorating or unforecast weather is reported to the pilot as soon as possible.
- Risk Analysis
  - Confirm/Verify all entries on risk assessment, filled out by pilot, before each HAA flight.
  - Assess weather conditions (departure, en route, and destination).
  - Acknowledge, Mitigate, or Decline the flight, in the OCS's professional opinion.
  - A written Acknowledgment from the OCC *must* be received by the pilot before the HAA flight may lift or FAA penalties may be imposed.

One principle frequently utilized by OCCs use is the "Advise, Recommend, Direct" concept:
- *Advise* pilots of any potential hazards along routes.
- *Recommend* possible mitigation strategies.
- *Direct* pilots to decline, divert, or terminate the flight.

The OCC is a vital aspect of the HAA process. This is especially true for single-pilot operations; the OCS is there to act as a "virtual copilot," putting an extra set of eyes on crucial flight data before and during a flight. They are an indispensable safety net giving every flight crew an added layer of protection.[8,10]

Alternative Sites/Backup Equipment

A well-designed CS center will have duplicity to its design. Sources of critical infrastructure must be well thought out as the program designs this space. Every building has a source of power that runs to the building. It has Internet services and traditional phone lines as well. Many of these are buried underground, coming into the building in a common room. Consideration of what happens when these lines are accidentally severed by a company digging a ditch to construct a building next door must be taken into account. While it isn't feasible to plan for and mitigate every possible situation, mitigation plans, such as alternative power supplies to the Communication Center, such as thoughts provided by an instant cutover generator that can power the center for considerable amounts of time, are of high importance. Designs that include Internet and phone lines coming into the building from more than one direction and provided by more than one service provider are another example of disaster mitigation. Each communication center must be able to continue operations at an alternative site with backup equipment, should the primary communication center become inoperable. An alternative site and backup equipment should be identified and prepared by every transport program. A plan of action to deal with such a scenario, should it ever occur, should be clearly documented and, at a minimum, be annually reviewed. Additionally, the plan and the CS staff should be tested routinely on utilizing the identified equipment to ensure the equipment and skill proficiencies meet the operational needs.

Plans should also be in place for rapidly repairing or replacing any piece of essential equipment in the communications center.

Telephones

Today, most communications center telephone systems are Internet Provider (IP) based. This technology allows immediate rerouting should the center have a failure or in some cases need to load balance with multiple other centers. Each communications center must have at least one dedicated number for the medical transport service. Like the design needs of power infrastructure, the center should also have multidirectional and independent service provider redundancy for Internet services.

All calls in which a request for services is made should be recorded, as well as any outgoing call that pertains to requests for assistance or notifications.

Both wired and wireless communication systems are routinely used. Cellular phones are used by many transport services. However, their use should be guided by Federal Communications Commission (FCC) regulations on air medical transport vehicles. The FCC prohibits the use of cell phones in flight per FCC Code of Federal Regulations, Part 22, subpart H, Section 22.925. Cell phone use during ground transport should never interfere with patient care or safe driving.

Satellite

Satellite phones may be available as independent handheld devices or as part of the aircraft. The satellite tracking systems come with satellite phone communication. Both CS and transport team members need to be educated on how to use them and should be trained on use before their potential need in an emergency.

Radios

The radio systems continue to be the key hardware element in medical transport communication systems. The crucial role of communication was especially recognized during responses to the September 11, 2001, attacks throughout the United States and during disasters such as Hurricane Katrina. These events, like so many others, have shown the overwhelming need for redundancy, interoperability, and multifrequency capabilities of a system. The radio frequencies on which a program operates are assigned by the FCC, based on recommendations by the state chapter of Associated Public Safety Communications Officers, to which it has delegated responsibility for frequency coordination. The FCC issues licenses and assigns call letters for radio communications systems. A program's assigned frequencies may be found in several radio bands (Box 7.4).

Included in the ultrahigh-frequency (UHF) spectrum are the so-called *MED channels,* which are a set of 10 paired frequencies set aside by the FCC for the exclusive use of EMS units. The channels from MED 9 to MED 10 are frequency allocation channels used in metropolitan regions where UHF traffic is high. To use

• BOX 7.4   Radio Bands

VHF high-band FM (148–174 MHz): The radio signal in this band follows a straight line.
VHF low-band FM (30–50 MHz): The radio signal in this band follows the curvature of the Earth and has the greatest range.
VHF AM (118–136 MHz): This band is typically used for aviation-related communications.
UHF (403–941 MHz): These ultrahigh frequencies have limited range and are most often used between ground units and base stations. They can be used for air-to-ground and ground-to-air communications for relatively short distances that fluctuate with the terrain.
800 MHz: Digital communication controlled by computers. They allow multiple agencies to communicate with each other and have higher frequency, less noise, and greater penetration outside of buildings.

AM, Amplitude modulation; *FM,* frequency modulation; *MHz,* megahertz; *UHF,* ultrahigh frequency; *VHF,* very high frequency.

• BOX 7.5   MED Channel Frequencies

463.000/468.000 MHz (MED-ONE)
463.025/468.025 MHz (MED-TWO)
463.050/468.050 MHz (MED-THREE)
463.075/486.075 MHz (MED-FOUR)
463.100/468.100 MHz (MED-SIX)
463.150/468.150 MHz (MED-SEVEN)
463.175/468.175 MHz (MED-EIGHT)
462.950/467.950 MHz (MED-NINE)
462.975/467.975 MHz (MED-TEN)

• BOX 7.6   New Mutual Aid Frequencies: Names and Renaming

Federal Standard
Mutual Aid 1: 866.0125
Mutual Aid 2: 866.5125
Mutual Aid 3: 867.0125
Mutual Aid 4: 867.5125
Mutual Aid 5: 868.0125

State of Ohio
Air Med 1: 867.0125
Air Med 2: 868.0125

Hamilton County, Ohio
I Call: 867.0125
I TAC 1: 866.5125
I TAC 2: 867.0125
I TAC 3: 867.5125
I TAC 4: 868.0125

such a channel, an EMS unit calls the frequency allocation center, usually located in an emergency services communications center, and requests assignment to a channel for the purpose of speaking with a specific hospital. The unit is then assigned an open channel or is told to stand by until one is available (Box 7.5).

The 800-MHz range has been assigned by the FCC because of overcrowding of other bands. These frequencies have a limited range because the signals are more line directed than the UHF and very high frequency (VHF) spectrums.

Some programs have their own private VHF channels. Others may choose to use one of the existing UHFs allocated for EMS use nationwide. Regardless, the same rules and principles apply when using any frequency spectrum.

Since September 11, 2001, and natural disasters such as Hurricane Katrina, a concerted effort has been made to make emergency and disaster management agencies interoperable. The advent of five mutual aid channels in the 800-MHz spectrum allows agencies from anywhere in the country to communicate to incident command or units on the scene when responding outside of their normal response area. One drawback has been that some agencies have given these frequencies different names, creating a myriad of names for the same channel (Box 7.6).

There are several basic types of radio systems[1,4,11,12]:
1. *Simplex system:* This system transmits in one direction at a time with a single frequency.
2. *Full duplex system:* This system transmits and receives simultaneously with two frequencies (typically UHF).
3. *Half-duplex system:* This system transmits or receives in one direction at a time with two frequencies (typically UHF high band).

4. *Multiplex system:* This system transmits from two or more sources over the same frequency.

A repeater system is a type of half-duplex system that involves a base station repeater at an elevated site remote from the communications center. This system is particularly useful in regions with mountainous terrain. A repeater system receives a signal on one frequency and instantly retransmits it on a second frequency to the other radios in the system, extending the communications center's range. The process is reversed when the repeater receives signals coming into the base station.

Radio Use

All members of the transport team must know how radios work. Each team member must know how to properly use radios under normal circumstances; how to troubleshoot a radio under abnormal circumstances; and how improper use of a radio could make a straightforward call complex, stressful, and potentially unsafe.[1]

Patch Use

With a phone–radio or radio–phone patch, special circuits in the radio console permit a radio and telephone to be linked together, one direction at a time, so that the medical crew can speak to a person who is not in the communications center and vice versa. This capability is useful for programs that require voice contact with a medical control physician and for occasions when a member of the medical crew needs to speak with the receiving physician.

Programs that use a phone–radio or radio–phone patch have found that radio-like procedures must be used because transmissions are simpler. At times, this presents problems when patched through to persons who may not understand the system. Cellular telephones and even satellite and Voice over Internet Protocol (VoIP) products have supplanted this feature in many programs.

Squelch Control

A continuous tone-controlled subaudible squelch (CTCSS) circuit acts as a filter for others who use the radio's frequency. Only users of radios with the same tone-control frequency setting normally hear each other. This feature may be disabled when the tone of a transmitting radio is unknown or different or the radio operator wishes to monitor the entire frequency. Private line and channel guard are proprietary names for CTCSS.

Pagers

Two-way paging with use of **satellite communications** allows voiceless pages to be sent and an acknowledgment to be received with use of data terminals. The push-to-talk (PTT) method provides a nationwide service that combines instant communications with bases that use multiple transmitters across the country. These units offer global positioning system (GPS)-enabled tracking to locate aircraft or staff should a precautionary landing need to be made and the staff leave the aircraft for some reason. The units can be left on the aircraft; they are not transmitting in the air, and they are being pinged by the transmitters in the service area.

An extremely detailed needs assessment should be undertaken by qualified technical personnel before the implementation of any radio system. It is ill advised for a program to purchase a system identical to that of another program based solely on its recommendation.

Headsets and Foot Switches

The use of headsets rather than stand-alone microphones should be considered in busy communications centers. When used in conjunction with a foot switch, a headset leaves the CS hands free, which is particularly desirable during busy operations for the CS on duty. With more centers moving to a computer-based radio system, the PTT feature of traditional radios is being replaced by selecting a channel with a simple mouse click on the radio computer. In these systems the foot switch is replaced entirely, and the radio system is integrated into the daily use of the computers for transmissions.

If used, stand-alone microphones should be able to filter out background noises. A microphone placed on a bracket or gooseneck fixture attached to the console is preferable because it leaves the desktop space clear. When a headset microphone is used, it should be close to the lips; proximity to the lips varies because of the varying speech characteristics of different people.

Communication Recorders

The CAMTS standards state that communication centers must have a system that records all incoming and outgoing telephone and radio transmissions with time recording and playback capabilities. These recordings should be kept for a minimum of 90 days.

In most communication centers the recorders that use physical tapes have been upgraded to keep digital copies of all communications that enter and exit the center. Because of the availability and low cost of modern-day storage devices, this information can be kept for an indefinite amount of time. Because those recordings are usually only accessed by certain individuals, many centers use an immediate playback feature so that the CS can review the last hour of transmissions in case he or she needs to double-check information or relisten to a report that was given over the radio. This protection has many benefits already discussed but is also a key component to a robust Quality Assurance process in a communications center.

Computers and Peripherals

Computers are an integral part of the well-equipped communications center. What a computer can do for a program is limited primarily by imagination and budget. Most communication centers operate multimonitor platforms on which a great deal of information can be displayed at a moment's notice. Depending on the individual program and the information technology infrastructure, most computer consoles are digitally backed up and can be accessed remotely, depending on the circumstances. Separate computers are generally used for each CS in the center, with an integrated setup on each computer that includes computer-aided dispatch (CAD), phone, and radio interfaces; this allows for an ideal communicator experience. Communication centers should have a backup PC built for quick replacement should you need to maintain business continuity.

Computer-Aided Dispatch Systems

The **CAD** is the heart of the dispatch software that is used in modern-day dispatching (Fig. 7.2). In the past, multiple systems had to be used simultaneously by the CS to accomplish a string of tasks, but now they can all be completed within one integrated program. For dispatch centers that remain at the forefront of technological advancement, one would be hard-pressed to find loose paper, reference manuals, and large Rolodex references sitting around. Modern-day communication centers and transport team environments rely heavily on the CAD to ensure that transport is accomplished safely and effectively.

The modern-day CAD often implements multiple systems into one functioning program; for example, it will usually have a built-in "library." This library can store information about agencies, locations, landing zones, hospitals, units, and any other data the CS may need to access. CAD systems are like many other computer systems today, finding new ways to leverage artificial intelligence (AI) to improve their functional products. If a transport is entered into the CAD from Point A to Point B, the library is readily accessed to show phone numbers, addresses, important hazard information, and relevant notes pertaining to those points, and all information is immediately accessible to the CS. Because CADs are usually network based and share a common server, when one CS changes information (like a phone number within the CAD), all the other users on the network that access that library will be receiving the most up-to-date information. Communication centers routinely back up their CAD in the event of an outage or routine maintenance. Backups are quite easy to print and store for a permanent reference should a center experience a complete power or Internet outage. Testing in the "old fashion" way of following a crew using skills such as departure bearing, time, and distance estimation is still a great way to validate the skills of the CS staff, should there ever be a total computer system failure.

In addition to the library feature, modern CAD software can transmit information to a crew-assigned cell phone in the form of a text, automatically alert the CS of critical updated information, and even incorporate mapping and distance features based on GPS points gathered from the units to determine which vehicle is the closest to a call. A modern flight CAD system can calculate the distance and heading that an aircraft must fly and where the closest airport is for fuel and even estimate the time it will take the aircraft to fly to the scene or hospital based on its current location.

The main feature of the CAD, however, is the management of transport resources and crews. It is a vital tool for providing the multiple CSs who are working within the center access to the same up-to-date information regarding the location and status of the various transporting units. This server-based software, as well as technological communication advancements, allows the center to

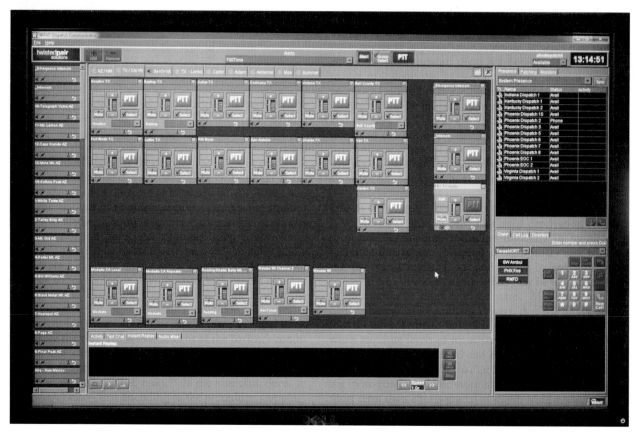

• **Figure 7.2** Modern Computer Radio Stack. (Courtesy Clayton Smith.)

be remotely located from any unit or location if the need arises. This is important because of the increasing need for disaster preparedness and evacuation procedures. A server-based CAD system allows the communication center to relocate and resume operations with nothing more than a bank of laptops and a high-speed Internet connection. Because of the vast degrees of complexity that a program may choose to implement with its CAD, it is important that transport team members understand the capabilities of their dispatch center and what they should expect as routine for the practices that have been implemented for their program.

Weather Radar

All pilots have access to FAA flight service weather information. Although the FAA generally does an excellent job, its reports may not be as current as desired at a given point in time. New weather tools are constantly being introduced. Great examples are available at https://www.aviationweather.gov/radar. Remember, a pilot can only base his/her weather decisions on an approved FAA weather information source.

Weather radar display systems are available through several commercial services. These systems may be connected to the National Weather Service radar site in the region via telephone line or computer modem. All weather radar display systems provide displays and printouts of excellent quality. The display should be installed where the pilots have access to it such as in the duty office or crew quarters, and of course, a similar display should be available to the communications center, but it is not essential. If the pilot needs an update while airborne, the CS may also have access to it. This situation may not be a problem

if the aircraft has its own weather radar. If a program has a computer-driven system, the CS can access the weather report from the communications center. An alternative to the phone-line system is to place a remote monitor in the communications center.[4] If the program does use an OCC, care must be taken so that the CS is taken out of the weather and risk analysis decision-making process; oftentimes, those conversations are for the pilot, crew, and OCC specialist only. This is not to discourage the CS from voicing an opinion if he or she feels something is wrong; instead, it is used to illustrate that weather decisions and discussions should be left to the trained OCC specialist, if the program uses them.

Closed-Circuit Television/Web Cameras

The CS should ideally have access to video scanning of the helipad or hangar ramp of the base location of each aircraft and, if possible, at their most frequently used referring facilities. Such scanning serves as a security system and enables the CS, who does not have direct visual contact with the program's parked aircraft, to see what is happening. Television monitors are available that may serve as a computer screen or as a video monitor by pressing a button, reducing the cost for the program. Web cameras also may be used to monitor aircraft and other areas of the transport service.

Maps

Technology has vastly improved "finding" EMS providers and referring hospitals. Mapping software that allows the CS to point and click on selected response sites is available, displaying coordinates for navigational purposes. GPS devices allow EMS to provide exact location information to both the communication center and the transport team. Many transport programs create websites with information about common destinations (hospitals and predesignated landing areas), which could save time and afford an opportunity to review helipads and landing areas.

It is important to remember that technology is generally only as good as the operator, so CS, pilots, and transport team members must know how to use a map. An aviation sectional map or maps of the program's normal area of operations should be available in the communications center and onboard transport vehicles. A compass radial overlay with a center string attached should be affixed to the map centered over the base of operations for backup if systems go down or are not functioning. A heavy dark line that radiates from base operations should be drawn on the map and marked off in 10-mile increments. This map enables the CS to rapidly obtain a heading and distance of a given point.

A street map should also be included of the metropolitan area around the base of rotary-wing operations. This map should be modified as previously mentioned. Topographic maps that show variations in terrain contour and various other maps that may be obtained from state or county highway departments prove useful in the communications center.

Policies and Procedures

A detailed policy and procedures manual is necessary for any organization that wishes to function in a systematically effective manner. The communications center manual must be a part of the program's overall policy and procedures manual. When the communications center manual is written, it should be carefully integrated with existing policies and procedures to minimize potential conflicting instructions to the CS.

The manual must cover all aspects of operation that have anything to do with communications. Each segment of the manual should be extremely detailed so that if a question arises about a specific item, it can be resolved by referring to the manual.

Communicating (Radio Language)

To effectively communicate within a program, standardized terminology should be used so that meanings are not lost or misinterpreted.

Generally, communication in plain language is preferable to using various codes; this precludes errors caused by misunderstanding a garbled coded transmission. Because of the broad area over which an air medical program operates, knowledge of codes for each of the many jurisdictions in the program's service area would be extremely difficult. Times should be communicated in the 24-hour clock format to ensure accuracy (Box 7.7).

When initiating a radio transmission, a transport team member should begin with the name or call sign of the unit being called, followed by the member's own name or call sign. When older radio systems and poorly maintained new systems are used, the speaker, when keying the microphone, should pause for a second before speaking to allow the radio to reach its maximal output level. This practice helps prevent the frequent problem of receiving incomplete messages. Another cause of this problem is speaking before keying the microphone.

BOX 7.7	24-Hour Clock		
AM		**PM**	
1:00	0100	1:00	1300
2:00	0200	2:00	1400
3:00	0300	3:00	1500
4:00	0400	4:00	1600
5:00	0500	5:00	1700
6:00	0600	6:00	1800
7:00	0700	7:00	1900
8:00	0800	8:00	2000
9:00	0900	9:00	2100
10:00	1000	10:00	2200
11:00	1100	11:00	2300
Noon	1200	Midnight	2400 (0000)

The speaker should talk at a normal level; yelling into the microphone distorts the transmission. The speaker should know what to say before keying the microphone; speak clearly and concisely without irrelevant comments; attempt to control the voice level and intonation even when under stress; try to avoid transmissions that reflect disgust, irritation, or sarcasm; and always avoid using profanity. Radio transmissions are a measure of a program's professionalism, and both the media and a large population of citizens with scanners hear every word.

Transport team members must know how to properly operate the two-directional radio-intercom switch commonly found on headset cords in aircraft or ground vehicles. Many transport team members have been embarrassed when personal conversations or comments less than socially acceptable were broadcast over a wide area. This problem occurs less often in programs that operate pressurized aircraft, in which transport team members do not use a headset system.

Communications between onboard crewmembers are also important. The pilot should keep the medical crew informed of any developments in a clear, complete message that leaves no doubt about what is happening.

The following two anecdotes illustrate this point. In the first incident, the crew experiences the helicopter making an abrupt and unexpected banking turn. The crew members looked at each other, concerned that the pilot had not communicated anything in advance, and were about to get upset when the aircraft resumed straight and level flight. The pilot came on the intercom and explained that he was not up on the intercom and that he had been speaking to approach control, and he was avoiding another aircraft. This highlights the need to have active communication in the aircraft. Proactive communication by the pilot to inform the crew the pilot would be off intercom temporarily and talking with air traffic control (ATC) about other traffic in the area. Advance warning on the intercom could have prevented a tense few moments for the crew.

In the second incident, the pilot of an outbound aircraft observed a transmission chip light blink on. In accordance with company policy, he immediately began a descent in preparation for landing. He told the crew, "We're going down." The crew prepared themselves for a hard landing. A normal landing was made, the mechanic arrived and corrected the problem, and the aircraft returned to its base. Once again, a more complete explanation such as, "I have a transmission chip light and I am declaring a precautionary landing and looking for a place to land," would have prevented these tense moments.

During a flight, the pilot of an airport-based aircraft communicates with ground control, airport tower departure control, air route traffic control center, approach control, airport tower, and ground control again, in addition to the CS.

Rotorcraft based at a hospital may or may not be near an airport but will be in communication with the appropriate segments of the air traffic control system and the program's own communications center. In either case, only the pilots should communicate with air traffic control. Aircraft on emergency scene flights also speak with units already on the scene or may be en route.

Sterile cockpit (not speaking except in case of an emergency) must be practiced during takeoff and landing and any other critical phases of flight. Radio traffic should always be kept to a minimum to avoid unnecessary distractions, whether transporting via air or ground.

Transport teams in programs with multiple aircraft should also be aware that nonessential radio conversations between aircraft may make a telephone conversation or receipt of an essential transmission from another unit difficult for the CS.

If a team member asks the CS to make a telephone call, sufficient time should be allowed to pass before transmitting again to avoid interrupting the call.

If either party is having difficulty making a word understood, then that person should spell it using the phonetic alphabet (Box 7.8).

Portable Units

A program may elect to provide transport members with portable handheld radios for use on the ground outside the aircraft. These radios are particularly useful for programs that do emergency scene flights and during transfer flights for alerting the pilot to the imminent return of the crew with the patient.

Cellular and satellite phones may also be used by transport team members for communication.

• BOX 7.8 Phonetic Alphabet and Numbers

Phonetic Alphabet

A: Alpha	T: Tango
B: Bravo	U: Uniform
C: Charlie	V: Victor
D: Delta	W: Whiskey
E: Echo	X: X-ray
F: Foxtrot	Y: Yankee
G: Gulf	Z: Zulu
H: Hotel	
I: India	**Phonetic Numbers**
J: Juliet	1: WUN
K: Kilo	2: TOO
L: Lima	3: TREE
M: Mike	4: FOW-ER
N: November	5: FIFE
O: Oscar	6: SIX
P: Papa	7: SEV-EN
Q: Quebec	8: AIT
R: Romeo	9: NIN-ER
S: Sierra	0: ZEE-RO

From Federal Aviation Administration. Accessed March 28, 2017. https://www.faa.gov/regulations_policies/handbooks_manuals/aviation/media/remote_pilot_study_guide.pdf.

Aircraft Radios

Aircraft radios are usually integrated with the avionics package within the cockpit of the aircraft. These radios have more power and can transmit larger distances than most handheld radios. The antennae for these radios are often mounted on the belly of the aircraft so that during flight the radio transmission is broadcast down toward the earth where there is nothing obstructing the signal from the repeater tower to the aircraft. These radios are also used to talk with other air traffic, air traffic control, and the ground agency or security unit that is assisting in the crew's arrival to a particular destination.

Effective Communication

The effectiveness of the transport team as well as the communication team to provide and deliver exceptional service in a safe and efficient manner is directly related to the quality of communication delivered. High-quality communication is the responsibility of every individual involved with the transport to ensure that their message is being conveyed clearly and concisely. Because of the routineness of the messages that are relayed between the CS and the transport team, their importance can easily be lost within the sheer number of transmissions that can occur during a transport. This can result in a "desensitization" of the information that is being relayed, and the importance of delivering a clear message may be lost. If left unchecked, this will lead to unsuccessful attempts at getting the message through, incomplete transmissions born out of frustration, and a general dysfunction in the overall communication atmosphere between the teams. In posttransport reviews of situations with unfavorable outcomes, the root cause can frequently be traced back to an issue with communication. Team members should:

1. Never assume the intent, content, or meaning of the message if it is unclear.
2. Believe in positive intent for everyone involved.
3. Be clear and concise in transmissions and ask for a repeat if the transmission is not clear.
4. Trust but verify the information received.

Sensitive Radio Traffic

When communicating information over the radio to the communications center, it is important to remember that these channels are oftentimes monitored by anyone who has access to a radio system and knows where the frequencies are published. Therefore, patient identifiers and protected patient information should never be shared over the radio for any reason. It is sometimes necessary for the transport team to relay patient information to the CS over the radio if they need to deliver a patient report to the receiving facility on behalf of the transport team. This is an acceptable and standard practice, but care must be used when delivering that information and it should never include any HIPAA-protected information including names, addresses, personal descriptions, or any other protected patient identifiers.

Additionally, the communications team must use discretion when dispatching their units for a call. It is common for the media and news organizations to scan the radio frequencies and receive information for breaking news based on publicly available dispatch transmissions. One helicopter transport service was surprised to hear an actual recording of their CS dispatching an aircraft played over the nightly news for a high-profile call.

When dealing with the communication of patient information, it will always be best practice to censor out the patient identifiers and deliver the information in a sterile, factual, and straightforward way. A good habit is to always assume that someone unaffiliated with the transport is listening to your radio traffic.

Telephones

Often a requesting party's first impression of a program is created by the CS who answers the telephone. A courteous manner combined with comprehensive knowledge of the program helps give the caller the impression that the program is staffed by competent professional personnel.

Electronic Communication

Advances in communication technology in recent years have opened the door for new ways to communicate between the transport team and the CS. With the implementation of VoIP radio communication, it is possible to integrate communications between a traditional radio frequency and the Internet. By transmitting the signal first via the Internet, the signal can then be broadcast locally to a unit or base once it is converted to a signal on a local frequency. With this technology, the communication center can communicate with aircraft or ground units potentially thousands of miles away. The voice message travels via the Internet for the majority of the distance, and then it is locally routed to a repeater that transmits the signal on a radio frequency that the unit is monitoring locally. When the unit responds back, the reverse process happens, and the transmission is heard in the communication center with only a small lag.

This advancement in Internet-based communication allows for the use of mobile phones and Internet-capable devices to transmit voice messages to a radio frequency even if they are out of the radio coverage area. With many different applications available for communicating on tablet and cell phone platforms, software companies are providing companion apps with their primary software packages that allow the users to utilize the features of the communication infrastructure that they have in place. Make sure you have a good understanding of the communication resources that your program provides (Box 7.9).

Satellite Communication

As the name implies, satellite communication uses an infrastructure of complex communication satellites orbiting the Earth to provide two-way tracking and communication capabilities between individuals. Because the signal to transmit and receive via satellite travels in a more vertical pattern instead of laterally across the Earth, it is far less prone to interruptions or coverage area issues caused by obstructions in the terrain. Satellite communication and the upgrade in features that it provides has improved the ability to communicate in locations in which radio coverage or traditional cell phone service does not exist. The technology has become easier and more cost-effective to implement within transport vehicles and mobile devices. Although conventional satellite tracking of transport vehicles has been around for many years, the ability to communicate and send messages through that same service is a newer advancement within the industry. Some units allow the transport team and the CS to communicate directly with either a text-based message or recorded voice transmission. This communication medium provides yet another outlet for expanding the service area and coverage for the transport vehicle. If the program incorporates such technology, it then must become familiar with the operation and transmission capabilities of the installed unit. There may come a time when that is the only possible way to communicate with the communications center.

Medical Direction

Programs that operate with nurses or paramedics are included under medical direction regulations that vary from state to state. Whether communicating with their medical direction physician via radio, radiophone patch, satellite, or cellular phone, the medical crew should follow the medical reporting format used in the region. All reports should be to the point. Any treatment orders received should be acknowledged by repeating the order verbatim. Medical direction that is delivered in the middle of a patient transport should be directly between the transport team and the physician. With the growing number of applications used for smartphones and tablets, some charting and reporting platforms allow for face-to-face video conferencing or for sharing of pictures with the physicians. These communication outlets can provide a valuable tool for sharing information from the field with medical control. As with all patient-related activities, care should be taken in respecting the patient's rights when sharing medical information through this medium. Although this method is more secure than radio transmissions alone, the same precautions must be taken in protecting the patient's identity.

Communicating With the Media

Local news media usually have a high level of interest in the activities of any transport program. The CS must be able to deal with their calls, politely but firmly, when they interfere with operations. He or she must be aware of program policy with respect to giving out information and should refer the caller to the appropriate person if this is dictated by policy. Most programs have a designated individual that is responsible for handling media requests for information. Ask your program management who this person is and how they would like requests to be delivered.

In addition to the media, there are times when other agencies or businesses may call requesting information regarding a transport that was done by the transport team. Care must be taken when giving out information to other agencies that request it. It may be tempting or sound quite persuasive to deliver information to a detective or state agent looking for information regarding a patient that was recently transported, but you can still violate the patient's rights and HIPAA by sharing information with agencies and individuals who are not privileged to hear it. The CS must become familiar with his or her programs' specific media and information request policies regarding these types of requests.

Emergency Procedures

The operational procedures section of the policy and procedures manual should include a subsection that deals with procedures to be followed in the event of any unscheduled incident that affects the use of the aircraft or directly involves the aircraft.

Post Accident Incident Plan

Every transport program must have a written plan in the event of an unexpected incident such as a vehicle accident. Each program should identify which incidents trigger this plan. The *Post Accident Incident Plan* (PAIP) must be easily identified, readily available, and understood by all of the transport team members. CAMTS[3] recommends that at a minimum, the plan should include the following: a list of personnel to notify in order of priority; notification plans including appropriate family members and support services; consecutive guidelines to follow in attempts to communicate with the aircraft or ambulance, initiate search and rescue or ground support, have a backup plan for transporting the patient or team, and have an aviation individual identified as the scene coordinator to coordinate activities at the crash site; a preplanned time frame to activate the PAIP for overdue vehicles; a method for ensuring accurate dissemination; coordination of transport of injured team members; a procedure to document all notifications, calls, and communications and to secure all documents and recordings related to the incident; a procedure to deal with releasing information to the press; resources available for critical incident stress management; and a process to determine whether the program will stay in service.

The program's specific utilization of the PAIP determines how frequently the CS and transport team will go through a PAIP situation. For some programs, the PAIP is limited to accidents and injuries, loss of communications with the aircraft, and overdue aircraft incidents. Other programs use the PAIP as a notification system for a wider variety of situations including weather turnarounds, flight path deviations, forgetting medical equipment at the sending or receiving facility, unscheduled landings, flight plan diversions for fuel, or changes in patient condition. For programs that run the PAIP frequently, it becomes a well-rehearsed action with the notification and activation of the plan and is often used for both ground and air units. For other programs, the PAIP is reserved for critical accidents and incidents only. Be sure to be familiar with the program's PAIP policy and procedures.

Drills

The program's PAIP plan should also allow for scheduled drills. These drills are an excellent opportunity for the communication staff and the transport team to become familiar with the program's emergency procedures and operations. The ways in which programs implement drills can be as specific or creative as warranted. Some programs used their drills to host a "Safety and PR" event day for local agencies.

These drills begin with the CS getting the indication that something is wrong and the PAIP is activated. The unit participating in the drill initiates emergency procedures and may involve the local responders in practicing for the emergency as well. Once the drill is complete, they can use that opportunity to review landing zone safety and important public relations information with the responders. The drill is then reviewed and critiqued by a designated board and changes are recommended based on the information that was learned from the drill. Many programs find that the success of the drill is dependent on proper planning so that it happens in a safe and effective way. Additionally, the review of the drill is critical in disseminating the information that was learned so that everyone within the organization can benefit and be better prepared should a real emergency occur.

Critical Incident Stress Management

Each program should have a critical incident stress management plan in place in the event of an incident that causes the CS or the transport crew to have a strong reaction. The CS on duty at the time must be included in this plan. Depending on the situation, the CS may feel just as involved and affected as the transport crew. The CS may believe that he or she could have done something more or failed to do something, taking on unwarranted feelings of guilt. In adapting to the recognized stresses inherent in these types of situations, it is imperative that those involved reach out to their program's affiliated critical incident response team to seek further assistance in dealing with these complex situations.

Summary

Effective communication begins long before the first dispatch is delivered to the transport team. Communication encompasses both the understanding of the physical equipment as well as the components of communicating on an interpersonal level. The job of the transport team and the CS can be tense, leading to situations in which stress and an urgency to complete the tasks at hand overwrite the ability to communicate what is important in an effective and efficient way. Using the new technology to its maximum potential and setting a precedent of making effective communication a habit will provide an atmosphere in which the exchange of information contributes to the success of the various teams and the program overall.

References

1. Kane D. Communications. In: York-Clark D, Stocking J, Johnson J, eds. *Flight and Ground Transport Nursing Core Curriculum*. 2nd ed. Air and Surface Transport Nurses Association; 2006.
2. American Academy of Pediatrics. *Air and Ground Transport of Neonatal and Pediatric Patients*. 3rd ed. American Academy of Pediatrics; 2007.
3. Commission on Accreditation of Medical Transport Systems. *Accreditation Standards*. 12th ed. CAMTS; 2022.
4. Federal Aviation Administration, Department of Transportation. 14 CFR 135.79. June 7 2007. Accessed July 30, 2023. https://www.ecfr.gov/current/title-14/part-135/section-135.79
5. International Association of Medical Transport Communication Specialists. June 2008. Accessed October 6, 2022. http://www.iamtcs.org
6. Rau W. 2000 Communications survey. *Air Med J*. 2000;6(2):22–26.
7. Yocum K. A new look at hiring communication specialists. *Air Med J*. 1999;5(2):132–134.
8. 14 CFR 135.619 Operations Control Center. Federal Aviation Administration. Updated Mach 8, 2023. Accessed March 10, 2023. https://www.ecfr.gov/current/title-14/chapter-I/subchapter-G/part-135/subpart-L/section-135.619
9. Federal Aviation Administration, Department of Transportation. Basic Requirements and Policy Applicable to All Air Carriers 8900.1, Vol.3, Ch25, Sec1. April 12, 2018. Accessed July 30, 2023 https://drs.faa.gov/browse/excelExternalWindow/DRSDOCID11071763852022121919I729.0001
10. AC 120-96A – Operations Control Center (OCC) for Helicopter Air Ambulance (HAA) Operations. Federal Aviation Administration. Updated January 7, 2016. Accessed December 4, 2022. https://www.faa.gov/regulations_policies/advisory_circulars/index.cfm/go/document.information/documentID/1028758
11. Sholl S, Morse AM, Broome R, et al. Communications. In: Blumen IJ, ed. *Principles and Directions of Air Medical Transport*. Air Medical Physicians Association; 2006.
12. Illman P. *Pilot's Communication Handbook*. 5th ed. McGraw-Hill; 1998.

8

Teamwork and Human Performance

PATRICK FALVEY AND B. DANIEL NAYMAN

COMPETENCIES

1. Identify the common types of errors that occur in transport medicine.
2. Understand the importance of teamwork and how to build effective teams.
3. Recognize the importance of Crew Resource Management and how it is designed to prevent errors and mitigate potentially harmful situations.
4. Understand how to effectively manage critical tasks in stressful environments.

Introduction

Knowing the Enemy: The Problem of Human Error

To understand the role of teamwork and human performance in the transport medicine setting, it is useful to begin with an understanding of the challenges that we seek to overcome. The fact is, human beings make errors. Regardless of the degree of automation, or the extensiveness of the rules and procedures we put in place, medicine, aviation, and the movement of critically ill patients is a human endeavor. It is therefore imbued with all the strengths and weaknesses that the human mind can bring to such challenges. These natural tendencies, rooted in our physiology, allow a consistent rate of error and mishap to continue despite our best attempts to engineer them out. As crew members and teammates, we are the source and the solution to many of these problems. The extent to which we understand how errors occur, and how we can apply principles of teamwork and human performance to identify, prevent, and stop them, will determine our ability to function and thrive in an unforgiving practice environment. It should be noted that although it is often discussed in just such a context, the consequences of these errors are not limited to the safe or unsafe operation of the vehicles. The problem of human error reaches into all aspects of transport medicine, both operational and clinical. We become better, safer clinicians by learning to master how we function as a team and how we master ourselves to manage errors before they reach a level of consequence.

When mistakes and mishaps occur in medicine or the transport environment, they can be categorized in a variety of ways. Helmreich et al.[1] developed a modal classification scheme that classified errors based on how the error occurred, resulting in five categories: procedural error, communication error, proficiency error, decision error, and intentional noncompliance. Other schemes have been contextually based and describe the timing or location of the error. The psychological approach, as described by Ferner and Aronson,[2] is used here because of its broad application and its ability to explain the causality of an event as opposed to merely describing one.

Slips and Lapses

A *slip* (sometimes referred to as a technical error) is an error caused by the failure of an individual to maintain the necessary attention on the task being performed. It results in performing a task incorrectly or in the wrong sequence. A *lapse* is caused by forgetting (and thereby omitting) a step in a planned sequence. Both slips and lapses are unintended and are skill-based mistakes. The error was not one of planning, but rather one of execution, because the person was correct in knowing what needed to be done but failed to perform that task correctly.[3]

Knowledge-Based Errors

Knowledge-based errors represent the ignorance of a fact that is required to respond appropriately to a given circumstance. Unlike slips and lapses, this is an error of planning; the course of action was incorrect, even though the incorrect act may have been performed correctly. One type of knowledge-based error is the loss of situational awareness (SA). In dynamic environments, the need to make timely and correct decisions requires that we not only observe our environment but correctly place our attention to understand what is happening around us and to our patients and formulate an expectation regarding what will happen in the immediate future.[4] When we fail to perceive appropriate cues from our environment, or we cannot correctly interpret the cues we have, we have a failure in our SA. Often, this can manifest as task fixation, resulting in the failure to perceive everything else happening in the environment.

Rule-Based Errors

A rule in this context is simply a course of action prescribed by a given policy or procedure for a familiar or expected situation. They can often be expressed in IF/THEN propositions. For example, IF the patient is in congestive heart failure, THEN fluids should be avoided. The adoption of rules like this reduces cognitive burden, but the problem remains that a subset of congestive heart failure patients would benefit from gentle fluid resuscitation. Add to this the natural tendency to force novel circumstances into the mold of previous events, and rule-based errors are born. Thus a distinction can be drawn between what is often described as good rules and bad rules. For a rule to be "good," it has to apply to the intended circumstance, and it must prescribe an appropriate course of action. A bad rule is one in which the situation at hand does not match the conditions the rule was intended to govern, or the action prescribed by the rule is unsuitable to the given situation.[5] When a rule-based error is committed, the individual fails to either apply or completely apply an appropriate good rule to the situation, or inappropriately applies a bad rule to the situation.

CASE STUDY

The Tenerife Disaster (KLM Flight 4805 and Pan Am Flight 1736)

On March 27, 1977, two Boeing 747 aircraft sat on the tarmac of Los Rodeos Airport in Tenerife on the Canary Islands. Both had been bound for Las Palmas Airport but had been forced to divert to their current location because of an unexpected closure of the Las Palmas Airport after a terrorist bomb explosion. Now both aircraft were sitting just off the departure end of the runway waiting. Unlike the KLM flight, the Pan Am flight had not deplaned its passengers and was ready for departure 15 minutes later when Las Palmas Airport had been reopened. The Pan Am flight was parked behind the KLM flight, however, and was forced to wait for over 2 hours while the KLM flight reboarded and refueled.

With poor visibility and a fog bank laying across the airport, dividing the runway in half, neither aircraft could see each other or the control tower once they began to taxi into position for takeoff; everyone was completely dependent on radio communication for coordination of their location on the airport and runways.[6] The control tower had instructed the KLM flight to back-taxi down the runway they intended to take off from, turn around at the end, and wait for takeoff clearance. The Pan Am flight was to follow behind the KLM flight on the same runway and turn off the active runway at about the halfway point. The Pan Am flight slowly back-taxied down the runway far behind and out of sight of the KLM flight. Meanwhile, the KLM aircraft had reached the other end of the runway and turned around.

On turning around, the KLM captain began to advance the throttles for takeoff, to which the KLM first officer said, "wait a minute we don't have clearance yet." The KLM captain, rather than acknowledge the mistake, retarded the throttles and said, "No, I know that, go ahead and ask."[7] The KLM first officer then requested both the ATC clearance (which specifies the routing the plane will take after departure) and takeoff clearance (required to take off from the runway). As the first officer of the KLM flight received the ATC clearance (not clearance for takeoff), the captain of the KLM flight, mistakenly believing he was cleared for takeoff, released his brakes and began his takeoff roll. The first officer (for whom English was a second language) then communicated with the tower stating with surprise, "we are now at takeoff," which the control tower interpreted as meaning that they were in position for takeoff, not that they were beginning takeoff.[6] The tower responded by saying "okay" with a pause, and then told KLM to

stand by for takeoff. The KLM first officer did not acknowledge the last message, and the control tower did not challenge him again.

At the same moment the tower was responding, the first officer of the Pan Am flight realized that the KLM flight may have interpreted the ATC clearance as takeoff clearance and quickly responded, "we are still on the runway." That transmission occurred simultaneously with the tower request to stand by for takeoff, resulting in both messages being barely audible and accompanied by a strong squeal heard in the KLM cockpit. The captain of the KLM flight commented on the quality of the radio transmission, and the collision killing 528 people in two fully loaded 747 aircraft occurred some 13 seconds later.

Combating Human Error

In the Tenerife disaster, all of the aircraft functioned properly and the crews were experienced. A series of miscommunications and errors of judgment compounded to bring about a tremendous loss of life. To combat human error and its effects, we must begin with the understanding that *error will occur*. Without acknowledging the possibility of error in our teammates and ourselves, we create an environment in which it becomes difficult to detect, confront, or learn from our mistakes. We may also create situations in which margins are so close that small mistakes can have significant and lasting consequences. If, however, we understand the inevitability of error, it becomes less personal and creates the mandate to be vigilant for error detection, requiring the formation of plans that do not require perfection. There are a host of measures used to accomplish this task, from how we engineer our technology and systems to how we build policy and procedures. For the ones out practicing in the transport environment, the team dynamic and the individual performances are the spheres in which we have the most impact and control. Teamwork and individual human performance are discussed together because, in the transport medicine environment, they are inseparable. The first prerequisite for effective team membership is individual development and competence, which is furthered and facilitated by effective coordination within a team. Without competent and effective individuals, teams are ineffective; without teams, the full potential of those individuals cannot be expressed.[7]

Teamwork

Value of Teamwork

The military theorist Charles Ardant D'Picq, writing on unit cohesion and adversity, said:

> *Four brave men who do not know each other will not dare attack a lion. Four less brave men, but knowing each other well, sure of their reliability and consequently mutual aid, will attack resolutely.*[8]

This idea, that the familiarity and confidence in the abilities of teammates allow individuals to complete tasks that capable individuals cannot, hints at how the creation of an effective team improves our effectiveness in the delivery of care and the safe operation within the transport environment. Effective team members contribute to the collective pool of knowledge that allows the synthesis of ideas, creating new options for the team. Within highly effective teams, individual strengths offset other teammates' weaknesses, allowing for the team to be stronger and higher performing than the individuals who make it up. The result is an increase in the reliability of performance and a higher rate of successful completion of critical tasks.

These benefits do not come without a cost, however, and the same quality that makes a team more effective can create traps that can weaken its performance. Interpersonal dynamics within the team, as well as personality and communication styles, can reduce performance or subject the team to the hazards of groupthink.

Teamwork is the process of working collaboratively with a team of people to achieve a goal.

Developing trusting, cohesive teams that are capable of operating effectively together can be a significant challenge. There must be trust between all the members, including supervisors and staff. Developing that trust, and cohesion must be intentional and ongoing. Trust and cohesion take time to build and are easily damaged.[9]

Character

Character is the cornerstone of trust. Integrity, perseverance, diligence, humility, confidence, courage, ethics, and altruism are a few of the character qualities that are needed to build relationships.[10] As relationships develop, respect is earned and given. This respect then leads to trust between members. By their example, members of strong character can encourage and mentor character development among other team members, thus improving the dynamics of the team.[9] Conversely, members of poor character can create fissures within the team and adversely affect team dynamics.

When building a team, leaders should consider hiring a person with high character and medium skills before a person with high skills and medium character. Skills are more easily acquired than character.

Foundation of Teamwork: Leadership and Followership

Teams are composed of leaders and followers, but within the dynamic context of transport medicine that distinction can shift quickly as circumstances change. It is possible within the span of a single call to have the roles of individuals shift. This may be because one crew member has more expertise in a given situation, or it may be because of the inclusion of different team members from outside the normal crew; for example, changes in the patient's condition may prompt the addition of an attending physician to the dynamic. These transitions of leadership do not absolve any of the team members from their responsibilities, but it does require a fluid and collaborative approach as the team encounters different spheres of authority in the course of a single call, moving between roles of leadership and followership. There are two compositions of teams in the operational transport team. First, there is the "crew," which is composed of clinicians and vehicle operators. This is what is typically described in the context of teamwork. There also is a second team composition at play. The "ad hoc team" is composed each time the crew goes out and interacts with the requesting agencies. One does not often receive patients in a vacuum, and often the transport team and the requesting agency work in cooperation or coordination for a period before the crew assumes full responsibility for the patient. Each time a new ad hoc team is formed, there is a critical point in the interaction when the boundaries of the relationship, the norms or culture of the group, and the scope of authority will be defined. Effective leaders typically address these three formative processes intentionally.[11]

Managing Boundaries

When a transport team arrives to receive a patient, they are almost always interacting with other services, clinicians, or institutions. Those entities will have their own rules, norms, values, and hierarchy. Entering and thriving in that realm requires respect for those systems; however, the boundaries that separate outsiders from insiders should be softened quickly so effective communication and actions can be facilitated.

Team Culture

A team's culture consists of unwritten, informal rules that influence the team's actions. Communication style, slang language, sharing gratitude, nonverbal communication, style of greetings, asking for help, seating arrangement, discussing ideas, and encouraging team members can all be part of a team's culture. It is important to note, however, that as these rules are unwritten, there are varying levels of rule knowledge in the team. It should never be assumed that one member has the same understanding of the culture as other members.[12]

Different organizations have different cultures. Different bases of the same organization also have different cultures or norms. It is important that leaders and team members alike are aware of and recognize those differences. When interacting with new teams, speak, listen, and act in a professional manner, and appropriately ask for clarity when needed.

Utilizing Appropriate Authority

When rapid action is required, an effective leader is capable of decisive unilateral action. That degree of decisive action is not frequently required, however, and an effective leader is capable of adjusting the tightness of control on the team depending on the capability of the members and the situation at hand.

As important as leadership is, equally important is the seldom-discussed role of followership. It is a commonly held fallacy that being a good follower is a temporary requirement on the way to a leadership position.[11] The truth is quite the opposite. Team membership in the transport medical environment means transitioning between leadership and followership roles quickly with adaptability and flexibility. The archetypal good follower is one with the ability to critically analyze the situation, who is not afraid to offer thoughts that contradict the prevailing opinions, and can communicate those thoughts in a respectful, effective, and timely manner.

In the patient transport environment, it is easy to become distracted and lose focus on the goal and priorities of the mission. Committees, training, equipment acquisition and maintenance, vehicles, weather, organizational needs, and other activities that, while important to supporting the mission, can easily become distractions. Leaders and team members should consistently evaluate potential distractions by asking "How does this activity help me take better care of the patient," or "how does this activity make transport safer and more efficient?"

Clear Leader Intent

The program leader should consider creating a clear mission intent. This intent is an expression of the purpose and focus of the mission and the desired outcome. This intent should serve to unify the efforts of the team and can be beneficial when the dynamics of the transport overwhelm the ability to communicate. Many patient care situations occur outside the boundary of our policies and protocols, and immediate communication for guidance is not always available. In those instances, the established mission intent can serve as guidance for prudent decision-making in the absence of other resources.

Know Your Team

Nobody cares how much you know, until they know how much you care

THEODORE ROOSEVELT

Building and maintaining a high-functioning team requires that leaders know the members of their team. Time and energy spent developing a relationship with team members will provide a great return on investment.[13] Leaders must take the time to not just know about individual team members, but get to know the team members on a personal level, while maintaining a professional relationship. To effectively utilize and inspire team members in their roles, leaders should seek to understand the motivations, values, interests, and future plans of each member of the team. In doing this, however, it is imperative that leaders avoid being too questioning or intrusive, and allow people to share only what they want to share. While the insight gained from taking the time to engage with and understand team members is often invaluable, simply ensuring that team members feel valued will allow them to achieve a level of engagement and commitment that would otherwise be unattainable.[13]

CASE STUDY

United Flight 173

On December 28, 1978, United Flight 173 had been flying from New York to Portland, Oregon, and was on the approach to land when the flight crew experienced a landing gear malfunction.[14] Electing to abort the approach, the crew climbed and entered a holding pattern about 20 miles from the airport and orbited for about an hour while troubleshooting the gear malfunction and preparing the cabin and passengers for the possibility of an emergency landing.

At 17:38 hours, the captain reported that he had 7000 pounds of fuel remaining with the intention of orbiting for 10 to 15 more minutes before returning to land. That estimation proved to be erroneous, and 8 minutes later at 17:46, the first officer asked the flight engineer, "how much fuel we got?" The flight engineer responded, "five thousand." The crew continued to discuss the landing gear until 2 minutes later when the captain asked for the fuel weight if they landed in about 15 minutes, specifying he would like to have about 3400 pounds at landing. The flight engineer replied, "Not enough. Fifteen minutes is gonna really run us low on fuel here." At 17:55, the flight engineer announced that the descent checklist was complete, at which time the first officer asked, "how much fuel you got now?" The flight engineer responded, "3000 pounds." At 17:57, the captain sent the flight engineer to check on preparation in the cabin for a possible emergency landing, and he returned at 18:01. The flight engineer then reported to the captain, "we have about three on the fuel and that's it."

At that time, the aircraft was only 5 nautical miles from the airport, turning away to continue holding. On hearing the flight engineer's report of the fuel, the captain said, "Okay, on touch down, if the gear folds..." never acknowledging the criticality of the fuel state. At 18:03, the captain told Portland approach they had, "about 4000" pounds of fuel. At 18:06, the captain announced his intention to turn back to the airport and begin the approach to land. He had just announced that intention to a flight attendant when the first officer announced, "I think you just lost number four..." followed by the flight engineer suggesting that they had better open the cross feeds. Ten seconds later, the first officer told the captain "We're going to lose an engine," to which the captain replied, "Why?" The first officer repeated himself, and the captain again asked, "Why?" The first officer responded, "fuel."

The first engine flamed out from fuel starvation at 18:07. At that point, the aircraft had traveled approximately 19 nautical miles from the airport. Six minutes later, the remaining engines flamed out and Flight 173 crashed 6 nautical miles short of the airport. Only 10 of the 189 people on board were killed because of absence of a postcrash fire. One of those fatalities was the flight engineer.

Teamwork Barriers in the Tenerife Disaster

In the Tenerife case study above, in the KLM cockpit, the captain was also the head of the Flight Training Department for the airline. In analyzing the crew management style of the KLM captain, Rotisch et al.[7] concluded:

> The KLM cockpit crew behavioral profile centered on a captain who gave the appearance to the rest of the crew that all factors had been considered and a safe takeoff was ensured. Such a posture was undoubtedly enhanced by the captain's position in the company as Head of Flight Training Department. Whenever upper management captains fly line trips, there is a natural subtle tension in the cockpit atmosphere that is not found between regular line crewmembers.

This subtle tension may have been the reason the KLM first officer failed to further challenge the KLM captain once takeoff was initiated when it is apparent that the KLM first officer was not expecting the commencement of takeoff, nor did he believe that they had received clearance. After the takeoff roll had commenced, the KLM flight engineer asked if Pam Am was clear of the runway. It was asked in a tentative and unsure manner and was curtly dismissed by both pilots.

Formation of Group Norms in the Tenerife Disaster

Although the aircraft were parked waiting for takeoff, the cockpit voice recorder on the KLM aircraft captured several concerns expressed by the crew that may have contributed to them feeling pressure to depart the airport quickly. These discussions, led by the KLM captain, established the cockpit crew's priorities and shaped the norms that would contribute to the accident. First, there was a question of duty time, which is the maximum number of hours a pilot can be on duty in a row. KLM's governing body in Belgium had recently changed the rules, making duty time more difficult to calculate, and with no discretion on the part of the pilots. The KLM captain and first officer discussed their concern about further delays encroaching on duty time and risking violation. Second, there was concern over the weather. With visibility so limited, it was a real concern that the airport would close, and the aircraft would be delayed much longer. Although these types of delays are common for line personnel, it is possible that a captain in upper management may have felt more responsibility for maintaining the airline's schedule.[7]

Task Saturation and Barriers to Teamwork in Flight 173

The risk associated with the crew's preoccupation with the emergency exceeded the risk the emergency itself posed. Despite having the fuel quantity information available to them, and having the means to calculate their remaining flying time, the information was not correctly understood by the captain and was not effectively communicated. Only once did the flight engineer express his concern about the low-fuel state and provide no additional information or details to the captain who, even as engines began flaming out, still believed he had sufficient fuel on board.

Origins of Crew Resource Management

In the 1970s, the airline industry had a problem. Several airline accidents had occurred with senior and experienced flight crews at the controls, and the accidents appeared to be caused by failures of interpersonal communications, decision-making, and leadership.[15] Throughout the latter half of the 1970s, the National Aeronautics and Space Administration's Aerospace Human Factors Research

Division had been tasked with studying the problems, and in 1979 it brought together the airline industry and key government agencies in a workshop to discuss their findings.[16] What was needed was improvement in teamwork, coordination, and an environment in which leadership encouraged subordinates' participation and critique. It was from here that the first generation of Crew Resource Management (CRM) was born.

CRM is a system that seeks to make optimum use of all available resources (equipment, procedures, and people) to promote safety and enhance the efficiency of flight operations.[11] Early CRM training emphasized the communication and managerial styles of the individuals to correct the under assertiveness of junior crew members, while reducing the excessively authoritarian behavior of senior crew members.[15] These efforts were bolstered by the National Transportation Safety Board (NTSB) in 1979. They included in their findings and probable cause of Flight 173's crash after running out of fuel that neither "the first officer nor the flight engineer conveyed any concern about fuel exhaustion to the captain." And the "failure of the other two crew members to either fully comprehend the criticality of the fuel state or to successfully communicate their concern to the captain" contributed to the cause.[14] For the first time, the NTSB had listed the failure of the crew's communication as a contributor to the accident. The greatest barrier to communication is the illusion that communication has occurred.

Throughout the 1980s, CRM continued to evolve. The emphasis on modifying management styles gave way to understanding cockpit group dynamics, emphasizing briefing strategies, SA, and breaking error chains. It was during this time that the name evolved as well. Recognizing that the concepts were really about the human interaction and not the equipment, the name changed to *crew resource management*. By the 1990s, CRM was spreading beyond the cockpit and including flight dispatchers, maintenance personnel, and cabin crew.

Operationalizing Teamwork: Crew Resource Management

Communication, teamwork, and an environment where all crew members have equal input, and their contributions are equally valued are the major tenets of CRM. Current concepts of CRM have at its center the acknowledgment that errors will occur, and all aspects of operation can be made safer by improving SA, communication, and decision-making through the efficient and timely use of all the available resources. CRM encompasses a wide range of assessment, communication, SA, problem-solving, decision-making, and teamwork.[11] Additionally, CRM is concerned with the interpersonal skills, interaction between members of the team, and standardization of procedures.

CRM's goals are not only to recognize and communicate that an error has occurred and to mitigate the effects of that error; but also to identify that an error is about to occur and prevent the error from occurring to begin with. To accomplish this, CRM seeks to address core problems of workload management and delegation, maintenance of SA, use of authority and assertiveness, utilizing all available resources including other crew members, and improving interpersonal communication.[17] CRM recognizes that very person on the team has a vested interest in the safe completion of the mission and ensures that every member has an opportunity, as well as an obligation, to voice their concerns and provide their assessment of situations, as well as provide courses of action the team should take. CRM values everyone's assessment, analysis, and suggestions. From the cockpit, medical crew,

communicators, and maintainers, every team member has a voice. Every team member is expected to respect and listen to the other members. As situations are assessed and decisions are being made, the team leader should actively seek input from all members. Policies such as "Three to Go, One to Say No" were implemented as a result of the move to CRM. Other improvements in communication include standardized handoffs during patient transfer, mission debriefs, standardized checklists, and standardized phrases and statements designed to reduce miscommunication.

CASE STUDY

Elaine Bromiley

On March 29, 2005, Mrs. Elaine Bromiley, a 37-year-old mother, underwent elective surgery to her nose.[18] In her preoperative anesthesia note, mouth opening was recorded as normal and neck movements as "slightly restricted" due to congenitally fused cervical vertebrae. No other note or particular concern was recorded, and the plan was for a general anesthetic with a laryngeal mask airway (LMA). At 0835, the anesthesia was induced with remifentanil and propofol, and an attempt was made to place the LMA. The muscular tone in the jaw proved to be too high and did not allow enough mouth opening. Believing that the patient was not deeply enough sedated, a repeat dose of propofol was given and a second attempt to place the LMA was made, as well as attempting placement with two smaller sizes of LMAs without success.

At 0837, Mrs. Bromiley's SpO_2 began to desaturate to 75%, and she became cyanotic and tachycardic. By 0839, her SpO_2 had fallen to 40% despite attempts to provide facemask ventilations with an oral airway. Shortly thereafter, her heart rate began to fall precipitously. Having already fallen to 69 beats per minute (bpm), it was now in the 40s. Around 0841, the decision was made to transition to endotracheal intubation, and Mrs. Bromiley was given atropine and succinylcholine. It was about this time that the anesthesiologist was joined in the operating room (OR) by a second anesthesiologist from an adjoining OR. On the first attempt at direct laryngoscopy (DL), a Connack-Lehane Grade IV (no laryngeal structure visible) was used. The SpO_2 remained less than 40%, although the heart rate had temporarily responded to the atropine and increased to the mid-60s.

Despite using a two-person technique, ventilation by facemask was described as extremely difficult and was ineffective at providing ventilation. The situation is now a can't-intubate-can't-ventilate emergency. Between 0847 and 0850, further attempts at DL intubation are made with a variety of instruments, without success. Fiberoptic attempts were made, but were unsuccessful because of blood in the airway.

At 0851, an additional anesthesiologist entered the OR and attempted DL intubations for an additional 4 minutes, and SpO_2 continued to remain less than 40%. At 0900, an LMA was placed successfully with a recovery of the SpO_2 to 90%. For the next 10 minutes, multiple additional attempts were made to intubate through the LMA with an occasional SpO_2 dipping as low as 49% but recovering to the 90s.

At 0910, it was decided to abandon the procedure and allow Mrs. Bromiley to awaken. At this point, Elaine Bromiley had been profoundly hypoxic in excess of 20 minutes. She did not regain consciousness, and after being transferred to the intensive care unit (ICU), she died a few days later.

Problem List That Crew Resource Management Had to Solve

Workload Management and Delegation

In a complex and technically advanced environment, how should workloads be managed and delegated to make the best use of the resources available to the crew? First, it must be understood that workload is not constant; rather, it is a constantly evolving state that shifts during different phases of a transport. Within a team, workload may impact different crew members at different times. The clinical crew has a very low workload en route to a patient and has a very high workload during a resuscitation. Similarly, the vehicle operator, be it an emergency medical technician (EMT) or pilot, may have a very low workload when the clinical team is preparing a patient for transport, but a very high workload during the transport phase. Understanding when the different team members have different workloads will help to properly time critical communication and tasking during the transport.

Different crew members are tasked with different workloads at different times, but not all work has the same priority. *Critical tasks* are ones that must be performed correctly at the right time to prevent harm to the team or the patient. Vehicle operation often involves critical tasking. Similarly, addressing apnea is a critical task in the clinical management of a patient and must precede other lower-priority tasks. One of the challenges of a transport environment is when there are multiple critical tasks occurring at the same time. A helicopter departing from an unsecured landing zone with a critical patient provides several critical tasks competing for attention, often referred to as Competing Priorities. When presented with such situations, they are managed in the following priority – safety of the team first and safety of the patient second. *Important tasks* will evolve into critical ones if they are not managed at the appropriate time. Replacing an intravenous vasopressor bag before it runs out is an important task because if it is not done, it will result in decline of the patient's hemodynamic status, prompting the critical task of resuscitating the patient to achieve an adequate mean arterial pressure (MAP). A *routine task* is a procedural step that, in and of itself, is neither important nor critical, but successful completion of the task is vital to recognize variations in the patient or the transport. The monitoring of blood pressure at a regular interval is a routine task that allows the identification of a situation that requires an important or critical task. Regardless of the timing of the workload, there are some consistencies in how individuals and teams react to different workloads.

Effects of High and Low Workloads

Response to workloads has a curvilinear bell-shaped relationship in which an optimum workload is in the center and performance trails off in either direction as workloads are underloaded or overloaded. During optimum workload, the individual or team is engaged and focused with enough reserve attention and energy to recognize and adapt to changes. This is in contrast to a team that is underloaded. In this state, the team has very little to challenge them; as a result, they have an overall lower level of attention, boredom may set in, and they may miss important environmental or clinical cues that the situation is changing or a new hazard is present. In an overloaded state, the team may begin to lose the larger picture as their attention begins to tunnel, SA begins to fail, and reasoning reverts to a pattern recognition mode in which team members return to old habits that have worked in the past. Additionally, overloaded teams may begin deviating from procedural standards and norms (Fig. 8.1).

Task Saturation

When a team or team member begins to have difficulty maintaining routine tasks or upholding procedural standards and norms because of an increased workload, that team or individual is task saturated. Any additional workload requires the displacement of a current task. Recognition of task saturation in yourself or your teammates allows the team to adjust to make the most of its resources. The signs that a teammate or team is task saturated vary based on the situation. They may include erratic errors or inconsistent performance, deviation from policy and procedure, indecision, fixation on a task or

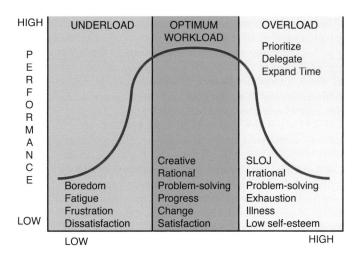

• **Figure 8.1** Effects of High and Low Workloads. (Redrawn from Smith D [n.d.]. CRM Resources, Workload Management, Briefings, Callouts, Checklist, Error Management, Darren Smith, Flight Instructor, CFI Homepage. Accessed March 10, 2017. http://www.cfidarren.com/crmworkload.htm.)

indication, distortion of time, or confused, halting speech. Scheduled tasks, medication doses, and record-keeping tasks may be missed. When task saturation is recognized, let the team know ("alright, we are task saturated right now"), and take steps to get caught up.

1. **Prioritize the critical tasks.** Ask the question: "What do we have to do now?" Then begin on those tasks. Set end points ("we need to start a heparin drip at 1000 units/hour") so that on its completion, you can reassess the priorities.

2. **Delegate tasks as able.** In specialized teams, there may be procedures or tasks that only particular team members can perform. Ensure those team members are free to complete their tasks by delegating tasks that others can perform to other team members. Appropriately use available people to perform tasks within their scope, so specialized team members are not prevented from completing tasks only they can perform.

3. **Expand available time.** Routine or less important tasks can be put off to free resources to manage the crisis or high tasking for the moment.

4. **Manage distractions.** Distractions are tasks or attention drains that have no bearing on the safe performance of the tasks at hand. They may be dealt with using some of the previously mentioned techniques, or they may be ignored outright. In error-prone situations, it may serve the team to develop a signal that the individual performing a task should not be interrupted for anything other than patient safety or crew safety. Similar to the use of a sterile cockpit during critical phases of flight, certain tasks have a high workload and high probability of error. Limiting communication to safety concerns prevents interruptions.

Task Saturation and Filtering Effects in the Tenerife Disaster

One of the earliest points the KLM crew could have intervened to prevent the accident was when the control tower said, "Okay ... standby for takeoff." That message, after the "okay," appears to never have been processed by the KLM crew. The reasons for their inability to process the message may have been task saturation at the time of takeoff and a filtering effect that prevented them from recognizing the transmission as coming from the control tower. Once the decision to take off had been made and the throttles advanced, the crew became absorbed in the task of taking off. Little attention was left for lower-priority information. To be processed, the message would need to overcome the attention filter that screens out lower-priority information while individuals are engaged in activities requiring high degrees of concentration. The transmission that followed, "hold for takeoff," was distorted by the simultaneous transmission from the Pan Am crew, thus removing the familiar voice that had been controlling them, making it sound distant and unrelated. The transmission failed to make it past the information filters of both pilots.

It is interesting to note the respective workload of the pilots and the flight engineers at the time the KLM flight engineer questioned if Pan Am was clear of the runway. When the flight engineer was "curtly dismissed," the pilots were at a peak workload accelerating down the runway, their attention was saturated, and their filters closed to anything but the most critical pieces of information. The KLM flight engineer had just completed the largest portion of his work and was less tasked, with a more open filter. Although it is apparent that the KLM flight engineer did not hear the tower's instruction to "standby for takeoff," he may have heard the Pan Am first officer respond to the tower shortly after with "okay, we will report clear." Questioning what they "will report clear" of may have prompted the KLM flight engineer to question where Pan Am was clear of the runway.

CASE STUDY

Blood Pressure Control Error

A ground-based critical care team consisting of an experienced team member and new team member were dispatched to a community hospital for a 59-year-old male with a subdural hematoma. The patient was hemodynamically stable, awake and alert, and nonintubated. Transporting this patient by critical care was a precaution and presented no complexity or challenge to the crew.

On arrival at the bedside, the newest team member went to obtain report, while the experienced team member assessed the patient and packaged him for transport. Both tasks were completed at the same time and when the new teammate returned to the bedside, the patient was ready to move to the ambulance as he asked, "did you get the story?" The experienced team member acknowledged his partner and said he had "gotten enough of it," but as they left the facility, both crew members had very different ideas about the cause of the head bleed. This was the first failure of CRM. They had an opportunity to share a mental model and make sure they were together in their thinking, but they did not take it. From report, the new teammate had learned that the head bleed was caused by a fall yesterday and was traumatic in nature, whereas his partner believed the head bleed to be spontaneous in nature. This misalignment would come into play during the course of the transport when the patient's blood pressure began to climb to a point when their standing orders required them to control the MAP as if it had been a spontaneous bleed. No such order existed for treating a traumatic head bleed.

After the blood pressure had cycled a couple of times and it was clear that the patient was in fact hypertensive, the more experienced crew member suggested starting nicardipine to lower the blood pressure. His teammate looked quizzical and suggested, "how about just some more fentanyl instead." It was clear to the experienced team member that his partner did not agree with the proposed treatment plan, but he did not question him about why. Instead, he dismissed his partner's hesitation without acknowledging it, allowing himself to believe he knew the reason for his partner's hesitation (his newness to the program, lack of familiarity with standing orders, etc.), and proceeded with his proposed plan of care. This was the second and third failure of CRM. The experienced team member recognized the concern of his partner but failed to act on it, and his partner failed to assert himself enough to be heard and understood when he believed an error was about to occur. Although in this case no harm befell the patient, it is easy to see how it may have been in a similar circumstance.

Maintaining Situational Awareness

In essence, SA is knowing what is happening around you in such a way that you are able to anticipate near-future events. There are several processes that take place as we develop an SA of our environment moment by moment and a host of pitfalls can be encountered as we do so. Individuals must perceive information from their environment, comprehend that information correctly, use that information to construct a model of what is about to happen in the near future, and base their actions off the results of that model. Each of those components – perception, comprehension, and projection – can have errors that render the individual's understanding of their situation incorrect and outdated, leading to impaired judgments and a potentially harmful outcome to the patient or team (see Fig. 8.1).

Situational Awareness and Decision-Making

For SA to exist within a team, the members that constitute it must feed information forward to build a comprehensive understanding without overwhelming or disrupting the decision-making process.[19] *When a team first encounters a challenge, whether clinical or operational, it begins a process of building its SA by observing and orienting to the environment and the challenges within which it is operating. This process, described by Colonel John Boyd as the "OODA Loop," describes how the individual cycles through a process of Observing, Orienting, Deciding on an action, and then Acting (Fig. 8.2).*[19]

The first task, observing, involves the team developing an awareness of those things around them that may impact the situation. Whether that team has a designated leader for a portion of the task or is responsible for all of the operations, the leader must develop this understanding using information fed to them from technology and teammates. The problem is that each of these data points is obtained from a different, although similar, point of view. In a clinical interaction, this observation phase may involve understanding patient assessment, laboratory data, vital signs, the anxiety of the sending staff, and the wishes of the patient. In an operational context, this may include vehicle type and availability, weather conditions (present and forecast), patient stability, out-of-hospital time, crew resources, crew experience, patient risks, and so on. Each one of these points is delivered through the sender's point of view. Information must be validated for its accuracy and its relevancy to the situation. More information is not necessarily good, as you must validate any additional information you acquire. You must learn to be specific and efficient as you gather information.

The second phase of the loop focuses attention on one or more discrepancies or challenges presented in the situation and establishes their priorities within the greater context. For example, in a clinical setting, there is a low systolic blood pressure reading that has been observed by a teammate. This fact in isolation does not give the leader the information required to act. Is the patient a penetrating trauma patient? Should lower blood pressure be accepted in the name of hypotensive resuscitation? Does the patient have low blood pressure at baseline, so this is not a deviation at all? Without orientation to make sense of the observation, meaningful intervention becomes difficult. Thus the leader must assemble these pieces using their previous experience, analysis, and organizational guidelines, as well as their own observations and the information from teammates to decide on an appropriate action.

It is now possible to see how information delivered by a teammate with poorly calibrated urgency, or poor timing, can skew the orientation process and disrupt a decision-making process. This is particularly true when the situation presents itself as a crisis requiring

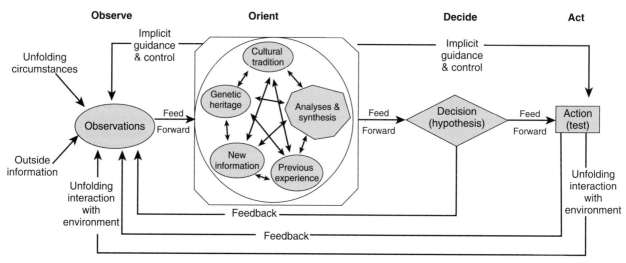

Observe   **Orient**   **Decide**   **Act**

• **Figure 8.2** The OODA Loop. (Redrawn from Boyd J. The essence of winning and losing. June 28, 1995. In: Brehmer B. *The Dynamic OODA Loop: Amalgamating Boyd's OODA Loop and the Approach to Command and Control.* The International Command and Control Institute; 2006.)

immediate and decisive action. In the previous case study United Flight 173, the pilot-in-command (PIC) had prioritized the troubleshooting of his landing gear light. The flight engineer knew the diminishing fuel supply was becoming an increasing hazard to the safe completion of the flight but pushed that information to the PIC in such a way that the urgency was not communicated and in language that allowed the PIC to misinterpret it as pounds of fuel instead of minutes remaining. In doing so, the flight engineer's information was given a low priority in the PIC's orienting process and not considered as decisions were made about when to land.

Thus when information is forwarded to a leader, it is imperative that the crew member advancing that information ensures both that it is correctly timed and that the appropriate degree of urgency is appreciated by the leader receiving it. Poorly timed information delivered in a crisis situation results in the attention of the leader being temporarily placed on something that not only does not contribute to the solution but detracts from the resources available to meet the challenge.

Recognizing Lost Situational Awareness, and Recovering It

In the case study about Elaine Bromiley, there was a fundamental loss of SA. There were sufficient staff and resources available, the procedure was elective, and the staff were experienced and well-trained. The initial failure was not one of technique, but of awareness, when the clinicians became fixated on completing the task and lost sight of the patient's safety. At no point did the two anesthesiologists or the ear, nose, and throat surgeon ever state out loud what was happening. Although the physicians seemed to have been late in realizing that the patient was in trouble, the nursing staff present was experienced and was aware of the risk to the patient early on. They independently brought in the surgical airway tray, announced its presence, and called for an ICU bed for the patient. What the nursing staff detected was a state in which the team was no longer meeting the planned goals, had an increasing fixation and tunnel vision, and was experiencing unresolved discrepancies in the information they were receiving. These are key moments when the team may be able to recognize that they have lost SA in the moment. The clues, however, are extremely difficult to detect by the individuals involved in the crisis. This is why each team member must be allowed to express their concerns, and be heard

by the team and its leader. Additionally, the team must have a practiced response to loss of SA, either in the operational or clinical realms. Those responses include the following:

1. **Announce the problem to the team.** State in clear terms what the problem or hazard is.
2. **Create time or space distance between the team and the hazard.** In a clinical setting, this may involve slowing or stopping the decline of a particular vital sign and providing temporizing care while the specific solution to the condition is sought or readied. In an operational setting, like in an aircraft, this may be increasing altitude in response to an accidental encounter with instrument meteorologic conditions.
3. **Stabilize the condition.** In addition to reversing the impact of the problem condition, stabilizing the condition also involves avoiding unnecessary complications to the situation and creating an increasing degree of margin allowing for latitude of action.
4. **Give the team enough time to get caught up to the situation.** Once the team is out of immediate danger, or the patient has been stabilized, time should be taken to assess if the original plan is still the correct one, or if a new plan is required.

Although the nursing staff in the Elaine Bromiley case recognized the loss of SA, they did not feel they had a mechanism with which to raise their concerns to the physician team, nor did they feel they would be heard if they had. How to communicate within the team during a crisis is the next problem that the principles of CRM seek to solve.

When and How to Communicate Within a Team

Each team member must have the skills and sensitivity to transmit information in an increasingly clear, bold, and concise manner as the team faces challenges and hazards. CRM seeks to improve safety of the team and the patient by emphasizing how to communicate effectively, recognize the barriers to effective communication, and overcome them. Communication within a team is a two-way process that begins with the sender encoding a message and transmitting it to the receiver. It is important when communicating within a team that both the content of the message and the tone with which it is delivered communicate the same meaning. Other considerations must be given to the volume that the situation

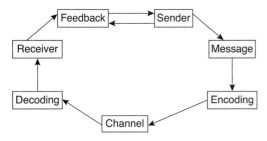

• **Figure 8.3** Effective Communication Cycle. (Redrawn from Patil M, Patil S. Process of Communication, Two Way Process of Communication. July 26, 2013. Accessed March 10, 2017. http://articles-junction.blogspot.com/2013/07/process-of-communication-two-way.html)

requires and to the timing of the message. Sending information when the intended recipient is unable to receive it or process it is ineffective. Once the message is encoded, it is transmitted across the medium. That may be just a spoken word in a room, or it may be across a radio, a phone, or an aircraft's intercom system. One of the challenges in communicating in a transport environment is that often, the nonverbal component of communication, responsible for expressing much of the message in routine face-to-face communications, is missing. This makes it even more important that the sender verifies that the message sent was the one received (Fig. 8.3).[20]

At the center of CRM's focus on communication is the mandate that *it is the responsibility of the person sending the message to ensure that they are understood.* All too often, what is intended by the sender is not what is understood by the receiver. Steps to ensure an effective message include the following:
1. Stating one idea at a time
2. Stating things simply
3. Encourage feedback
4. Repeat and explain as required

In times of crisis, when immediate action from the team is required, the order of communication also becomes important. For example, an air medical crew member sees an immediate hazard to the helicopter as it lands on a country road. There is a barbed wire fence obscured by high grass that poses a risk of striking the tail rotor if the aircraft continues to land in the direction it is currently moving. Time is short, and the first thing the crew member needs to express is the action that is required to avoid the accident; this is *directive communication.* "Abort!" or "Go around!" delivered with the appropriate degree of urgency and at an appropriate volume gives direction to the pilot to avoid the impact. Only then, after the aircraft is free of the hazard, does the crew member use *descriptive communication* to describe the reason for the direction given, "fence line, at 6 o'clock." There are times when certain hazards may be anticipated, either operationally or clinically. In those circumstances, it can serve the team to brief specific language to be used if that hazard is encountered. If, for example, a team is moving a patient on an intraaortic balloon pump and the pump is being pulled behind the patient, it improves patient safety if, before moving the patient, the team states, "if at any point someone sees a problem during movement, say the word *stop,* and everyone immediately will stop movement." This seems intuitive, but often people will use more causal language, such as "hold on," "just a second," or even "ok" to indicate the need to stop. In a situation in which a snag or a stumble could result in the displacement of the device sitting in the aorta, the delay while the team decodes the intent of the message could have dire results. Once the message is encoded by the sender and transmitted across the medium, a variety of barriers may exist between the sender and the receiver. Understanding these barriers will aid the crew member in overcoming them.

Barriers to Communication

Identifying barriers to communication and mitigating their effects is key to successful communication. In the transport medicine environment, physical barriers to communication are commonly encountered. These may include environmental factors such as walls or other physical objects, excessive noise, poor lighting conditions, the distance between the sender and the receiver, or safety equipment, such as masks. Different languages or even different dialects of the same language can skew or block the intended information or prevent effective communication.[21] Words, phrases, gestures, and body language from one location or culture often have different meanings in different locations or cultures.[21] Poor diction, font, penmanship, and even ink color can make the deciphering process very difficult for the receiver.

Lack of attention or interest from sender or receiver will often result in inaccurate information being sent or received. When the words of the sender are different than their nonverbal communication, a level of uncertainty is created.[22] Each person sends and receives information through their own filter, which is created based on experiences. We are each responsible for awareness of our internal filters, as well as the barriers and distortions those filters may put on information that is sent or received.[23] Distractions frequently impair the ability to concentrate on the task of communication. Examples of distractions that may impair effective communication may be other people talking, cell phone or radio use, time constraints, task overload, activities occurring in the environment that may capture the sender or the receiver's attention, and fatigue.

Optimize Communication

Face-to-face communication is best, as it enhances the clarity of the message being sent by allowing for immediate feedback and requests for validation, as well as the pairing of verbal and nonverbal communication. Written communication has the advantage of being stored, to confirm the words and timing of a prior message. Mixing varied types of communication can effectively strengthen the message being received. Simple examples of mixing various types of communication are verbal and nonverbal communication, or visual and verbal communication in a conference or presentation setting. The delivery of a message is an important variable in communication. Messages should be simple, concise, and clear; communicating one concept at a time, confirming the message has been accurately received, then moving on to the next concept.

When the safety of the vehicle or patient is imminently threatened, the crew should have a predetermined word that communicates the urgency of the threat. Instances would include an intraaortic balloon pump tubing that is caught and threatens to dislodge the balloon, or an obstacle that threatens the safe landing at a landing zone. "STOP" is often used, and all activity is halted, the threat is clearly communicated and is able to be managed.

Another technique is to clearly announce the name or title of the intended recipient, state your specific concern, state the threat that is posed, and your proposed solution. "Annie, the balloon tubing is hanging off the side of the stretcher, we may catch it on a door handle, we must stop and better secure that tubing."

Task Fixation

The relationship between workload and available attention for effective communication was discussed in the previous section. This behavior may be evident in tasks requiring a high degree of concentration or ones that have high stakes attached to them. The act of intubating a critically ill patient serves as a good example. This is a high-risk activity that also has a great deal of social pressure on the person instrumenting the airway; as, typically, the majority of the team stops and waits while this task is completed. Task preoccupation may be avoided by empowering the team to intercede at a designated point if a team member goes beyond it; for example, the briefing at the beginning of the airway procedure states, "if the saturations fall below 95%, stop me, we will back out and bag the patient." Doing this makes it clear to the team that not only is it okay to stop you, but you are asking them to do it.

When a team member is task fixated and is not hearing a message, using the person's proper name, title, or rank helps break through their focus and ensure the message is heard. There may be times when a teammate's task fixation is severe enough to prompt more assertive behavior. The *two-challenge rule* is an agreement within a team. When an unsafe condition is present, the team will advise the team leader, or person performing the procedure, of that hazard or condition, e.g., "the saturations are falling." If that message is not acknowledged, then the team member repeats the message using the name or title of the individual, with increased urgency and with a recommended action: "John, the sats are falling below 80%, we have to bag the patient." If the individual does not acknowledge the second message, then the teammate takes action to correct the problem. In this case, they begin bagging the patient.

Rank and Experience Differences

When there is a significant difference in rank or experience between teammates, there can be a reluctance to challenge plans or question actions for fear of the consequences extending beyond the momentary situation. The experienced or ranking member expressly stating their openness to questions and their ability to make mistakes can overcome this barrier. The other pitfall of rank and experience can be *excessive professional courtesy*, which is a hesitancy of less senior or lower-ranking teammates to challenge or insult the more experienced or higher-ranking teammate's skills. Communication patterns in these situations tend to be passive and avoid direct confrontation.

Overcoming the Barriers: The Practice of Assertiveness Within a Team

Assertiveness is the ability of a teammate to state and maintain a position even if that position is contrary to the prevailing opinion of the group. Further, that individual maintains their position until they are persuaded by the facts and is not swayed by the authority or personality of the other team members. Within the context of CRM, effective leaders expect and advocate for open and questioning communication from their crewmates. At the heart of assertiveness is the belief that each individual on the team has the right to express ideas and feelings, the right to be heard by the team, the right to be taken seriously, the right to ask for clarification, and the right to be treated with respect. *Teammates must speak up when they are unsure of instructions or a plan of action, when they believe they have a solution to the problem, or when they believe the crew or patient is in danger.*

How we practice assertiveness in a high-stress environment, particularly with a high task loading, is as important as when we practice it. There are four key elements to communicating a concern in this setting:

1. Use the intended recipient's proper name or title.
2. State a specific concern.
3. State what you believe the consequence of that concern will be if it is not addressed.
4. Propose your solution.

In all of the case studies presented thus far, one member of the respective teams following this procedure may have prevented disaster. In the Tenerife disaster, had the flight engineer stated, "Captain (stating proper title) I am not sure we have been cleared for takeoff (stating specific concern) Pan Am may still be on the runway (perceived consequence), abort the takeoff (proposed solution)," the disaster may have been averted. In the case of Elaine Bromiley, had the nursing staff stated, "Doctor, the patient's saturations are below 50%, we are in a can't-intubate can't-ventilate situation, we need to move to a surgical airway," her death may have been avoided.

Often, when time is less critical, a fifth step should be included: seeking feedback from the team. Conflicts within a team should be viewed as differences of opinion and approached open-mindedly with a focus on finding the solution as opposed to defending positions.

When team members are called to act, and assertiveness is required, two factors often influence the decision to speak up and be heard. The first factor is anticipation of the team's reaction, and the second is the perceived difference in experience, rank, or authority. Often, in a team setting, when something appears to be going wrong, team members look to the rest of the team and judge their reaction to the situation. If other team members do not appear to be concerned, then the individual with the concern is less likely to speak up. The second factor that may prevent speaking up is the belief that in doing so we would be questioning authority. *It is imperative that the senior crew empower the junior crew to speak up and question plans and actions.* Each of these factors is amplified in effect when an individual lacks confidence, believes a teammate is not approachable or is disinterested, fears reprisal, or is hesitant to invite conflict.

Sharing the Mental Model

A shared understanding of a task and the context of why it is being performed is the idea behind a shared mental model. This may take the form of recapping events, defining where the team is at in a problem, and deciding what the next steps are; this approach has been demonstrated to improve team performance.[24] This sharing of a mental model is often undertaken by the team leader but may be initiated by any member of the team as a means to bring some clarity to the situation. Additionally, mental model sharing provides the team leader the opportunity to invite alternate ideas and perspectives from the team.

Lack of Shared Mental Model in the Blood Pressure Control Error

In the case of Emily Bromiley, both crew members recognized the change in the patient's status and the change in blood pressure. However, because of a lack of a shared understanding of the patient's condition, the significance of that change held different meanings for the respective crew members, which promoted contradictory actions.

Recognizing Decision-Making Hazards

Strength of an Idea

When confronted with a time-sensitive emergency, there is a tendency for an individual to grasp the first seemingly appropriate explanation or action without considering the alternatives. This is particularly true if the person offering up the solution is perceived to have expertise or authority. Once the group has grasped that one solution, it can be extremely difficult to change directions, even when contradictory evidence is presented.

Groupthink

Groupthink can be described as a situation where the team decides to pursue an action without consideration of alternative solutions. Additionally, the team may continue to rationalize the decision, even when evidence that is contrary to the current action is presented or identified.[25] When a team has a high task loading, or during an emergency, voicing a perspective that is contrary to the prevailing thoughts of the team may be perceived by an individual as increasing the stress of the group and something that should be avoided. Consequently, the single team member may not be comfortable providing information that conflicts with the group consensus, even if that information may be vital to the safe treatment or movement of the patient or the safety of the crew. Research has suggested that the more cohesive the group, the more likely it is that individuals will prioritize group harmony over the introduction of alternative perspectives or the exploration of additional options.[25] This effect is intensified if the team leader is the person promoting the preferred solution.[25] It is critical that team members actively seek to identify and avoid groupthink and, when it is recognized, notify the team of what is believed to be happening: "We may be experiencing groupthink," and ask for any alternative ideas or perspectives.

Seeking the Perfect Solution

Seeking the perfect solution is a characteristic often found in newer team members. It is a tendency to seek the perfect solution or diagnosis at the exclusion of other appropriate and safe actions. This tendency may prevent any action from being taken and may allow the emergency to worsen. This tendency can be dealt with by first looking for safe, workable solutions and then improving on those solutions as time allows.[11]

Leadership

Most of what has been discussed in this chapter applies to the roles of leadership. The CRM principles of leadership seek to balance the authority of the team leader with the previously mentioned assertiveness of the team, thus allowing for decisive action when required and an environment open to input. As important as it is for the team to speak up when required, the team leader mustn't hinder or withhold team input. They need to encourage crew member input during planning and task completion, clearly stating the team's goals or intentions, and be flexible enough to change those plans if the team provides feedback that should be used.

Use of All Available Resources

Throughout all of this, the central theme has been that when confronting a challenge or a routine tasking, an effective team uses all available resources to ensure the safe care and movement of a patient. The principles applied here shape the interactions, regardless of the team makeup, to provide the safest possible means of moving a sick or injured patient.

Human Performance

Human performance in times of crisis is a matter of how well an individual or a team is prepared to meet the emergency, how well-equipped that team is, and how well it manages acute stress. While environmental stressors, such as a high workload, heat, cold, noise, vibration, and sleep deprivation, are inherent in the transport medicine environment, the acute stress of unique situations or patients is a compounding factor.

Acute stress is the result of situations that involve a novel situation, an unpredictable outcome, or a threat to the ego of an individual or team. The acute stress response is mediated by the sympathetic nervous system and is driven by the flight, fight, or freeze response. Individuals must understand how external stressors affect their abilities, and recognize the effects of acute stress so it can be managed appropriately to ensure maximum performance in this challenging environment.

Task Performance and External Stress

In 1908, Yerkes and Dodson developed a model that described how separate tasks require various degrees of arousal to complete but, at a certain point, tasks requiring high-order thinking begin to fail as arousal increases, and simple tasks remain intact.[26] These findings have evolved to suggest an optimal stress-performance zone, in which performance was enhanced at a moderate stress level and degraded as the individual became either under-stimulated (low stress) or overwhelmed (high stress). This theory has evolved to be described as the "Inverted U" of performance under stress (Fig. 8.4).

This curvilinear representation of stress and performance suggests performance increases as stress levels increase, until it is impaired by excessive states of stress. Although this model is useful and explains aspects of individual performance at different stress levels, the problem with the model extrapolated from the work of Yerkes and Dodson is that different stressors affect performance differently, suggesting that there is no universal stress response.[27] For example, Broadbent described how the loss of sleep affected speed but not accuracy of simple tasks, whereas heat stress affected accuracy but not speed and only typically at the beginning of a task. In his latter works Broadbent demonstrated that increasing stress narrowed attention and limited the range of information that was being perceived and processed.[28] What we are left with is a nonlinear effect of stress on performance. The evidence suggests

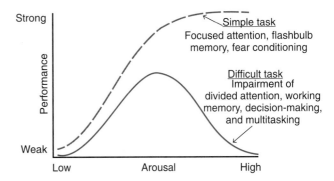

• **Figure 8.4** Stress and Performance. (Redrawn from Diamond DM, Campbell AM, Park CR, et al. The temporal dynamics model of emotional memory processing. *Neural Plast*. 2007. doi:10.1155/2007/60803)

that, as opposed to higher arousal states leading to improved performance until stress reaches a point where performance declines, the stress response is dependent on the type of stressor.[28]

Responses to External Stressors

Effects of Workload

Workload can be understood as the relationship between the amount of work needing to be done (often referred to as task loading), the time available, and the amount of cognitive resources committed to the task (work capacity). It represents the cost to an individual's team as they attempt to adapt to that work with limited attention and concentration. The cost of high workloads can be identified in the form of increased fatigue, stress, and errors[29] as the amount of resources required exceeds the amount of resources available. Common errors during high workloads include slower reaction times and communication errors. When multiple concurrent demands are placed on a crew member, those tasks may interact in one of several ways. Tasks may interfere with each other by either confusing or competing with other tasks. For example, placing a central line competes and interferes with the task of maintaining SA of the patient's condition. The greater the requirement for attention (in this case to place a central line), the more likely the clinician is to lose sight of the patient's condition. When the clinician attempts to simultaneously perform both tasks, the limited resource of attention will result in a degradation of one or both of the tasks.[30] If the clinician elects to switch between tasks – first attending to the procedure, stopping, then attending to the understanding of the patient's condition – before returning to the procedure, they may be more effective. The ability to effectively task switch is dependent on the degree of similarity among the tasks. The more dissimilar a task is, the more effectively an individual can switch between them without seeing degradation in one of the tasks. Thus in the previously mentioned case, the more motor-based skill of placing a central line is significantly different from the primarily cognitive task of assessing the patient's condition. Furthermore, the more practiced a task is, or the more expertise present in the individual, the less negative the effect is when switching behaviors or simultaneously performing both tasks.[31]

Thermal Stress

The effect of thermal stress, both heat and cold, on crew performance is related to the severity of those conditions, with the majority of cognitive impairment occurring in extremes of cold.[26] If a breakdown in thermal regulation is excluded from consideration, the predominant source of cognitive impairment involving information processing is a result of the distraction caused by the extremes of temperature. In terms of heat, initial exposure has been found to have little effect on strength. However, as exposure time increases, evidence of increased levels of fatigue,[32] decreases in vigilance,[33] and decreases in accuracy[34] is found.

Effects of Noise

Understanding the effect of noise on performance requires that first, we describe the temporal characteristics of that stimulus (i.e., is the noise continuous or intermittent). Continuous noise seems to have little effect on simple task performance,[35] at even relatively high decibel (dB) levels. As tasks become increasingly complex, however, continuous noise, especially above 95 dB, induces increasing numbers of errors, occasional slow responses, and some impairment of memory, often occurring after approximately 30 minutes of exposure.[36]

Intermittent noise, however, appears to be significantly more disruptive than continuous noise, specifically if the intermittent noise comes at unpredictable intervals. When a new noise is present in the environment, there is a notable decline in the performance of individuals, as the intermittent noise causes additional cognitive load and performing additional tasks is more difficult.[36] This effect will be minimized as the individual adapts to the noise and the task. As long as the tasks being performed are well practiced and the noises are familiar, there should be little effect on performance. The performance of a new task, paired with the introduction of a novel noise, however, could result in a marked, although temporary, reduction in performance.

Effects of Fatigue

It will come as little surprise that sleep deprivation results in performance degradation, including difficulty in monitoring data, increased distraction, focusing on the primary task while neglecting peripheral information, and delays in response and consistency.[37] Some of those fatigue effects may be moderated by failures of motivation in sleep-deprived states. Matthews and Desmond demonstrated, while studying drivers, that when task demands are low, the effort to perform well is found to be low as well; however, when requisite levels of stress are introduced, many of the effects of fatigue can be mediated and performance preserved.[38] The authors went on to suggest that interventions geared toward enhancing motivation would be more effective in mitigating fatigue in the short term than efforts geared at minimizing attention demands.

The degree of sleep deprivation has a linear relationship to the degree of impact on performance. In an experiment performed by Van Dongen et al., the authors investigated the extent to which sleep can be restricted before the development of cognitive deficits. Two groups were assigned either 4 hours or 6 hours of sleep for a period lasting 3 days. Both groups demonstrated a linear reduction of cognitive performance but differed greatly in their ability to recognize their impairment. After 3 days, the group limited to 6 hours of sleep per night functioned at an equivalent level to an individual deprived of all sleep for 2 days, but they tended not to be aware of their inability to perform at normal levels.[39] The effects of fatigue seem to be less evident when the tasks being performed are self-paced, but more apparent when the tasks are externally paced.[34]

Responses to Acute Stress

Acute stress is driven by fear, which is the recognition by an individual that something in the environment poses a danger to their emotional well-being or their physical self. Imagine an experienced clinician responding to a cardiac arrest caused by an intentional overdose. There is likely very little acute stress in that circumstance. It is not a novel situation for the experienced clinician, and they expect to perform well. Now imagine the same circumstance but the cardiac arrest immediately followed the administration of an overdose of a medication given by this same clinician. The patient's condition is no different, his physiology has not changed, but the stress level of the clinician has increased monumentally. What is different in the circumstance? The clinician in the second scenario is attached to the outcome and consequences of the resuscitation, resulting in an acute stress reaction to the event.

When acute stress presents itself, the sympathetic nervous system adapts the body for a physical response; adrenal glands release adrenalin, muscles tense, blood pressure rises, and heart rate increases. This increase in heart rate correlates with performance and is a marker of the degree of stress the individual is under.

Stress and Heart Rate

As stress levels increase, the sympathetic surge drives heart rates higher with effects on our mentation and motor skills that are significantly different from high heart rates obtained during exercise. There are predictable points in this escalation when our performance begins to alter. Grossman and Christensen[40] described that when we first identify a threat, or are faced with a potential threat, our heart rates increase to between 90 and 115 bpm as our bodies begin to respond by increasing awareness, but we have not begun to prepare ourselves for the full flight or flight response yet. When faced with greater stress, or more immediate danger, the authors described how our heart rates climb between 115 and 145 bpm, preparing us to make the most of our gross motor skills and enhance our rapid visual and cognitive reaction time. The cost of this preparation is degradation in our fine motor skills, which is observed above a heart rate of 115 bpm. Beyond 145 bpm, our performance begins to drop off, with loss of peripheral vision, depth perception, and near vision, as well as auditory exclusion (Fig. 8.5).

After the Adrenaline

It is common after an acute stress reaction and a resolution of the emergency for there to be a period of almost giddiness. For example, after a particularly difficult or dicey intubation, there is a collective release of the tension in the resuscitation bay or ambulance. Staff may start joking or talking about weekend plans. This is the result of the parasympathetic surge that follows the high-stress encounter. It is also a time of danger for the patient and crew because SA is lowered.

Improving Performance Under Stress

Emotional Awareness

The ability of an individual's emotional awareness to mitigate stressor states is summarized by a document on Stress, Cognition, and Human Performance, published by NASA:

> There is some evidence to suggest that individuals with greater awareness of their emotional states—the ability to label their current feelings—perform better under stress than those unable to do so. Worchel and Yohai (1979) found that individuals who were able to label or identify the novel physiologic reactions they experienced under stress were less distressed by them and they performed better. Similarly, Gohm, Baumann, and Shiezak (2001) noted that individuals who are able to label or identify their emotional reactions to stressful events appear to have more attentional resources (perhaps due to engaging in fewer ruminations) to devote to tasks. The result is improved performance compared with those who are not able to label their emotional experience. It seems reasonable to conclude from these findings that cognitive appraisal is at least one explanatory mechanism. Those who can introspect and cognitively frame their experience are likely to feel better and improve their sense of control and predictability over their reactions than those unable to do so. These factors have previously been shown to be of value in reducing the negative effects of stress exposure.[26]

Stress Inoculation

To fortify an individual or a team against some of the effects of stress, training can be developed to simulate those conditions in an otherwise safe and controlled environment. The increasingly realistic nature of the simulated encounters makes stress inoculation different from rehearsal and other psychomotor training. Stress inoculation, through an iterative approach, helps individuals or teams that are exposed to it, become more familiar with stressful situations, learn what can generally be expected in those situations, and how outcomes can be influenced by changing variables. This process allows participants to reframe their paradigm of stressful situations into a more positive perspective while developing confidence and a sense of mastery.[26] Furthermore, this approach helps build a routine around what might have been an anxiety-producing situation.

Training Fine Motor Tasks With Stress in Mind

When training for tasks or new procedures, repetition under increasing stress will develop a motor pattern that will remain intact despite higher levels of stress. How a provider anchors their hand while holding an instrument to perform a critical procedure should be rehearsed in a manner that resembles a high-stress environment and assumes fine motor skills will be impaired. This can be mimicked by practicing skills and procedures immediately following strenuous physical activity.

Tactical Breathing

Designed by the military, tactical breathing allows for a targeted reduction in heart rate and stress level during times of acute stress. Also referred to as box breathing, it involves breathing in for 4 seconds, holding the breath for 4 seconds, exhaling for 4 seconds, and holding the exhale for 4 seconds. Doing this several times before or during a stressful situation will help regulate your sympathetic surge and keep you in a heart rate range appropriate for the situation in which you find yourself (Fig. 8.6). More information on stress and stress management can be found in Chapter 24 of this text.

Conclusion

The key to operating in the dynamic, high-stress environment of transport medicine safely and effectively is to develop a team of people that are united in a common goal, can maintain SA, and are who effectively communicate with each other and other stakeholders to safeguard each other and the patient. This requires

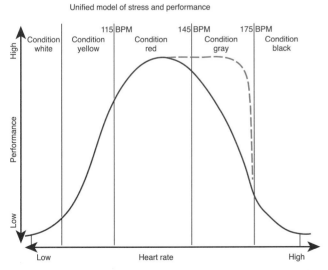

• **Figure 8.5** Stress and Heart Rate. (Redrawn from Grossman D, Christensen LW. *On Combat: The Psychology and Physiology of Deadly Conflict in War and Peace.* Warrier Science Publication; 2008.)

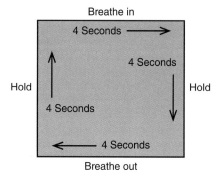

Breathe in

4 Seconds

4 Seconds

Hold

4 Seconds

Hold

4 Seconds

Breathe out

• **Figure 8.6** Tactical Breathing.

that we understand how we communicate in a team, what barriers may get in the way, and how to overcome them in stressful situations. By leveraging each team member's experience and expertise, we can better prevent errors and more effectively manage challenges.

References

1. Helmreich RL, Klinect JR, Wilhelm JA. System safety and threat and error management: The line operations safety audit. *Proceedings of the Eleventh International Symposium on Aviation Psychology.* The Ohio State University; 2001.
2. Ferner RE, Aronson JK. Clarification of terminology in medication errors: Definitions and classification. *Drug Saf.* 2006;29(11):1011–1022.
3. Aronson JK. Medication errors: Definitions and classification. *Br J Clin Pharmacol.* 2009;67(6):599–604.
4. Endsley MR. Toward a theory of situational awareness in dynamic systems. *Human Factors.* 1995;37(1):32–64.
5. Reason J. *Human Error.* Cambridge University Press; 1990.
6. McCreary J, Pollard M, Stevenson K, Wilson M. Human factors: Tenerife revisited. *J Air Transp World Wide.* 1998;3(1):23–32. Accessed July 30, 2023. https://rosap.ntl.bts.gov/view/dot/13937
7. Rotisch PA, Babcock GL, Edmunds WW. Human Factors Report on the Tenerife Accident. 1977. Accessed January 29, 2023. www.project-tenerife.com; http://www.project-tenerife.com/engels/PDF/alpa.pdf
8. Ardant D'Picq C. *Battle Studies: Ancient and Modern.* Military Service Publishing; 1947.
9. Rego A, Owens B, Yam KC, et al. Leader humility and team performance: Exploring the mediating mechanisms of team PsyCap and task allocation effectiveness. *J. Manag.* 2019;45(3):1009–1033. doi:10.1177/0149206316688941
10. Koohang A, Paliszkiewicz J, Goluchowski J. The impact of leadership on trust, knowledge management, and organizational performance: A research model. *Ind Manag Data Syst.* 2017;117(3):521–537. doi:10.1108/IMDS-02-2016-0072
11. Buljac-Samardžić M, Dekker-van Doorn CM, Maynard MT. What do we really know about crew resource management in healthcare?: An umbrella review on Crew Resource Management and its effectiveness. *J Patient Saf.* 2021;17(8). doi:10.1097/pts.0000000000000816
12. Grover E, Porter JE, Morphet J. An exploration of emergency nurses' perceptions, attitudes and experience of teamwork in the emergency department. *Aust Emerg Nurs J.* 2017;20(2):92–97. doi:10.1016/j.aenj.2017.01.003
13. Lee K. Simple ways to make your team feel valued. *Harvard Business Review.* July 20, 2022. Accessed February 1, 2023. https://hbr.org/2022/07/simple-ways-to-make-your-team-feel-valued
14. National Transportation Safety Board. *Aircraft Accident Report: United Airlines Inc., Douglas DC-8-54, N8082U, Portland, Oregon, December 28, 1978 (NTSB-AAR-79-7).* Government Printing Office; 1979.
15. Helmreich RL, Merritt AC, Wilhelm JA. The evolution of crew resource management training in commercial aviation. *Int J Aviat Psychol.* 1999;9(1):19–32.
16. Cooper GE, White MD, Lauber JK, eds. *Resource Management on the Flight Deck: Proceedings of a NASA/Industry Workshop (NASA Conference Publication 2120).* Government Printing Office; 1979.
17. Kanki BG, Helmreich RL, Anca J. *Crew Resource Management.* Academic Press; 2010.
18. Michael H. The case of Elaine Bromiley: Independent review on the care given to Mrs. Elaine Bromiley on March 29, 2005. 2005. Accessed July 30, 2023. http://s753619566.websitehome.co.uk/wp-content/uploads/2018/06/ElaineBromileyAnonymousReport.pdf
19. Brehmer B. 10th International Command and Control Research and Technology Symposium. In *The Dynamic OODA Loop: Amalgamating Boyd's OODA Loop and the Approach to Command and Control.* Symposium conducted at the Department of War Studies, Stockholm, Sweden; 2006. Accessed February 2, 2023. http://www.dodccrp.org/events/10th_ICCRTS/CD/papers/365.pdf
20. Endsley MR, Garland DJ. *Situation Awareness Analysis and Measurement.* CRC Press; 2008.
21. Norouzinia R, Aghabarari M, Shiri M, Karimi M, Samami E. Communication barriers perceived by nurses and patients. *Glob J Health Sci.* 2015;8(6):65. doi:10.5539/gjhs.v8n6p65
22. Wanko Keutchafo EL, Kerr J, Jarvis MA. Evidence of nonverbal communication between nurses and older adults: A scoping review. *BMC Nursing.* 2020;19(1). doi:10.1186/s12912-020-00443-9
23. Padilla Cruz M. Interlocutors-related and hearer-specific causes of misunderstanding: Processing strategy, confirmation bias and weak vigilance. *Res Lang.* 2017;15(1):11–36. doi:10.1515/rela-2017-0006
24. Westli HK, Johnsen BH, Eid J, et al. Teamwork skills, shared mental models, and performance in simulated trauma teams: An independent group design. *Scand J Trauma Resusc Emerg Med.* 2010;18:47.
25. Janis IL. *Groupthink.* Houghton Muffin Company; 1982.
26. Staal MA. Stress, cognition, and human performance: A literature review and conceptual framework. 2004. Ames Research Center, Moffett Field. http://human-factors.arc.nasa.gov/flightcognition/Publications/IH_054_Staal.pdf
27. Broadbent DE. Differences and interactions between stresses. *Q J Exp Psychol.* 1963;15:205–211.
28. Broadbent DE. *Decision and Stress.* Academic Press; 1971.
29. Hart SG. Task Loading Index. 2006. Human Factors and Ergonomics Society. http://www.stavelandhfe.com/images/TLX_20_years_later_2006_Paper.pdf
30. Hitch GJ, Baddeley AD. Verbal reasoning and working memory. *Q J Exp Psychol.* 1976;28:603–621.
31. Spelke E, Hirst W, Neisser U. Skills of divided attention. *Cognition.* 1976;4(3):215–230.
32. Enander AE. Effects of thermal stress on human performance. *Scand J Work Environ Health.* 1989;15:27–33.
33. Grether WF. Human performance at elevated environmental temperature. *Aerosp Med.* 1973;44(7):747–755.
34. Driskell JE, Johnson B, Hughes S, Batchelor C. *Development of Quantitative Specifications for Simulating the Stress Environments* [Report No. AL-TR-1991-0109]. 1992.
35. Stevens SS. Stability of human performance under intense noise. *J of Sound Vib.* 1972;21(1):35–56.
36. Broadbent DE. Human performance and noise. In: Harris CM, ed. *Handbook of Noise Control.* 2nd ed. McGraw-Hill; 1979.
37. Bartlett FC. Psychological criteria for fatigue. In: Floyd WF, Welford AT, eds. *Symposium on Fatigue.* H.K. Lewis; 1953.
38. Matthews G, Desmond PA. Task-induced fatigue states and simulated driving performance. *Q J Exp Psychol.* 2002;55(2):659–686.
39. Van Dongen HP, Maislin G, Mullington JM, Dinges DF. The cumulative cost of additional wakefulness: Dose-response effects on neurobehavioral functions and sleep physiology from chronic sleep restriction and total sleep deprivation. *Sleep.* 2003;26(2):117–126.
40. Grossman D, Christensen LW. *On Combat: The Psychology and Physiology of Deadly Conflict in War and Peace.* Warrior Science Publications; 2008.

9

Patient Safety

KRISTA HAUGEN, KEVIN SCHITOSKEY, AND PATRICIA FRANCES CORBETT

"It may seem a strange principle to enunciate as the first requirement in a hospital that it do the sick no harm."

FLORENCE NIGHTINGALE, 1863[1]

Strange, indeed, but clearly necessary both then and now. In the year 1999, the Institute of Medicine's (IOM's) *To Err Is Human* report using information from the Harvard Medical Practice study estimated that at least 44,000 to 98,000 Americans die each year from medical errors and compared that total to a "jumbo jet" crashing every day.[2,3,4,5] Later publications in 2008 suggested these numbers are much higher: up to 400,000 deaths annually with associated costs of at least $17.1 billion for measurable medical errors.[2,6] Other sources argue that these economic costs are severely underestimated and that if the "quality adjusted life years (QALYs)" of the deceased are considered, the economic costs may rise to around $1 trillion.[7] It is also important to note that these figures are referring to mortality from medical error and don't include morbidity statistics.

The noneconomic costs, namely pain, suffering, and the less tangible, but no less important, impacts on those who have entrusted their or their loved one's care to healthcare systems and providers only to have something go wrong, are even more difficult to measure. In any case, it is clear that adverse medical events are extraordinarily costly from both economic and noneconomic perspectives and are difficult to accurately measure. It should also be noted that this data refers to healthcare in general – there is a paucity of data on the incidence of adverse medical events specific to the medical transport realm and how patients view the transport experience (Box 9.1).[8,9]

The Patient Safety and Quality Improvement Act (PSQIA) was introduced in 2005 to address patient harm as a result of medical error and to create systems to better understand why harm is occurring and how to prevent it.[10] The PSQIA "establishes a voluntary reporting system designed to enhance the data available to assess and resolve patient safety and health care quality issues. To encourage the reporting and analysis of medical errors, PSQIA provides Federal privilege and confidentiality protections for patient safety information, called Patient Safety Work Product."[10] The legislation also allowed for the creation of Patient Safety Organizations (PSOs), which partner with healthcare agencies to reduce adverse medical events by collecting deidentified data, helping to review and analyze events, and provide protection from discoverability for the organization's Patient Safety Work Products (PSWP), thus allowing for transparency

and learning to occur within the organization to help prevent future adverse events.[10] Multiple organizations have also been instrumental in the improvements in patient safety, including the Agency for Healthcare Research and Quality (AHRQ), the Institute for Healthcare Improvement (IHI), Institute for Safe Medication Practices (ISMP), and the National Patient Safety Foundation (NPSF). Some research shows "a modest reduction in the mortality rate associated with AEMT [adverse effects of medical treatment] in the United States from 1990 to 2016."[15]

However, in their 2020 book, *Still Not Safe*, Robert Wears and Kathleen Sutcliffe suggest that "...hazards from medical care seem just about as prevalent as they were in 2000 and earlier" and that the "modern patient safety movement" is an "important social movement which has seemingly lost its way."[1] As there is minimal data on this subject in the medical transport realm, it's difficult to present a counterargument to this assertion and it is reasonable to assume that there is much work to be done to ensure patients who are being medically transported consistently receive high quality, compassionate care in the safest way possible.

> *"Risk management is a more realistic term than safety. It implies that hazards are ever present, that they must be identified, analyzed, evaluated and controlled, or rationally accepted."*
>
> **JEROME LEDERER, FLIGHT SAFETY FOUNDATION AND NASA AVIATION SAFETY EXPERT[16]**

Air and surface medical transport occurs at the intersection of two overly complex, high-risk industries: healthcare and transportation, whether transport occurs by air or by ground. Hazards are certainly ever-present, and harm can come to patients in innumerable ways. "Patient safety" may be best summed up as "clinical risk-management" to capture the complexity and variability of risks in air and surface medical transport and connote that this is an ongoing, dynamic process.

We know that humans are fallible and even the best of the best can err. The same is true for organizations – even highly reputable medical centers have experienced high-profile adverse events. Historical approaches of "blaming & shaming" individuals who err have been shown to be counterproductive, as it has been demonstrated that system failures are at the heart of most harm-causing events in hospitals.[2] Therefore, focusing exclusively on individuals does not mitigate future risks, as latent system failures are allowed to continue. As Drs. Wiegmann and Shappell point out, "The human is rarely, if ever, the sole cause of an error or accident. So, if your goal is to reduce accidents ... efforts must focus on the system as a whole, not just the human component."[17]

With the focus on systems and how humans function within a system, clinical risk management requires a concerted, intentional effort from the organizational leadership and the organization as a whole. It should not be the responsibility of a singular position or department; rather, it is the responsibility of everyone in the organization, requiring cross-departmental collaboration. The ability of transport teams to provide high-quality clinical care during transportation of patients in a way that mitigates risks to the highest degree possible is the result of everyone in the organization working in concert to that end.

Because of the innumerable hazards and potential risks ever-present in the dynamic and complex realm of medical transport and the lack of data available, how do we begin to understand our current reality with regard to incidence and nature of patient harm events and how to prevent them? How do we move from being reactive to more predictive risk management? We can begin by exploring models and principles from other industries, such as the safety sciences and aviation safety. While there are numerous philosophies, models, and strategies from a number of disciplines related to safety and managing risk, considering a combined approach may be the most useful path forward.

Organizational Underpinnings of Clinical Risk Management

Principles of Prevention

One overarching model of clinical risk management to consider comes from a public health model of prevention (Box 9.2)[19]:

- Primary prevention: prevent harm events from occurring to begin with the maximum extent possible.
- Secondary prevention: respond to events in a way that minimizes damage and maximizes learning, to include individual and organizational recovery.
- Tertiary prevention: apply lessons learned and improve processes to mitigate future risk.

Building a Clinical Safety Management System

In air medical transport, SMSs have been instituted to help decrease risk of aviation incidents and accidents. SMS is comprised of four foundational components (Fig. 9.1)[20]:

- Safety policy
- Safety risk management
- Safety assurance
- Safety promotion

Bringing the precepts of aviation SMS to the clinical arena would potentially positively influence clinical risk management for both air and ground operations.

The Four SMS Components

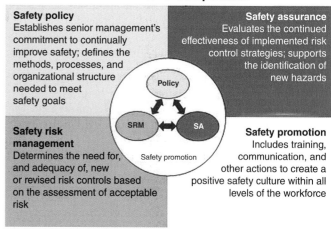

Safety policy
Establishes senior management's commitment to continually improve safety; defines the methods, processes, and organizational structure needed to meet safety goals

Safety assurance
Evaluates the continued effectiveness of implemented risk control strategies; supports the identification of new hazards

Safety risk management
Determines the need for, and adequacy of, new or revised risk controls based on the assessment of acceptable risk

Safety promotion
Includes training, communication, and other actions to create a positive safety culture within all levels of the workforce

• Figure 9.1 The Four SMS Components. (From US Department of Transportation. Federal Aviation Administration. https://www.faa.gov/about/initiatives/sms/explained/components)

Striving for High Reliability

High-Reliability Organizations (HROs) are those that "operate in complex, high-hazard domains for extended periods without serious accidents or catastrophic failures."[21]

Organizations that are considered HROs include commercial aviation, air traffic control, and the nuclear industry. It is important to note that the success of these organizations is not based on the absence of human error; rather, these organizations recognize that humans err and have developed systems to capture error before it results in catastrophe.

HROs operate utilizing the following principles:[21]

- Preoccupation with failure: all team members constantly scan for what could potentially go wrong and proactively develop mitigation strategies.
- Reluctance to simplify: team members recognize the complexity and dynamic nature of their work. They look beyond the easy answers and deploy critical thinking strategies, are mindful of biases, and seek out the actual, but often not easy, solutions.
- Sensitivity to operations: team members maintain "situational awareness" and understand the "big picture."
- Deference to expertise: team members recognize that the people who do the work typically know where the problems are and likely what solutions are as well. A culture of psychological safety is created, where team members feel free to voice concerns and are responded to in a constructive way.
- Commitment to resilience: team members recognize the inherent risks of system failures and strive for the development of resilient and reliable systems as well as continuous improvement.

Building a Culture of Learning – Just Culture

A Just Culture is a culture of learning with an emphasis on shared accountability between the organization that designs the systems and the individuals who work within the system.[22,23,24] In a Just Culture:

- It is recognized that errors most often occur because of defects in systems
- The organization recognizes and is accountable for its role in building the systems team members work within
- Team members are responsible for their own behaviors and choices made within the system and for alerting the organization to system defects or weaknesses

- System contributing factors and context are evaluated before humans when there is a mishap
- Team members are treated consistently and fairly
- Human error is not subject to discipline unless it becomes repetitive
- The organization understands that errors and at-risk behavioral choices may be influenced by human factors, drift, and normalization of deviance
- Transparency, reporting errors, whether or not harm occurred, and voicing concerns are encouraged
- Lessons learned are shared and applied forward to mitigate future risk.

With the emphasis on system evaluation, the question as to how to approach systems arises.

How to Look at Systems

British psychologist James Reason developed the Swiss Cheese Model of risk management, an incredibly useful model to illustrate the concept of systems and upstream risks that may contribute to a mishap.[23,24] Each layer of cheese represents a barrier separating various hazards becoming potential losses. Weaknesses or flaws in these barriers are represented by a hole in the Swiss cheese. Reason's theory was that if the holes line up, the hazards are allowed to slip through and result in a loss. The model presents a clear depiction of the upstream contributing factors to any given event, beyond just the individual, and demonstrates the potential roles of system contributing factors in adverse events. The "active failures (errors)" occur at the pointy end of the model, while the "latent failures" are the system weaknesses that lie in wait, "setting up" the individual for potential error.[4,24] While the image of the Swiss cheese is static, it is important to remember that reality is highly dynamic (Fig. 9.2).

Human Factors Analysis and Classification System[17]

Drs. Shappell and Wiegmann applied the Swiss Cheese Model to hundreds of aviation incidents and accidents and developed the Human Factors Analysis and Classification System (HFACS). While there is some criticism in the industry regarding the language

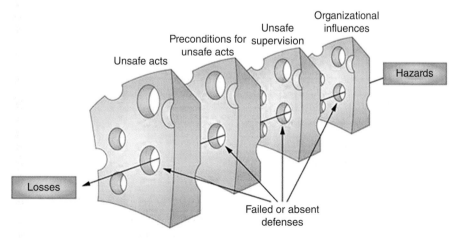

• **Figure 9.2** Reason's Swiss Cheese Model.

used in the HFACS model (i.e., "lack of," "failure to," "inadequate"), it is a useful guide in looking at systems and is essentially a roadmap to potential "holes in the Swiss Cheese" for any given system. In that respect, it can be used both reactively and proactively. It is important to note that if an organization looks exclusively at the individual team member(s) involved in a mishap and doesn't look at itself in the mirror, evaluating the organizational systems and processes that contributed to the mishap, then there is no shared accountability. This results in the marginalization of a Just Culture, as shared accountability is a primary tenet of a Just Culture. The HFACS model helps to demonstrate this notion as, if an event review focuses exclusively on the "Unsafe Acts" portion of the model where the human error occurred, then the opportunity to identify and potentially correct the upstream "holes in the Swiss Cheese" is lost. Therefore, the same latent conditions would persist, lying in wait for the next fallible human. If we truly wish to solve problems in healthcare and medical transport, it is essential to address the weaknesses in our systems (Fig. 9.3).

In the medical transport realm, there are societal systems issues that may be beyond the control of the organization. These types of issues may require a PESTLE Analysis:

PESTLE Analysis

- Political
- Economic
- Social
- Technological
- Legal
- Environmental

With these methods for evaluating systems in mind, systems can be constructed, as well as evaluated and refined, using these models as templates. One goal of the organization should be to make every attempt to set their team members up for success by optimizing the systems and environments within which they work (Box 9.3).

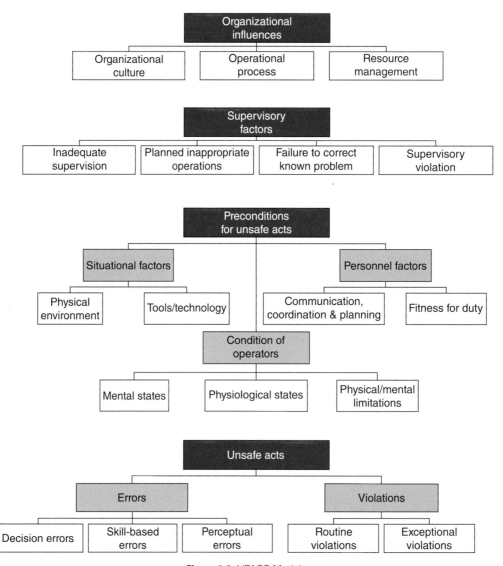

• **Figure 9.3** HFACS Model.

• **BOX 9.3** **Suggestions for Setting Team Members Up for Success From a Systems' Perspective**

- Evaluating organizational culture and priorities – emphasizing team member well-being and patient safety
  - Team member wellness/combatting burnout (not just frontline – all team members)
    - Context of pandemic
    - Civil/social/political unrest
    - Address criminalization of error in recent cases
  - Identifying and managing competing/conflicting priorities
  - Researching, developing, and disseminating evidence-based policies/protocols/guidelines
  - Effective communication of expectations
- Providing appropriate equipment/tools
- Engineering controls and eliminating single points of failure for critical processes
- Ensuring high-quality education/training
  - Initially and at regular intervals
  - Including high-risk/low-frequency clinical events
  - Determining competency/proficiency
  - Including instruction on documentation
  - Training leaders and supervisors on leadership principles, strategies, and communication
- CRM training
  - Integrate into clinical arena
  - Integrate into organization as a whole

Using principles from public health models of prevention, HRO, Just Culture, HFACS, and PESTLE analysis can help organizations build systems, processes, and ultimately a culture focused on reducing risk of harm to patients, team members, and the organization itself. Further, when clinical mishaps occur, these models can be utilized to evaluate the systems and context team members were working within, and weaknesses within the system can collaboratively be identified and addressed through process improvement to mitigate future risk.

Human Performance Underpinnings in Clinical Risk Management

Human and Organizational Performance

In her June 24, 2021, National Safety Council presentation, "Human & Organizational Performance (HOP): A Path to Improvement for All Organizations," Lisa Brooks defines HOP as a "risk-based operating philosophy which recognizes that error is part of the human condition and that an organization's processes and systems greatly influence employee actions and choices, and consequently, their likelihood of success." She then goes on to describe the HOP principles as[25,18]:

"1. People are fallible, and even the best make mistakes
2. Workers are masters at adaptive problem-solving
3. Context drives worker actions and behaviors
4. Leadership's response to failure matters
5. Blame fixes nothing
6. Improvement happens through learning"

While these concepts are consistent with Just Culture and the systems approaches to risk management, this model also emphasizes the dynamic nature of systems and humans and the constant interplay between them. This is summed up well by a quote about aviation mishaps from a US Navy Pilot: "In aviation you rarely get your head bitten off by a tiger – you usually get nibbled to death by ducks."[26] This can be applied to harm events in healthcare as well in that there is typically not one catastrophic factor that leads to an event; rather, there are usually a number of smaller factors within dynamic conditions creating circumstances in which even a seemingly benign action or inaction at the pointy end can lead to catastrophe as the "margin of safety [was] previously eroded."[26] The degradation of these safety margins can be insidious and subtle, setting up the humans at the pointy end for error.

Pursuing Individual Accountability and Peak Performance

Shared accountability is a two-way street. While it is essential to evaluate systems when reviewing and analyzing an adverse or untoward event, it is also essential that shared accountability occurs and that individuals involved are accountable for their choices and behaviors. As the pendulum swings away from blaming individuals toward the systems approach, it is important to be mindful of not allowing the pendulum to swing too far. Deploying an exclusively systems approach defeats the notion of shared accountability. Thus, the intent would be for the pendulum to stop in the middle, between the system and the individual. While it is true that human error is ubiquitous, we cannot use that as an excuse and must always strive to reach our peak performance potential and be accountable for our behaviors and choices within any given system. In his book *Blue Threat* Tony Kern discusses the notion of "personal error control," that with self-awareness, practice, and discipline, humans can improve their performance significantly.[26] Imagine how powerful the combination of a robust systems approach and individuals striving for peak performance within the system would be in the context of managing risks and decreasing harm.

Understanding Human Performance

Human Factors

"Human Factors focuses on human beings and their interaction with each other, products, equipment, procedures, and the environment. Human Factors leverages what we know about human behavior, abilities, limitations, and other characteristics to ensure safer, more reliable outcomes."

— **FRANK FEDERICO**[27]

Team Member Health and Wellness (See Chapter on Wellness)

At the heart of a robust risk management model lies the health and well-being of the individual team members. The ability to manage the complex factors that impact human performance, execute CRM well, identify and manage risks effectively, maintain sustainability in a career, and be able to continue to find joy in one's life in spite of the nature of the work depends on the wellness of each team member and the health of the collective team.

Research shows that "disruptive and unprofessional behaviors" are "significantly associated with poorer safety climate."[28] Further, the emotions induced by difficult patient encounters may impact decision-making and ultimately patient care. This warrants interventions to heighten awareness of the issue and arm team members with the tools to help them manage the impact of their emotions on their practice and be emotionally regulated.[29,30] Evidence also shows that burnout negatively impacts the ability of team members to "provide optimal and compassionate care for patients, to recover from stressful and emotional events, and to innovate in their daily work."[31,32] Current research demonstrates that the health and well-being of team members is a critical aspect of patient safety and team members experiencing burnout are "more likely to make errors, provide poor quality of care, lack work-place engagement, and ultimately leave their jobs."[33,32]

Not only does the ability to manage stress and to be self-regulated help team members manage human factors and execute CRM, thereby helping to mitigate risks during patient transport, but it also promotes a positive culture as intraorganizational communications and interactions may be more professional and respectful than otherwise. It is helpful to utilize a standardized approach to assist with objectively identifying potential risks related to personal human factors and readiness/fitness for duty, such as the IMSAFE tool (Box 9.4).

Human Factors Engineering[23]

Human factors engineering evaluates all of the aspects of a system, along with the capabilities of the humans, who are fallible, working within the system, and try to create systems that enhance safety, decrease hazards, and capture human error before it results in harm. The IHI and NPSF outlined engineering principles specific to patient safety (Box 9.5):

Managing Human Factors – Applying Lessons From Aviation

Many risk reduction principles in healthcare began in aviation. An important concept that belongs in the clinical realm as well as in an aircraft is Crew Resource Management (CRM) (Box 9.6).

• BOX 9.4   Human Factors Risk Assessment

IMSAFE mnemonic[27]:
- I – Illness
- M – Medication
- S – Stress
- A – Alcohol
- F – Fatigue
- E – Eating & elimination

From Federico F. *Human Factors.* Institute for Healthcare Improvement; November 2016. https://app.ihi.org/Events/Attachments/Event-2926/Document-6124/Day_1e_Human_Factors.pdf

---

• BOX 9.5   Patient Safety Engineering Principles[27]

- Simplification
- Standardization
- Avoiding reliance on memory
- Improving access to information
- Taking advantage of habits and patterns
- Exploiting the power of constraints and forcing functions
- Promoting effective team functioning
- Ensuring accessibility of protocols and checklists
- Creating redundancies
- Eliminating environmental factors that degrade performance
- Creating systems that are better able to tolerate the occurrence of errors and eliminating single points of failure for critical processes
- Reducing interruptions and distractions

• BOX 9.6   Human Factors Support

- Fatigue risk management systems
- Support for team members
  - Psychological/emotional/spiritual
  - Second Victim Experience
- Utilizing checklists and job aides
  - Transport related (i.e., equipment checks, challenge, and response)
  - Clinical care related (i.e., medication cross-check, preintubation checklists)
- Managing alarms and alarm fatigue
- Encouraging timeouts and procedural pauses
- Providing resources
  - Protocol apps
  - Medical control/supervisor accessibility

Crew Resource Management (See Chapter on CRM)

CRM evolved out of Cockpit Resource Management to provide education, training, and tools to help manage human factors and reduce adverse events in aviation.[34] As the utilization of CRM leads to a decrease in aviation incidents and accidents, it follows that applying the same principles in the clinical context would be useful in reducing harm events. We could begin deploying CRM by defining, describing, and applying the following CRM concepts in the clinical arena, including in scenario-based training:
- Authority gradient
- Stress/fatigue
- Complacency/normalization of deviance
- Workload
- Situational awareness/managing distractions
- Communication
- Threat and error management
- Leadership
- Teamwork
- Decision-making/judgment, including:
  - Cognitive biases
  - System 1 vs. System 2 thinking

While the following illustrations of the FAA's "Dirty Dozen" common factors for human error are specific to aviation and maintenance, the applicability to the clinical context is clear (Fig. 9.4).[35]

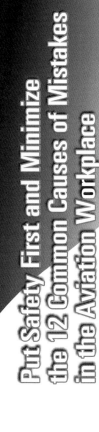

Federal Aviation Administration

Avoid the Dirty Dozen

12 Common Causes of Human Factors Errors

Put Safety First and Minimize the 12 Common Causes of Mistakes in the Aviation Workplace

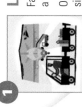

1

Lack of Communication

Failure to transmit, receive, or provide enough information to complete a task. Never assume anything.

Only 30% of verbal communication is received and understood by either side in a conversation. Others usually remember the first and last part of what you say.

Improve your communication—

- Say the most important things in the beginning and repeat them at the end.
- Use checklists.

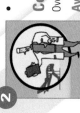

2

Complacency

Overconfidence from repeated experience performing a task.

Avoid the tendency to see what you expect to see—

- Expect to find errors.
- Don't sign it if you didn't do it.
- Use checklists.
- Learn from the mistakes of others.

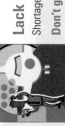

3

Lack of Knowledge

Shortage of the training, information, and/or ability to successfully perform.

Don't guess, know—

- Use current manuals.
- Ask when you don't know.
- Participate in training.

About **80** Percent of Maintenance Mistakes

Involve Human Factors

. . . and if Not Detected. . .

Would Lead to Accidents.

FAASTeam
FAA SAFETY TEAM

www.FAASafety.gov   YOUR SOURCE FOR AVIATION SAFETY

- **Figure 9.4** Examples From Aviation: Dirty Dozen. (From The Human Factors "Dirty Dozen." SKYbrary Aviation Safety; 2022, February 12. https://skybrary.aero/articles/human-factors-dirty-dozen)

Avoid These Common Causes of Mistakes in the Aviation Workplace

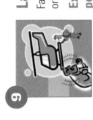

4

Distractions

Anything that draws your attention away from the task at hand.

Distractions are the #1 cause of forgetting things, including what has or has not been done in a maintenance task.

Get back in the groove after a distraction—

- Use checklists.
- Go back 3 steps when restarting the work.

5

Lack of Teamwork

Failure to work together to complete a shared goal.

Build solid teamwork—

- Discuss how a task should be done.
- Make sure everyone understands and agrees.
- Trust your teammates.

6

Fatigue

Physical or mental exhaustion threatening work performance.

Eliminate fatigue-related performance issues—

- Watch for symptoms of fatigue in yourself and others.
- Have others check your work.

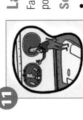

7

Lack of Resources

Not having enough people, equipment, documentation, time, parts, etc., to complete a task.

Improve supply and support—

- Order parts before they are required.
- Have a plan for pooling or loaning parts.

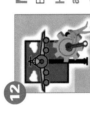

8

Pressure

Real or perceived forces demanding high-level job performance.

Reduce the burden of physical or mental distress—

- Communicate concerns.
- Ask for extra help.
- Put safety first.

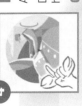

9

Lack of Assertiveness

Failure to speak up or document concerns about instructions, orders, or the actions of others.

Express your feelings, opinions, beliefs, and needs in a positive, productive manner—

- Express concerns but offer positive solutions.
- Resolve one issue before addressing another.

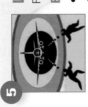

10

Stress

A physical, chemical, or emotional factor that causes physical or mental tension.

Manage stress before it affects your work—

- Take a rational approach to problem-solving.
- Take a short break when needed.
- Discuss the problem with someone who can help.

11

Lack of Awareness

Failure to recognize a situation, understand what it is, and predict the possible results.

See the whole picture—

- Make sure there are no conflicts with an existing repair or modifications.
- Fully understand the procedures needed to complete a task.

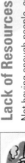

12

Norms

Expected, yet unwritten, rules of behavior.

Help maintain a positive environment with your good attitude and work habits—

- Existing norms don't make procedures right.
- Follow good safety procedures.
- Identify and eliminate negative norms.

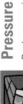

Visit us at:
www.FAASafety.gov
Your Aviation Safety Web Site

• **Figure 9.4,** cont'd

"Critical Phases" of Clinical Care

Another concept from aviation that would be beneficial in the clinical arena is the notion of "Critical Phases of Flight." These are the critical phases of aviation where all crew members must be engaged as a team to ensure safe operations. In some instances, a sterile cockpit is required so that the pilot can focus on the tasks at hand without unnecessary distractions and interruptions. Some examples of critical phases of flight include take-off, landing, operations in high-traffic areas, and in-flight emergencies. A similar approach of focused teamwork is also applicable to patient care. "Critical Phases of Clinical Care" are situations in which there may be considerable risk for errors, requiring the minimization of distractions and interruptions as well as robust communication and teamwork. These include, but are not limited to, invasive procedures, loading/unloading patients, medication dosing and administration, and handoffs.

Operationalizing a Culture of Learning

Once organizations and teams realize that reducing iatrogenic harm to patients and team members needs to be a priority, focus can shift to how to communicate about clinical risks within the organization. These are often difficult conversations, as it can be highly uncomfortable to discuss a clinical error one has made, even if there was no harm. Further, with burnout being prevalent in the postpandemic era, taking the time to communicate a near-miss, incident, or unsafe condition may not be high on a team member's priority list. This requires building a culture in which team members understand the importance of reporting; the collaborative nature of event reviews and process improvement initiatives to address the risks they have identified; and a culture in which they can be vulnerable because they know they will be supported and treated fairly, with dignity, respect, and professionalism – this creates psychological safety.

When an organization recognizes the value of near-miss reporting and creates a culture where clinicians feel appreciated for sharing these "almost events" a window of opportunity opens up for error prevention. Showing appreciation and celebrating the reporting of these types of events will encourage increased communication from frontline team members. The insights provided and shared experiences can be used to make system changes and be disseminated as learning opportunities systemwide.

Communicating Within a Culture of Learning – Reporting Incidents, Near-Misses, and Unsafe Conditions

In his book *Just Culture* (second edition), Sidney Dekker advises that there are two major considerations in getting people to report[22]:
- Maximizing accessibility
- Minimizing anxiety

Maximizing Accessibility

Those closest to the work usually know what the issues are and likely have ideas regarding solutions as well. It is essential that frontline team members have a voice and the means to share it. Sharing with teams the "why" behind reporting, along with helping them understand systems and the potential to work collaboratively to enhance their work environment, may help to encourage reporting.
- Desired qualities of a reporting platform:
  - Accessibility
  - Ease of use

1. Understand that your response to an event matters
2. Are the people okay?
3. Is the facility (or equivalent) safe, secure, and stable?
4. Tell me the story of what happened
5. What could have happened?
6. What factors led up to this event?
7. What worked well? What did not work?
8. Where else could this happen?
9. What else do I need to know about this event?

- Routing to relevant stakeholders
- Central venue for patient safety work
- Communicating progress
- Process improvement tracking
- Loop closure
- Tracking and trending
- Risk register
- Data analytics

Minimizing Anxiety: Understanding the Second Victim Experience

Trauma-informed organizations understand what traumatizes people and how to support them. Making an error, whether or not harm occurs, can be highly traumatizing to team members. The Second Victim Experience encompasses the psychological and emotional impact being involved in clinical mishaps has on team members.[36–38] The toll can be highly detrimental to those involved and can, in some cases, be career ending. A critical component of developing a culture of learning is understanding the Second Victim Experience, along with how to identify team members that are impacted as Second Victims, how to support them, and developing accessible resources such as professional clinicians who specialize in this type of trauma to refer team members to (Box 9.7).

A Roadmap to Managing Reports

- Respond in a timely manner when a report is received
- Conduct fact-finding and event reviews (vs. "investigations")
- Reviews should be conducted respectfully, with support systems in place for team members
- Evaluate systems and context before humans
- Identify lessons learned collaboratively
- Develop process improvement initiatives – ensuring completion and loop-closure occurs
- Audit process improvement strategies

Managing Events

While there are many methods for reviewing and analyzing events, a robust approach is the "Root Cause Analysis and Action," or "RCA[7]."[39] A collaboration between the NPSF and the IHI, the RCA[7] provides a more consistent and thorough approach than a traditional RCA and many other methods used historically. Recognizing that there is almost never a singular "root cause" for events, the RCA[7] emphasizes the identification of system contributing factors and requires "action" to create sustainable system fixes. The RCA[7] model is "risk-based" rather than "outcome based."[39]

The AHRQ advocates for the "Communication and Optimal Resolution (CANDOR)" approach.[40] Described as a "timely, thorough, and just" way to approach adverse events, the CANDOR approach includes early disclosure of errors to patients and families and facilitates "amicable and fair resolution" for all involved.[40]

There is likely no singular model, framework, or approach that meets all of the needs of an organization and those impacted by a given event. Utilizing a combination of approaches is useful, keeping the emphasis on supporting all of those involved, ensuring systems issues are identified and mitigated, and completing and auditing process improvements.

Event Classification

Historically, transport programs have used subjective terms to describe critical events which have impacted patients, such as "sentinel" or "never" events. These terms are borrowed from hospital quality assessment programs which list adverse events associated with inpatient admissions, such as iatrogenic infection or surgical mishaps.[41,42] Using these classifications in transport medicine is highly subjective, as the programs have no corresponding crosswalk for adverse or sentinel events which occur outside of a hospital setting.

Evaluation of preventable harm or adverse events in the transport medicine environment can be more readily accomplished by utilizing a research-based tool that provides for objective classification of safety events through a standardized decision-making tool to evaluate for process deviation along with a formal taxonomy to define different levels of impact to the patient, ranging from minor to extremely serious. There are many different formats; examples of such tools include the *Healthcare Associated Preventable Harm Level Classification Tool*, developed by the American Society for Healthcare Risk Management,[43] and the *Common Formats for Event Reporting (CFER)*, developed by the AHRQ.[44]

Shifting the focus of a safety event investigation to determine the impact of the event upon the patient centers on the patient and their experience of healthcare, which is an approach consistent with the healthcare priorities established by the IOM[45] and IHI.[46] Safety events which have a negative impact on patients should rise in priority for mitigation and corrective action through system evaluation and process improvement to protect patients and reduce preventable harm.

Applying Lessons Learned – Process Improvement

Process improvement can be complex and require extensive resources when it comes to solving systems issues. It is important to include the perspectives of all relevant stakeholders and evaluate any unintended consequences that may arise from proposed solutions. Laying the appropriate groundwork in terms of communicating change, educating and training, and setting clear expectations for stakeholders is essential prior to implementation of solutions. Auditing solutions to ensure they are doing what they were intended to do is critical.

Data Collection and Analysis

It is difficult to manage what we don't understand and what we don't measure. Obtaining and analyzing data related to reported incidents, near-misses, and unsafe conditions will help us better

---

• BOX 9.8   Select Patient Safety Priorities

- Airway management
- Ventilation
- Pediatric/neonatal
- OB/HROB
- Bariatric
- Behavioral health/combative patients
- Equipment issues
- Delays
- Falls/drops, including stretcher tips/drops
- Medication administration
- Handoffs/transitions of care
  - SBAR
  - I-PASS
- Aircraft/vehicle crashes
- Complications during invasive procedures
- Device dislodgements
- Patient injuries
- Deviation from Patient Care Guidelines or protocols

---

understand the realities of clinical risk and help drive targeted solutions (Box 9.8). Team members may not recognize risks and likely underreport errors.[26] Thus, the incidents that do get reported represent the proverbial "tip of the iceberg." It is important to ensure that the organization is
- Collecting "good" data
- Ensuring that definitions of data points are standardized and clear, i.e., organizations should provide definitions, preferably aligned with national and federal entities such as the AHRQ, to classify reports:
  - Error
  - Incident
  - Near-miss
  - Unsafe condition
  - Adverse event
  - Sentinel event
- Asking the right questions
- Making data meaningful

Conclusion

The thought of inadvertently harming those who have entrusted us with their care is difficult and painful. It takes courage to face the fact that iatrogenic harm is occurring, and it is incumbent upon all of us to understand, learn, and manage the risks that lead to harm. Managing risk and preventing harm to patients and team members in the medical transport realm takes commitment and resolve from everyone who works for medical transport organizations and not just those with "boots on the ground." Empowering our team members, patients, and families to speak up about their observations and experiences related to safety and risk and strongly encouraging reporting of near-misses and no-harm events is critical to harm reduction efforts. Taking a systematic approach to understanding events utilizing models like High Reliability, Just Culture, HFACS, RCA[7], and CANDOR can help us better understand why events happen and how to manage them in a way that minimizes damage and maximizes learning to mitigate future risks. The industry as a whole would benefit from collaboration, sharing data, lessons learned, and risk-reduction strategies. Building an industry-wide culture of learning and transparency will lead to improved care for those whom we serve.

References

1. Adair KC, Rehder K, Sexton JB. How healthcare worker well-being intersects with safety culture, workforce engagement, and operational outcomes. In: Montgomery A, Leiter M, Panagopoulou E, eds. *The Triple Challenge: Connecting Health Care Worker Well-Being, Patient Safety and Organisational Change*. Springer; 2019.

2. Andel C, Davidow SL, Hollander M, Moreno DA. The economics of health care quality and medical errors. *J Health Care Finance*. Fall 2012;39(1):39–50. PMID: 2315574.

3. ASTNA. *Patient Transport Principles & Practice*. 5th ed. Elsevier; 2018.

4. Bergman L. *In Safe Hands*: Patients' Experiences of Intrahospital Transport During Intensive Care. Science Direct; August 2020. https://pubmed.ncbi.nlm.nih.gov/32223920/

5. Brooks LM. *Human & Organizational Performance (HOP): A Path to Improvement for All Organizations* [Slides]. NSC/ORCHSE; June 24, 2021. https://www.nsc.org/getmedia/72bb8904-013d-46c9-88fa-e9b72d9e0f4c/hop062421.pdf

6. *Communication and Optimal Resolution (CANDOR)*. Agency for Healthcare Research & Quality; n.d. https://www.ahrq.gov/patient-safety/capacity/candor/index.html

7. Conklin T. *Pre-Accident Investigations: An Introduction to Organizational Safety*. 1st ed. CRC Press; 2012.

8. Dekker S. *Just Culture: Balancing Safety and Accountability*. 2nd ed. CRC Press; 2012.

9. *Do It for Drew Foundation*. Do It for Drew; 2019. https://www.doitfordrew.org/

10. FAA. *Safety Management System – Components*. Federal Aviation Administration; n.d. https://www.faa.gov/about/initiatives/sms/explained/components

11. Federico F. *Human Factors*. Institute for Healthcare Improvement; November 2016. https://app.ihi.org/Events/Attachments/Event-2926/Document-6124/Day_1e_Human_Factors.pdf

12. Frankel A, Haraden C, Federico F, Lenoci-Edwards J. *A Framework for Safe, Reliable, and Effective Care. White Paper*. Institute for Healthcare Improvement and Safe & Reliable Healthcare; 2017.

13. PSNet. *High Reliability*. Agency for Healthcare Research & Quality; September 8, 2019. https://psnet.ahrq.gov/primer/high-reliability

14. Josie King Foundation. *Home*. Josie King Foundation; 2016. https://josieking.org/home/

15. Institute of Medicine, Committee on Quality of Health Care in America, Donaldson MS, Corrigan JM, Kohn LT. *To Err Is Human: Building a Safer Health System*. Illustrated ed. National Academies Press; 2000.

16. Isbell LM. What do emergency department physicians and nurses feel? A qualitative study of emotions, triggers, regulation strategies, and effects on patient care. *BMJ Qual Saf*. October 1, 2020. https://qualitysafety.bmj.com/content/29/10/1.5

17. Isbell LM, Tager J, Beals K, et al. Emotionally evocative patients in the emergency department: A mixed methods investigation of providers' reported emotions and implications for patient safety. *BMJ Qual Saf*. 2020;29:1–2.

18. *There's More to the 60 Minutes Story on Heparin Errors*. Institute For Safe Medication Practices. https://www.ismp.org/resources/theres-more-60-minutes-story-heparin-errors

19. Lavietes S. *J. F. Lederer, 101, Dies; Took Risk Management to the Sky*. New York Times. February 9, 2004. https://www.nytimes.com/2004/02/09/us/j-f-lederer-101-dies-took-risk-management-to-the-sky.html

20. Leape L. *Making Healthcare Safe: The Story of the Patient Safety Movement*. Springer Publishing; 2021.

21. Kern T. *Blue Threat: Why to Err Is Inhuman*. Pygmy Books; 2022.

22. MacDonald R, Banks B, Morrison M. Epidemiology of adverse events in air medical transport. *Acad Emerg Med*. 2008;15(10):923–931.

23. Office for Civil Rights (OCR). *Patient Safety and Quality Improvement Act of 2005 Statute and Rule*. HHS.Gov; June 28, 2021. https://www.hhs.gov/hipaa/for-professionals/patient-safety/statute-and-rule/index.html

24. *Patient Safety 101*. PSNet. December 1, 2015. https://Psnet.Ahrq.Gov/Primer/Patient-Safety-101. https://psnet.ahrq.gov/primer/patient-safety-101

25. Pietravoia N. *Emily Jerry Foundation – For Patient Safety and Safe Medication Practices*. Emily Jerry Foundation; 2022. https://emilyjerryfoundation.org/

26. *Primary, Secondary and Tertiary Prevention*. Institute for Work & Health; 2015. https://www.iwh.on.ca/what-researchers-mean-by/primary-secondary-and-tertiary-prevention

27. *RCA2: Improving Root Cause Analyses and Actions to Prevent Harm*. Institute for Healthcare Improvement; 2015. https://www.ihi.org/resources/Pages/Tools/RCA2-Improving-Root-Cause-Analyses-and-Actions-to-Prevent-Harm.aspx

28. Reason J. *Managing the Risks of Organizational Accidents*. 1st ed. Ashgate; 1997.

29. Rehder K, Adair KC, Sexton JB. The Science of Health Care Worker Burnout. *Arch Pathol Lab Med*. 2021;145:1095–1109.

30. Rehder KJ, Adair KC, Hadley A, et al. Associations between a new disruptive behaviors scale and teamwork, patient safety, work-life balance, burnout, and depression. *Jt Comm J Qual Patient Saf*. 2020;46(1):19–26.

31. Scott S. *Second Victim Support: Implications for Patient Safety Attitudes and Perceptions*. Patient Safety & Quality Healthcare. October 12, 2015. https://www.psqh.com/analysis/second-victim-support-implications-for-patient-safety-attitudes-and-perceptions/

32. *Second Victims: Support for Clinicians Involved in Errors and Adverse Events*. PSNet. September 8, 2019. AHRQ. https://psnet.ahrq.gov/primer/second-victims-support-clinicians-involved-errors-and-adverse-events

33. Sexton JB, Adair KC, Profit J, et al. Perceptions of institutional support for "second victims" are associated with safety culture and workforce well-being. Joint Commission journal on quality and patient safety. 2021;47(5):306–312. doi:10.1016/j.jcjq.2020.12.001

34. *Study Suggests Medical Errors Now Third Leading Cause of Death in the U.S.* Johns Hopkins Medicine; May 3, 2016. https://www.hopkinsmedicine.org/news/media/releases/study_suggests_medical_errors_now_third_leading_cause_of_death_in_the_us

35. Sunshine J, Meo N, Kassebaum N, Collison M, Mokdad A, Naghavi M. Association of adverse effects of medical treatment with mortality in the United States: A secondary analysis of the global burden of diseases, injuries, and risk factors study. *JAMA Netw Open*. 2019. https://jamanetwork.com/journals/jamanetworkopen/fullarticle/2720915

36. Tawfik DS, Scheid A, Profit J, et al. Evidence relating healthcare provider burnout and quality of care: A systematic review and meta-analysis. *Ann Intern Med*. 2019;171(8):555–567. doi: 10.7326/M19-1152

37. *The Human Factors "Dirty Dozen."* SKYbrary Aviation Safety; February 12, 2022. https://skybrary.aero/articles/human-factors-dirty-dozen

38. van den Bos J, Rustagi K, Gray T, Halford M, Ziemkiewicz E, Shreve J. The $17.1 billion problem: The annual cost of measurable medical errors. *Health Aff*. 2011;30(4):596–603. doi: 10.1377/hlthaff.2011.0084

39. Wears R, Sutcliffe K. *Still Not Safe: Patient Safety and the Middle-Managing of American Medicine*. 1st ed. Oxford University Press; 2019.

40. Wiegmann DA, Shappell SA. *A Human Error Approach to Aviation Accident Analysis: The Human Factors Analysis and Classification System*. 1st ed. Routledge; 2003.

41. The Joint Commission. *Joint Commission Resources: Sentinel Event*. 2022. Accessed October 4, 2022. https://www.jointcommission.org/resources/sentinel-event/

42. Agency for Healthcare Research and Quality. *Patient Safety Network: Patient Safety 101 – Never Events*. 2019. Accessed October 4, 2022. https://psnet.ahrq.gov/primer/never-events

43. American Society for Healthcare Risk Management. *White Paper Series – Serious Safety Events: A Focus on Harm Classification: Deviation in Care as Link Getting to Zero™ White Paper Series – Edition No. 2*. 2014. Accessed October 4, 2022. https://www.ashrm.org/sites/default/files/ashrm/SSE-2_getting_to_zero-9-30-14.pdf

44. Agency for Healthcare Research and Quality. *Common Formats: What Are the Common Formats for Event Reporting (CFER)?* 2021. Accessed October 4, 2022. https://pso.ahrq.gov/common-formats/overview

45. Agency for Healthcare Research and Quality. *Six Domains of Health Care Quality*. 2018. Accessed October 4, 2022. https://www.ahrq.gov/talkingquality/measures/six-domains.html

46. Institute for Healthcare Improvement. *Triple Aim for Populations*. 2022. Accessed October 4, 2022. https://www.ihi.org/Topics/TripleAim/Pages/Overview.aspx

10

Operational Safety and Survival

AMI BESS AND KAREN ARNDT

COMPETENCIES

1. Identify the safety risks related to air and surface patient transport.
2. Integrate methods to reduce safety risks related to air and surface transport.
3. Integrate safe operations around helicopters, fixed-wing aircraft, and ground transport vehicles.
4. Understand emergency procedures for transport vehicles.
5. Understand basic survival skills, including shelter building, fire building, water procurement, and signaling.

Most chapters in this book contain information intended to help the air medical or ground transport crew members provide care for the critically ill or injured patient. This chapter is different; its purpose is to encourage the development of a safety attitude. It seeks to foster an active awareness and commitment to safety in every aspect of every vehicle movement. In short, it is devoted to taking care of the transport team members.

A safety culture exists within every transport program. Some safety measures are good, and some are not. For a strong positive culture, each member of the program must accept that they contribute directly to a safe environment. Every individual, whether they are a nurse, paramedic, physician, respiratory therapist, emergency medical technician (EMT), pilot, mechanic, communication specialist, or administrator, must accept personal responsibility for safety and be a safety advocate.

Definition of Safety

Webster's dictionary defines *safety* as "... the state of being safe from the risk of experiencing or causing injury, danger, or loss." Few human endeavors are completely safe from risk. The medical transport environment by its nature presents a wide range of potential risks. Medical transport exists at the unique interface of aviation, public safety, emergency medicine, and critical care medicine, all of which are complex technologic and human systems. In any complex system, human errors inevitably occur.[1] Effective risk management and safety programs recognize this and focus efforts on both reducing the rate of errors and, more importantly, reducing the consequences of the errors that do occur.

Safety may best be defined in the medical transport setting as identifying risks and managing them to eliminate or significantly reduce the possibility of accident or injury. The following sections explore some of the significant risks associated with air and ground medical transport and identify what has been, and is being, done to manage these risks and improve safety in the transport environment.

Air Medical Safety Survey

In 2015, Coons and Zalar[2] conducted the most recent Air Medical Safety Survey, and found the following:

- Three-fourths of the programs offer multimedia transport including helicopter, fixed-wing, and ground transport.
- Sixty percent of the aircraft have autopilot capabilities.
- The primary staffing configuration is nurse–paramedic.
- Sixty-four percent of the programs have a fatigue management system.
- Eighty-four percent of the respondent programs conducted formal air medical resource management (AMRM) programs annually.
- Respondents reported that 98% of the pilots and medical crew participate in a debriefing process.
- Sixty-three percent reported participation from communication specialists.
- Eighty-nine percent of the programs had a safety officer.
- Fifty-three percent of the programs used their Part 135 operator's safety management systems (SMS).
- Eighty-five percent of the programs did a preflight walk-around.
- Ninety-six percent of the programs report the use of night vision goggles (NVGs).
- All respondents reported that pilots can always cancel a flight; 99% of participants reported that the crew can cancel a flight, 75% of the participants reported that the maintenance technicians can cancel, 66% of participants reported that operational control can cancel, and 59% of participants reported that the communication specialist can cancel a flight.

Historical Perspective on Air Medical Accidents

The use of the term *accident* in the following discussion reflects its use by the National Transportation Safety Board (NTSB) for an event "... in which any person suffers death or serious injury, or in which the aircraft receives substantial damage."[3] This does not suggest that these tragic events are or were unavoidable. Most, if not all, of the accidents discussed had controllable factors that could have potentially prevented the occurrence or lessened the severity of the event.

The first hospital air medical program was established in 1972. Following that, the air medical industry underwent tremendous growth, from that one program in 1972, to 32 in 1980, to 101 by 1985.[4–7] With this growth came the realization that air medical helicopters had an accident rate far greater than that of helicopters engaged in general aviation.

From 1980 to 1985, the Helicopter Emergency Medical Services (HEMS) industry had an estimated accident rate of 12.3 accidents per 100,000 patients transported. The accident rate for nonscheduled turbine-powered air taxi helicopter operators, a comparable non-HEMS population, was 6.9 accidents per 100,000 patients for the same period.[4–8] In 1988, the NTSB concluded that weather-related accidents were the most common and most serious type of accident experienced by Emergency Medical Services (EMS) helicopters.[4–8]

The 1990s showed continued growth in the air medical industry, from an estimated 174 HEMS programs operating 232 helicopters in 1990 to 225 programs operating 360 helicopters in 1999.[4–8] From 1998 to 2001, the accident rate increased sharply to an average of 10.8 HEMS accidents per year, still with weather-related accidents as the most common, and with an increase of 10% in weather-related crashes in the studied time period.[4–8]

In 2002, the Air Medical Physician Association (AMPA) released "A Safety Review and Risk Assessment in Air Medical Transport," which examined HEMS accidents from 1980 to 2001.[3] The analysis showed a decreasing trend in number of HEMS accidents per 100,000 patient transports from the high in 1982 of 24.9 per 100,000 (a higher rate than that calculated by the NTSB in 1988) to a low in 1996 of 0.57 per 100,000. The average for the last 5 years of the study (1997–2001) was 4.6 per 100,000 patient transports. The most common factors in HEMS accidents were again found to be poor weather conditions and operations at night.

In January 2006, the NTSB released an "Aviation Special Investigation Report" that examined 55 EMS aircraft accidents that occurred between January 2002 and January 2005 of which were helicopter accidents.[9] The investigation identified these recurrent safety issues:

- Less stringent requirements for EMS operations conducted without patients on board
- A lack of aviation flight risk evaluation programs for EMS operations
- A lack of consistent comprehensive flight dispatch procedures for EMS operations
- No requirements to use technologies such as terrain awareness and warning systems (TAWS) and night vision imaging systems (NVIS) to enhance EMS flight safety

Also in 2006, Baker et al.[1] reviewed HEMS accidents from 1983 to 2005 to determine the factors related to fatal outcomes. They concluded that accidents that occur at night or in bad weather or that result in a postimpact fire have a higher risk of being fatal.[1] Blumen[3] conducted a focused analysis of HEMS accidents from

1998 to 2022 and found there were 267 accidents, of which 257 were dedicated HEMS aircraft and 10 were dual-purpose aircraft (e.g., combined police work and patient transport). Of the 267 accidents, 81 resulted in at least one fatality, with a total of 206 individuals killed. Among the people who died, 170 were crew members, 7 were dual-purpose crew members, 22 were patients, and 7 were "others" (family member, ride-along, etc.). In addition to the fatalities, 90 individuals suffered serious injuries, 92 had minor injuries, and 420 were listed as no injuries in the NTSB reports, for a total of 770 individuals involved in these accidents since 1998.

Hon et al.[10] reported that from January 2003 to the end of July 2015, there were 59 air medical incidents: 52 occurred with helicopters and 7 with fixed-wing aircraft. There were 104 fatalities. Factors identified that contributed to incidents included impaired visibility, equipment failure, pilot error, weather, and undetermined causes. The researchers found that postincident fire was related to a higher incident of fatalities. They did note a significant decrease in the number of accidents, but this was offset by an increase in fatalities. Table 10.1 summarizes an analysis for factors associated with fatal crashes or injury.

The NTSB examined more than 3000 EMS and non-EMS helicopter accident records from 1999 to 2018[11] (Fig. 10.1). The study found that fatal accident rates for EMS were twice those of non-EMS accidents (Fig. 10.2). Additionally, the study found two prevalent factors that determined EMS accident fatality: visibility/darkness and pilot decision-making/judgment (Fig. 10.3).[11] However, the study also found that the rates for fatal helicopter accidents did not differ between EMS and non-EMS (Fig. 10.2). While only 14% of non-EMS helicopter accidents resulted in at least one death, this rate was 34% for EMS helicopters.[11]

This data does not pretend to paint the whole picture of accident risk in air medical transport. The actual rates and the causes of air medical accidents are continuing topics of intense study and debate.[1] Although specific numbers and root causes may not always

TABLE 10.1 Univariate Analysis for Factors Associated With Fatal Crash or Injury

Category	No Injury or Fatality	Injury or Fatality	Significance*
Abnormal weather conditions	1/9	21/50	P = 0.057
Impaired visibility	1/9	23/50	P = 0.035
Aircraft make/type			
Agusta model	0/7	7/7	
Bell model	5/21	16/21	
Eurocopter model	2/20	18/20	
Other helicopter	2/4	2/4	
Fixed-wing aircraft	0/7	7/7	P = 0.096
Postincident fire	1/9	22/50	P = 0.045
Time of incident (7 pm–6 am)	2/9	35/50	P = 0.007

*Variables reaching statistical significance (P < 0.20) for inclusion in multivariate analysis.
From Hon H, Wojda TR, Barry N, et al. Injury and fatality risks in aeromedical transport: Focus on prevention. *J Surg Res.* 2016;204(2):297–303.

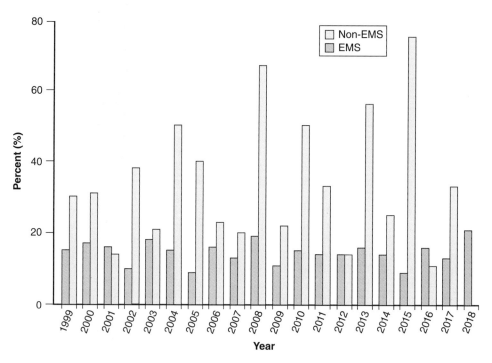

• **Figure 10.1** FAA medical helicopter accident review: Causes and contributing factors. *EMS, Emergency medical service.* (https://www.faa.gov/data_research/research/med_humanfacs/oamtechreports/2020s/media/202119.pdf)

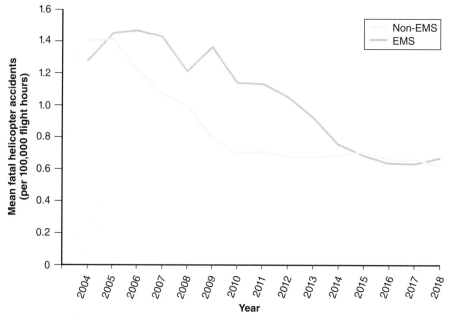

• **Figure 10.2** FAA medical helicopter accident review: causes and contributing factors, p. 20. *EMS, Emergency medical service.* (https://www.faa.gov/data_research/research/med_humanfacs/oamtechreports/2020s/media/202119.pdf)

be clear, what is clear is that there continue to be accidents and that patients and flight crews continue to be injured and killed. Also clear is that recurrent factors continue to be involved in air medical accidents, most notably operations at night and in inclement weather. Air transport crews need to maintain a respect for these hazards and promote (and use) every tool and practice available to reduce the risks of flight in the air medical environment.

Fixed-Wing Accidents

Fixed-wing air medical accidents have not been as well studied as HEMS accidents. In 2015, 111 air medical programs listed in the Atlas and Database of Air Medical Services operated 362 fixed-wing aircraft.[12] Seventy of these programs operated both fixed-wing aircraft and helicopters. A review of accident data from 2002

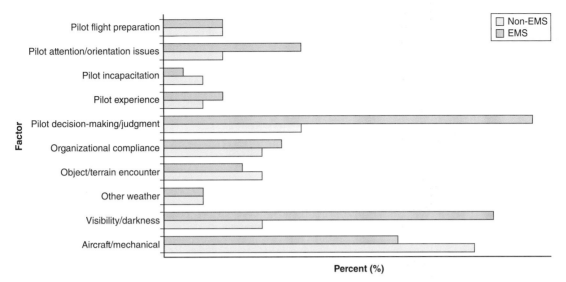

• **Figure 10.3** Contributory and causal factor groups in EMS and non-EMS fatal helicopter accidents, 2008 to 2017. FAA medical helicopter accident review: causes and contributing factors, p. 22. *EMS, Emergency medical service.* (https://www.faa.gov/data_research/research/med_humanfacs/oamtechreports/2020s/media/202119.pdf)

to November 2008 showed 14 accidents from 2002 to 2006, 6 of which were fatal. In 2007 six fixed-wing air medical accidents occurred, four of which were fatal; none were found in 2008.[13]

A study on factors associated with fatal outcomes in fixed-wing aeromedical flights, using the National Transportation Safety Board Aviation Accident Incident Database from 1984 to 2009, found fatal outcomes were significantly higher in medical flights (35.6% vs. 19.7%), with more aircraft fires (20.3% vs. 10.5%) and on-ground collisions (5.1% vs. 2.0%) compared with commercial flights. Aircraft fires occurred in 12 of the 21 fatal crashes (57.1%), compared with only 2 of the 38 nonfatal crashes (5.3%). In the multiple logistic regression model, the only factor with increased odds of a fatal outcome was the presence of a fire.[14] Most fatalities occurred during cruise flight with landing and take-off being the lesser causes. The major causes of crashes were related to loss of control on the ground, system malfunction (nonpowerplant related), abnormal runway contact, and unintended flight in instrument meteorologic conditions (IMC).[14] However, most fatalities were due to system malfunction (nonpowerplant related), controlled flight into terrain (CFIT), loss of control inflight, and loss of separation/midair collision.[14] These results are new to our safety culture of heightened awareness of critical phases of flight (ground taxi, take-off, and landing) and suggest that all phases of fixed-wing flight are critical to our safety (Figs. 10.4–10.7).

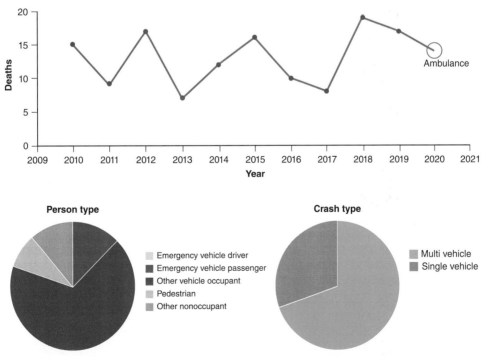

• **Figure 10.4** Ambulance deaths involving lights and sirens use, 2010–2020. (https://injuryfacts.nsc.org/motor-vehicle/road-users/emergency-vehicles/)

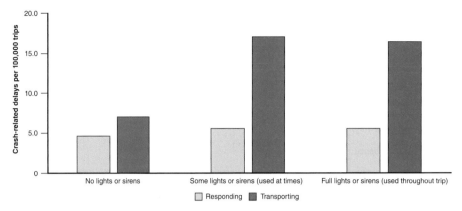

• **Figure 10.5** Ambulance deaths with lights and sirens and patient vs. nonpatient transports. (https://injuryfacts.nsc.org/motor-vehicle/road-users/emergency-vehicles/)

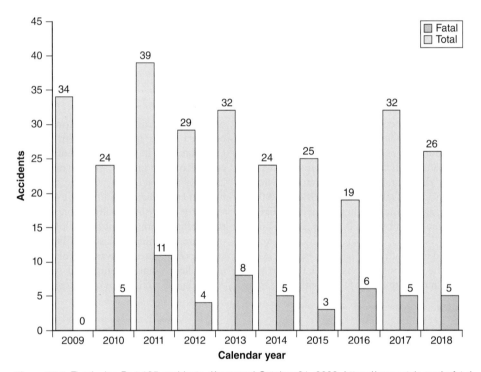

• **Figure 10.6** Fixed-wing Part 135 accidents. (Accessed October 31, 2022. https://www.ntsb.gov/safety/data/Pages/AviationDataStats2018.aspx)

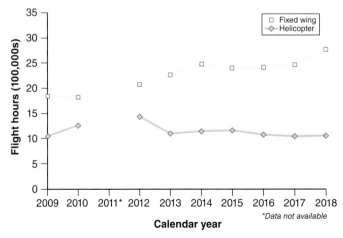

• **Figure 10.7** Flight hours Part 135 accidents. (Accessed October 31, 2022. https://www.ntsb.gov/safety/data/Pages/AviationDataStats2018.aspx)

Ground Ambulance Accidents

The same level of attention paid to air medical accidents has not been paid to ground ambulance accidents. Unlike air medical accidents, which must be reported and investigated by the NTSB, ground ambulance crashes are monitored on a state or local level, which makes consistent nationwide data difficult to obtain. In 2014, the National Highway Traffic Safety Administration (NHTSA) reported an estimated mean of 4500 motor vehicle crashes involving an ambulance between 1992 and 2011.[15] Sixty-five percent resulted in property damage only, thirty-four percent resulted in an injury, and less than one percent resulted in a fatality. Sixty-three percent of the fatalities were occupants in other vehicles. In both fatal and nonlethal crashes, most crashes occurred while the ambulance was in emergency use. From 2010 to 2014, there were 133 ambulance-related deaths (see Fig. 10.8) and from 2015 to 2020, there were 185 ambulance-related deaths (see Fig. 10.9).[16] This represents a 39% increase in ambulance-related deaths.

In 2019, Watanabe et al.[17] showed that crash risk increases when ambulances operate with lights and sirens. When an ambulance responds to an emergency call without using lights and sirens, the crash rate is 4.6 per 100,000 transport responses. The crash rate increases to 5.5 per 100,000 transports when lights and sirens are used. The increase in risk is even greater when the ambulance is transporting a victim. The crash risk without lights and sirens is 7.0 per 100,000 transports and increases to 16.5 per 100,000 transports when lights and sirens are used throughout the transport (Figs. 10.10 and 10.11).[17]

The Federal KKK-A-1822F (KKK) standard was initially the only existing standard and was written for federally purchased ambulances. A major focus of the KKK standards was ambulance construction. A recent focus on safety has led to new standards: the Commission on Accreditation of Ambulance Services (CAAS) Ground Vehicle Standard (GVS) v3.0[18] and the National Fire Protection Agency (NFPA) 1917.[19] NHTSA published the "Model Minimum Uniform Crash Criteria,"[20] which includes a uniform way for police to collect data about an ambulance crash. Examples of data to be collected are shown in Box 10.1. CAAS and NFPA 1917 safety recommendations are excerpted in Box 10.2.[18–20]

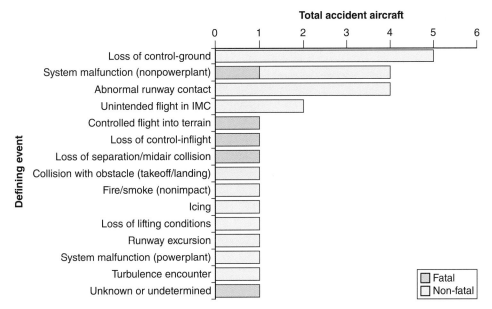

• **Figure 10.8** Defining events for Part 135 fixed-wing accidents, 2018. (Accessed October 31. 2022. https://www.ntsb.gov/safety/data/Pages/AviationDataStats2018.aspx)

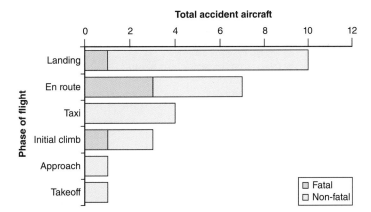

• **Figure 10.9** Phase of flight for Part 135 fixed-wing accidents, 2018. (Accessed October 31, 2022. https://www.ntsb.gov/safety/data/Pages/AviationDataStats2018.aspx)

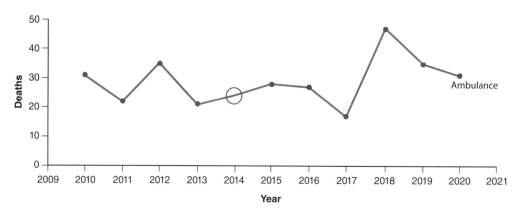

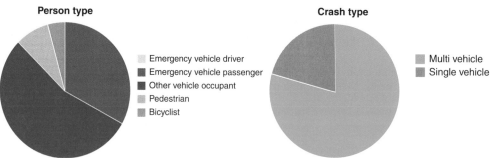

• **Figure 10.10** Deaths in crashes involving emergency vehicles, 2010–2014. (https://injuryfacts.nsc.org/motor-vehicle/road-users/emergency-vehicles/)

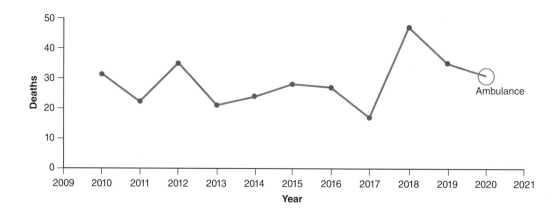

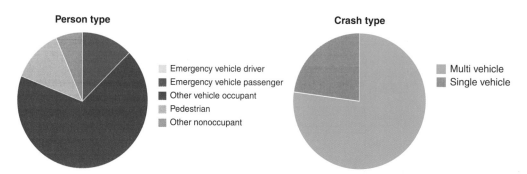

• **Figure 10.11** Deaths in crashes involving emergency vehicles, 2010–2020. (https://injuryfacts.nsc.org/motor-vehicle/road-users/emergency-vehicles/)

• BOX 10.1   Recommended Ground Ambulance Crash Data Collection

- Emergency transport
- Nonemergency transport
- Emergency operation
  - Warning equipment in use
  - Warning equipment not in use
- Ambulance seating/positioning
- Crash location
- Weather conditions

- Contributing circumstances
- Roadway surface conditions
- Motor vehicle body type
- Vehicle configuration
- Air bag deployed
- Alcohol and drug testing
- Driver distracted by

• BOX 10.2   Ground Ambulance Safety Recommendations

Design Specifications
- Enlisting the help of crew to design the interior for functionality and safety.
- Seat access that allows access to the patient, equipment, and vehicle controls while remaining in seatbelts.
- All heavy equipment (e.g., monitors, oxygen cylinders, mechanical CPR devices, computers, and medical kits) should be restrained or kept in a secure cabinet.
- NFPA 1917 recommends that all equipment weighing more than three pounds be mounted in a bracket that can withstand up to 10 Gs of force. This prevents it from becoming a deadly missile in an accident or evasive maneuvers.

Chassis and Suspension Selection
- An undersized, overloaded ambulance chassis moving down the road with lights and siren is an accident waiting to happen.
- Inventory all equipment and supplies you typically carry and carefully estimate the total weight. Always weigh your ambulance as it leaves the factory and again when it is fully loaded with the crew inside.
- To add a margin of safety, select a chassis that exceeds your estimated payload. If you do not do this, you may find that your chassis exceeds the recommended GVWR (gross vehicle weight rating is the maximum operating weight of your vehicle).

Structural Components
- Visit ambulance factories to see how each company builds their bodies.
- Educate yourself, ask the builder about their construction techniques, visit factories, and network with other users before you make a purchase.

Safe Seating
- Make sure your seats meet dynamic testing requirements[18–20] (NFPA 1917, SAE J2917: Occupant Restraint and Equipment Mounting Integrity-Frontal Impact System-Level Ambulance Patient Compartment; and J3026: Ambulance Patient Compartment Seating Integrity and Occupant Restraint).
- The standards also address seat belts, head clearance, patient access, child restraints, and seat belt warning systems.
- One recent study emphasizes that forward- or rear-facing seats provide better protection in the event of an accident or evasive maneuver than side-facing seats.[48,49]

Cot Lifting Systems
- An electric stretcher, hydraulic cot lifting system, or lift gate system will help reduce back injuries and extend the careers of crew members.
- If your scope of service includes bariatric patients, cot lifting weight abilities should be considered.

Warning Devices
- Emergency lighting, scene lighting, loading lights, and ground lighting increase the visibility of your ambulance and improve safety both day and night.
- Lighting packages that meet the new standards focus on warning zones, signaling modes ("calling for the right of way" or "blocking the right of way"), flash rates and patterns, lighting zones, and power requirements.
- Chassis-mounted LED ground lights can also add a greater margin of safety for anyone entering and exiting the ambulance and help you see items placed or left on the ground.
- A siren should have ample power, produce a wide spectrum of frequencies, and have multiple signaling modes. Several new siren types emit low-frequency sound waves that penetrate and shake solid materials. These are highly effective in urban environments with heavy vehicle and pedestrian traffic.

Vehicle Visibility
- Crew safety depends on other motorists quickly identifying your approaching ambulance in any environmental condition: day and night, rain, snow, or low light conditions. New standards recommend increasing retroreflective striping by 25% on the front and 50% on each side.[36]
- The rear of the vehicle should be equipped with retroreflective striping that forms a downward-sloping chevron pattern and covers 50% of rear-facing surfaces. For maximum visibility, red with alternating fluorescent yellow or yellow-green stripes are the recommended colors.

Training and Procedures
- A well-designed training program should include classroom time, behind-the-wheel training, and testing. Drivers should have an annual refresher training and baseline medical exam to verify their ability to physically operate an ambulance.
- Establishing standard operating procedures (SOPs) for emergency vehicles is a must. Written guidelines should include intersection approach, maximum response speeds, driver responsibilities, backing guidelines, warning device usage, and vehicle limitations.
- Each accident and near miss should be fully investigated by a safety committee to establish the root cause and determine what corrective action is needed to avoid future injuries or damages.

Maintenance
- A comprehensive maintenance plan is essential to the safety of the occupants.
- A proactive maintenance plan can prevent emergency run breakdowns, prolong the life of the vehicle, avoid costly repairs, and reduce costly vehicle downtime.

These studies show that ground ambulance accidents also have recurrent contributing factors. Safety training programs should focus on the awareness of these risks, safe driving, and proper use of safety equipment, such as seat belts. Ground transport programs need to establish the same safety culture and have the same commitment to safety and risk reduction as air medical programs.

Risk Mitigation

Since the 1980s, efforts have been made to reduce the risks of flight in the air medical environment and ground transport environments. These efforts at risk reduction have taken many forms, from safety policies/procedures, enhanced training, advancing technologies, and regulations.

Critical Thinking, Decision-Making, and the Human Factor

The probable cause for many of the accidents described previously is listed as *pilot error*, which is another way of saying the pilot made a bad decision, or a series of bad decisions, which resulted in the accident. Decision-making in the aviation environment is a complicated process, with many factors that need to be considered. To be able to make good decisions, pilots and flight crew members need to have training in critical thinking and decision-making in the HEMS environment and have access to decision-making tools.[21,22] These tools may be technologies, policies, algorithms, or other processes. No single tool or practice ensures a good decision but used together they can be effective in helping pilots and crews make safe decisions. The human factor, the ability of the pilot and crew to make informed safe decisions, remains the single most crucial factor in ensuring safety in the medical transport environment.

Weather Minimums

From the beginning of the industry, weather and impaired IMCs have been recognized as a significant cause of accidents.[23] Each program's weather minimums must comply with Federal Aviation Administration (FAA) regulations, meet CAMTS requirements, and address the specific needs and hazards of the program's operating area. Once a program's weather minimums have been established, they need to be followed; "pushing the envelope" on minimums has been implicated in many weather-related HEMS accidents.

Another weather-related concern noted in the 2006 NTSB report was the lack of reliable information regarding weather conditions in many areas in which HEMS programs operate, which increases the risk of an inadvertent entry into IMCs (IIMCs). To find ways to reduce this risk, representatives of the HEMS industry, the FAA, and the University Center for Atmospheric Research conducted a HEMS Weather Summit in 2006. One result of this summit was the development of the Aviation Digital Data Service (ADDS) experimental HEMS Low Altitude Flight Tool.[24] The FAA met again with industry representatives to fine-tune the tool in 2013. This online application is designed to enhance the safety of flight in the low-altitude environment used by HEMS aircraft. It provides a visual representation of ceiling, visibility, convection, radar information, and geographic information system data in areas between established weather-reporting sites.

Planning and Risk Assessment

The safe completion of any medical transport operation starts with premovement planning. The first step in planning is an assessment of the potential risks involved, which leads to a decision about whether the transport request should be accepted. Once the decision has been made to accept the transport request, other aspects of planning must occur, including weight and performance planning, fuel management, destination considerations, pilot and crew duty time, and clinical factors.

Operational risk assessment begins with a daily or shift evaluation, which considers factors that remain constant during the day. These factors can include prevailing weather patterns, pilot and crew experience, and the availability of safety technologies (discussed subsequently). Another risk assessment should be performed during each request, evaluating the time of day, current weather conditions, weather forecasts, pilot and crew fatigue, and other variables. Some programs have established operational control centers to assist pilots in assessing the risks of certain missions by having the request reviewed and any identified risks evaluated by another individual (typically a senior pilot) before the request is accepted. Fig. 10.12 shows an example of a risk assessment tool.[26]

Risk assessment should be a fluid, dynamic process. If conditions change as the operation progresses, so should the risk assessment. Pilots and flight crews need to continuously observe and evaluate the operational environment and the potential risks. If changes in the operational environment can be anticipated, then decision thresholds and alternative plans can be discussed and decided on ahead of time.

Declined Missions

Although the pilot-in-command (PIC) has the ultimate responsibility for accepting or declining any request, all members of the transport team have the right, and the responsibility, to refuse to accept any transport request in which there is a legitimate safety concern. This includes both air and surface transport. Each program should have a written policy for declining or aborting missions, so that individual crew members do not have to worry about disciplinary action or other negative action because of refusing to participate in an operation for safety concerns. The safety culture of the program should support the "All to say go, one to say no" philosophy.

Air Medical Resource Management

AMRM is the operational practice of involving all members of the flight team (pilot and clinical crew members) in planning, decision-making, and safety. It is the air medical industry's adaptation of *crew resource management* (CRM), which is used in the commercial aviation industry and by the US Air Force. CRM grew out of several significant accidents that resulted from poor decision-making on the part of airline pilots, and in some cases, over the objections of other flight crew members. CRM involves communication skills, situational awareness, problem-solving, decision-making, and teamwork.

The PIC was traditionally the sole decision-maker in an airline cockpit. The rest of the crew followed the PIC's instructions and did not offer input or question decisions. By encouraging crew members to pay attention, make suggestions, and voice concerns, CRM involves all the crew members in the decision-making process. The PIC still has the ultimate authority and responsibility for the aircraft, but other crew members can offer suggestions or, more importantly, question decisions they feel are unsafe or unwise.

The essence of AMRM/CRM is teamwork, based on effective communication between all crew members and the use of all available resources to maximize safety. Mutual respect, trust, and an organizational culture that supports safety provide the

Operations Compliance Form (Risk Analysis)

GENERAL:

This form is used to comply with the requirements of 14 CFR 135.617 and 14 CFR 135.621.

INSTRUCTIONS:

General Information

1. Enter one or two digit day of the month in the DAY field.
2. Enter the three letter abbreviation for the month (ie, JAN, FEB, MAR, etc.) in the MONTH field.
3. Enter the time, in military format (ie, 0800, 1621, 1945, etc) that the form was completed.
4. Circle either "NA" or "YES" for each of the four major categories, as appropriate.
5. When required, enter the name of the person providing approval for the operation.
6. When required, enter the final risk score, as provided by the OCS.
7. Sign the form as shown.
8. The completed form must be kept at the base where the operation originated from for a minimum of 90 days. Lead pilots will organize and maintain a system for management of these forms at their respective bases.

Crew Briefing

The **PEOPLE** briefing is used to meet the requirement of 14 CFR 135.621 for medical personnel who have not been trained.

Additional Fields

1. Remaining fields are for administrative purposes only and are not required.

Operations Control Specialist (OCS) Entry Form

Also included is the OCS Entry Form, an Excel spreadsheet based form used by the OCS to determine risk scoring and level of approval.

Sample Pilot Form (front)

OPERATIONS COMPLIANCE FORM

RISK ANALYSIS

WEATHER (All Legs, Current and Forecast) **NA/YES**
Ceiling < 3,000' AGL **OR**
Visibility < 5 sm **OR**
Temp/Dewpoint Spread < 3 deg **OR**
Surface Wind > 20 kts

FLIGHT CONSIDERATIONS **NA/YES**
LZ Density Altitude > 8,000' **OR**
Unimproved LZ **OR**
MSCA > 7,000' MSL

AREA FAMILIARITY **NA/YES**
Unfamiliar Base (less than 20%) **AND**
Unfamiliar Destination / Scene (past yr)

HUMAN FACTORS **NA/YES**
SLEEPY (any element) **OR**
More than Two Flights **OR**
Personal Issues

Score | Approved by

CREW BRIEFING

P hysiology
Route / altitude / environmental

E mergency Procedures
In-flight / landing / evacuation

O perational Differences
Day / night / NVG

P atient
Type / loading / hot on-off

L Z Safety
Helipad / scene / general

E ffective Communications
CRM / sterile cockpit

Route / Notes

DAY
MONTH
TIME

Flight #:________
Aircraft ID:________
Call Arrive:________
Dispatch:________
Liftoff:________
Patient Miles:________
Total Miles:________

Hobbs Stop:________
Hobbs Start:________
Total:________

T/O	LDG

Pilot's Signature

Intermountain Life Flight *FQA-0103 Rev 16-02*

• **Figure 10.12** An example of a risk assessment tool: The Operations Compliance Form (Risk Analysis). (Courtesy Intermountain Life Flight, Salt Lake City, Utah.)

Continued

Sample Pilot Form (back)

FATIGUE SELF-EVALUATION	**VFR MINIMUMS**

FATIGUE SELF-EVALUATION

SLEEP More than two hours short?[1]

LOST SLEEP More than four hours in debt?[2]

EARLY MORNING Flying between 0200 and 0600?

EXTENDED DAY Awake longer than 16 hours?

PUSHING IT More than 5-7 straight shifts?

YOU personal signs of fatigue[3]

1 You likely need 8 hours every 24 hours
2 The difference between the sleep you need and the sleep you get accumulates over time. It takes two consecutive full nights of sleep to get out of debt.
3 Delayed reaction time, problems focusing, moodiness, fixation, inattention, feelings of sleepiness degraded judgment, missed cues,etc.

VFR MINIMUMS

Use 14 CFR 91.155 when more restrictive

	DAY		NIGHT	
	Clg	Vis	Clg	Vis
Local	800'			3 sm
Non Local	1,000'	3 sm	1,000'*	5 sm

1,500' without NVGs

PRE / POST FLIGHT

W	**EATHER**
	Ceiling / Visibility / Winds
	MECA
A	**IRCRAFT & EQUIPMENT**
	Non-Std Conf (LR Med, Trauma, Neo)
	Final Equipment Requirement Check
	Fuel
	NVGs
I	**NDIVIDUALS**
	Pilot – Risk Assessment
	Medical Team – Concerns & Questions
	Patient – Status & Weight
T	**IME & TRACK**
	Confirm Destination
	Route / Altitude /Airspeed / ETE
S	**AFETY**
	As Briefed / Unexpected
	Reportable Concerns (QA Report?)
M	**EDICAL**
	Concerns (Crew/Referring or Receiving)
	QA Report?
A	**VIATION**
	Weather
	Maintenance Issues
C	**OMMUNICATIONS**
	Flight Team / Comm Center
	EMS/Outside Agencies
O	**THER**

Sample OCS Entry Form (with supporting point assignments)

ROTOR WING RISK ANALYSIS

EXPERIENCE
Low ☑

TIME OF DAY
Night Shift ☑

WEATHER (all points, current/forecast)
Ceiling < 3,000' AGL ☐
Visibility < 5 sm ☑
Temp/Dewpoint Spread < 3 degrees ☐
Surface Wind > 20 kts ☐

FLIGHT CONSIDERATIONS
LZ Density Altitude > 8,000' ☑
MSCA (Min Safe Cruise Alt) > 7,000' ☐
Unimproved LZ ☐
Reserve Fuel < 30 Minutes ☐

AREA FAMILIARITY
Outside Local Area ☑
Unfamiliar Base ☐
Unfamiliar Destination / Scene ☐

HUMAN FACTORS
Fatigue (SLEEPY) ☐
More than Two Flights (91/135) ☐
Health ☐
Distracting Life Events ☐
Other Stressors ☐

ADDITIONAL RISKS
Prior Turn Down (wx related only)* ☐
Complicated Flight ☐

*Prior Turn Down past 60 minutes is automatic Ops consult

25
Consult? **Ops Only**

NOTE: Are there contingencies that should be considered?

Mitigations: When Ops Controllers, pilots and managers consider high risk flights they should review mitigation strategies that would lower associated risks. For example, if human factors is deemed a high risk area, consider using another pilot who would not be subject to those same factors.
Or, if another program turned down the flight because their only available aircraft was at a location with IFR conditions but our own aircraft and the planned route were VFR, then the flight could be accepted.

Low Experience	1.5	Multiplier
Night Shift	1.3	Multiplier
Ceiling	5	
Visibility	5	
TempDew	5	
Wind	5	
DA	5	
MECA	4	
Unimproved LZ	6	
Fuel	4	
LocalArea	3	
UnfamiliarBase	5	
UnfamillarDestination	5	
Fatigue	8	
TwoFlights	7	
Health	5	
Distractions	5	
OtherStressors	5	
PriorTurnDown	10	
ComplicatedFlight	5	
Second Pilot Consult	40	
Manager Consult	60	

• Figure 10.12, cont'd

best environment for effective communication and use of AMRM. AMRM classes should be a part of initial and recurrent training and should involve all members of the transport team, including the medical transport team, specialty teams, program administration, maintenance technicians, and communication specialists.[27]

Helicopter Shopping/Selective Resource Management

Fatal HEMS accidents occurred when a HEMS program accepted a transport request declined by another provider. In 2019, ASTNA partnered with the Emergency Nurses Association (ENA) and the International Association of Flight and Critical Care Paramedics (IAFCCP) updated their joint position statement on the subject.[28] In the interest of working together with a shared goal of increasing the safety of flight operations, the author team agreed that the phrase "helicopter shopping" does an injustice to not only the problem but also to the hospital- and EMS-based staff who request air medical services. The phrase conveys that the problem is that hospitals and EMS agencies "shop" for helicopters. Patricia Corbett, ASTNA's team leader on the project,

describes the conversation, "We chose the phrase 'selective resource management' over 'helicopter shopping' because we wanted the statement to focus on the shared accountability to communicate vital information to mitigate risk." This new phrase acknowledges the importance and inclusion of a closed-loop feedback for all parties involved in patient transport. Selective resource management emphasizes that patient transport is a *shared* responsibility, whereas "helicopter shopping" may seem to attribute responsibility or even blame solely on a requestor.[28]

Safety Technologies

In 2014, the FAA released "Initiatives to Improve Air Ambulance Safety." The basic recommendations are focused on stricter flight rules and procedures, improved communications and training, and additional onboard safety equipment. These recommendations are summarized in Box 10.3.[29]

All reviews of air medical accidents have identified the same two environments as significant contributing factors: operations at night and during harsh weather. These two environments have

---

• BOX 10.3 Summary of Federal Aviation Administration Recommendations for Helicopter Emergency Medical Services

Year	Recommendations
January 2005	Publication of a notice providing guidance for safety inspectors to help operators review pilot and mechanics decision-making skills, procedural adherence, and crew resource management practices
August 2005	Guidelines issued to inspectors promoting improved risk assessment and risk management tools to all flight crews including medical staff
September 2005	Guidance issued to operators to establish minimum guidelines for Air Medical Resources Management training
	All personnel involved in operations are included: pilots, maintenance technicians, flight nurses and paramedics, medical directors, specialty team members, communication specialists, program directors, and any other identified transport team members
September 2005	Revised standards issued for inspection and surveillance of air ambulance operators with special emphasis on operations control, risk assessment, and facilities and training, especially at outer facilities away from the certified holder's principal base of operations
December 2005	The FAA-established On-Demand Training Center Branch to work the 135 and 142 policy issues
	Inspectors with "helicopter only" experience were hired
Formed in 2005	International Helicopter Safety Team to promote safety and prevent accidents worldwide
January 2006	LOC and CFIT handbook released with description of acceptable models to develop LOC and CFIT Accident-Avoidance Programs
March 2006	Guidance issued to inspectors on surveillance and oversight of public aircraft operators for air ambulance operations
March 2006	Weather summit in Boulder, Colorado, hosted by the FAA and University Cooperation for Atmospheric Research
	Developed and implemented a graphical flight planning tool for ceiling and visibility assessment along direct flights in areas with limited available surface observations capability (revised in 2013)
June 2006	Special Committee to develop H-TAWSS
	In the 2015 Safety Survey, 67% of the surveyed programs reported H-TAWSS installed in aircraft[3]
August 2006	Aeronautic Information Manual revised to provide guidance to pilots on assessing ambient lighting for night visual flight rules operations and/off airport/heliport landing operations
May 2008	FAA's Flight Standards Service issued an advisory highlighting "best practices" for establishing operational control centers and training their specialists
November 2008	FAA published a notice in the Federal Registry that advised operators of important mandatory changes to air ambulance flights including encouraging the use of night vision goggles TAWSs (Terrain Awareness and Warning Systems); all air ambulance operators will comply with Part 135 weather minimums, including repositioning flights with medical crew onboard
	The flight crew was required to determine a minimum safe altitude and obstacle clearance before each flight
January 2009	FAA established a task group to focus on surveillance of large helicopter emergency medical services operators, which resulted in an increase of inspectors and the organization of these inspectors into operator-specific oversight teams
February 2014	Helicopter Air Ambulance, Commercial Helicopter, and Part 91 Helicopter Operations; Final Rule. 135-all rotorcraft must have radio altimeter by 2017, operations over water require additional safety equipment. Revision of alternate airport weather minimums and requiring pilot testing in flat-light, whiteout, and brownout conditions. Demonstrate competency in recovery from IIMC any air operations with medical personnel onboard but operate under Part 135 rules. Operators with 10 or more helicopters must establish an operational control center (OCC), equipped with HTAWS, install flight data monitoring, and perform preflight risk assessments, amongst other safety initiatives

CFIT, Controlled flight into terrain; *FAA*, Federal Aviation Administration; *H-TAWSS*, helicopter terrain awareness and warning systems standards; *LOC*, loss of control. From the Federal *Aviation Administration*. 2014. Fact Sheet-FAA initiatives to improve helicopter air ambulance safety. Accessed July 16, 2010. https://insurancenewsnet.com/oarticle/FAA-Initiatives-to-Improve-Helicopter-Air-Ambulance-Safety-a-463889; Coons J, Zalar, C. Air medical safety survey. *Air Med J.* 2016;35:120–125; https://www.govinfo.gov/content/pkg/FR-2014-02-21/pdf/2014-03689.pdf

one major factor in common: reduced visibility. A variety of technologies can reduce the risk of operating during reduced-visibility conditions by supplying additional information about potential hazards in the flight environment. One of the recurrent safety issues identified in the 2006 NTSB report was the lack of requirements that air medical aircraft make use of these safety technologies to enhance flight safety.[30]

In the 2015 safety survey conducted by Coons and Zalar,[3] the use of the following equipment is advocated, based on the NTSB 2009 HEMS recommendations.[31]

Instrument Flight

Flight operations under instrument flight rules (IFR) are a customary practice for fixed-wing aircraft but have historically been less common in helicopter aviation. Many older helicopter models used in air medical transport were not approved for instrument flight, except in emergency conditions. Many newer HEMS aircraft are IFR capable, and more programs are using this added capability.

When operating under IFR, the pilot is flying under the guidance of the FAA air traffic control (ATC) system. The controller monitors the position of the aircraft on radar and provides routing instructions that keep the aircraft away from terrain and other air traffic.[31] IIMC is always an emergency, but for an IFR-capable aircraft and pilot, encountering reduced-visibility conditions can present less risk of unexpected entry into IMC because the pilot has the option of planning the flight under IFR or of transitioning to IFR flight en route.

Night Vision Goggles

NVGs, also called NVIS, use an electronic system to amplify visible light and provide improved visibility during night operations. NVGs have been used by the military for many years and have seen a rapid acceptance in the HEMS community recently. In 2008, the National EMS Pilots Association released a survey of 382 active HEMS pilots about NVG usage in the HEMS environment. The responses were overwhelmingly in favor of the use of NVGs in night HEMS operations.[2,5,6,10,30–32,40] In the 2015 safety survey, 96% of the programs that responded reported NVG use. In most programs (64%), both the pilot and transport team members wear NVGs.

Terrain Awareness and Warning Systems

One of the common scenarios in air ambulance accidents is loss of adequate visibility and subsequent CFIT. A TAWS provides the pilot with a visual display of the terrain along the flight path and alerts the pilot with visual and audible alarms if the aircraft flies too close to the terrain. Some of these systems also include a *traffic collision avoidance system*, which provides information about the location of other nearby air traffic.[31,33]

Satellite Tracking and Position Reporting

Automated flight following with a satellite-based tracking system provides the flight communication center with up-to-the-minute information regarding the position and status of the aircraft. In an emergency, the aircraft's exact position is always known. Many of these systems also permit satellite-based voice and data communications.[31]

Crashworthy Aircraft and Vehicle Systems

Design changes to improve the crashworthiness of the airframe, fuel system, and seats in US military aircraft have shown improved crash survival rates.[34] Newer civilian and military helicopters are equipped with crashworthy landing gear, crashworthy fuel systems, and crash-attenuating seats that absorb energy and reduce the g force applied to the occupant in a hard impact to improve occupant survival in a crash.[4,34,35] In November 2015, the Air Medical Operators Association, in cooperation with helicopter manufacturers Airbus Helicopters and Bell Helicopter, announced their commitment to the installation of crash-resistant fuel systems (CRFS) in all new aircraft and equipping current aircraft with CRFS as those products become available. On October 3, 2018, the US Senate passed the long-awaited FAA Reauthorization Act 2018.[36] An important safety improvement in this act mandates CRFS in newly manufactured helicopters; improved oversight for the air ambulance industry and clarity over its billing practices. The CRFS provision flows from the legacy of the 2015 crash of an Airbus H125 in Frisco, Colorado. A pilot lost his life in the postcrash fire, and the flight nurse and paramedic were severely injured. Since the bill was enacted, all H125 aircraft are required to have the CRFS, and retrofit kits for the AS350 models were certified by the FAA.

Changes in ground ambulance design to enhance safety have included improved seat and seat belt/harness restraint systems for occupants of the rear compartment, ergonomic interior designs that permit easier access to the patient and supplies while remaining restrained, padded ambulance interiors, and backup camera systems.[37]

Safety Management

An effective comprehensive SMS[26] should be a major part of all transport programs. The commitment to safety must include all disciplines and processes of the organization, and needs to be a core component of the organizational culture of every transport program, from the chief executive officer (CEO) to the newest front-line employee. An SMS is composed of four functional components, also known as the four pillars of safety (Fig. 10.13). The CAMTS Accreditation Standards include their list of SMS components, summarized in Box 10.4.

A *Safety Policy* establishes senior management's commitment to continually improve safety; defines the methods, processes, and organizational structure needed to meet safety goals. This policy establishes management commitment to safety performance, clarifies safety objectives and a commitment to management by those objectives, and establishes cross-organizational communication

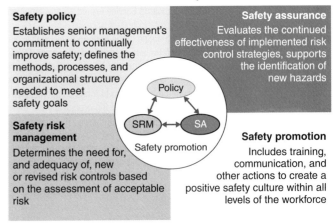

The four SMS components

Safety policy
Establishes senior management's commitment to continually improve safety; defines the methods, processes, and organizational structure needed to meet safety goals

Safety assurance
Evaluates the continued effectiveness of implemented risk control strategies, supports the identification of new hazards

Safety risk management
Determines the need for, and adequacy of, new or revised risk controls based on the assessment of acceptable risk

Safety promotion
Includes training, communication, and other actions to create a positive safety culture within all levels of the workforce

Policy
SRM — SA
Safety promotion

• **Figure 10.13** The four safety management system (SMS) components.

CAMTS Elements of Safety Management System

- A statement of policy commitment from the accountable executive
- A risk identification process and risk management plan that includes a non-punitive system for employees to report hazards, risks, and safety concern
- A system to track and document root cause analysis
- A system to track, trend, and mitigate errors or hazard
  - A safety manual (electronic or hard copy)
  - A system to audit and review organizational policy and procedures, ongoing safety training for all personnel (including managers), a system of pro-active and reactive procedures to insure compliance, etc.
- Operational risk-assessment tools
- Ongoing safety training for all personnel (including managers)
- A system to audit and review organizational policy and procedures
- A system of proactive and reactive procedures to ensure compliance

From *Commission on Accreditation of Medical Transport Services. Accreditation Standards.* 12th ed. Sandy Springs, SC: CAMTS; 2020.

and cooperation to facilitate meeting safety goals. The policy defines the methods, processes, and organizational structure needed to meet safety goals. Importantly, the safety policy also establishes transparency in management of safety, including structures for employee reporting and resolution system and accountability processes for employees at all levels of the organization.[26]

Safety Risk Management structures determine the need for, and adequacy of, risk controls based on the assessment of acceptable risk. The work of patient transport is not, and cannot be, risk free, so it requires careful assessment of risks and evaluation of acceptable risk. The safety risk management process describes the system, identifies hazards, assesses identified risks, analyzes the risks, and identifies measures for risk mitigation.[26]

Safety Assurance evaluates the continued effectiveness of implemented risk control strategies and supports the identification of new hazards. These SMS process management functions, including information acquisition, data analysis, and systematic assessment, provide continuous evaluation to provide confidence that organizational outputs meet or exceed safety requirements. They also provide insight into opportunities and new methods for minimizing risk. Aviation safety elements of the SMS additionally ensure compliance with FAA orders, standards, policies, and directives.[26]

Safety Promotion includes training, communication, and other actions to create a positive safety culture within all levels of the workforce. These activities include:
- Providing SMS training
- Advocating/strengthening a positive safety culture
- System and safety communication and awareness
- Matching competency requirements to system requirements
- Disseminating safety lessons learned

Safety Committee

The safety committee should be composed of representatives of all disciplines involved in the transport program: aviation, clinical, maintenance, communications, and administration. The committee should meet at least quarterly to address safety issues, practices, concerns, or questions. Reports of the committee's discussions and actions should be easily accessible and communicated to all participating in the transport process.

The safety committee should be linked to the program's quality management committee and risk management. Aviation and surface-related events are identified and tracked to minimize risks. There should be a policy as to what safety issues or incidents should be reported and to what agency. The policy should also identify who would be responsible for reporting.[26,27]

Safety Training

Operational Safety Training

All regular transport team members and members of specialty teams who may also participate in transport should receive regular operational safety training. Operational safety training should include AMRM, operational planning, use of the program's operational risk-assessment tools, aircraft and ground vehicle safety, emergency scene operations, and survival. In addition to scheduled didactic sessions, operational safety training should include regular aircraft or ground vehicle emergency drills.[8–11,18,22,25–27,29,31,38,39]

Clinical Safety Training

Clinical safety training should review flight physiology and the stressors of flight, hazardous materials and items (HAZMAT) recognition and response, infection control, and the management of combative or violent patients. These subjects are addressed in detail in other chapters of this textbook. Other safety training topics may include employee wellness, injury prevention, and specific topics required by state, federal, or local statutes.[27,38]

Aircraft Safety Training[8–11,18,22,25–27,29,31,38,39]

All flight crew members must be familiar with the aircraft in use by their program, including all regular and backup aircraft operated by the program in which the crew member may be expected to fly. Specific items with which all crew members must be familiar for all aircraft include the following:
- Operation of seat belts or harness
- Operation of all doors and emergency exits
- Emergency egress procedures
- Emergency egress of patients both with and without a backboard
- Emergency engine shutdown
- Emergency communications
- Oxygen and medical gas shutoff
- Location and operation of onboard fire extinguishers
- Location and use of other onboard emergency equipment, such as the survival kit, personal flotation devices (PDFs), and aviation emergency oxygen systems
- Hot loading and unloading procedures and policies

Ground Ambulance Safety Training[15,16,18–20,27,37,40,41]

Ground ambulance safety should be a part of the training presented by both ground and air transport providers. Air medical crews often are expected to transfer patients from an airport or other landing site to the hospital via ambulance. Ground vehicle safety[18] training should include the following:
- Driver training (where applicable)
- Use of seat belts by all crew members while the vehicle is in motion
- Avoiding standing or kneeling in the patient compartment
- Oxygen and medical gas shutoff
- When to use red lights and siren (RLS) response
- Securing equipment in the ambulance
- Gurney operations and back/lifting safety

Occupational and Workplace Safety Training

All crew members must be familiar with the safety procedures and requirements of the assigned workplace, whether in a hospital, at an airport, or at another location. Items with which all staff need to be familiar include the location and type of fire extinguishers; use of the fire extinguishers; the process for refueling aircraft or vehicles; HAZMAT or fuel spill response; electricity and gas shut-off; occupational injury or illness reporting; and site-specific procedures or practices, such as emergency evacuation routes.[27]

Outreach Safety Education

Along with safety training for transport program staff, safety training and practice must be provided for first responders, hospital personnel, and others who may be asked to work around EMS aircraft. These personnel may include fire service, law enforcement, EMS, and park rangers or game wardens.[27,42]

Safety in the Transport Environment

Personal Safety

Personal safety is an important aspect of the safety attitude. For the individual crew member, personal safety is the mindset, habits, and daily practices that keep that individual safe. Each member of the transport team also bears the responsibility for the personal safety of others, including partner, pilot, patient, and fellow responders. For the transport service, personal safety means providing a safe work environment, appropriate personal protective equipment, and safety training. It also involves establishing and following safety standards and policies. The best safety training and equipment in the world are of little value if not used properly, and safety standards cannot be effective if they are not followed.[27,38,43,44]

Fitness Standards

The transport environment is physically challenging and requires that transport team members maintain a high personal level of both physical and emotional fitness. The requirements of each program vary, and no industry-wide formal guidelines exist. Minimal physical requirements of any person working in the medical transport environment should include the ability to work within the space limitations of the transport aircraft and vehicles operated by the program; to lift and carry a reasonable amount of weight; and to function in the typical work environments encountered by the program, such as scene calls. Transport team members must not have any preexisting conditions that could interfere with flexibility, strength, or cardiovascular fitness. Transport team members also must not have any condition that could cause altered mental or neurologic function.[27]

Fatigue Policies[8,14,15,18,23,26,27,31,45]

Studies on the effects of fatigue on performance have shown that they are similar to the effects of alcohol. Fatigue is a factor in many aviation mishaps and accidents. It should be addressed in the same fashion as other risks, especially during night operations. Transport programs need to have policies in place to address crew fatigue. These should include reliable and/or valid fatigue and sleepiness survey instruments should be used to measure and monitor fatigue, avoiding shifts of 24 hours in duration (if napping is not allowed), having access to caffeine as a fatigue countermeasure, having the opportunity to nap while on duty to mitigate

fatigue, and receiving education and training to mitigate fatigue and fatigue-related risks annually. The NASEMSO risk assessment tool can be found at https://emsfatiguerisk.ibrinc.org/risk.ibrinc.org/.[46]

Sleep[47]

Adults need 7 to 9 hours of sleep per night, and variations may be based on overall health and activity levels. Meeting that goal requires planning especially within the confines of EMS shift work. Some strategies that mitigate risk due to lack of sleep include:
- Maintaining a sleep schedule on and off duty
- Having a nightly sleep routine
- Maximizing the comfort of your bed – mattress, bedding, and pillows
- Minimizing potential disruptions from light and sound while optimizing your bedroom temperature and aroma
  - Set the room thermostat set between 60°F and 67°F
- Disconnecting from electronic devices like mobile phones and laptops for a half-hour or more before bed
- Monitoring your intake of caffeine and alcohol and trying to avoid consuming them in the hours before bed

Crew members should have the right to call a time-out from any flight or ground transport duties if they or a fellow flight team member feel that continuing duty is unsafe because of fatigue, no matter what the shift length. No adverse personnel action or undue pressure to continue should occur.

Pregnancy[27,48]

Many women of childbearing age work in the transport setting. No existing industry standard is found regarding pregnancy employment policies. The effects of high altitude, high noise levels, and vibration and the increased risk for injury in mishaps have been identified as potential risks to the fetus and maternal health. Transport team members who are considering pregnancy should discuss these risks with their personal physician and program administration.

Personal Protective Equipment[27,38,43,44,49]

The 1988 NTSB study recommended that air medical personnel who routinely fly EMS helicopter missions wear protective clothing and equipment to reduce the chance of injury or death in survivable accidents. The ASTNA position papers have also endorsed the use of protective equipment, which consists of helmets, fire-resistant uniforms, and boots.

Helmets[49]

In the military, the use of flight helmets has been shown to protect significantly against head injuries. Despite the obvious advantages afforded by flight helmets, acceptance in civilian air medical programs was not initially widespread. Reasons cited for not wearing helmets included excessive cost, uncertain benefit, and negative public relations. However, a survey performed to determine the public's perception of helmet usage found that patients and family members positively viewed the use of helmets by air medical personnel.[50] The use of helmets by EMS pilots and flight crew members has become the accepted standard. CAMTS now requires that all helicopter transport team members wear a helmet, including specialty team members.[27]

The flight helmet must be approved for use in helicopters. The chinstrap should hold the helmet firmly in place, and the liner needs to fit comfortably. Some manufacturers use customized liners that are molded to the individual's head. The helmet visor should be kept in the down position as much as possible during flight. Helmets should receive routine maintenance. They should also be routinely evaluated for appropriate fit.

Fire-Resistant Clothing[27]

The goal of fire-resistant clothing is to minimize skin exposure to the intense heat of an aircraft fire. The uniform should have long sleeves and be made of a flame- and heat-resistant materials like Nomex. Flame-resistant fabrics are designed to withstand high temperatures for a brief period, usually less than 20 seconds, which permits the wearer to evacuate a burning aircraft or vehicle.[10,27,38] The fabric can reduce the risk or severity of tissue damage but does not prevent thermal injury to the skin.

Undergarments worn under the fire-resistant flight suit (including briefs, T-shirt, or long underwear) should be made of natural fibers, such as cotton, silk, or wool.[50] When exposed to flames, synthetic materials such as polyester or polypropylene melt and become embedded into the skin. The uniform should fit to allow a 0.25 inch of air space between the flight suit and undergarments. Nomex gloves protect the hands and should be considered by people who wear fire-resistant uniforms.

Protective Footwear[27,38,50]

Boots should protect the foot from punctures, lacerations, and thermal injuries and provide stability to the ankle on rough or uneven ground. Boots should be constructed of leather, or leather and Nomex, and extend several inches above the ankle. The sole should be thick and oil resistant, and the boot should have a safety toe and shank. It should also have adequate ventilation to prevent moisture from being trapped.

Hearing Protection[27,38,50]

The average sound level produced by a running helicopter is between 90 and 100 decibels (dB). The Occupational Safety and Health Administration regulations require employers to provide hearing-conservation programs for employees exposed to time-weighted average sound levels of 85 dB or greater. Hearing protection, such as earplugs, earmuffs, or the flight helmet, should be worn during high-decibel exposures such as engine startup, hot loading and unloading, extreme noise levels at some scenes, and around running aircraft at airports. Earplugs are smaller and less expensive, but noise protection varies with fit; custom-fitted earplugs provide the most noise reduction. Earmuffs offer more uniform protection but are more expensive, are not as easily carried or stored, and may be less comfortable than earplugs. A properly fitted flight helmet provides adequate hearing protection for most individuals and should be worn while in flight. Active noise reduction (or noise canceling) circuitry or communications earplugs can be added to most flight helmets to provide further noise attenuation.

Patient Safety

Along with the safety of the transport team, the safety of the patient being transported must be ensured. The patient should be properly restrained in the transport vehicle and provided with appropriate hearing and thermal protection. All patient care should be performed in a safe manner. Clinical decision-making, patient treatment, and error reporting are all discussed elsewhere in this textbook, but each has a significant impact on patient

safety. Keeping the patient safe should be an equally important part of the safety attitude. Family members or other passengers who accompany patients must be properly identified and listed by name (in compliance with HIPAA regulations) in the communications center by the transport coordinator and be listed on the manifest. All riders must receive a safety briefing and be properly restrained during transport.

Helicopter Safety

The most obvious component of the helicopter that presents a risk is the rotor system. The main rotor blades turn at approximately 400 rpm, with the rotor tips moving at more than 500 mph. At full speed, the main rotor blades create a disk that can be seen above the cabin. When the main rotor is spinning at lower speeds, such as during the startup and shutdown phases, the blades can flap or sail with wind gusts, which may allow the blades to drop below shoulder level. The degree to which this presents a hazard varies by aircraft model and design, but the best precaution is to never approach or depart any helicopter during startup or shutdown. The crouch position is advised for anyone approaching or departing the aircraft at other times while the blades are turning. When a helicopter lands on uneven ground or on a slope, the rotor disk comes closer to the ground on the uphill side. In this situation, the aircraft should always be approached and departed from the downhill side in the crouched position, with constant attention paid to the terrain and the rotor disk. Program policy dictates whether patients are loaded into the aircraft with the rotor system turning, which is commonly referred to as *hot loading*. When loading or unloading patients and equipment, nothing should ever be carried above the head.

The tail rotor is potentially the most hazardous component of the helicopter. At a speed greater than 2000 rpm, it is invisible. Aircraft manufacturers have worked to reduce the risks presented by the tail rotor by developing safer designs, such as the shrouded fenestron and no-tail-rotor systems. A safety person should be designated at all unsecured landing sites to ensure that no one inadvertently walks near the tail rotor.

All persons who approach the helicopter must do so in full view of the pilot and should not proceed under the rotor disk without the pilot's permission. The safest approach zone for most helicopters is from the sides, at the 3 o'clock or 9 o'clock position (12 o'clock is the nose of the aircraft; (Fig. 10.14). Some aircraft models permit a safe approach from the front, depending on rotor or skid height and aircraft design. Flight crew members must be familiar with the safe approach zones for their program's aircraft. Those who work around the aircraft, such as EMS personnel, must be instructed to remain back from the aircraft after it lands and to approach only after being directed to do so by the pilot or a flight crew member and to never approach the aircraft from the rear.

The wind created by the moving rotor blades, referred to as *rotor wash,* can exceed 50 mph. In a hover and on the ground during the warm-up or cool-down stage, a rotor wash of approximately 25 mph can occur. Crew members should keep helmet visors down or wear protective glasses when operating around the running aircraft. All loose objects near the helicopter must be secured to prevent them from being blown away or ingested into the air intake of the helicopter's engine. Rotor wash also increases the wind-chill factor. An air temperature of 10°F combined with a 25-mph rotor wash creates a wind-chill temperature of −11°F.[52] Transport team members need to consider this and take steps to protect the patient before loading. Other hazardous areas that

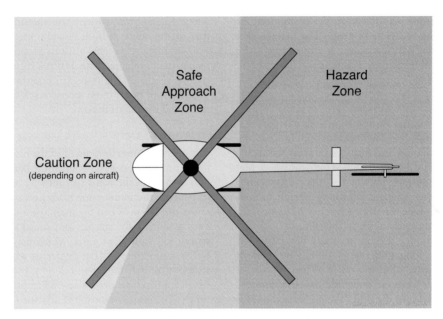

• **Figure 10.14** Typical safe helicopter approach zones.

should be avoided include the engine exhaust ports (the exhaust temperature is approximately 400°C) and the pitot tubes, used to measure the aircraft's airspeed and heated to prevent ice formation, which presents a burn hazard.

Fixed-Wing Aircraft Safety

Fixed-wing aircraft have their own set of safety requirements. The propellers carry the same risk of injury as the rotors on a helicopter, and jet engines present risks from both the engine exhaust and the possibility of aspiration into the engine intakes. No one should be allowed to approach the aircraft until the engines have been shut down. Many fixed-wing aircraft used as air ambulances have pressurized cabins, which permit flight at higher altitudes. All crew members need to be familiar with how to ensure that the hatches are properly sealed and with emergency procedures in the event of cabin depressurization.

Ground Ambulance Safety

Study results of ground ambulance crashes described previously show that the high-risk environments for ground ambulance operations are emergency responses and intersections. Regulations for emergency response with the use of running lights and sirens vary from state to state, but the decision is left to the transport team with all in agreement with the level of response to ensure the safety of all on board. Program operational and safety policies in addition to driver training should guide when running emergent is acceptable. Air transport programs should educate their crews about ground ambulance safety and appropriateness of emergency response using lights and sirens. This is especially important if the medical crew/patient are using a ground ambulance service that is not part of their organization or not known to the air medical crew. A discussion between all team members should take place with all in agreement with the level of response. The use of appropriate safety equipment and procedures in ground vehicles should be just as important as it is in rotor or fixed-wing modes of transport. Seat belts must be worn by all people in the ground ambulance, and all equipment must be properly secured.

Daily Shift Safety Procedures

At the beginning of each shift, the pilot/driver and medical crew should complete a vehicle safety inspection. This inspection should include an overall walk-around inspection of the vehicle and a check of onboard medical and safety equipment. The pilot/driver and medical crew should perform their respective daily checklists to ensure the vehicle and equipment are operation ready. The daily risk assessment should be performed, and the pilot/driver should brief the medical crew and the communications center regarding weather concerns/road conditions, expected maintenance, equipment issues or other issues related to the aircraft, and any specific-planning needs.

Dispatch/Communications

The 2006 NTSB report recommended that air medical programs be dispatched from a dedicated flight dispatch center, separate from any hospital or public safety dispatch center. The report also recommended expanding the role of the flight dispatcher/communication specialist to include specialized training in aviation weather, navigation, aircraft weight and balance planning, instrument approaches, and other aviation topics. These recommendations were not to take any decision-making authority away from the pilot or flight crew but to provide a resource to the pilot for informed safe decisions. Communications and the role of the communication specialist are discussed in detail in Chapter 6.

An important safety consideration during the notification of a transport request is that the communication specialist should only provide the pilot/ambulance driver with the information needed to decide whether the operational request can be safely accepted. Before the pilot/driver makes the decision, no patient-specific information should be shared. Initial notification of the pilot/driver should include:
• Nature of the request (scene call vs. interfacility transfer)
• Location of the request
• Destination (if known)

- Patient weight (if known)
- Whether another aircraft or program has declined the request, and the reason for any such decline
- Known weather, road conditions, or other hazards

Once the pilot/driver has evaluated the request and decided that the operational request can be safely accepted, additional patient information may be communicated. An alternative method is to have the communication specialist contact the clinical crew separately and provide them with the patient information. The clinical crew should not discuss the patient with the pilot until a decision has been made that the operational request can be safely accepted. The clinical crew should not pressure the pilot/driver to accept an operational request based on patient needs if it has been declined for safety reasons.

Helipad/Airport Safety

Hospital and off-site helipads should be designed to meet all applicable FAA and local regulations and should be able to safely accommodate the weight and size of the largest helicopter expected to use the helipad. Other helipad planning considerations include approach and departure routes, the location of the helipad relative to patient care areas, the provision of emergency exits, fire protection equipment, and helipad lighting. Provisions also need to be made for snow removal, fuel/HAZMAT/biohazard spills, and general cleaning. The helipad should be secured and monitored to prevent access by unauthorized persons. All flight crew members should be trained in fire safety and should know the location of fire alarm boxes and fire extinguishers. Smoking should be prohibited around or near the aircraft.

Crew members of aircraft based at airports need to be familiar with the safety and security requirements of the airport; the location of fire extinguishers and other emergency equipment at the base; and the methods of reporting an emergency to the FAA control tower (if present), airport administration, and local authorities. Other safety considerations at airports include access to restricted areas, awareness of runway/taxiway safety, and operations around other aircraft.[42]

In-Flight Safety

In-flight safety begins with preliftoff checks of the aircraft to ensure that all doors and outside cowlings are secure, that engine and other covers/tie downs have been removed, that shoreline electric cords have been disconnected, and that the aircraft is ready for departure. It also includes safety equipment such as helmets, seat belts, and shoulder harnesses during all flight phases. At times, patient needs may necessitate that a crew member come "out of belt," but this should be done only while in level flight and with the approval of the pilot; the belts should be reapplied as soon as possible.

Situational Awareness

Situational awareness refers to the maintenance of an active awareness of all aspects of the flight environment. This awareness includes scanning for other aircraft, listening to radio traffic, maintaining a sterile cockpit during critical phases of flight, and observing for hazards on approach to scenes or other unfamiliar landing areas. Crew members should always advise the pilot when they need to be "eyes in," with their attention focused inside the aircraft for patient care or other reasons.

Crew members should scan for other air traffic as much as possible, especially when no patient is onboard. They need to report any obstacle or other air traffic, even though the pilot may have already seen it. Traffic or other hazards should be reported with use of clock position, with 12 o'clock being the nose of the aircraft and 6 o'clock being the tail. The location should further be identified as high, level, or low. One effective technique for scanning is the front-to-side method. This method involves starting with a fixed point in the center of the front windshield, slowly moving the field of vision leftward, returning to the center, refocusing, and then moving the eyes to the right. Other scanning techniques are available, and selection of one is a matter of preference, but the technique should involve some series of fixations. When the head is in motion, vision is blurred, and the mind does not register targets as easily.

The use of unmanned aerial vehicles (UAVs) and unmanned aerial systems (UAS) (also often called drones) has seen a significant increase over the last few years, and the growth is just beginning. The size of the drones can vary from as small as a hummingbird to as large as a regular aircraft. The FAA has issued regulations in the Small Unmanned Aircraft Rule (Part 107) about the use of drones.[53] Transport team members must always remain vigilant to prevent any potential incidents related to these aircraft.

Use of lasers in construction, speaker presentation, and general entertainment has presented a safety hazard to flight teams. Although it is illegal to point a laser at an aircraft, it still happens frequently. This can disorient the pilot and cause eye damage, especially when wearing NVGs. Programs should have policies in place to immediately report near UAVs and UAS (unmanned aircraft systems) and laser hits to the local authorities and the FAA.[54]

Sterile cockpit refers to restricting all nonessential communications over the aircraft intercom system. Federal aviation regulations (FAR 135.100) require the observance of a sterile cockpit during all critical phases of flight, including taxi, takeoff, landing, and all other flight operations except cruise flight. Flight crew members should also attempt to maintain an awareness of the location of the aircraft along its flight path. Should a sudden emergency arise, quick communication of the aircraft's position may be necessary.

Flight Following

A crucial component of transport safety is having the location of the aircraft or vehicle always known, which is a process known as *flight following*. If an aircraft has any type of mishap that requires an emergency landing and the crew is unable to make a distress call, the flight following information permits the aircraft's position to be estimated with a high degree of accuracy. Typically, the communication specialist keeps abreast of the progress of the transport with periodic scheduled communications with the pilot or driver. Some programs use satellite-based real-time tracking systems that display the aircraft or vehicle location on a computer screen or map. Cellular telephones should not be used while in flight but may be used by ground transport teams to provide position/status reports.

When direct communications are not available, the pilot, driver, or crew should contact other transport program communication centers, emergency dispatch centers, airports, or hospitals along the flight or transport path and ask them to relay status reports. Flight following can also be requested from the FAA ATC system. Flight following with ATC has the added advantage of the aircraft being followed on radar by the controller.

Securing Patients and Equipment

The CAMTS[27] accreditation standards specify that patients must be secured with at least three cross straps that restrain the patient to the litter at the chest, hips, and knees. Patients who are loaded head forward should also be restrained with a shoulder harness. The belts need to be adjustable to accommodate patients with specific needs or injury locations. The patient must also be secured so they are isolated from the pilot and the controls. Pediatric patients should be restrained with an appropriately sized securing device. If a car seat is used, it must have an FAA approval sticker.

Combative or potentially violent patients should be evaluated for the need for physical or chemical restraint before loading into the aircraft or vehicle. Physical restraints should be applied before takeoff or departure of the ground unit. Physical or chemical restraints should be guided by periodically reviewed and updated program policies. All patients and baggage should be checked for weapons and dangerous objects (this may include items that may deteriorate in flight) prior to being placed in a transport vehicle.[27]

All bags and equipment must be secured while the aircraft or vehicle is in motion to prevent these objects from becoming projectiles and inflicting injuries to the patient or crew. Confirmation that all bags and equipment are properly secured should be a part of the preliftoff checks.

Scene Safety

The EMS scene call environment is one of the most potentially hazardous aspects of air medical operations.[3] The number of variables is huge, and the flight crew has direct control over only a small portion of the operation. Situational awareness, attention to detail, communications skills, critical thinking abilities, and knowledge of program and local EMS policies all come into play during each scene response. Flight crew members who operate in the scene call environment should be familiar with the Incident Command System (ICS, also called the Incident Management System) because it is used in their service area.[55]

Landing Zone Selection and Safety

Landing a helicopter at an unfamiliar location presents a variety of hazards. Each program should establish requirements for a suitable LZ for the program's aircraft. The LZ should be at least 75 × 75 feet for daytime use and 125 × 125 feet or larger at night. Larger is always better. A useful way to determine whether a proposed LZ is suitable is the mnemonic HOTSAW (hazards, obstructions, terrain, surface/slope/nature of the surface, animals, and wind/weather) (Box 10.5).

Although the pilot makes the ultimate decision about landing at any site, the initial selection and preparation of the LZ are often the responsibility of the local fire department or EMS provider. LZ selection and preparation should be a part of routine outreach education provided to first responders. Training should also include a discussion of radio and visual communications procedures, use of eye and hearing protection, hot-loading procedures, and an aircraft-specific orientation.

Two-way radio contact should be established with the LZ coordinator as early as possible before arrival. The usual preference is to use a dedicated air-to-ground frequency for LZ communications (one that is not in use for other on-scene radio traffic). If a hazard is identified during approach or landing, the LZ coordinator needs to be able to notify the aircraft immediately. The pilot

---

• BOX 10.5   HOTSAW: A Tool for Evaluation of Potential Landing Zones[50]

Hazards
Potential Hazards Within the Landing Zone
Rocks
Downed timber
Vegetation
Fences, loose debris
Vehicles

Obstructions
Overhead Obstructions Along the Flight Path Into or Out of the Landing Zone
Trees
Hills
Power lines
Flag poles
Buildings

Terrain
Nature of Landing Zone and Nearby Terrain Features
Elevation
Uneven ground
Creeks or ditches
Surrounding terrain (mountains, cliffs, water, etc.)

Surface/Slope/Nature of Surface
Character of Surface
- Hard
- Soft/muddy (risk of landing gear sinking)
- Icy

Loose Surface Materials That May Blow in Rotor Wash
- Sand
- Snow
- Dirt
- Dry vegetation
- Slope of ground

Animals
Domestic animals (horses, cows, dogs, etc.)
Wild animals
Humans (bystanders and responders)

Wind/Weather
Wind speed and direction
Overall weather conditions (clouds, fog, height of cloud ceiling, precipitation, air)

---

should perform a high reconnaissance, followed by a low reconnaissance, which allows the pilot and flight crew to observe for hazards before the final approach. If the pilot or crew detect a problem with the LZ, the landing should be aborted, and the LZ coordinator informed of the issue. If the concern can be immediately corrected, then the site may be used. If the situation cannot be easily resolved, then a new LZ may need to be chosen.

An awareness of activities in and around the LZ is always important when the aircraft is on approach, on the ground, and departing. Ground personnel should only be allowed to approach the aircraft when directed to do so by the pilot or a flight crew member. On departing the scene, the flight crew should provide the LZ coordinator with a final report. A "thank you" to the ground crew for their help is always a good idea.

Multiple Aircraft Response[27]

When more than one helicopter is on scene, or other aircraft are expected to land, clear communications must be maintained between the pilots of all aircraft and with the LZ coordinator. All air medical personnel on scene should remain in communication with their own pilot via radio and with the pilot or crew of any other helicopter on scene via direct radio contact, relay via their own pilot, or hand signals. Crew members should never approach or pass under or near the rotor disk of another aircraft without the knowledge and approval of the pilot of that aircraft.

On-Scene Safety

Crew members must maintain an awareness of the hazards present in the prehospital setting. Unless specifically trained and authorized, transport team members should not participate in vehicle extrication or specialized rescue efforts. The extrication process should only be interrupted if immediate life-saving measures are needed, and then only if the procedure can be performed without unnecessary risk to the crew member or other rescuers. When responding to a violent crime scene, transport teams should always consult with law enforcement personnel to ensure the scene is safe before entering. When caring for a victim of a violent crime, care should be taken to disturb the scene no more than necessary to preserve evidence.[27]

Hazardous Materials[27]

Response to HAZMAT scenes must be done cautiously. The priority is always the safety of the flight crew and aircraft. The LZ should be upwind of the incident and at a safe distance. Air medical personnel should not participate in the decontamination process for HAZMAT-exposed cases, regardless of any skills or experience the individual crew members may possess. HAZMAT-exposed cases should never be placed onboard the aircraft until they have undergone complete decontamination by a qualified HAZMAT team.

Postoperation Debriefings

A preflight briefing is an important part of operational safety. A postoperation debrief is equally, if not more, important. It permits the crew to come together and review the evolution and identify issues or concerns about any aspect of the flight, including adequacy and accuracy of planning, operational safety and decision-making, and clinical care of the patient. Debriefings can help identify recurrent issues and event-specific occurrences that need to be addressed. They may also identify risk factors that should be considered in the planning of subsequent missions. When communication-related issues are identified, the communication center should also be included.

In-Flight Emergencies

An *in-flight emergency* is "a sudden unforeseen occurrence or incident requiring immediate action." These events can range from the catastrophic failure of a critical aircraft component to a malfunction in an aircraft system that does not present an immediate risk but indicates that prompt action must be taken to prevent further problems. A common aviation description of how to manage an in-flight emergency is to *aviate, navigate, and communicate*. The priorities are to maintain (or regain) control of the aircraft, decide on the next step, select an appropriate emergency landing site (if indicated), and then report the emergency to the program communication center, ATC, or the local emergency dispatch center.

The transport team member's key role in an in-flight emergency is to serve as a resource to the pilot. Once the pilot has announced an emergency, the crew members should[8,50]
- Ensure sterile cockpit
- Assist the pilot as needed or requested
- Prepare self for an emergency landing: helmet strap tight, visor down, seat belts snug
- Prepare the patient for an emergency landing: position properly, secure/tighten seat belts
- Prepare the cabin for an emergency landing: secure equipment, shut off oxygen and inverter
- Look for suitable emergency landing sites
- Initiate emergency communications as directed by pilot

Training in emergency procedures should be part of the safety training program, and proficiency should be demonstrated annually. Regularly scheduled emergency drills permit practice and increase familiarity with emergency procedures.

Aircraft Mechanical Emergencies

Mechanical emergencies involve a malfunction in some aspects of the aircraft's systems. Sensors are in all the aircraft's important systems to provide the pilot with a visual or audible warning if a problem occurs in that system. Some of these conditions can be managed in flight, and others require that the aircraft land to ensure safety. The pilot should inform the crew as soon as a potential mechanical emergency is identified and advise them if an emergency landing is necessary.

Aircraft Fire Emergencies

Aircraft fires can be divided into two broad categories: those that involve the engines and fuel system and those that occur within the aircraft cabin. Engine fires usually trigger a warning light on the pilot's instrument panel and produce visible smoke. To confirm the presence of an engine fire on a helicopter, the pilot may put the aircraft into a gentle turn and ask the crew member on the side facing the inside of the turn to look back for a smoke trail. A confirmed engine fire is a serious emergency and requires that the affected engine be shut down. On twin-engine aircraft, emergency procedures should dictate that the pilot requests visual confirmation from the crew that the correct engine is being shut down before doing so. Some aircraft have built-in fire extinguishers in the engine compartments.

Smoke from an aircraft cabin fire can fill the cabin quickly and potentially incapacitate the crew. Fire extinguishers should be within easy reach of all crew members. On larger aircraft in which the medical crew is separated from the pilot, a fire extinguisher should be in each compartment. In the event of a cabin fire, the crew members should shut off the oxygen source, turn off the inverter, and close the windows and vents to prevent acceleration of the fire. If the fire is caused by medical equipment plugged into the aircraft power supply, the equipment should be turned off and unplugged and the inverter turned off. If smoke and heat become excessive, the crew should open windows or doors with discretion, fight the fire aggressively with the fire extinguisher, and prepare for an emergency landing.[38,50] Aircraft fire extinguishers are typically filled with halon, an inert gas that extinguishes fire by displacing oxygen. Halon extinguishers present the risk of asphyxiation when discharged in a closed space and should only be used in ventilated spaces. Fire extinguishers should only be discharged in the aircraft cabin at the pilot's direction.

Emergency Communications

Emergency communications are the responsibility of the pilot but may be delegated to a crew member, depending on program policy. If a crew member is expected to make emergency radio calls, this responsibility should be clearly defined in the program's emergency procedures. Emergency radio calls should only be made at the direction of the pilot. All members of the flight team should be familiar with radio operations.

In the event of an emergency landing because of a serious situation (engine fire, etc.), the term *Mayday* is used to ensure that the severity of the situation is clear to the receiving party and to indicate the need for additional assistance to respond to the emergency landing site (fire department, etc.). A Mayday call indicates immediate serious distress and should only be used in a true emergency. The typical way to declare an emergency over the radio is Mayday, Mayday, Mayday; (aircraft tail number/identifier) is making an emergency landing at (location) due to (nature of emergency).

In less serious situations that necessitate a precautionary landing, the appropriate description should be used, rather than a Mayday call. Include the location of the landing site and as much additional information as the circumstances dictate. In some situations, initial radio calls should be made to the local 911 emergency dispatch center, which may be easier to contact than the program's dispatch center and can rapidly mobilize any needed resources (fire department, ambulance, etc.).

Emergency Locator Transmitter

All EMS aircraft are required by the FAA to carry an emergency locator transmitter (ELT). The ELT is activated by an impact that exceeds $4g$ (four times the force of gravity) and broadcasts a signal on one of the universal distress frequencies: 121.5, 243, or 406 MHz as of February 1, 2009, the COSPAS-SARSAT satellite system no longer monitors the 121.5 and 243 MHz frequencies. The 406-MHz ELTs transmit a digital signal that identifies the aircraft and contains global positioning system position information. The signal is received by the international COSPAS-SARSAT satellite system, and the information relayed to search and rescue (SAR) personnel. The 406-MHz ELTs also transmit a signal on the 121.5-MHz emergency frequency that may be used by radio direction-finding equipment to pinpoint the location of the beacon.[52]

Transport team members should know the location of the ELT on all their program's aircraft and how to ensure that it has been activated. If an impact does not automatically activate the ELT, it can be activated manually by following the directions on the front of the unit. Each crew member should know the location and how to activate the ELT.

Emergency Landings

In an emergency or precautionary landing situation, in which a hard landing may be anticipated, flight crew members should assume the survival position before impact. They should sit upright with knees together and feet approximately 6 inches apart. In forward-facing seats equipped with shoulder belts, one should

hold the arms across the chest, forming an X with the forearms and grasping the shoulder harness. In forward-facing seats without shoulder belts, one should bend forward at the waist and encircle the knees with the arms. In aft-facing seats, one should sit upright with the head held against the seat headrest and the arms in an X across the chest. Crew members should keep a point of reference inside the cabin to maintain spatial orientation in case the aircraft comes to rest on its side or inverted.

Emergency Egress

All crew members need to be prepared to manage the emergency evacuation of the crew and patient from all the aircraft used by their program. After an emergency landing, disorientation is common, particularly if the aircraft is not upright. The only available route of egress may involve climbing up to a door or window, into the cockpit, over seats, or over other occupants of the aircraft. One should make a quick survey to reestablish spatial orientation and assess the condition of the aircraft, other crew members, and the patient. In night conditions or in smoke-filled cabins, spatial orientation can be maintained with the hand-over-hand method, during which one hand is kept on a known reference point while a new reference point is selected with the other hand. After the aircraft has come to a complete stop, crew should exit the aircraft by normal means when possible or by jettisoning doors, opening emergency exits, or using forcible means if necessary.[50]

Individual crew members should evacuate to a predesignated position away from the aircraft, typically the 12 o'clock position off the nose of rotor-wing aircraft and the 6 o'clock position off the tail for fixed-wing aircraft. Crew members should evaluate the risk of fire and other hazards before attempting the rescue of injured or entrapped fellow crew members or the patient. After a forced landing, a significant danger is fire. All crew members should be familiar with the emergency shutdown procedure for all aircraft in which they may be asked to operate and how to operate the fire extinguishers carried on the aircraft.

Emergency egress, aircraft evacuation, and emergency shutdown should be part of initial training for all crew members and should be practiced regularly. Crew members should keep in mind that they may need to perform postcrash emergency egress and evacuation when they are injured. Practice and drills should include consideration of how to open emergency exits or perform emergency shutdown with only one arm and with other disabilities.

Forced Water Landings[38,50]

Air medical programs that frequently operate over large bodies of water need to ensure that all crew members are familiar with emergency egress procedures in the event of a forced water landing, or ditching. When flying over water, all flight team members should wear a PFD. Aircraft PFDs should have an attached strobe light that automatically activates upon contact with the water. Flight team members may consider wearing additional survival gear and signaling devices in a vest system. The ability to swim should be mandatory, and water egress procedures and open-water survival should be part of the training received by all flight team members. Each program should evaluate its risk of a water landing and provide specialized open-water survival equipment where appropriate.

In a ditching situation, jettisoning of doors and other emergency procedures should be performed under the pilot's direction. The sequence for emergency escape from an aircraft after a water landing is as follows.

Before Impact With the Water

1. Try to keep calm and concentrate on how you are going to get out.
2. Know which way the closest door is from your position.
3. Open or jettison doors as directed by the pilot.
4. Place one hand on a known reference point within the cabin.
5. Disconnect your ICS cable.
6. Place your other hand on the seat belt buckle (do not release).

After Impact With the Water

7. Do not attempt to exit the aircraft until the rotor or propeller has stopped moving.
8. Helicopters almost always capsize after striking the water; do not attempt to exit the cabin until the aircraft is upside down.
   - Wait for the helicopter to all but fully fill with water.
   - Take a deep breath.
   - Release your buckle; you will immediately float.
   - Pull yourself toward the closest door and out.
   - Do not swim or kick; this increases the chance of becoming entangled and you may unintentionally kick other crew members.
   - Exhale slowly during ascent to the surface to reduce the risk of pulmonary barotrauma.
   - If necessary, observe your air bubbles to determine which way is up.
9. Fixed-wing aircraft float for a few minutes.
   - Locate the safest exit route.
   - Open the appropriate door and crawl through.
   - Assist others in exiting.
   - Enter the water and move away from the fuselage before it sinks.
10. Do not inflate your life vest until outside and away from the aircraft.
11. If a helmet is worn, keep it on for insulation and visibility.
    Open-water survival is discussed later in the chapter.

Ground Vehicle Emergencies[18,19]

All people riding in the front seat of a ground transport vehicle should always wear their seat belts. Everyone in the patient compartment should remain in seat belts as much as possible during patient care and stay in their seats with seat belts secured at all other times. Programs should have response plans to address ground vehicle and aircraft accidents. All vehicles should be equipped with fire extinguishers, and emergency egress and evacuation training should be a part of the annual training.

Postcrash Responsibilities

Crew Responsibilities

After any crash or other accident, the crew should first ensure the safety of all on board the aircraft or vehicle. Then, the crew members should attend to any injuries that have occurred and attempt to contact help. Help may be the local emergency dispatch center, the program communication center, or the FAA. A 911 call from a cellular phone may be the easiest and most expedient way to accomplish contact help if a cellular signal is found.

Missing or Overdue Aircraft or Ground Vehicle Procedure

The practice of flight or ground transport following should be standard operating procedure in all transport programs. The communication specialist should maintain a constant awareness

of the location of each aircraft or vehicle for which they are responsible. If a scheduled check-in is missed, or arrival is overdue, the communication specialist should initiate the *postaccident incident plan* (PAIP).

Postaccident Incident Plan

The PAIP is a program policy document outlining the communication specialist and program administration's responsibilities. See Chapter 25 for a full treatment of this important resource.

Safety Attitude Revisited

The preceding sections of this chapter have discussed the historic and current safety records of the air medical industry and the initiatives, practices, and tools available to improve safety. These resources alone are not enough to prevent future tragedies. The vital component is the human factor. Every individual involved in medical transport must commit themselves to the development of a positive safety culture within their own program and throughout the industry. Everyone must stay informed about new safety practices and technologies and maintain an open mind about their use. Most importantly, all those involved in medical transport must make good, safe, informed decisions about every aspect of every operational request as well as develop, maintain, and spread a safety attitude.

Ed MacDonald,[22] an experienced HEMS pilot and safety advocate, in a paper titled "Dumb Down for Safety" published in the *Air Medical Journal* in 2008, summarized how to keep safe in the transport environment by following these three lessons:
- Lesson 1: My crew and I are responsible for making good decisions that will cause no harm.
- Lesson 2: I will not operate in any conditions wherein I cannot see and avoid every hazard or have a way out.
- Lesson 3: Not dealing with internal and external pressure can push me to where I do not belong.

Survival Basics[18,27–29,34,38,43,50,56,57]

All medical transport crew members need to be prepared to face the possibility of a survival situation. The situation may result from an emergency landing in a remote location because of weather or mechanical issues or changes in the operational environment (such as weather deterioration while at a remote scene LZ). Ground transport vehicles may break down or be stranded by weather. Regardless of the cause, the essentials of survival remain the same.

The goal in a survival situation is survival until a rescue can be accomplished. Flight-following procedures provide the flight communication center with the general location of the incident. The ELT on the aircraft assists rescuers in locating the aircraft and crew. All air medical aircraft should be equipped with a complete survival kit, and all crew members should receive training in its use. Ground transport vehicles that operate in remote areas should also carry survival equipment. Crew members should be prepared to spend an unexpected 24 to 72 hours outdoors and be able to look after their own needs for that period.

Preparation and Priority Setting

Successful survival strategy is based on two equally important concepts: preparation and priority setting. In a survival situation, individuals who are both psychologically and physically prepared to survive and who can establish and address the priorities for their own survival needs have a much higher chance of surviving the situation.

Psychological Preparation

The biggest threat to survival in any emergency is panic. Panic reduces the mind's ability to respond properly to a threat and leads to actions that may worsen the situation. Fear, anxiety, anger, and denial are all normal reactions to an emergency, but they need not lead to panic. Preparing oneself psychologically for a survival situation means developing a positive attitude about one's own abilities to manage such a situation. Practice and familiarity with the tools and skills necessary in a survival situation help to build self-confidence and develop a positive "I can do this" attitude. The most valuable tool in one's survival kit is a mind that possesses a positive outlook.

Psychological preparation also involves preparing oneself for the possibility of being in a survival situation while injured or when others have been injured or killed in a crash. Practice and familiarity with survival skills, faith in the SAR system, personal beliefs, and introspection can all help crew members function and manage under such circumstances.

Physical Preparation

Physical preparation for survival consists of two primary areas: keeping oneself in good physical condition and selecting and carrying the items needed for a survival situation. A good physical fitness routine is important for everyone, but the demands of a survival situation make good physical condition even more important.

Clothing and Personal Equipment

Clothing is the first line of defense against the environment and needs to be selected based on the nature of that environment.

Clothing should protect the wearer, be comfortable and practical, and meet the fire safety guidelines described previously. Garments should be layered; this method traps dead air, provides the best insulation, and allows adjustment as environmental conditions change. Even if the weather appears mild, a jacket should be taken on all transports. Gloves and a warm hat or cap should be carried during cold weather. Warm-weather clothing should protect against the sun. Long sleeves and pants legs, together with head and eye protection, diminish water loss and heat exposure.

Personal equipment includes a personal survival kit and other items carried by the crew member. The most well-designed and comprehensive aircraft or vehicle survival kit is not of much use if it is not accessible because of damage to the aircraft, fire, or injury. Each crew member should carry basic survival items on their person (see Box 10.6).

Priority Setting

To establish the priorities in a survival situation, follow the *rule of threes*. The average person can survive 3 minutes without oxygen, 3 hours without shelter in extreme conditions, 3 days without water, and 3 weeks without food.[34,43] Once safety and immediate medical concerns have been addressed, the rule of threes should guide priority setting. The two biggest killers in the outdoors are inadequate thermoregulation (lack of shelter) and dehydration (lack of water).[34] With this in mind, the immediate priorities should be finding or creating shelter, building a fire, taking steps to maintain hydration, and signaling by whatever means possible.

Survival Skills

The subject of emergency survival cannot be covered fully in this brief section. Transport programs should conduct annual survival

---

• BOX 10.6 Survival Kits[56]

Basic Personal Survival Equipment (Minimum Recommended List)
Flashlight or headlamp
Water bottle
Knife
Nylon cord
Plastic whistle
Sunglasses
Waterproof matches in match safe or other reliable method of fire starting
Space blanket or large heavy-duty plastic trash bag
Compass
Energy bars

Basic Aircraft Survival Kit
Flashlight or headlamp
Water-purification tablets or water filter
Plastic whistle
Water container
Waterproof matches in match safe
Nylon cord or rope
Second reliable method of fire starting (metal match, etc.)
Space blankets or large heavy-duty plastic trash bags
Dry tinder (cotton balls/petroleum jelly)
Aluminum foil
Candle
Knife
Signal mirror

Compass
Signal flares
Maps
Ax or saw
Insect repellant
Duct tape
Sunscreen
Pocket survival guide or card

Additional Aircraft Survival Kit Items (Depending on Operating Environment and Aircraft Type)
Tent
Appropriate additional clothing
Sleeping bags and pads
Tarps or plastic ponchos
Cook kit
Snowshoes
Stove
Snow shovel
Foodstuffs
Inflatable raft
Handheld global positioning system unit
Fishing kit
Strobe light
Canned smoke or smoke flares

training to ensure that all crew members have the necessary knowledge and skills. Survival training should include hands-on practice with all the items in the aircraft or vehicle survival kit and a review of survival strategies for a variety of environmental conditions, with emphasis on how to prepare for those that exist in the program's service area. Transport team members are encouraged to consult other sources of information to improve their individual survival knowledge and skills, including the references listed at the end of this chapter, other survival manuals, and outside survival classes.

Shelter

An emergency shelter should be as simple to construct as possible and provide protection from wind, rain, snow, sun, extremes in temperatures, and animals. It should be big enough to protect all survivors and their survival equipment but not large enough to be difficult to construct or to heat. Shelter building should be practiced during survival training.

The aircraft or vehicle should be the first choice for an emergency shelter. If the aircraft or vehicle is used for shelter, ensure that it is stable and will not roll or tilt on the terrain or during adverse weather. Any holes should be patched with sheets, tarps, or space blankets. All windows and exposed metal should be insulated to reduce heat loss. Avoid sleeping or placing the injured on exposed metal or directly on the ground. Aircraft are usually poorly insulated; in cold weather, construction of a shelter near the aircraft that can be heated with a fire may be a better choice.[34,43]

If the aircraft or vehicle is not available or safe, a shelter must be located or constructed. Natural shelters such as caves, rock overhangs, or large trees may be available. Look for potential hazards such as dead trees or tree limbs that may fall in a strong wind, rockslides, caves with other inhabitants (such as bears, skunks, or cougars), and tall trees or rocks that may conduct lightning. If a shelter needs to be constructed, the first step is locating a suitable site. When selecting the site, attempt the following:
1. Stay as close to the aircraft or vehicle as possible.
2. Find a spot that is protected from the prevailing wind.
3. Avoid natural hazards such as overhanging tree branches, avalanches or rock fall chutes, and steep terrain.
4. Find a level spot that will stay dry; avoid dry streambeds that could flood.
5. Avoid low-lying areas that collect cold air.
6. Orient the door of the shelter toward the east so that the morning sun will warm the shelter.

Shelters can be constructed with a variety of natural materials, supplies from the survival kit, and items from the aircraft or vehicle. Examples are shown in Fig. 10.15. Natural materials that may be used for shelter construction include trees, branches, brush, logs, and rocks. In snow country, trench shelters are quick and easy to construct. Aircraft and vehicle parts that may be useful include doors (shelter panels), foam from seats or litter (insulation), and wiring (for tying or lashing). Large heavy-duty plastic trash bags are useful for constructing shelters. An individual can

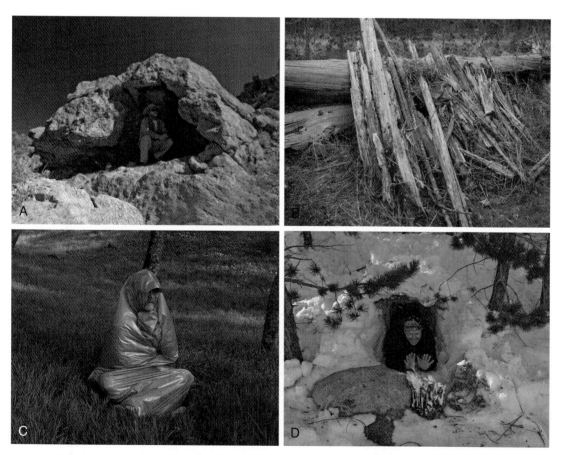

• **Figure 10.15** Simple shelters. **A.** Natural shelter: shallow cave in the desert. **B.** Lean-to shelter made from natural materials. **C.** Large heavy-duty plastic garbage bags may be used as a bivy sack. **D.** Snow trench shelter.

use one bag as a bivy sack, or bags can be opened and used as a tarp to build a lean-to. They can also be used to waterproof shelters constructed from brush or branches or to create a roof for a snow shelter. Mylar plastic space blankets are compact to store and effective at reflecting heat but tear easily and are noisy in windy conditions.[34,43,50] Corners, edges, and stress points on space blankets or plastic bags can be reinforced with duct tape.

Fire Building

A fire provides warmth, light, and a sense of security. If adequate clothing and shelter are available, a fire may not be needed for warmth. When the need is recognized, prepare the materials, and start the fire before dark. Gather enough firewood to last through the night. Locate the fire so that it provides as much heat to the inside of the shelter as possible and contain it within some type of boundary to prevent its spreading by accident. In high fire danger conditions, exercise caution when building any fire.

There are many methods of fire building and many ways to start a fire, including waterproof matches, lighters, and "metal matches," which create a shower of sparks when scraped with a steel edge (Fig. 10.16). Fire steel is available commercially. These consist of a steel rod $1/4$ to $1/2$ inch in diameter and a striker that can produce a shower of sparks and can work in wet conditions. At least two reliable methods of starting a fire should be packed in the survival kit. Matches (even waterproof matches) should be stored in a waterproof match safely. Transport team members need to be familiar with the use of all the fire-starting tools carried in the survival kit.

The simplest way to build a fire is to create a teepee of small sticks or kindling over a pile of fine dry tinder. On damp ground or snow, build the teepee on top of a platform of large dry sticks. Use the available fire-starting equipment to create a flame in the tinder. A few dry cotton balls and a few impregnated with Vaseline are excellent as fire starters and can produce a good flame for up to 8 minutes. As the tinder ignites and begins to set the small sticks on fire, slowly add small and progressively larger kindling to the fire. As the fire grows, larger pieces of wood may be added. Practice with the techniques of fire building should be a part of all survival training.[43]

Hydration

Maintenance of adequate hydration is important in the survival setting. Each person should drink at least 1 to 1.5 L of water daily in temperate conditions. Extremes of temperature (hot or cold) and exertion can dramatically increase water requirements. A good rule of thumb is to drink enough water to produce at least 1 L of urine every 24 hours. Conserve available water stores by rationing until a water source is located. All surface water must be purified before drinking by boiling, filtration, or using water-purification tablets to prevent gastrointestinal (GI) infection from bacteria, viruses, or parasites. GI infections can lead to vomiting and diarrhea and cause significant water loss and worsening dehydration.

In woodland environments, water can be collected with a transpiration bag (Fig. 10.17). Place a plastic bag over a tree branch, ideally in the sun, with a small clean rock in one corner of the bag. The leaves or needles transpire water vapor, which then condenses and collects on the inside of the bag. Dew can be collected from leaves, plastic sheets, or the outside of the aircraft. If rain is expected, set up a method of catching the rainfall. Do not eat snow; this can cause substantial heat loss. Snow may be melted over a

fire or by placing a canteen filled with snow in the sun or between the outer and inner layers of one's clothing. Protect water from freezing by keeping the container inside the shelter or under the outer clothing. In the desert, efforts to find and collect water may return less water than the amount that is lost in sweat. If rescue can be expected shortly, conserve water by resting in a shaded location and minimizing water loss from sweating.[34,43]

Signaling

Once basic needs have been met, signaling becomes the next priority. As soon as an aircraft is reported overdue, SAR resources are mobilized. SAR aircraft initially searches for transmissions from the aircraft radio and ELT. If the aircraft radio and the ELT are not operational, other methods of signaling must be used. Signals in groups of three are recognized internationally as distress signals.[34,43] Visual signals should have as much movement and contrast with the environment as possible.

1. *Portable radios and cell phones:* Aviation portable radios should be tuned to the last known ATC frequency or the emergency frequency (121.5 MHz). Conserve the batteries, turning on the radio to transmit only when an aircraft is heard. Cellular phone service now covers an extensive area in North America; a cellular signal may be obtainable even in remote locations.

2. *Smoke and fire:* Besides providing warmth, fire is a valuable signaling tool. At night, a fire can be visible for many miles. Smoke is an effective way to signal SAR aircraft during daylight. The addition of green leaves, grass, or water to the fire creates white smoke. The addition of oil, rubber, plastic, or pitchy wood creates black smoke. A can filled with sand and oil burns and generates black smoke for a long time. Use the color of smoke that provides the most contrast with the background.

3. *Flashlights, strobes, and flares:* A flashlight or a small, lightweight strobe light can be an effective signal at night. Flares can be used if they are available in the aircraft but should be used with caution during high fire danger conditions. Many SAR aircraft are now equipped with NVG technology. Even the smallest light is visible for many miles to searchers with NVGs. It should be noted that "rescue lasers" are now approved by the FAA for the emergency signaling of searching aircraft and so forth. They are compact and battery operated.

4. *Signal mirror:* All crew members should practice signaling with the signal mirror. The preferred type of mirror is one made of laminated safety glass with a sighting hole in the center. Flash the mirror in the direction of any aircraft that can be heard, even if it cannot be seen. Other shiny objects such as CDs, cans, foil, or aircraft parts may be used as improvised signal mirrors.

5. *Clothing and other colored objects:* Brightly colored parkas, space blankets, plastic garbage bags, signal panels, or other items that provide a contrast with the colors of the surrounding environment are useful signals. These may be placed on the ground in a geometric pattern or waved to create maximal visibility.

6. *Whistle:* A plastic whistle provides an effective way to signal ground SAR units. Use of a whistle is much more efficient than shouting. The standard signal is three blasts, pause, three more blasts, and then listen for a reply.

7. *Ground-to-air signals:* Signals may be created by piling debris, digging trenches, or stamping out patterns in snow or sand. The most easily recognized patterns are a large X or the letters S-O-S.

8. *Dyes:* Dyes are effective in water and on snow. Fine dyes should be used downwind.

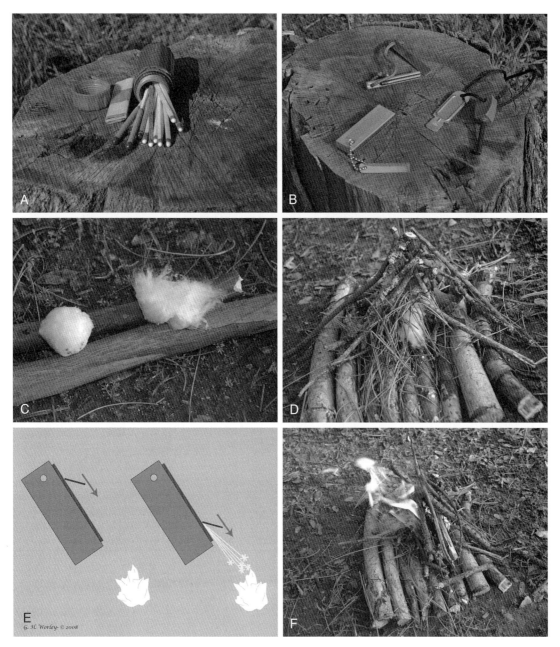

• **Figure 10.16** Fire building. **A.** Commercial stormproof matches *(left)* and strike-anywhere kitchen matches, waterproofed with clear nail polish *(right),* in a waterproof match safe. **B.** A variety of metal matches are available; all incorporate a piece of mischmetal that creates sparks when scraped with a steel edge. **C.** A cotton ball smeared with petroleum jelly makes effective tinder *(left);* six to eight will fit into a film can. To use, pull the cotton ball apart to expose the inner fibers *(right),* which ignite easily. **D.** Basic fire teepee with cotton ball tinder in the center. The tinder can be ignited with matches or a metal match. **E.** Hold the tip of the metal match about an inch from the tinder and scrape the mischmetal insert with the striker, directing the shower of sparks onto the tinder. **F.** As the fire builds, slowly add small and progressively larger kindling. (**C,** From Model Minimum Uniform Crash Criteria. 2016. Accessed July 16, 2010. http://www.mmucc.us/)

Food

The need for food is a low priority during a survival situation of fewer than 4 to 5 days. Although not a direct threat to survival in the short term, depleted energy stores can have other negative effects, including depression and diminished problem-solving capabilities. In cold weather, lack of calorie intake can increase the risk of hypothermia.

Overland Travel and Navigation

The first rule in a downed aircraft situation is to stay with the aircraft, because it is what searchers are looking for. Consider overland travel only in case of a clearly identified need, such as an injured person who needs immediate medical attention. Land navigation skills require training and practice. Cross-country travel should only be attempted by individuals who possess the

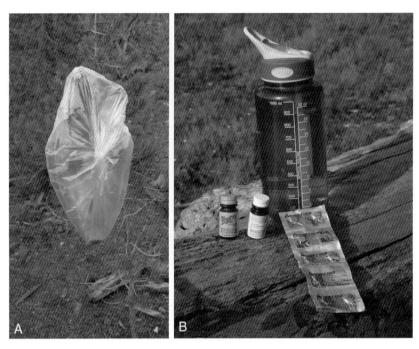

• **Figure 10.17** Hydration. **A.** Transpiration bag tied around a tree branch. **B.** Water-purification tablets. Be sure to follow the manufacturer's instructions for each type.

necessary experience and skills and who have a clear picture of the route they need to follow to reach a location where help may be obtained. Programs may want to consider adding a good compass to the survival kit to aid in land navigation. Personnel should be trained in their use.

If the decision is made to leave the aircraft, leave a detailed note listing the number of survivors, their condition, the intended route of travel, and the intended destination. Mark the outbound route with visible markers, such as strips of brightly colored cloth or surveyor's tape, to permit retracing the route of travel (if necessary) and aid searchers in following the trail. In most situations, the best decision is to stay put and devote one's energy to shelter building, water procurement, and signaling.[34,43]

Specific Environmental Considerations[27,34,43]

Transport programs that operate in regions that have specific environmental conditions or seasonal weather patterns should conduct specialized survival training focused on those environments.

Water Landings and Open Water Survival

The process for emergency aircraft evacuation after a water landing was described previously. After impact with the water, the priorities are to evacuate the aircraft, account for all persons who were on board, and move to a safe location away from the sinking aircraft. A prearranged rendezvous spot should be part of the emergency evacuation plan. If the accident occurs close to shore, consider swimming toward the shore. Distances can be hard to estimate, and one can easily become exhausted when swimming against waves or current.

If the distance does not seem to be within the survivor's capabilities to swim, or if one of the survivors is injured, the best option may be to minimize heat loss with the heat escape–lessening posture (HELP) shown in Fig. 10.18. Remain still and assume the

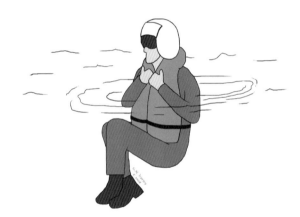

• **Figure 10.18** Heat escape–lessening posture.

fetal position, cross your arms over your chest, and bring your knees up to your chest. A PFD must be worn when assuming the HELP to stay afloat.[34,43] Surviving flight team members should huddle together to decrease heat loss. The flight helmet should be worn in the water because it provides insulation and improved visibility to searchers. Protect against salt and sun exposure by covering any exposed skin surface. Protection against hypothermia, care of the raft (if used), and signaling are the primary objectives in open-water survival.

Desert Survival

Desert areas can reach ambient temperatures of more than 120°F (50°C) during the day and drop to below freezing at night. Maintain an awareness of heat exposure and illness, minimize exertion, and rest in the shade as much as possible. Sheltering in the shade of the aircraft may be preferable to the interior during the daytime. Wear long sleeves and long pants, along with head and neck protection, sunglasses, and sunscreen. Water collection, hazardous plants and animals, and desert shelter construction should all be part of desert survival training.

Cold Weather Survival

Transport programs that operate in areas that have significant snowfall should conduct specialized winter survival training, including snow shelter construction, water procurement, fire building in winter conditions, and the use of any specialized equipment in the survival kit (tents, snowshoes, etc.). Adequate clothing, sunglasses, and sunscreen should be worn or carried when operating in cold weather conditions.

International Survival Concerns

Transport teams who may cross international boundaries need to consider international survival concerns. Air medical team members should be aware of the climate and terrain of the areas they fly over and of the planned destination. Recognition of the need for additional survival equipment and food stores should be part of planning. In some countries, SAR resources are limited, and in many others, they are nonexistent.

Patient Care in a Survival Situation

In addition to looking after their own needs, a stranded transport team may also need to care for a patient or an injured team member. The priority is to ensure the safety of everyone involved before starting medical care. Providing shelter and warmth for the injured should be a high priority and take precedence over everything except interventions to address life-threatening conditions. Ration patient care supplies, such as oxygen and intravenous fluids, and use battery-powered equipment to monitor the patient intermittently to conserve battery life. Mental and emotional preparation for an unfavorable patient outcome is also important, particularly if rescue is delayed.

Survival Equipment

Survival equipment should be carried on all air medical aircraft and on ground transport vehicles that operate in remote or severe weather settings. The specifics of the service area, climate, type of aircraft or vehicle, and time of year should all be considered in the selection of survival equipment and supplies. The survival kit should be assembled and stored in a manner that affords easy access, ideally in the aircraft cabin. Transport team members should carry basic survival equipment on them in case the aircraft survival kit is damaged or inaccessible. Box 10.6 lists recommended items to be included in personal and aircraft survival kits. Survival training should include hands-on use and practice of each item contained in the survival kit(s).

Summary

Safety should be the number one priority of all transport services. Safety is a pervasive attitude that must be supported by all transport team members.

Just as transport team members must be safe, they must also be prepared to survive. The goal in a survival situation that involves a medical transport team and patient is to survive until a rescue can be accomplished.

This chapter has provided an overview of two important transport concepts. Every individual, whether nurse, paramedic, physician, respiratory therapist, EMT, pilot, mechanic, communication specialist, or administrator, must accept personal responsibility for safety and be a safety advocate.

References

1. Baker SP, Grabowski JG, Dodd RS, et al. EMS helicopter crashes: What influences fatal outcome? *Ann Emerg Med.* 2006;47(4):351–355.
2. Coons J, Zalar C. 2015 Air medical safety survey. *Air Med J.* 2016;35(2016):120–125.
3. Blumen I. *The Wizard of Odds: A Statistical Analysis of HEMS Accidents and Risk.* Presented at the Air Medical Transport Conference, Tampa, FL, October 2022.
4. Frazer R. Air medical accidents: A 20-year search for information. *Air Med J.* 1999;8(5):33.
5. Frazer R. Air medical accidents involving collision with objects. *Air Med J.* 2001;20(3):13.
6. Frazer R. Weather accidents and the air medical industry. *Air Med J.* 2000;6(6):49.
7. Aerossurance. US HEMS Accident Rates 2006–2015. 2016. Accessed August 23, 2016. http://aerossurance.com/category/air-accidents-incidents/
8. Blumen I. (Editor in chief). *Principles and Direction of Air Medical Transport.* 2nd ed. Air Medical Physicians Association; 2015.
9. NTSB. Special Investigation Report on Emergency Medical Services Operations. Adopted January 2006. Accessed October 31, 2022. https://www.ntsb.gov/safety/safety-studies/Documents/SIR0601.pdf
10. Hon H, Wojda T, Barry N, et al. Injury and fatality risks in aeromedical transport: Focus on prevention. *J Surg Res.* 2016;204:297–303.
11. FAA Medical Helicopter Accident Review: Causes and Contributing Factors. https://www.faa.gov/data_research/research/med_humanfacs/oamtechreports/2020s/media/202119.pdf
12. Atlas and Database of Air Medical Services. https://www.cubrc.org/index.php/data-science-and-information-fusion/adams
13. NTSB. Aviation: Data and Stats. https://www.ntsb.gov/safety/data/Pages/AviationDataStats2018.aspx
14. Handel DA, Yackel TR. Fixed-wing medical transport crashes: Characteristics associated with fatal outcomes. *Air Med J.* 2011;30:149–152.
15. National Highway Traffic Safety Administration and Ground Ambulance Crashes. 2014. Accessed July 7, 2022. https://www.naemt.org/Files/HealthSafety/2014%20NIITSA%20Ground%20Amubulance%20Crash%20Data.pdf
16. Deaths in Crashes Involving Emergency Vehicles 2010–2020. https://injuryfacts.nsc.org/motor-vehicle/road-users/emergency-vehicles/
17. Watanabe BL, Patterson GS, Kempema JM, Magallanes O, Brown LH. Is the use of warning lights and sirens associated with increased risk of ambulance crashes? A contemporary analysis using national EMS information system (NEMSIS) data. *Ann Emerg Med.* 2019;74(1):101–109.
18. CAAS. Ground Vehicle Safety v3.0. Accessed October 31, 2022. https://www.groundvehiclestandard.org/wp-content/uploads/2022/06/CAAS_GVS_V3_Final_07_01_2022_2.pdf
19. National Fire Protection Association. 1917 Standard for Automotive Ambulances 2019. Accessed October 31, 2022. https://statefirecommission.delaware.gov/wp-content/uploads/sites/103/2019/08/2019-NFPA-Edition-NFPA-1917.pdf
20. Ambulance Patient Compartment Human Factors Design Guidebook. February 2015. United States Department of Homeland Security. Accessed May 15, 2017. http://www.naemt.org/docs/default-source/ems-health-and-safety-documents/health-safety-grid/ambulance-patient-compartment-human-factors-design-guidebook.pdf?sfvrsn=2
21. Krebs MB, Guohua L, Baker SP. Factors related to pilot survival in helicopter commuter and air taxi crashes. *Aviation Space Environ Med.* 1995;66(2):99–103.

22. MacDonald E. Dumb down for safety. *Air Med Saf.* 2008;27(6): 73–275.

23. Crognale, Michael, Krebs, William. Performance of helicopter pilots during inadvertent flight into instrument meteorological conditions. *Int J Aviat Psychol.* 2011;21:235–253.

24. NOAA and National Weather Service. Aviation Weather Testbed. 2016. Accessed July 10, 2016. https://aviationweather.gov/hems

25. An Example of a Risk Assessment Tool: The Operations Compliance Form (Risk Analysis). (Courtesy Intermountain Life Flight, Salt Lake City, Utah.) https://www.semanticscholar.org/paper/Intermountain-life-flight-preflight-risk-assessment-Thomas-Groke/6566fdb1cc7554aa1865ade56f055ba4afa37cb4

26. Safety Management System. Accessed November 17, 2022. https://www.faa.gov/documentLibrary/media/Order/Order_8000.369C.pdf

27. Commission on Accreditation of Medical Transport Services. *Accreditation Standards.* 12th ed. Sandy Springs, SC: CAMTS; 2020.

28. Emergency Nurses Association (ENA) and the International Association of Flight and Critical Care Paramedics (IAFCCP). Responsible "Helicopter Shopping" Through Selective Resource Management. 2018. Accessed October 19, 2022. https://www.airmedicaljournal.com/article/S1067-991X(19)30038-0/fulltext

29. Aviation Safety Action Program. Accessed November 18, 2022. https://www.faa.gov/about/initiatives/asap

30. NTSB. Special Investigation Report on Emergency Medical Services Operations. Adopted January 2006. Accessed October 31, 2022. https://www.ntsb.gov/safety/safety-studies/Documents/SIR0601.pdf

31. NTSB Most Wanted List of Transportation Safety Improvements for HEMS. https://www.ntsb.gov/safety/safety-recs/recletters/A09_87_96.pdf

32. National EMS Pilots Association November. Helicopter Emergency Medical Services (HEMS) NVG Utilization Survey, 2008. Accessed August 18, 2017. https://verticalmag.com/press-releases/nemspa-releases-survey-on-nvg-usage-in-air-medical-services-html/

33. Greenhaw, Richard. Medical Helicopter Accident Review: Causes and Contributing Factors. May 2021. Accessed October 31, 2022. https://www.faa.gov/data_research/research/med_humanfacs/oamtechreports/2020s/media/202119.pdf

34. Department of the Army. *The Official US Army Survival Guide, FM 3–05.70, FM 21-76.* Washington, DC: US Government Printing Office; 2017.

35. Xianfeng Yang, Jingxuan Ma, Dongsheng Wen, Jialing Yang. Crashworthy design and energy absorption mechanisms for helicopter structures: A systematic literature review. *Prog Aerosp Sci.* 2020;114. https://eprints.whiterose.ac.uk/169313/1/AAW_Yangxianfeng_JPAS_2020.pdf

36. FAA Reauthorization Act of 2018. Accessed October 16, 2022. https://www.congress.gov/bill/115th-congress/house-bill/302/text?q=%7B%22search%22%3A%5B%22PL+115-254%22%5D%7D&r=1

37. Ambulance Patient Compartment Seating Integrity and Occupant Restraint. Accessed October 31, 2022. https://www.sae.org/standards/content/j3026_201611/

38. Air and Surface Transport Nurses Association. Transport Nurse Safety in the Transport Environment. 2018. Accessed November 15, 2022. https://cdn.ymaws.com/www.astna.org/resource/collection/4392B20B-D0DB-4E76-959C-6989214920E9/ASTNA_Safety_Position_Paper_2018_FINAL.pdf

39. Isakov AP. Souls on board: Helicopter emergency medical services and safety. *Ann Emerg Med.* 2006;47(4):357–360.

40. 10 Things to Consider When Improving Ambulance Safety. October 2017. Accessed October 3, 2022. https://www.jems.com/operations/10-things-to-consider-when-improving-ambulance-safety

41. SAE J2917: Occupant Restraint and Equipment Mounting Integrity-Frontal Impact System-Level Ambulance Patient Compartment. Accessed October 31, 2022. https://standards.globalspec.com/std/14520821/j2917

42. Heliport Safety Course, OSHAcademy. https://www.oshatrain.org/courses/mods/180e.html

43. Hudson J. *How to Survive: Self-Reliance in Extreme Circumstances.* W. W. Norton; 2021.

44. de Anda HH, Moy HP. *EMS Ground Transport Safety.* StatPearls Publishing; May 15, 2022. https://www.ncbi.nlm.nih.gov/books/NBK558971/

45. Nix S, Brunette S. Rest, shift duration, and air medical crew member fatigue. *Air Med J.* 2015;34(5):289–291.

46. Fatigue in EMS. Accessed October 31, 2022. https://nasemso.org/wp-content/uploads/Fatigue-in-EMS-January-5-2022.pdf

47. How Much Sleep Do We Really Need? August 2022. Accessed October 31, 2022. https://www.sleepfoundation.org/how-sleep-works/how-much-sleep-do-we-really-need

48. Drew K. Should a pregnant flight nurse be allowed to fly? *J Air Med Transport.* 1991;10(7):11.

49. Safety Helmets for Rescue Workers: Certifications and Ideas to Buy the Good One by Emergency Live. Last updated June 18, 2020. Accessed November 18, 2022. https://www.emergency-live.com/civil-protection/protective-helmets-for-rescue-workers-a-selection-of-certified-models-often-multi-functional/

50. Holleran RS. *Patient Transport Principles and Practice.* 5th ed. Mosby; 2017.

51. Cooper D, ed. *Fundamentals of Search and Rescue.* Jones & Bartlett Publishers; 2005.

52. COSPAS-SARSAT. Farewell to 121.5 MHz COSPAS-SARSAT Bulletin. 21. 2009. Accessed August 23, 2016. https://www.cospas-sarsat.int/images/stories/SystemDocs/Current/Bul%2021ENG_%2010Feb2009_small.pdf

53. Small Unmanned Aircraft Systems (UAS) Regulations (Part 107). October 6, 2020. Accessed Nov 1, 2022. https://www.faa.gov/newsroom/small-unmanned-aircraft-systems-uas-regulations-part-107

54. Laser Incidents. Accessed Nov 18, 2022. https://www.faa.gov/about/initiatives/lasers

55. FEMA Emergency Management Institute. *IS-100 Introduction to Incident Command System.* Washington, DC; 2013. Accessed October 7, 2016. https://training.fema.gov/emi.aspx

56. Auerbach PS. *Wilderness Medicine.* 7th ed. Elsevier/Mosby; 2017.

57. Bowman WD, Kummerfeldt P. Essentials of wilderness survival. In: Auerbach PS, Cushing TA, Harris NS, eds. *Auerbach's Wilderness Medicine.* 7th ed. Elsevier; 2017. https://www.clinicalkey.com/#!/browse/book/3-s2.0-C20130134915.

11

Patient Assessment

JACOB A. MILLER

COMPETENCIES

1. Obtain initial, focused, and comprehensive subjective and objective data through history taking, physical examination, and the review of records, pertinent laboratory values, and radiographic and other diagnostic studies.
2. Effectively communicate with the patient, bystanders, prehospital providers, referring personnel, and other healthcare providers.
3. Recognize and anticipate critical signs and symptoms related to the patient's illness or injury.
4. Perform critical patient interventions as indicated by the patient's illness or injury.
5. Anticipate potential situations associated with the patient's condition during transport that may arise, and prepare interventions accordingly.
6. Identify operations specific to air or ground transport that may impact the delivery of care and the safety of the patient and team.
7. Prepare the patient for transport via ground or rotor-wing or fixed-wing vehicle.
8. Identify and prepare for issues related to international transport.

Preparation

The transport process begins with the identification of the need to transfer a patient. This step is usually initiated by members of the referring agency, such as prehospital care providers or healthcare providers in the referring hospital. Part of performing a detailed patient assessment includes receiving clear communication about the indication for transport, the care the patient has already received, what will be needed from the transport team, and the specialty care available at the receiving facility. This information should be confirmed by the transport team and included in patient handoff and documentation of care.

An adequate patient assessment provides the transport team with an opportunity to identify potential problems or interventions that may be needed before transport. It also allows the transport team to anticipate and prepare for events that may occur during transport. Patient assessment and preparation for transport are composed of multiple elements including primary and secondary assessment; prioritization and performance of critical interventions; anticipation and preparation of potential changes in the patient's condition that may occur during the transport; and treatment of specific problems, such as pain management.

The dynamic and complex nature of the transport environment may not always permit the completion of a full patient assessment and all preparatory steps. The transport team must be familiar with all the components of a complete patient assessment and the necessary preparation to make appropriate decisions and perform the appropriate interventions for safe and successful patient transport. Findings identified during the

patient assessment may also be useful in determining the most appropriate receiving facility.

Indications for Patient Transport

Currently, there is no universal agreement on the indications for interfacility transport, specialty critical care transport (CCT), or air medical transport. Although key professional organizations have proposed indications for CCT, particularly helicopter air ambulance (HAA) transport, it would be impractical to attempt to cover the nuance of every possible patient scenario.[1-7] Interfacility transfer requirements may include a lack of necessary resources at the referring facility, availability of higher-level care with improved outcomes at other facilities, or the desire to move the patient to facilities closer to home or support systems for continued care. With the regionalization of specialty and complex care, transfer from a scene via CCT team or HAA may be required to access specialty resources not available at closer rural or community hospitals when a specific indication is identified by first responding EMS crews (e.g., major trauma, stroke, occlusive myocardial infarction (OMI), or a complex critically ill medical patient).[2] Identifying the need to transfer a patient, and determining the most appropriate mode of transport, is based on several factors, including the following:

- The severity of the patient's illness or injury
- Transport time, traffic, distance, geographic terrain, and weather[8]
- The need for nursing and medical expertise, diagnostic procedures, or other specialty services not available at the referring (or closest) healthcare facility

- A request by the patient's family that the patient be transferred to another facility

Another key consideration in transport decisions is the level of care provided by the transport team. EMS systems – including ground, helicopter, and fixed-wing assets – are heterogenous and different agencies may have different levels of care, specialty expertise, and/or specialized therapeutics and equipment available to care for certain patient populations that other assets in the region may not have. For example, it may be preferential (or, in some systems, required) to have a dedicated neonatal transport team provide care for a critically ill neonate[4] or have a team with a physician or advanced practice provider care for a patient with a complex critical illness at high risk for deterioration in transport.[6,9] Similarly, it may be wise to request an ambulance or HAA equipped with blood products to respond to the scene of a trauma patient in hemorrhagic shock.[10,11]

Specialty Patient Populations

Within the United States, the American College of Surgeons' trauma triage guidelines provide indications for preferential transport to trauma centers from the scene of a traumatic event.[3] In some situations, transport from the scene or a referring facility to a Level I or II trauma center may be indicated, which may require either ground CCT or HAA transport due to the acuity, time, and/or distance to reach the destination trauma center.[2,3,12]

Similar transport considerations exist for patients with time-sensitive cardiovascular disorders.[2] Patients experiencing acute OMI, including ST-elevation myocardial infarction (STEMI), are recommended to have a *first medical contact* –including EMS providers – to device time of less than 90 minutes.[13] Acute stroke patients suspected of having large vessel occlusion (LVO) should also be transported preferentially to interventional-capable centers.[14] The peri-transfer period for patients with diagnosed acute aortic syndromes has been recognized as a high-risk area of transport medicine and necessitates careful consideration for CCT team composition, resources, and management protocols during transfer.[15]

Neonatal, pediatric, and obstetrical patients may also require primary scene response and/or interfacility transport to reach specialty centers of excellence.[2] These patients may be transported by dedicated specialty teams or by cross-trained providers that also provide care for other populations. Regardless of team composition, these populations often require additional equipment to accommodate the differences in patient anatomy, physiology, and monitoring requirements.[4,5]

In addition to specialized destination facilities, field response itself is becoming increasingly specialized. Mobile stroke units, equipped with computed tomography (CT) scanners, point-of-care laboratory machines, and thrombolytic or fibrinolytic medications are gaining traction as a venue for ground CCT medical crews to provide rapid care for time-sensitive neurologic emergencies.[16] Specialty units capable of field cannulation onto extracorporeal membrane oxygenation (ECMO) for refractory cardiac arrest represents another unique area of CCT medicine.[17]

Specific considerations related to the care of each of these specialty populations will be discussed in subsequent chapters.

Interfacility Considerations

In 1986, Congress enacted the Emergency Medical Treatment and Labor Act (EMTALA) as a part of the Consolidated Omnibus Reconciliation Act (COBRA). This legislation, coupled with the

1990 Omnibus Reconciliation Act amendments to COBRA, furnishes guidelines, regulations, and penalties that govern patient transfer and transport.[18,19] The implications of this law and its revisions are discussed in Chapter 21.

Transport teams, whether air or ground, providing interfacility transport should have personnel with the experience necessary to perform an adequate patient assessment; stabilize the patient's condition to the extent possible prior to transport; provide ongoing monitoring, care, and indicated interventions during transport; and use the equipment and technology necessary to deliver care during transport to specific groups of patients.[1,20] Guidelines for appropriate patient transfer have been issued by the American College of Emergency Physicians (ACEP), American College of Critical Care Medicine (ACCM), Society of Critical Care Medicine (SCCM), American Academy of Pediatrics (AAP), and American College of Obstetrics and Gynecology (ACOG).[4–7] Box 11.1 provides a summary of these guidelines.

Decision to Transport

Several factors must be considered by referring personnel when they decide to transport a patient via CCT, whether this is initiated by first-responding EMS personnel or a referring healthcare facility. Identification of an appropriate receiving facility must be considered. When choosing a receiving facility, referring personnel must consider the resources available at the receiving facility, such as specialized care staff, equipment, bed availability, and expertise. It may be beneficial to transport patients with complex medical or surgical history to the facility where they regularly receive care, especially if the patient's current condition is related to that aspect of their history. Preplanning is an important step in any patient transfer. The existence of written policies and transfer agreements between receiving and referring agencies can speed up the transfer process and save time when it is the most precious.

Those responsible for making the decision to transfer a patient should also consider the safety of the transport. The location and accessibility of the receiving facility is also an important consideration when determining the mode of transport. Although air medical transport may be indicated in some situations, the concept of "helicopter shopping" should be avoided whenever possible, and must be completed responsibly if necessary. It is incumbent upon the requested transport agencies to provide a factual reason for declining any transport request (e.g., specific weather details, mechanical issues, or staffing shortages), and requesting agencies and facilities must pass this information along to subsequent agencies contacted for the same transport.[2,21]

Equipment used in transport continues to advance, offering monitoring in transport that has not been previously available. Selection criteria should consider the cost and benefit to the patient in the transport setting. For advanced technology and improved processes, Continenza and Hill[22] recommended that the equipment should:

- Be useful in the transport setting
- Be lightweight, portable, and perhaps fulfill several functions
- Be easy to clean and maintain
- Have a battery life or power source that lasts the length of the transport
- Have the ability to be used both inside and outside the transport vehicle
- Be able to withstand the stresses of transport, such as movement, altitude changes, physical durability, water or fluid contamination, and temperature extremes

• BOX 11.1 Summary of Professional Society Guidelines for Appropriate Interfacility Transfer

- The optimal health and well-being of the patient should be the principal goal of patient transfer. The benefits of transfer must outweigh potential risks, and the transferring facility is responsible for obtaining and documenting informed patient consent for transfer prior to the transfer whenever possible.
- Transferring facility personnel should abide by applicable laws regarding patient transfer, including providing an MSE and stabilizing treatment within the capacity of the facility before transfer. The medical facility's policies and procedures and/or medical staff bylaws should identify the individuals responsible for and qualified to perform MSEs and who is responsible for accepting and transferring patients on behalf of the hospital.
- Agreement to accept the patient in transfer should be obtained from a responsible individual at the receiving hospital in advance of transfer. When a patient requires a higher level of care other than that provided or available at the transferring facility, a receiving facility with the capability and capacity to provide a higher level of care may not refuse any request for transfer. When transfers occur as part of a regional plan to provide optimal care at a specialized medical facility, written transfer protocols and interfacility agreements should be in place.
- The mode of transportation and level of care provided during transfer should be at the discretion of the treating physician, PA, or NP and based on the individual clinical situation, available options, needed equipment, and patient preference. For critically ill patients, there should be at least

two medical personnel in attendance with the patient, at least one of whom should be a registered nurse. A physician, PA, or NP should be considered as part of the transport team for acutely unstable patients.
- Transport crews must have the equipment and medications necessary to manage the patient's airway, breathing, and circulation. Communication equipment should also be available to communicate with providers at referring and/or receiving facilities.
- Continuous monitoring should take place during transport. Critically ill patients should receive at least the same level of basic physiologic monitoring they had at the transferring facility. Patients with specific problems may require additional monitoring, such as capnography, invasive hemodynamic monitoring, or maternal-fetal monitoring.
- Transport crews must be able to safely accommodate patient size and positioning in transport (e.g., appropriate methods of securing pediatric patients, use of neonatal isolette, and ability to properly position a gravid patient).
- All pertinent records and copies of imaging studies should accompany the patient to the receiving facility or be electronically transferred as soon as is practical.
- Payment for transport should not be retrospectively denied by insurance companies.

MSE, Medical screening exam; *NP*, nurse practitioner; *PA*, physician associate/physician assistant.

Medical equipment carried on the transport vehicle is often dictated by state or local EMS regulatory bodies, vehicle/aircraft type, patient populations served, mission profile, and anticipated time to be spent with the patient. The Association of Critical Care Transport's recommended equipment list for critical care teams is outlined in Box 11.2.[23]

Communication

Communication is among the most important components in the preparation of the patient for transport. While communication is a multifaceted concept, this section focuses on the communication process among personnel between the referring facility or EMS agency, the transport team, and the receiving facility.

Communication begins before the transport team's arrival. The initial communication may be made physician to physician, directly to the transport communication center, or via EMS dispatch centers. The transport communication center should have a written guideline regarding what information is minimally required before dispatching a team, and what information is ideal to obtain when available and/or after the team has been dispatched. This information may include patient age, reason for transport, requested mode of transport, receiving facility and accepting physician, specialty equipment needed (such as mechanical circulatory support [MCS] devices, specialty medications, and ventilator), patient weight, and whether family are requesting to travel with the patient. This information must include details necessary to ensure that an appropriately trained team is dispatched, and specialty personnel and equipment are added before departure. Transport teams can improve speed, efficiency, and safety with requesting entities through outreach and education regarding preparing a patient for transport, information to have available for the dispatch center, landing zone safety, and team capabilities.

When the transport team arrives at the patient's location, the team should identify the lead medical provider and ask if there are any immediate concerns and/or perform their own evaluation to rapidly identify and address life threats. A report from the medical team at the referring facility or scene is obtained and should include the history of events, initial physical and diagnostic assessment, interventions provided, response to treatment, and concerns or outstanding needs identified. Handoffs in patient care are a high-risk activity, providing opportunities for critical information to be lost or misunderstood. A structured handoff report can prove beneficial in capturing pertinent information in a potentially chaotic environment.[24–26]

For interfacility transports, there should be direct communication between the physician/provider treating the patient and the accepting provider at the receiving facility. The reason for the patient transfer, the treating physician's name and contact information, the accepting physician's name, bed assignment at the receiving facility, and all other pertinent contacts at both the referring and accepting facilities should be clearly identified and documented. Some transport programs require signed documentation by the treating or accepting physician to certify the need for transport before they transfer the patient due to potential reimbursement issues, particularly from Medicare.

The transport team should be cognizant of how their interactions with referring personnel may be interpreted. The referring team is often invested in the care of the patient and may take offense at what they perceive as the transport team taking over and not communicating with them. Communicating directly, providing eye contact, asking for their input and concerns, and thanking them for the work they put in to prepare the patient for transport can go a long way in establishing a professional and respectful interaction.

Before departure from the referring location, any laboratory, radiographic, and diagnostic findings should be copied and sent with the patient. Radiographic and diagnostic study results may be transmitted electronically or by means of telemedicine before the

•BOX 11.2 Recommended Critical Care Equipment[23]

Monitoring Equipment
- Cardiac monitor, including:
  - 12-lead ECG
  - Pulse oximetry
  - Continuous waveform capnography
  - Noninvasive and core temperature monitoring
  - Noninvasive blood pressure
  - Minimum of two invasive pressure monitoring ports
  - Cardiac defibrillation, cardioversion, and transcutaneous pacing
- Doppler ultrasound
- External fetal monitoring (for HROB teams)
- Endotracheal cuff pressure manometer
- Glucometer
  - Additional POC labs (e.g., electrolytes, blood gas, hemoglobin/hematocrit) strongly recommended for teams performing extended transports
- Appropriately sized stethoscope(s)

Respiratory Support Equipment
- Multimode transport ventilator, including:
  - Noninvasive positive pressure ventilation, including ability to adjust inspiratory and expiratory pressures, FiO_2 (from 21% to 100%)
  - Volume and pressure control ventilation, including conventional modes (Assist Controlled and Synchronized Intermittent Mechanical Ventilation with Pressure Support available) with the ability to regulate positive end-expiratory pressure, FiO_2, and inspiratory time
  - Means for clinicians to assess respiratory values (actual delivered pressures, volumes, etc.)
  - Ventilator circuits for all transported patient populations
- Complete selection of airway management equipment, including:
  - Laryngoscope (direct, video, or both)
  - Endotracheal tubes and means to secure them
  - Airway adjuncts (oral and nasal airways)
  - Supraglottic airway devices
  - Surgical and needle cricothyroidotomy supplies
- Needle, tube, and/or finger thoracostomy supplies
- Pericardiocentesis kit
- Meconium aspirator, bulb syringe, and suction catheters
- Fixed oxygen cylinder or liquid oxygen with at least 2 flow meters and a source to provide 50 psi oxygen
  - Minimum gas volume must support any ventilated patient for the longest possible transport plus a 30-minute reserve
- Portable oxygen
- Vehicle/aircraft-powered suction
- Portable suction unit capable of continuous suction

Hemodynamic Support Equipment
- Transvenous/epicardial pacemaker
- Consider mechanical chest compression device
- Intravenous pump(s) capable of administering multiple, concurrent infusions
  - Pumps should have a medication formulary and dose calculation software
- Intravenous access equipment
- Intraosseous access equipment
- Pressure infusion device

Other Equipment
- Patient restraint or immobilization devices
- Obstetrical delivery kit
- Gastric decompression tubes
- Bleeding control devices (tourniquets, gauze, hemostatic agents, etc.)
- Pelvic stabilization device
- Escharotomy supplies
- Patient thermoregulatory devices appropriate for geographic area and weather conditions
- Provisions to initiate or continue targeted temperature management
- Provisions for isolation and manage patients with highly infectious disease
- System to maintain vehicle cabin within approved limits for pharmaceuticals, blood, or other temperature-sensitive supplies
- Communications equipment with ability to consistently access medical oversight at all times

Medications, Including
- Vasoactive agents
- Muscle relaxants/paralytics for emergent intubation
- Anxiolytics/sedatives
- Antiinflammatory/steroids
- Anticonvulsants
- Opioids/analgesic agents
- Alpha and beta 2-adrenergic agonist
- Antiemetics
- Antibiotics
- ACLS medications: epinephrine, atropine, antiarrhythmics, etc.
- Electrolytes: potassium, magnesium, calcium
- Tocolytic medication to manage preterm labor
- Vitamin K
- Hyperosmolar agents (hypertonic saline/osmotic diuretics)
- Blood glucose control agents
- Blood products
- Crystalloid fluids

HROB, High-risk obstetrics; *POC*, point-of-care.

---

patient leaves the referring facility. If the receiving facility is able to directly access the electronic health record from the referring facility, key portions of the patient's past history, allergies, medications, and diagnostic workup should still be copied for the transport team to reference while providing care during transfer.

If the patient has any valuables, then they must be accounted for. Valuables are sometimes easier left with a family member, whenever possible. Documenting what was transported with the patient and to whom it was given at the receiving facility is necessary to establish a chain of custody. Many hospitals require signed documentation of any valuables by both the transport team and the receiving personnel. Clothing or other valuables are sometimes considered evidence and should be treated as such in accordance with forensic or evidence preservation protocols.

Consent

The transport team should attempt to communicate with the patient and/or responsible party to obtain informed consent for treatment and transport. Written or verbal consent for transport and for emergency treatment is not always possible to obtain directly from the patient or family. Consent for transport may be implied, particularly in the prehospital setting or when the patient has a clear life-threatening emergency that requires interfacility transfer. Even if the patient's consent is implied, the transport team should always explain to the patient and available family members the transport process and any anticipated procedures that will occur during transport. It may be helpful for the transport team to obtain the name and direct contact information for any legal next-of-kin or decision-maker, if available, to expedite necessary consent processes at the receiving facility.[20,27,28] Patient consent is also discussed in Chapter 21.

A Twenty-First-Century Patient Transport Challenge

During the last few years, the closing of rural and community hospitals, the decrease in nursing and other healthcare providers, the need to recognize critical access hospitals, and the lack of funds to provide healthcare have made the interhospital transfers of patients from rural and community hospitals to other facilities routine.[29–31] Many facilities that in the past accepted patients without question have now adopted diversion policies, usually specific to select patient populations or acuity, which means a decrease in available beds, longer waits for transfer, longer transfer distances, refusal of some patients, transfer of patients that were not typically transferred in the past (psychiatric, ortho, etc.), and diversion. ACEP has developed guidelines on the interface between EMS and healthcare systems as it relates to regionalization of care and ambulance diversion.[32] Similarly, the National Association of EMS Physicians (NAEMSP) has authored a position paper and resource document on ambulance diversion and offload delays.[33,34]

Transport programs need to ensure that the patient is eligible for transfer based on the condition and capabilities of both the transferring and receiving facilities, that the patient has been accepted at the receiving facility, has a confirmed bed assignment, and has an accepting physician. Diversion notification should also include all services that provide patient transport to prevent any undue delay in patient transfer and transport.

Patient Assessment

Primary and secondary assessment, identification of patient problems, and initiation of critical interventions provide a framework for preparing a patient for transport. Each of these tasks must be performed in an organized, rapid, and complete manner. Patient assessment is a continuous process that occurs before, during, and after transport.

The general order for patient assessment includes establishing scene safety, completing a primary survey concurrent with initiating immediate resuscitative measures, then conducting a secondary assessment which may include subjective information, objective data, and any additional diagnostic workup.[35]

Scene Assessment

The prehospital assessment begins with assessment of the area in which the aircraft or ambulance will be staged (i.e., on scene or at a facility). This is particularly important when in a helicopter, where hazards exist within the landing zone radius, debris may be present that can fly up in the rotor wash, and people on the ground can be unpredictable. The transport team should assess the surrounding environment for hazards, the number of patients present, and any clues to what has happened (number of vehicles, type of damage, etc.). Box 11.3 summarizes some of the hazards that may be encountered.[36,37] Remember that scene safety may be dynamic and hazards can change over time.

Upon arrival at the referring facility or with the referring EMS agency, the transport team should survey the available resources to assist in preparing the patient for transport. In many cases, the

> **• BOX 11.3 Potential Environmental Hazards**
>
> **Hazards at a Scene**
> Vehicles
> Fire or toxic substances
> Electrical hazard (downed power lines)
> Uneven surfaces
> Unstable structures
> Hazardous materials
> Confined spaces
> Animals or livestock
> Machinery
> Violent or unpredictable bystanders
> Active threat situations
> Explosive devices
>
> **Hazards at an HAA Landing Zone**
> Uneven ground or cracks in pavement
> Obstructions (trees, poles, buildings)
> Wires
> People
> Vehicles
> Stumps
> Brush
> Rocks
>
> *HAA,* Helicopter air ambulance.

transport team brings a higher level of care on arrival to small or rural facilities or to first-responding EMS teams. Equipment and supplies necessary for patient stabilization may have limited availability; thus the team should be independently supplied with the tools and knowledge to administer life-sustaining care until delivery to definitive care.

The principles of patient assessment used by the transport team are no different than those used when patients are assessed within the walls of a hospital. However, the prehospital environment dictates that the assessment be organized, direct, and rapid. Adaptation and flexibility are necessary when patient assessment is performed. Clinics and smaller hospitals may be limited in their diagnostic capabilities and resources. In the prehospital setting, confined space, lack of light, noise, hostile environment (such as weather extremes), and limited diagnostic equipment can present challenges to a thorough patient assessment.

Primary Assessment and Critical Interventions[1,35,38–40]

The hands-on assessment of every patient begins with the primary assessment. This assessment may be done at the same time as the scene survey and obtaining the history. Primary assessment is a rapid assessment following one of two mnemonics:
- A-B-C-D-E mnemonic for medical patients, assessing:
  - **A**irway
  - **B**reathing
  - **C**irculation
  - **D**isability (neurologic status), and
  - **E**xposure of the patient
- M-A-R-C-H-E mnemonic for trauma patients,[41,42] addressing:
  - **M**assive hemorrhage
  - **A**irway
  - **R**espiratory status
  - **C**irculation

- **H**ead injury, and
- **E**nvironment (hypothermia prevention)

During the primary assessment, as life-threatening problems are identified, critical interventions are initiated. The basic steps remain the same, whether at a scene or an interfacility transport; the only variance is for unresponsive medical patients suspected to be in cardiac arrest, for whom chest compressions should be started immediately before evaluating airway and breathing, in a "C-A-B" order.[43]

Massive Hemorrhage[35,41,44]

Hemorrhage remains a leading cause of preventable prehospital trauma death.[45,46] Upon arrival at the patient, the patient is evaluated for any signs of significant, life-threatening hemorrhage (Box 11.4).

Pulsatile or briskly flowing bleeding must be immediately controlled based on anatomic location. Injuries located on an extremity that are anatomically amenable to tourniquet application should have a tourniquet applied at least 2 to 3 inches above the wound. Bleeding from a junctional site (e.g., groin or axilla) should be managed with a junctional tourniquet if one is available and the transport provider is trained in its use. Tourniquets must be tightened until bleeding stops and distal arterial flow (i.e., distal pulse) is absent; tourniquets applied too loosely so they only impede venous return without adequately occluding arterial flow may worsen hemorrhage and increase complications.

If a tourniquet is unavailable or the wound is located at an area not amenable to tourniquet application, the wound cavity should be packed with either hemostatic (preferred) or regular gauze. The medical provider must do this carefully to avoid injuring themselves on any broken bones or embedded foreign body and quickly minimize ongoing blood loss. Once the wound has been packed, continued pressure must be held for several minutes through either manual direct pressure or with application of a suitable pressure dressing.

If neither tourniquet nor wound packing is available, hemorrhage control can be attempted using direct pressure.

Airway[1,35,38–40]

The patient's airway is assessed to determine whether it is patent and maintainable (Box 11.5). For any patient who may have a traumatic injury, cervical spine precautions should be used while the airway is evaluated. Assessment of the patient's level of consciousness, in concert with assessment of the airway status, provides the transport team with an impression of the effectiveness of the patient's current airway status and potential for deterioration.

If an airway problem is identified, appropriate interventions should be initiated, which may include suctioning, airway adjuncts, extraglottic airway placement, endotracheal intubation, or front-of-neck access. The decision to use an intervention depends on the nature of the patient's problem and the potential for complications or deterioration during transport. Airway interventions are addressed in greater detail in Chapter 12.

Pharmacologic Adjuncts for Airway Management

Specific pharmacologic agents have been found to be useful in rapidly establishing an airway. These agents include those that provide sedation, amnesia, and neuromuscular blockade to facilitate intubation. An in-depth discussion of the use of these medications is provided in Chapter 12.

Neuromuscular blocking agents will eliminate a patient's ability to express pain or discomfort, and the transport team should always, with rare exception, provide sedation or analgesia in concert with the paralytic. The team should also assess for signs of pain, such as elevated blood pressure (BP) and heart rate – although the absence of these vital sign abnormalities should NOT be misinterpreted to suggest the patient does not have any discomfort.[47] Special care should be taken to ensure that the patient is positioned in a way that does not put pressure on extremities or decrease circulation. Heat or cooling should be considered depending on environmental and patient condition.[48]

Breathing[1,35,38–40]

The evaluation of breathing includes visual inspection of effort, rate, accessory muscle use, and equal rise and fall of the chest (Box 11.6). Standing at the foot of the bed with the patient's chest exposed gives the best visual view of unequal chest rise. Palpation is useful in identifying subcutaneous air that may alert to the presence of a pneumothorax. Auscultation of the chest will help identify equality across the lung fields or the presence of any adventitious, diminished, or absent breath sounds. The presence of tachypnea may indicate a critical cardiac, pulmonary, or metabolic disturbance and must always be further investigated.

If the patient's breathing is compromised, intervention may be needed. The transport team must consider the immediacy of intervention and weigh it against complications and transport time. For example, if a chest tube is placed in a patient with severe chest trauma, they may require immediate blood transfusion for severe

---

• BOX 11.4 **Summary of Massive Hemorrhage Control**

- Control extremity hemorrhage with tourniquet (2–3 inches above wound)
- Control junctional hemorrhage with wound packing and direct pressure, ideally with hemostatic gauze
- Control other major bleeding using direct pressure

• BOX 11.5 **Summary of Primary Airway Assessment**

- Level of consciousness
- Airway clearance
- Vocal disturbance (e.g., hoarse or muffled)
- Preferred posture to maintain airway
- Sounds of obstruction
- Anatomic concerns (e.g., expanding neck hematoma)

• BOX 11.6 **Summary of Primary Breathing Assessment**

- Rate, depth, and patterns of respirations
- Presence of obvious injury or deformity
- Work of breathing
- Use of accessory muscles
- Flaring of nostrils
- Cyanosis
- Auscultation of bilateral breath sounds
- Symmetry of chest movement
- Position of the trachea
- Palpation of crepitus
- Integrity of chest wall
- Oxygen saturation measured with pulse oximetry

hemorrhage. Unless the team carries blood products, they may want to alert the trauma team to prepare for the procedure and transport rapidly. However, immediate life-threatening conditions must be addressed during the primary survey as they are identified. If the patient is apneic or in severe respiratory distress, immediate interventions are indicated; the transport team must identify the most likely cause of the compromise and proceed with the appropriate interventions. Emergent interventions may include basic life support (BLS) airway maneuvers, bag-mask ventilation, or advanced airway management (discussed in further detail in Chapters 12 and 13).

Tension pneumothorax should be decompressed using needle, finger, or tube thoracostomy as soon as it is suspected. The most sensitive sign of tension pneumothorax is progressively worsening dyspnea; hypotension and hemodynamic instability are rare findings in the spontaneously breathing patient, but may be observed more frequently in patients receiving positive pressure ventilation. Traditionally taught signs like tracheal deviation and jugular venous distension are often incredibly late signs and may not present until the patient is peri-arrest, if at all.[49] An open pneumothorax should be covered with a vented or occlusive dressing. If a simple (i.e., nontension) pneumothorax is suspected to be the cause of respiratory distress, a thoracostomy should be considered before intubation, because positive-pressure ventilation may push a simple pneumothorax into a tension pneumothorax.

Although not traditionally considered part of the primary survey, point-of-care ultrasonography (POCUS) may be helpful in identifying pneumothorax, with a higher sensitivity and similar specificity to plain radiographs.[50] Supplemental oxygen should also be considered for all patients during transport and initiated when necessary, understanding that higher flows or positive pressure ventilation may be required to correct hypoxia in complex patients. Hyperoxygenation is generally not indicated, except in preparation for intubation; in most patients, oxygen should be titrated to maintain an oxygen saturation of 92 to 96%.[51] Specific equipment, such as a pulse oximeter and capnography, helps provide continuous respiratory evaluation during transport. The indications and the procedures for use of these devices are included in Chapter 13.

Circulation[1,35,38–40]

Circulatory assessment (Box 11.7) should begin with evaluation and management of any active external bleeding. This includes re-evaluating any previously applied tourniquet, wound packing, or dressing to ensure adequate hemostasis is still achieved. Any ongoing bleeding should be quickly identified and controlled.

The transport team should observe the patient for indications of circulatory compromise. Palpation of central and peripheral pulse to note quality, rate, and bilateral equality should be assessed to both establish a baseline and identify perfusion competence. Skin color and temperature, diaphoresis, and capillary refill are appraised during circulatory assessment. Delayed capillary refill identifies poor distal perfusion, whether from inadequate perfusion pressure or from hypothermia. Visual inspection of the skin, both centrally and peripherally, detects pallor, mottling, diaphoresis, and discoloration that suggest inadequacy of perfusion. Observation of the level of consciousness further evaluates the patient's cerebral perfusion.

Although vital signs are not classically measured quantitatively during the primary assessment, recent vitals are often available to the transport team from the requesting EMS agency or healthcare facility. In addition to evaluating for signs of frank hypotension or tachycardia, it may also be helpful to calculate a shock index (heart rate divided by systolic blood pressure). An elevated shock index, above 0.9 for adults, has been associated need for aggressive resuscitation, such as blood product transfusion, or indicates peri-intubation cardiovascular collapse, and overall mortality.[52,53] Table 11.1 provides validated shock index values for pediatric patients over age 4.[54]

Adequate vascular access should be obtained for administration of fluid, blood, and/or medications as indicated by patient condition. Depending on the patient's location and the accessibility of veins, vascular access can be secured using peripheral veins, intraosseous access, or, if within the transport team's scope of practice, central venous access. Fluid resuscitation must be guided by the etiology of the patient's shock and the patient's response to incremental fluid administration and should be administered with consistent re-assessment. Point-of-care ultrasound (POCUS) can be a useful resource to differentiate shock states when the cause of shock is not readily apparent and is discussed more in Chapter 20. A detailed discussion of interventions for shock management is discussed in Chapter 14.

Disability: Neurologic Assessment[1,35,38,39]

Neurologic assessment includes assessment of the level of consciousness; the size, shape, and response of the pupils; and motor sensory function (Box 11.8). The following simple method using the mnemonic AVPU may be used to evaluate the patient's level of consciousness:

A: Alert
V: Responds to verbal stimuli

TABLE 11.1	Elevated Shock Index Values[54]	
Patient Age	**Shock Index Cutoff**
4–6 years	>1.2
7–12 years	>1.0
13 years and older	>0.9

• BOX 11.7 Summary of Primary Circulatory Assessment

- Control of any bleeding
- Pulse rate and quality
- Central and peripheral pulses
- Skin color
- Skin temperature
- Level of consciousness
- Urinary output
- Blood pressure
- Cardiac rhythm

• BOX 11.8 Summary of Primary Disability Assessment

- Level of consciousness (AVPU)
- Glasgow Coma Score (GCS)
- Pupillary response
- Gross sensorimotor function
- Stroke screening, when indicated

TABLE 11.2	Adult Glasgow Coma Scale[55]	
Eye Opening	**Verbal Response**	**Motor Response**
4 – Spontaneously open	5 – Oriented	6 – Follow commands
3 – To voice	4 – Confused	5 – Localizes pain
2 – To pain	3 – Incoherent words	4 – Withdrawal to pain
1 – No response	2 – Incomprehensible sounds	3 – Abnormal flexion (decorticate)
	1 – No response	2 – Abnormal extension (decerebrate)
		1 – No response

TABLE 11.3	Pediatric Glasgow Coma Scale[59]	
Eye Opening	**Verbal Response**	**Motor Response**
4 – Spontaneously open	5 – Coos/babbles	6 – Spontaneous movement
3 – To voice	4 – Irritable/cries	5 – Withdrawal to touch
2 – To pain	3 – Cries to pain	4 – Withdrawal to pain
1 – No response	2 – Moans	3 – Abnormal flexion (decorticate)
	1 – No response	2 – Abnormal extension (decerebrate)
		1 – No response

Note: Although other pediatric versions of the GCS have been developed,[56] this is the only version to have been validated in a large cohort of pediatric patients.[58]

TABLE 11.4	Full Outline of Unresponsiveness Score[61]	
Eye Response	**Brainstem Reflexes**
4 – Eyelids open; tracking or blinking to command	4 – Pupil and corneal reflexes present
3 – Eyelids open but not tracking	3 – One pupil wide and fixed
2 – Eyelids closed but open to loud voice	2 – Pupil or corneal reflexes absent
1 – Eyelids closed but open to pain	1 – Pupil and corneal reflexes absent
0 – Eyelids remain closed with pain	0 – Absent pupil, corneal, and cough reflex
Motor Response	**Respiration**
4 – Following command (thumbs-up, fist, or peace sign)	4 – Not intubated, regular breathing pattern
3 – Localizing to pain	3 – Not intubated, Cheyne–Stokes breathing pattern
2 – Flexion response to pain	2 – Not intubated, irregular breathing
1 – Extension response to pain	1 – Breathes above ventilator rate
0 – No response to pain, or generalized myoclonus	0 – Breathes at ventilator rate or apnea

---

• BOX 11.9 Possible Causes for Altered Mental Status

Alcohol
Epilepsy, Electrolytes
Insulin (hypoglycemia), Inborn Errors of Metabolism
Overdose, Oxygen (hypoxia)
Uremia
Trauma
Infection
Psychiatric, Poisoning
Stroke (ischemic or hemorrhagic), Shock

P: Responds to painful stimuli
U: Unresponsive

The Glasgow Coma Scale (GCS; Table 11.2)[55–57] or, for preverbal children younger than 2 years of age, the pediatric GCS (Table 11.3)[57–59] is commonly used in the CCT environment to assess and communicate the patient's level of consciousness and motor function. When calculating the verbal component of the GCS, the patient must be oriented to person, place, and time to obtain an "oriented" score; disorientation to any one component is considered confused.[57] Within the GCS, the motor score has been found to be most predictive of morbidity and mortality after brain injury,[60] but importantly, the patient's *best* effort should be scored; if a patient is able to localize pain on one-half of the body, but exhibits abnormal extension on the other, the score reflects the better (i.e., localization) of the two responses. Additionally, Teasdale recommends that *localizing* pain should require the patient to bring their hand above the clavicle (thus, necessitating a central noxious stimulus above that level to elicit a response as may be produced with trapezius squeeze or supraorbital pressure), adding that "bringing a hand to the opposite side of the body is not sufficient."[57]

The GCS is not always practical because of the need for verbal response, which is challenging in patients with artificial airways. The Full Outline of UnResponsiveness (FOUR) Score (Table 11.4)[61] has been shown to provide a more accurate assessment and prognosis of the intensive care or intubated patient's status in contrast to the GCS.[62] Patients suspected of having an ischemic stroke should have a rapid stroke screening assessment completed, especially in a primary scene response.[14]

If the patient has an altered mental status (AMS), the transport team needs to consider possible etiologies for the AMS. If a clear cause of the patient's AMS is not apparent, the mnemonic AEIOU-TIPS can help determine possible causes (Box 11.9).[63] The transport team should also consider that a patient with AMS may pose a safety problem during transport. Use of physical restraints, chemical sedation, or paralytics (if intubated) may be necessary to ensure safe transport.

For patients with suspected head trauma, early steps must be taken to prevent any secondary brain injury. Preventing and aggressively treating the three "H-bombs" of traumatic brain injury (TBI) has been shown to have a meaningful improvement on patient survival:[64]

- **H**ypoxemia: Maintain an oxygen saturation >90%
- **H**ypotension: Maintain a systolic blood pressure of at least 90 mm Hg, although the optimal target remains a topic of debate[65]
- **H**yper- or Hypoventilation: Target a normal respiratory rate and normal $EtCO_2$ (40 mm Hg, 5.3 kPa)

Summary of Primary Exposure Assessment

- Appropriate tube placement:
  - Endotracheal tubes
  - Chest tubes
  - Naso- or orogastric tubes
  - Urinary catheters
- Intravascular access:
  - Peripheral
  - Central
  - Intraosseous
- Skin color, temperature, and condition
- Rashes or other discoloration
- Identifications of injury

For both medical or trauma patients with suspected increased intracranial pressure (ICP), noninvasive steps should be taken as soon as possible to reduce ICP. Noninvasive means to reduce ICP include maintaining the neck in neutral alignment, preventing occlusion of the jugular veins, elevating the head of bed to 30° to 45° (or the extent possible if a long backboard is used), ensuring adequate analgesia and sedation, and minimizing stimulation to the greatest extent possible.[40,66] More detailed management of head trauma and TBI is discussed in Chapter 16.

Exposure and Hypothermia Prevention[35,38,39]

With environmental conditions in mind, the body should be fully exposed for examination (Box 11.10). Injury, rashes, bruising, and skin discoloration can be obscured by clothing, and important clues to underlying illness or injury can be missed. Although exposure for examination is emphasized most frequently in the care of the trauma patient, it is equally important in the primary assessment of the patient with a medical illness to identify rashes, perfusion indicators, sources of infection, swelling/distention, and so forth. In addition, IV sites should be assessed for location, patency, and adequacy of securing for transport. Clothing can also hide bleeding that occurs because of thrombolytic therapy or rashes that may indicate potentially contagious conditions.

Once patient assessment has been completed, the patient needs to be kept warm. Hypothermia can lead to cardiac arrhythmias, increased stress response, and hypoxia. Medications such as neuromuscular blocking agents interfere with the patient's ability to maintain a stable body temperature. If extended transport times are necessary, the team should reassess the patient's temperature during the transport. Consider continuous core body temperature (e.g., via urinary catheter, esophageal probe, or rectal probe) or surface body temperature (e.g., via skin electrode) monitoring, especially for neonates or critically ill/injured patients and for those transported over long distances where there is greater opportunity for hypothermia to manifest.

Prevention of hypothermia, actively and passively, should be considered a critical intervention, and methods to reduce heat loss should be initiated during the primary assessment. These interventions may include the following[41,67,68]:

- Removing any wet clothing
- Covering the patient with blankets or an insulated layer; consider using an active warming blanket when indicated
- Limiting exposure when examinations are needed
- Preventing heat loss through conduction or convection by shielding the patient from the elements and away from metals,

such as up against the aircraft doors, ambulance walls, or on a metal scoop stretcher
- Shielding the patient from wind and rotor wash
- Using warmed IV fluids or a fluid warmer for crystalloid or blood products
- Using warmed humidified oxygen if possible, or for ventilated patients, at least use a heat and moisture exchanger (HME) in the ventilator circuit

Secondary Assessment[1,35]

Once the primary assessment has been completed and necessary stabilization/resuscitation strategies undertaken, the transport team may move on to the secondary assessment. The secondary assessment includes the history of present illness/injury, past health history, additional subjective details, and either a detailed or focused physical examination. A complete set of vital signs should be obtained if not already completed. Acquisition or review of diagnostic testing may also be considered here as appropriate.

The ability to perform a detailed secondary assessment is influenced by patient condition and transport time. If the illness or injury is time dependent, then the secondary assessment should occur during transport and not delay the departure from scene or bedside. However, space limitations, reduced lighting, and noise may interfere with the ability to perform a complete secondary assessment during transport.

History[35,38]

The history of the events surrounding illness or injury, as well as comorbidities that may affect the condition, provides a guide for critical interventions and clinical decision-making, raises the level of suspicion for occult issues, and helps in preparing the patient for transport. The history may also inform and prepare the transport team of the need for ongoing assessment and possible interventions related to the sequela associated with an illness or injury. For example, the history of a patient who has multiple rib fractures alerts the transport team to the potential of developing a tension pneumothorax or worsening oxygenation caused by pulmonary contusions. Although the transport team may be given some patient information before arrival or while en route to the patient, it is often limited and can devolve before arrival. The team should be prepared to revise initial perceptions and course of action after their assessment.

General Principles of History Gathering

The transport team should keep in mind that the history provides the basis for everything that occurs afterward. It will guide treatment and transport decisions and can alert transport team members to potential problems that may develop during the transport. It is important to follow an organized pattern when gathering a patient history, understanding that in time-critical situations, it may only be possible to obtain a rapid, focused history based on the most likely cause of the patient's condition.

The first step is to establish the patient's chief symptom or problem. If the patient is unable to provide this information, the transport team may obtain it from others at the scene (prehospital care providers, police, family, or other bystanders), referring healthcare personnel, or any persons who may be with the patient. A survey of the scene by the transport team can also provide valuable information about what may have happened. Information about the mechanism of injury (MOI), such as vehicle damage or the height of a fall, can suggest possible injuries. If the patient is unconscious, the transport team should look for medical alert jewelry, syringes, medications, pill bottles, or information in the patient's wallet or purse.

The history then progresses on to the history of the present illness or injury, a review of the pertinent body systems, and their general medical history. A common mnemonic used to collect history information is SAMPLE:

S: Signs (objective) and symptoms (subjective) reported

A: Allergies, alcohol, or substance abuse

M: Medications, including immunizations, over-the-counters, and herbal supplements

P: Past medical and surgical history, including pertinent illnesses and injuries

L: Last meal or oral intake

E: Events that led to the emergency and everything that has been done before the arrival of the transport team

If the patient's chief symptom or problem is related to pain, the OPQRST method can be used to collect information for the history, but many of these questions can also be adapted to other complaints:

O: Onset – What were the circumstances surrounding symptom onset? Was the onset abrupt or gradual?

P: Provoking and palliating factors – Does anything cause the symptoms to worsen? Does anything provide any symptom relief?

Q: Quality of symptoms – Most applicable to pain, but this elicits subjective descriptor words from the patient. Ideally, this should be provided without prompting from the examiner to prevent reporting bias. Some symptom descriptors may provide the transport team member with clues to the underlying etiology. For example, chest pain described as "heavy pressure" or "like an elephant sitting on my chest" paints a different picture than a "sharp, tearing pain."

R: Region and radiation – The patient should be asked to identify the primary area of symptoms and any secondary areas to which the symptoms radiate.

S: Severity – A rating scale from 0 to 10 can be used to describe the intensity of symptoms.

T: Time – Determine the time of onset, the duration of the symptoms, and whether the symptoms have been constant or fluctuating.

As much information as possible should be collected and communicated with the receiving facility. When patients are transported directly from a scene, information may not be as readily available, but requesting EMS agencies should be asked if family is available or if their contact information had been obtained to be passed on to the receiving facility. Obstacles such as the patient's inability to communicate because of their illness or injury, language barriers, the lack of witnesses to a particular event, or the absence of family members or significant others may limit the history information available.

Transport personnel should always assume that there are holes in the patient's history and that there may be potentially important pieces of information of which they are unaware. They may not be able to identify what these missing pieces are, but they should always have an awareness that in the chaos of a scene call or critical interfacility transport, important pieces may be missing and always be on the lookout for new information.

The transport of a patient from a scene or health facility involves multiple transfers of patient care, also referred to as a patient pass-down or handoff. This has been identified as one of the highest-risk aspects of emergency and critical care. It is very easy

for important details about the patient's condition or other key bits of information to get lost in the chaos. It is important that the transport team follow an organized process for obtaining and subsequently relaying information. One simple step toward this is to write down as much as possible about the patient report. As previously mentioned, using a structured handoff report can also prove beneficial in relaying critical information during handoff.[24–26]

Trauma History

Assessment of the traumatically injured patient includes gathering information on the MOI. Information on when, where, and how the patient was injured can guide the transport team in their assessment. A complete description of the event is often limited. However, a general idea of the MOI provides clues regarding additional injuries and complications associated with mode of injury. Box 11.11 describes predictable injuries that may occur because of motor vehicle crashes, which is an example of taking a trauma history.[36]

With the growing and nearly ubiquitous availability of digital photography, obtaining images of patient injuries, MOI characteristics, unique scene circumstances, and other pertinent information has grown in popularity. Importantly, however, these

---

• BOX 11.11 Predictable Injury Patterns by Mechanism of Injury[36]

Frontal Impact
- Traumatic brain injury
- Cervical spine injury
- Facial injuries
- Myocardial contusion
- Pneumothorax/hemothorax
- Aortic injury
- Spleen or liver laceration
- Posterior hip dislocation

Lateral Impact (T-bone)
- Cervical spine injury
- Pneumothorax/hemothorax
- Pulmonary contusion
- Spleen, liver, or kidney lacerations
- Pelvic fracture
- Extremity injuries on the side of impact

Rear Impact
- Cervical spine injury

Pedestrian vs. Car
- Traumatic brain injury
- Abdominal visceral injuries
- Spleen or liver laceration
- Lower extremity and pelvic fracture

Small-Vehicle Crashes (e.g., motorcycle, all-terrain vehicle, etc.)
- Traumatic brain injury
- Facial fractures
- Pneumothorax/hemothorax
- Extremity and pelvic fractures
- Spinal fractures
- Degloving injuries
- Clothesline injuries with airway compromise
- Rectal and vaginal trauma

photos must only be obtained for legitimate medical reasons, and transport personnel must be careful when obtaining, storing, disseminating, and deleting images to prevent violation of patient privacy laws or Health Insurance Portability and Accountability Act (HIPAA) privacy regulations.[69,70] Photographs should include only the information and context necessary to convey the MOI or other critical details to the receiving facility. Transport services opting to permit photography should have strict privacy policies regarding obtaining, storing, transmitting or disseminating, and destruction of photographs. Patient privacy and HIPAA is discussed in greater detail in Chapter 21.

When obtaining the history of a trauma patient, the transport team should also attempt to gather information that describes the kinematics of the injury. For motor vehicle crashes, this includes speed and type of vehicle(s) involved, patient position in the vehicle, trajectory of crash (head-on, rear-end, side impact, rollover, etc.), use of protective devices (e.g., seatbelts, airbag deployment), need for any extrication, and other fatalities in the same vehicle. For other types of traumatic injuries, information that should be obtained about the scene should include the height of a fall and the surface impacted, type and caliber of firearms (if known), size and type of a knife blade (again, if known), use of protective equipment such as helmets, and the size and weight of objects that may have fallen on or struck the patient.

Detailed Physical Assessment[1,35,38,39]

Secondary assessment is done after the primary assessment is completed and involves a head-to-toe evaluation. Patient data are collected by means of inspection, palpation, and auscultation during secondary assessment. Whether the patient has had an injury or is critically ill, the evaluator should observe, touch, and listen to the patient.

Secondary assessment begins with an evaluation of the patient's general appearance. The transport team should observe the surrounding environment and evaluate its effects on the patient. Is the patient aware of the environment? Is there appropriate interaction between the patient and the environment?

Additional systems that should be assessed include the integumentary (color, presence of wounds, and temperature); head and neck (deformities, crepitus, and pain); eyes, ears, and nose (drainage); thorax and lungs (chest movement and heart and breath sounds); abdomen; genitourinary; and extremities and back. Box 11.12 details many components of the secondary physical exam that could be considered as time, access, and patient circumstance allows.

• BOX 11.12 Summary of Secondary Physical Exam[35]

Skin
- Presence of petechiae, purpura, abrasions, bruises, scars, and birthmarks
- Rashes
- Abnormal skin turgor
- Signs of pressure injury
- Signs of abuse and neglect

Head
- Deformities, contusions, abrasions, lacerations, and/or penetrating injuries
- Tenderness, bony crepitus, and/or subcutaneous emphysema
- Skin and mucosal trauma, swelling, ecchymosis, hematoma, and burns
- In the infant, examination of the anterior fontanel

Eyes, Ears, and Nose
- Integrity of globe and eyelid
- Pupil size and shape
- Presence of contact lenses
- Gaze and extraocular motions
- Hemorrhage of the conjunctiva or fundi
- Scleral discoloration
- Drainage from the nose, mouth, and ears
- Gross assessment of vision and hearing

Mouth and Throat
- Loose teeth, artificial teeth, malocclusion, or oropharyngeal foreign bodies
- Mucous membranes
- Breath odor
- Drooling

Neck
- Deformities, penetrating and/or surface trauma, changes in skin color (e.g., ecchymosis, hematoma), and edema
- Instability or step off of the cervical spine and tenderness or pain, as well as adequacy of any spinal motion restriction devices already in place
- Presence of lymphadenopathy or neck masses
- Carotid pulse quality and auscultation (e.g., for bruit)
- Position of the trachea
- Neck veins

- Swallowing difficulties
- Nuchal rigidity

Thorax, Lungs, and Cardiovascular System
- Deformities, asymmetry or instability, areas of tenderness or pain, bony crepitus, or the subcutaneous emphysema
- Symmetry of chest wall movement
- Accessory muscle use and/or retractions
- Lung sound auscultation
- Heart sound auscultation

Abdomen/Pelvis
- Gross abdominal shape and size
- Surface trauma, changes in skin color, rash, or purpura
- Bruising, especially flank or periumbilical bruising
- Tenderness or pain, rigidity and guarding, masses, pulsatile masses, enlarged organs, and/or subcutaneous emphysema
- Bowel sounds
- Aortic or renal bruits
- Percussion
- Femoral pulses
- Pelvic stability and tenderness

Genitourinary
- Blood at meatus
- Rectal bleeding
- Color of urine in catheter

Extremities and Back
- Bilateral symmetry
- Generalized or point tenderness, obvious deformities, or injuries
- Digital clubbing
- Edema
- Gross motor and sensory function
- Peripheral pulses
- Equipment is appropriately applied (e.g., splints)
- Vertebral column, flank, and buttock

Pain Assessment

Determination of the amount of pain the patient has because of illness or injury is an important component of patient assessment. Physiologic indicators of pain may include tachypnea, controlled respirations (splinting), tachycardia, hypotension, hypertension, nausea and vomiting, and diaphoresis. Behavioral indications of pain are crying, protective behavior, guarding, moaning, and self-focusing. Importantly, however, the absence of physiologic and/or behavioral signs does not necessarily indicate the absence of pain. Pain should be evaluated preferentially using a patient's self-reported pain score or, if the patient is unable to provide a pain score (e.g., nonverbal or preverbal), through use of a validated pain scale.[47,71] Baseline data are collected about the pain the patient has so that the effectiveness of pain management can be assessed during transport. Pain management remains an important consideration for CCT teams and transport clinicians should work collaboratively with their administrative and medical direction staff to facilitate resources for optimal pain control in the transport setting.[72,73]

Additional Assessment Data[35]

In addition to the history and physical examination, the transport team should evaluate, as applicable, patient agitation and sedation, the condition of monitoring devices and invasive lines, and the results of any available diagnostic data. Vital signs should be obtained including, at minimum, heart rate, respiratory rate, BP, pulse oximetry, and temperature. Trends in patient vitals should be noted and re-evaluated as additional vitals are measured.

Sedation Assessment

Evaluating a patient's level of agitation or sedation can help to determine the patient's level of comfort and objectively guide the management of pharmacotherapy, especially for intubated patients. Transport teams should use a reliable and validated score to evaluate the patient's level of sedation. One of the most commonly used scales is the Richmond Agitation and Sedation Scale (RASS; Table 11.5), but the Ramsay Sedation Scale or Riker Sedation-Agitation Scale (SAS) may also be used.[74] Patients without adequate sedation should be first managed by means of addressing potential pain or discomfort before sedatives are administered or increased.[47,71]

Equipment Assessment

Although the concept of an "equipment assessment" is not routinely included in descriptions of patient assessment, it is an important step to ensure a safe transport. Before departure with the patient, the transport team should check that equipment, such as cardiac monitors, ventilators, external pacemakers, infusion pumps, drainage systems, MCS devices, and any other therapeutic equipment that is carried, are functioning correctly. All equipment should have airworthiness approval if transporting by rotor-wing or fixed-wing vehicle, or approved for transport outside of the hospital setting for ground transports. An adequate supply of oxygen should be calculated using patient demand, ventilator requirements, tank size, and transport time (including any transfers to/from the transport vehicle) to ensure an adequate supply is available. The transport team should consider the possible need for additional oxygen demands if transporting at altitude, and anticipate delays in transport in these calculations, and factor in a buffer.

The transport team should be aware of the battery life of each piece of equipment in use and that backup batteries or a power

TABLE 11.5	Richmond Agitation and Sedation Scale[75]	
Score	Title	Description
+4	Combative	Violent, immediate danger to self or others
+3	Very agitated	Aggressive; pulling at or removing tube(s) or catheter(s)
+2	Agitated	Frequent nonpurposeful movement; ventilator dyssynchrony
+1	Restless	Anxious, apprehensive, but not aggressive
0	Alert and calm	
−1	Drowsy	Not fully alert; makes sustained (>10 seconds) eye contact to voice
−2	Light sedation	Brief (<10 seconds) eye contact to voice
−3	Moderate sedation	Movement or eye opening to voice (but no eye contact)
−4	Deep sedation	Movement to physical stimulation; no response to voice
−5	Unarousable	No response to voice or physical stimulation

source are available. For both oxygen and power requirements, the transitional phase of vehicle-to-handoff time should be considered.

An important first step is noting the depth of any invasive lines or percutaneous devices (e.g., endotracheal tubes, MCS devices, pulmonary artery (PA) catheters, thoracostomy tubes, etc.) and recording this information to identify any inadvertent migration in transport. Ensure all lines, tubes, and devices (including monitoring or defibrillation electrodes and other sensors) are securely connected to the patient and are positioned so they can be accessible during transport but not easily disconnected or dislodged as patients are moved. Cervical collars should be appropriately sized, and the patient should be adequately secured and positioned so there are no pressure points. This assessment of equipment helps prevent complications during transport that could potentially leave the patient at risk of harm.[76]

Scoring Systems

Scoring systems were initially developed to identify patients who needed critical care that was not available at referring facilities, such as patients who needed to be transported to a Level I trauma center. Scoring systems can be used in the field and for evaluation of patients who may need interfacility support. Scoring systems have routinely been used for the trauma patient, but are now used in the evaluation of critical patients, regardless of illness or injury. These scoring systems include the Sequential Organ Failure Assessment (SOFA), and its abbreviated "quick SOFA," or qSOFA; Acute Physiology and Chronic Health Evaluation (APACHE) I, II, III, IV; Revised Trauma Score; National Early Warning Score (NEWS); Rapid Acute Physiological Score (RAPS), Cardiac Arrest Risk Triage (CART); and others. Although these do help to classify patients retrospectively and have some use in the in-hospital environment, their applicability to CCT and prehospital care is questionable.[77–79]

Diversity Assessment

Although the focus of patient care during the transport process is generally on critical needs, a patient's age, class, culture, beliefs, attitudes, customs, ethnicity, gender identity, nationality, race, religion, and sexual orientation may influence response to illness and injury. The transport team must take into consideration these factors as well as the patient's concept of illness and health when providing care and respect and, when possible, adapt the care to include the impact of diversity on response to illness, injuries, and the need to be transported.[80,81]

Awareness and knowledge of all patient diversity is impossible; however, the transport process can be made to be a little less stressful for the patient, the family, and the transport team when the multiple factors that influence a patient's response to illness and injury are not ignored. Transport team members should become familiar with the patient populations they may interact with and learn about the special healthcare needs of these populations, while being careful to avoid stereotyping patients based on "classic" cultural profiles. Additionally, transport team members should develop cultural humility in which they recognize their own biases and limitations and use that insight to avoid making assumptions about other cultures.[82]

Laboratory and Diagnostic Testing Interpretation

Laboratory and diagnostic tests can provide additional information about patient illnesses and injuries that may necessitate interventions before and during transport. Some diagnostic workup may have been obtained prior to arrival of the transport team, especially for interfacility transfers, and may be pertinent to review when able in the transfer process. If there are data points that the transport team feels may be particularly useful, it may also be possible to discuss with the transferring physician or practitioner the feasibility and risk/benefit ratio of obtaining those tests prior to transport (e.g., it may be prudent to obtain a portable chest x-ray (CXR) prior to departure in an intubated patient with a recently placed central line to exclude pneumothorax). Increasingly, CCT teams may have their own point-of-care laboratory devices and/or POCUS units that enable these diagnostics to be obtained at any time during the transport process by properly credentialed medical crew.

Laboratory Tests[35,40,74,83]

Laboratory values can provide insight into the cause or progression of a patient's condition as well as the overall function of vital organs and their current metabolic state. For interfacility transports, the team should be prepared to review pertinent laboratory tests before transport at the transferring facility if time and condition allow. While not an all-inclusive list, common laboratory tests that may be of use during the patient care and transport are summarized in Table 11.6.

Chest X-Ray Interpretation[39,84,85]

The CXR can identify important information to support or direct care during transport (Fig. 11.1). A CXR assists in the confirmation of endotracheal tube placement, central line position, and chest tube effectiveness in evacuating air and/or blood. It may also identify pulmonary and cardiac abnormalities or thoracic injuries that may guide clinical decision-making. Altitude and positive pressure ventilation both present risks of extension of a simple pneumothorax into a life-threatening tension pneumothorax, and

TABLE 11.6 Common Laboratory Values[74,83]

Diagnostic Group	Laboratory Test	Normal Reference Range
Chemistry and electrolytes	Sodium	136–145 mEq/L
	Potassium	3.5–5.0 mEq/L
	Chloride	98–106 mEq/L
	Bicarbonate (total carbon dioxide [CO_2])	23–30 mEq/L
	Blood urea nitrogen (BUN)	10–20 mg/dL
	Creatinine	0.5–1.1 mg/dL
	Glucose	74–106 mg/dL
	Anion gap (*without potassium)	8–16 mEq/L
	Calcium, total	9.0–10.5 mg/dL
	Calcium, ionized	4.5–5.6 mg/dL / 1.05–1.3 mmol/L
	Magnesium	1.3–2.1 mEq/L
	Phosphate (PO_4) (phosphorus)	3.0–4.5 mg/dL
	Lactic acid (lactate)	5–20 mg/dL / 0.6–2.2 mmol/L
Liver function	Alanine aminotransferase (ALT)	4–36 units/L
	Aspartate aminotransferase (AST)	0–35 units/L
	Alkaline phosphatase (ALP)	30–120 units/L
	Bilirubin, total	0.3–1.0 mg/dL
	Bilirubin, direct (conjugated)	0.1–0.3 mg/dL
	Bilirubin, indirect (unconjugated)	0.2–0.8 mg/dL
Hematology and coagulation	Hemoglobin	M: 14–18 g/dL / F: 12–16 g/dL
	Hematocrit	M: 40–52% / F: 36–47%
	White blood cells (total)	$5–10 \times 10^3/\mu L$
	Platelets	$150–400 \times 10^3/\mu L$
	Prothrombin time (PT)	11–12.5 seconds
	International normalized ratio (INR)	0.8–1.1
	Activated partial thromboplastin time (aPTT)	30–40 seconds
	D-dimer	<250 ng/mL / <0.4 mcg/mL
	Fibrinogen	200–400 mg/dL
Cardiovascular	Troponin-I	<0.03 ng/mL
	High-sensitivity troponin T (HS-TnT)	M: <22 ng/L / F: <14 ng/L
Blood gas	pH	7.35–7.45
	$PaCO_2$	35–45 mm Hg
	Bicarbonate (HCO_3-)	21–28 mEq/L
	PaO_2	80–100 mm Hg
	Base excess	0 ± 2
	Carboxyhemoglobin (COHb)	Nonsmoker: <3% / Smoker: ≤12%
	SvO_2 (from pulmonary artery catheter)	60%–80%

Note: Reference ranges presented are for adult patients and may vary for pediatrics or elderly. While these represent commonly used reference ranges, individual laboratories may have different normal ranges and/or may use different units when reporting results. Verify any abnormal results against the testing laboratory's reference ranges.

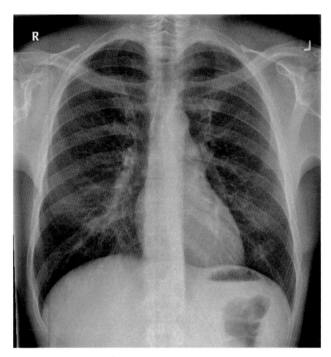

• **Figure 11.1** Normal Chest X-Ray. The hemidiaphragms, cardiac border, and gastric bubble are clearly visualized. (From Scott S, Messer B. Critical care chest radiography. *Surgery (Oxford)*. 2018;36:694–698. doi:10.1016/j.mpsur.2018.09.020)

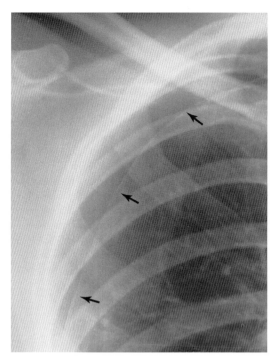

• **Figure 11.2** Apical Pneumothorax. A thin line caused by the visceral pleura is seen separated from the lateral chest wall *(arrows)*. Note that no pulmonary vessels are seen beyond this line, and the line is curved. Notice also that the pleural line is white and is almost equally dark on the side of the pneumothorax and the side of the lung. (Figure 3.70 from Mettler JA, ed. *Essentials of Radiology*. 4th ed. Elsevier; 2018:81.)

the transport team should either perform or prepare for chest decompression (Fig. 11.2).

CXR interpretation takes education and practice. Transport team members should take every opportunity to practice reading CXRs. They should be familiar with lung and thoracic anatomy. The Transport Professional Advanced Trauma Course[39] provides an opportunity to interpret and discuss CXRs.

Much like interpreting a 12-lead ECG, there are many methods for systematic CXR review, and the specific tool used is not as important as following a set structure for interpretation. Critical care patients may have multiple findings, including disease or injury pathology, invasive lines and devices, and other incidental findings, that must be accounted for on x-ray review (Fig. 11.3). A systematic approach to CXR interpretation ensures that more subtle findings are not overlooked. Once the film is identified for viewing, either electronically or in hard copy, proceed in a systematic fashion. Below is one example using the four Ps of study quality, then the ABCDEFGHI approach to interpretation:

- **P**: Patient – Always begin by verifying that the imaging study is of the correct patient.
- **P**: Position – Identify if the patient is rotated, which can often be done by locating the proximal ends of the clavicles and identify that they are equidistant from the vertebral bodies. A rotated film may hide or make more prominent certain anatomic features.
- **P**: Projection – Determine the direction the x-ray beam passed through the patient. For frontal views, this is either front-to-back (anteroposterior, or AP) or back-to-front (posteroanterior, or PA). Radiographs tend to exaggerate structures on the side closest to the beam, or furthest from the x-ray plate or film; think of it this way: Your shadow appears larger when you stand closer to a light source, and smaller as you get closer to the surface onto which your shadow is being cast. Because of

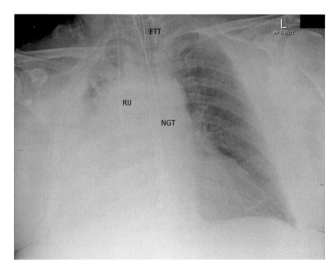

• **Figure 11.3** Multiple Findings on X-Ray. AP erect CXR showing large right-sided pleural effusion. An endotracheal tube (ETT) is present and terminates at the level of the clavicles. A nasogastric tube (NGT) can be seen traversing below the left hemidiaphragm. And a right internal jugular (RIJ) central line can also be seen terminating near the right atrium. (Figure 3 from Scott S, Messer B. Critical care chest radiography. *Surgery (Oxford)*. 2018;36:694–698. doi:10.1016/j.mpsur.2018.09.020)

patient acuity and complexity, CXRs for patients encountered in the CCT setting are almost always obtained by portable machine, and in that case are almost always obtained in AP projection, causing more anterior structures (e.g., the heart) to be exaggerated. This exaggeration can be variable with portable views because the distance from the x-ray beam to the cassette varies with positioning. PA projections are more standardized, but must be obtained in the radiology suite, so they are often impractical in critically ill patients.

- **P**: Penetration – A sufficient film is one in which, at a minimum, the bronchovascular structures can be identified through the heart. An overpenetrated or underpenetrated CXR will obscure bone structure or soft tissues, respectively.
- **A**: Airway – This refers to the trachea position. It should be midline, but may be shifted away from a space-occupying pathology (air, blood, and fluid) or shifted toward collapse/atelectasis. Also, look for narrowing indicative of stenosis, edema, or masses.
- **B**: Bones and tissue – Examine clavicles, ribs, sternum, and thoracic spine. Look along the edges of the bone for interruptions that could indicate a fracture. Be sure to evaluate all bones imaged, even if outside of the chest. Increased intercostal distance can signify air trapping which may indicate chronic lung disease or an acute obstructive process. Look in the surrounding soft tissue for evidence of subcutaneous air, suggesting a possible pneumothorax.
- **C**: Cardiac – Look at size, shape, and borders of the heart. The borders of the heart and mediastinum should be well-defined. Abnormality in structures that border the heart may suggest specific lung lobe abnormality. For example, if the right border of the heart is not clear or is obscured, then there is a suggestion of a right middle lobe abnormality. In relation to heart size, it should take up less than half of the thoracic diameter (although, as mentioned, portable AP films may make the heart look falsely enlarged). A widened mediastinum might suggest aortic dissection or aneurysm.
- **D**: Diaphragm – The outline of the diaphragm should be dome-shaped and visible on both sides. The right hemidiaphragm should be slightly higher than the left because of the location of the liver. Flattened diaphragms suggest hyperinflation, as might be seen in chronic lung disease or an acute obstructive process. Absence of the diaphragm may indicate diaphragmatic rupture. Also, look for air below the diaphragm, which may indicate bowel perforation, although a "gastric bubble" may normally be seen beneath the left hemidiaphragm.
- **E**: Edges – Costophrenic and cardiophrenic borders should be visible. Haziness may indicate pleural effusion or hemothorax, and a deep costophrenic sulcus may be evidence of a pneumothorax.
- **F**: Fields of the lung – Examine the lung sections individually and as a whole, using a standard pattern (e.g., top-down, left-to-right). Look for bilateral symmetry, opacity, shadows, and vasculature. Vascular marking should be visible from the cardiac border to the chest wall. Loss of markings may indicate a pneumothorax (Fig. 11.2). Prominent markings may suggest volume overload. Assess for infiltrates, masses, or air bronchograms.
- **G**: Gastric bubble – Gastric air should be under the left hemidiaphragm, and is present in about 70% of normal films. Note any gastric distension which, if extreme, may affect cardiac function. A nasogastric (NG) tube should be placed whenever possible and should be visible traversing below the diaphragm.
- **H**: Hilum – The hilum consists of the main bronchus and the pulmonary arteries. In the great majority of the population, the left side should be slightly higher than the right. Space-occupying or space-eliminating pathologies can pull the hilum up or down. Increased congestion at the hilum is suggestive of pulmonary edema associated with cardiac failure.
- **I**: Instrumentation – Note any additional instruments, tubes, lines, or foreign bodies. Note the depth of artificial airways (e.g., an endotracheal tube should terminate approximately 3–5 cm above the carina in an adult) and the presence and location of any central venous catheters, chest tubes, gastric tubes, and MCS devices. If the patient has an implanted device, evaluate for the continuity of any lines or wires. The presence of sternotomy wires, mechanical heart valves, surgical clips, or other hardware might provide evidence of a patient's history.

Computed Tomographic Scan Interpretation[39,84]

The most common CT scans evaluated by the transport team are cranial CT scans. CT scans of the head can assist with the diagnosis of neurologic injury and evaluation for the etiology of neurologic deficits or symptoms. Just as with CXR interpretation, evaluation of cranial CT scans takes education and practice. The CT scan should always be used in conjunction with a physical assessment.

A CT scan is created when radiographs pass through the body and are recorded in terms of different absorption values; a denser body part absorbs more radiation. A CT scan can detect bleeding, fractures, and soft tissue injury.

CT scan interpretation requires familiarity with the basic anatomy of the part of the body that is being scanned. For example, a healthy head CT scan shows the skull as white and the brain as gray in color. Dark areas within the brain indicate areas filled with fluid. These areas include the ventricles, cisterns, and the sagittal and transverse tissues. The cisterns are four fluid spaces in the brain and are visible on the CT scan.

A systemic review of cranial tomography includes the following:
- Is this scan for the correct patient?
- Is this a contrast or noncontrast scan? (Note that contrast is the same density as blood and can obscure hemorrhage)
- Is there artifact that may influence ability to interpret?
- Is the scout film available for overview?
- What window level (brain, soft tissue, and bone) is being viewed? Different windows accentuate different densities and each may be better for viewing different types of tissue.

As with CXR interpretation, evaluation of the head CT should be systematic, and a knowledge of cerebral anatomy is necessary. The following is one example of a systematic approach using the *Blood Can Be Very Bad*[86] mnemonic (Fig. 11.4), which prompts the evaluation of (B) Blood, (C) Cisterns, (B) Brain, (V) Ventricles, and (B) Bone:

Blood:
- Look for the presence of blood, which appears hyperdense (white) in the acute phase, and darkens with age as the clot retracts. The age of the hemorrhage can be estimated by whether it is hyperdense, isodense, or hypodense.
- Evaluate for hemorrhagic lesions including epidural, subdural, subarachnoid, intraparenchymal, intraventricular, and extracranial hemorrhage.
- Figs. 11.5 to 11.7 show examples of epidural, subdural, and subarachnoid bleeds.

Cisterns:
- Cisterns are structures that collect cerebrospinal fluid, which surrounds and protects the brain. Cisterns become effaced, fluid filled, and asymmetric with cerebral pathology such as edema.

Brain:
- Sulci and gyri: Look for effacement and asymmetry.

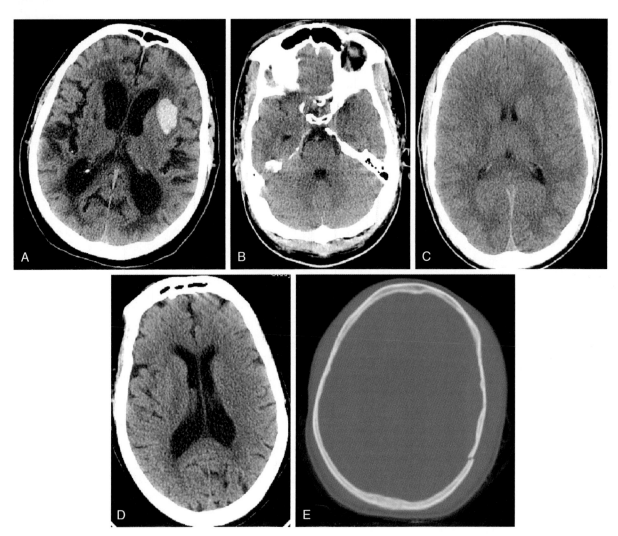

• **Figure 11.4** "Blood Can Be Very Bad." **A.** Acute intracerebral blood in the left front lobe appears as a hyperintense (*bright white*) lesion. **B.** Cisterns are CSF collections jacketing the brain; suprasellar and circummesencephalic cisterns on NCCT. **C.** Appearance of normal brain on Non-contrast computed tomography (NCCT) scan. **D.** Lateral ventricles on NCCT. **E.** Left parietal skull fracture on bone windows of NCCT. NCCT = Non-contrast computed tomography scan. (Figure 9 from Nentwich LM, Veloz W. Neuroimaging in acute stroke. *Emerg Med Clin N Am.* 2012;30:659–680. doi:10.1016/j.emc.2012.06.005)

- Gray–white matter differentiation: Loss of differentiation is associated with cerebral edema.
- Areas of hypodensity (air and edema), hyperdensity (blood and calcification), and structural shift.
  Ventricles:
- Examine the lateral, third, and fourth ventricles for asymmetry, dilation, and effacement.
  Bone:
- The bones of the skull are best viewed using the bone window setting on the CT viewer. Look for fractures.

Point-of-Care Ultrasonography[87,88]

Ultrasound is an ideal initial imaging modality because it can be performed simultaneously with other resuscitative interventions and provide vital information without the time delay caused by radiographs or CT. Various ultrasound protocols have been described for different situations, and facile sonographers can obtain a wealth of information about patient condition and potential etiologies for shock. As POCUS devices are becoming more durable and cost-effective, they are being used increasingly in the prehospital and transport environment to assist with a variety of clinical assessments and to guide patient management. The role of POCUS in CCT is discussed in greater detail in Chapter 20.

Preparing the Patient for Transport

This section summarizes patient preparation for transport. More in-depth discussions about patient preparation are contained in the various clinical care sections of this book. The patient is prepared for transport based on the information obtained from the primary and secondary assessment, mode of transport, estimated transport time, and anticipated complications that may arise during transport. Anticipating and planning for potential complications or worsening of patient condition will better prepare the transport team to either prevent or minimize complications and to facilitate rapid and efficient intervention should compromise occur.

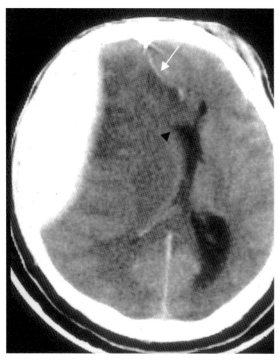

• **Figure 11.5** Epidural Hematoma. Large right epidural hematoma. Epidural hematomas are typically elliptical or lentiform in shape and do not cross suture lines. (From Mirvis SE, Shanmuganathan K. *Imaging in Trauma and Critical Care.* 2nd ed. Saunders; 2003.)

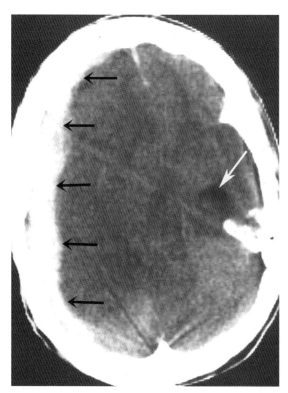

• **Figure 11.6** Subdural Hematoma (SDH). CT scan image of large right convexity SDH *(dark arrows)*. Subdural hematomas are typically crescent-shaped and cross suture lines, as seen here. (From Mirvis SE, Shanmuganathan K. *Imaging in Trauma and Critical Care.* 2nd ed. Saunders; 2003.)

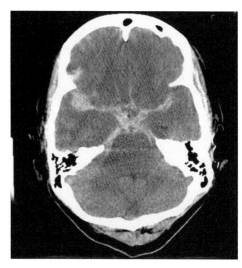

• **Figure 11.7** Subarachnoid Hemorrhage. Acute SAH as seen on noncontrast brain CT. Subarachnoid blood may develop anywhere in the subarachnoid space, depending on the location and etiology of the underlying bleed. (Figure 8 from Nentwich LM, Veloz W. Neuroimaging in acute stroke. *Emerg Med Clin N Am.* 2012;30:659–680. doi:10.1016/j.emc.2012.06.005)

The transport team must consider their differential diagnosis and any indicated interventions. These interventions may be direct orders from a physician, physician assistant, or advanced practice nurse or may arise from agency standing orders, guidelines, or protocols. When multiple interventions are indicated, they must be prioritized, and the crew must carefully determine which must be performed prior to transport and which may be safely deferred until transport is underway.

Airway Management

Patient preparation begins with the assessment and management of the patient's airway, if not already controlled during the primary assessment. The team will first need to determine whether the patient can maintain their airway for the duration of the transport. The patient's neurologic status, facial or airway injury, swelling, and hemorrhage all influence airway maintenance. If equivocal, it may be safer to intubate the patient at a referring facility with additional personnel, resources, and physical space than risk the patient deteriorating during transport and requiring intubation in the back of an ambulance or aircraft.

If intubation is, or has been, performed, tube placement and security must be evaluated and continuous waveform monitoring initiated and maintained throughout transport. An unsecured endotracheal tube may be inadvertently dislodged. A tube that is positioned too high in the airway may also lead to dislodgement with patient movement or cause vocal cord damage if the balloon is inflated in the vocal cords. A tube that is too low, such as one located in the right mainstem, can lead to pulmonary injury from high airway pressures delivered to a single lung or collapse of the nonventilated lung. In addition, movement of the endotracheal tube can cause mucosal damage, induce gagging and coughing, and increase the patient's intracranial or intraocular pressure.

Ventilation Management

A focused assessment of the patient's ventilatory status should be performed as the patient is prepared for transport. If a CXR has been obtained, it should be viewed to determine whether any pathology exists as well as appropriate positioning of devices. The transport team should assess the CXR using a systematic approach to interpretation as discussed previously. Interventions are based on clinical need and transport time. Breath sounds should be auscultated before transitioning to the transport vehicle when possible because of noise interference.

If a pneumothorax is suspected or is present on CXR, appropriate interventions should be initiated. It should be noted that a CXR, particularly supine, may not identify a pneumothorax, and other assessments should be used to support the need for chest tube placement. If a chest tube or tubes are already in place, the team should check that connections are secure; check that the tube is not kinked, occluded, or clamped; and assess for air leak and drainage as well as the adequacy of the system to evacuate air or fluid. The drainage system may need to be changed so that it continues to function during transport.

If an advanced airway is in place, a ventilator should be used for transport for consistent and safe delivery of ventilatory support. If the patient is on a ventilator when the transport team arrives, the team should identify and evaluate current settings, including minute ventilation, fractional concentration of inspired oxygen (FiO_2), positive end-expiratory pressure, tidal volume, and set, as well as spontaneous respiratory rate. If the patient is being bag ventilated, the team will need to select settings depending on clinical condition. Patients with severe respiratory compromise may take time to recover on transitioning to a transport ventilator because of alveolar derecruitment, and the team should resist the urge to remove the patient from the ventilator. Ventilation management and techniques to reduce derecruitment are discussed in Chapter 13.

Circulation Management

Initial care related to circulatory management is directed at controlling any active bleeding and support of cardiac function and output. Bleeding can be controlled with direct pressure with application of gauze pads and elastic tape or bandages or hemostatic gauze. The source, cause, and degree of the bleeding should be carefully evaluated before transport. The patient should be prepared for transport so that sheets or blankets do not inhibit regular visualization of wounds that may start, or restart, bleeding during transport. If blood is available and the need exists, transfusion should be initiated, ideally with a blood/fluid warmer. The receiving facility should be notified of uncontrolled hemorrhage potentially requiring damage control resuscitation and mass transfusion on arrival. Consider the use of antifibrinolytic therapy (e.g., tranexamic acid [TXA]) or anticoagulant reversal agents if clinically appropriate and available.

Cardiovascular support by defibrillation, cardioversion, or cardiac pacing may be required to provide sufficient cardiac output during transport. Pads used for therapeutic intervention can be placed before transport for easy and quick access in patients at risk of lethal arrhythmia. IV or IO access must be established, but it should not delay transport in patients with a time-dependent condition. Sufficient access to provide fluid replacement, blood infusions, and medication delivery may call for more than one IV. This is particularly important in patients dependent on IV therapy or who could deteriorate if an IV/IO line is lost during transport.

When medications are infused, infusion pumps should be used to ensure the appropriate delivery and titration of medication and are essential when vasoactive agents are used. Medication concentrations and dosages should always be double-checked

when initiating or transitioning onto transport pumps. Infusion pumps should be equipped with concentration and dosing calculators[23,89] and other technological safeguards, such as dosing "guardrails" programed into the pump's software should be considered. In an attempt to reduce error, the transport team may elect to mix its own infusions rather than transfer the medications mixed at the referring location. If invasive lines such as central, pulmonary, or arterial catheters are in place, the transport team needs to check the patency and functioning of these lines. The lines must be appropriately maintained and secured so that their functioning is not impaired and to prevent accidental dislodgement. If a service transports patients with invasive lines, they should use a monitor that can provide continuous observation of transduced ports. PA catheters must always have the distal (PA) waveform monitored to ensure the catheter does not migrate into the right ventricle or wedged position, both of which can have lethal consequences if not promptly identified and corrected.[90–93] Air should be evacuated from all infusion bags unless they are placed on an infusion pump with an air alarm. This is done to prevent air from entraining in the line when the bag is positioned in a nonupright position when moving the patient. This is particularly important in central and arterial line flush bags to prevent an accidental power flush of air directly into the circulation.

Urinary catheters must be appropriately placed and affixed so that they can drain and are not pulled or dislodged with patient movement. It is recommended that catheter bags are emptied before the patient leaves the referring facility. The amount of urine emptied from the bag and its color should be recorded. This allows accurate assessment of urinary output for longer transports, which can help monitor renal perfusion and function.

Gastric Decompression

A gastric tube should be inserted for intubated patients or those with acute GI disorders to prevent aspiration and allow for gastric decompression during transport. This procedure should be considered for scene patients as well, particularly when the patient has undergone extended bag-valve-mask (BVM) ventilation.

As with the urinary catheter, the gastric decompression tube must be appropriately placed and secured to prevent it from being removed or repositioned outside the stomach. If the tube is not going to be placed on suction during transport, it should be capped so that it does not leak gastric contents. If not connected to suction on fixed-wing transports with potentially higher altitudes, opening the gastric tube to gravity at fixed intervals may be necessary to prevent gastric distention. When possible, the patient's stomach should be drained before the tube is plugged. The amount of the drainage and its color should be recorded.

When patients undergo treatment for massive upper gastrointestinal bleeding, a balloon tamponade device (e.g., Sengstaken-Blakemore tube or Minnesota tube) may be in place. Traction must be maintained so that the tube continues to function properly. When this tube is present, the patient may be at risk for aspiration, asphyxia, gastric rupture, and erosion of the esophageal wall; the pressure inside the esophageal balloon should be monitored frequently with altitude changes and should never exceed 45 mm Hg. When the patient is transported with a gastric tube that may compromise the airway, the airway should be secured with intubation, and the transport team must be prepared to intervene if any complications occur and to provide continued traction on the tube.

Wound Care and Splinting

Wounds and splinting devices should be surveyed quickly, before the patient is moved. Hidden wounds may cause the patient discomfort and increase the risk of bleeding and long-term complications. Improperly placed splints or lack of splinting when indicated may cause additional injury.

Several types of splints and splint devices are available for transport. The transport team must be familiar with the type of equipment that is used. The team should be well practiced in the placement of the splint, potential complications of the device, and indications for removal. The neurovascular status of the extremity to which the splint is applied should be assessed and documented. Musculoskeletal, soft tissue, and vascular emergencies are discussed in Chapter 18. Wound care is provided for patient comfort and protection. Dressing the wound helps control bleeding and keep it free of debris. If concern exists about additional bleeding or neurovascular compromise, the wound should be dressed in such a manner that continuous assessment is possible during transport. Any wet dressings are replaced with dry sterile dressings to prevent heat loss during transport. Care must be taken when changing dressings to not dislodge any clot that may have formed.

The need for infection control is important when tending to the wounds of the patient being prepared for transport. Many patients being transported may have infected wounds that create a risk for the transport team and anyone else who may need to be transported in the vehicle. Appropriate personal protective equipment (PPE) and decontamination procedures should be followed for both the transport team members and the vehicles.

Pain Management[72,94,95]

Prehospital pain management is quite variable, with several factors influencing the use or lack of use of pain medications in the field, including the location of the patient, the nature of the patient's illness or injury, the possible masking of symptoms, and the effect of pain medications on the patient's vital signs.[72] Importantly, however, care must be taken to ensure any reason for avoiding analgesia is evidence-based (e.g., there is no evidence that providing analgesic medications to patient with abdominal pain will "mask" symptoms or delay definitive diagnosis, despite this being cited as a reason to defer pain medications).[96,97] Movement, noise, changes in temperature, and fear may be contributing factors that cause or increase the patient's pain during preparation and transport.

The transport team should assess and document a pain score appropriate to the patient population to measure the intensity of a patient's pain. The OPQRST mnemonic previously described helps provide a baseline description of the patient's pain. If the patient received medication before the team's arrival, information about the medication used and its effect on the patient should be included in the pain assessment.

Both the American Academy of Emergency Medicine[94] and the European Society for Emergency Medicine[95] have developed guidelines for the management of pain in the emergency and acute care setting. These guidelines broadly involve combining the use of nonpharmacologic interventions (splinting, hot/cold therapy, etc.) with pharmacotherapy, which may include nonopioids and opioids.

Pain medications used for analgesia in the prehospital care environment need to be rapid in onset, short in duration, easy to administer, allow for multiple routes of administration, and easy to

store. The IV route is the quickest method of administration and has a rapid onset. However, IV access may not always be available; several medications, including fentanyl and ketamine, can also be safely administered via intranasal (IN) route when vascular access is not available. The transport team needs to be familiar with specific medications that can be used during transport to provide analgesia and sedation. Adjuvant medications, such as antidepressants, antiemetics, anxiolytics, corticosteroids, and others, have been found to be effective in pain management when used in combination with analgesics. This knowledge must include appropriate medication dosage, possible drug interactions, adverse reactions, and management of these adverse reactions.

Also, during transport, some patients may have received neuromuscular blocking agents for safe transport, management of specific problems, or both (although neuromuscular blocking agents should be used sparingly and not as a first step unless immediate safety precautions need to be implemented without delay). The transport team should pay attention to the needs of these patients for sedation and pain management because verbal and visual indicators of pain are eliminated.

Consideration of nonpharmacologic methods combined with conventional methods of pain management is also recommended for treatment of acute pain relief. Nonpharmacologic methods that may be used by the transport team to help with pain management during transport include the following:

- Distraction: Encourage patients to look out the window if they are alert enough to do so. A security object such as a stuffed toy may be of help to a child. Music via headset or built-in DVD players are also helpful distractors.
- Talk to the patient.
- Comfort: Attend to warmth, air, positioning, and nausea.
- Reduce fear: Describe everything that is going to occur. Wheels coming down, turbulence, loading/unloading, and alarms may be routine to the medical team, but they may create anxiety and fear in patients and family.
- Allow a family member to accompany the patient.
- Therapeutic touch: Be cognizant that some people and cultures do not welcome touching.

Regardless of the method of pain management provided, the CCT team must perform an ongoing reassessment of pain, especially after any interventions, and determine whether pain is adequately controlled or additional interventions are warranted.

Patient Safety

Chapters 6 and 9 have been devoted to safety issues. This section concerns safety measures that must be taken into consideration by the transport team when preparing the patient for transport. Placing a combative or psychologically unstable patient in a moving vehicle, in air, or on ground can pose a danger to the patient and a threat to team members, and may require physical or chemical restraint to ensure the safety of all.

The NAEMSP has a policy addressing the prehospital use of patient restraints[98] and their use may also be addressed in agency policy, or state or local laws. Additionally, the use of patient restraints is covered in the Code of Federal Regulations[99] for hospitals, which likely extends to hospital-based transport teams. In accordance with NAEMSP's recommendations, each CCT or HAA program should have a clear protocol or guideline developed, in consultation with legal counsel and other stakeholders, that addresses the use of restraints by transport clinicians. Use of physical or chemical restraints should only be a last resort; the least-restrictive method of restraint should always be employed, and clinicians must consider protecting the patient's dignity. Restraint guidelines should outline the need to clearly document the necessity of restraint use, the application of restraints, and ongoing monitoring of the patient's condition and the neurovascular status distal to the restraint location. Whenever restraints are applied, care should be taken to ensure that skin integrity is not compromised; that the patient is positioned for comfort; and in the case of chemical restraint, the patient is assessed frequently for signs of pain or anxiety. All local and state laws regarding the use of restraints must be known and followed. Additionally, it is paramount that reversible causes of the patient's agitation that led to the use of restraints be sought and corrected, including hypoxia, hypoglycemia, intoxication, postictal state, TBI, etc.

When transporting a child, the child's size, weight, and state laws necessitate that restraint systems appropriate for a child be used. Devices that may be used include care beds, car seats, restraint systems, and transport boards. Any equipment that is used during transport needs to meet both federal and state standards.

Patient Preparation: The Family

Families react to trauma and acute illness of their loved ones differently. Some families are resilient; however, others may feel overwhelmed because of high stress, ongoing burden, and limited resources that quickly deplete coping mechanisms. Culture, ethnicity, religious beliefs, and the patient's age may influence coping ability. The transport team should be supportive, nonjudgmental, and engage the family as much as possible, given limited exposure time. They should provide some detail of the transport process and what they will experience when they arrive at the referring facility. They should instill a sense of safety and professional competence. Engaging the family can simply involve obtaining a patient history and asking a few personal questions, such as how the patient responds to heat or cold, or it may include taking a family member along on the transport whenever possible and as program policies allow. The transport team should recognize that the family's ability to retain information can be limited and should alert the receiving facility staff of the need for social service support.

A discussion about family needs, how to care for the family, and when transport of a family member is appropriate is contained in Chapter 21.

Cardiopulmonary Arrest During Transport

A cardiopulmonary arrest during transport poses a unique challenge to the transport team. Prior to departure from the referring facility, the transport team should confirm the patient's current code status with the referring physician and family, if present. The family should be apprised of the risks of transport and be aware of the condition of the patient before team departure. If there is a possibility of diversion to another facility, the team should make the family aware and get a phone contact number from them so the transport team can advise them of any changes.

The transport team must address four essential issues if a patient has a full cardiopulmonary arrest during the transport: (1) the service's policies and procedures for in-transport codes; (2) the decision to return, divert, or continue to proceed to the destination; (3) the availability of resuscitation equipment and medications; and (4) the endurance of the transport medical personnel. After these issues have been weighed and deliberated, the transport

team will make the final decision, in conjunction with medical direction or agency policies and procedures on whether to continue resuscitative efforts.

Transport team members need to be well-versed in the service's policies and procedures for cardiopulmonary arrest during transport. Every state has specific laws that deal with terminating resuscitation efforts in the prehospital arena. The program should have policies and procedures in place to direct the decision options and any medical control communication required should cardiopulmonary arrest occur.

In addition, legal aspects of interstate and international transport may complicate the decision to terminate resuscitation en route or before reaching the destination. Some locales require pronouncement of death be performed by provincially recognized, licensed, and credentialed professionals. Therefore, some air medical services have a policy that a patient cannot be pronounced dead until the aircraft has landed and required notification of local authorities has been completed and documented, especially if the transport takes place outside the United States.

Second, if the patient's condition deteriorates into a cardiopulmonary arrest during any portion of the transport, the transport team must weigh distance and time factors to determine in which direction to transport. This decision may be based on the distance and time to return to the referring facility or to the closest appropriate facility, on the availability of ground ambulances (if air transport), on resources at the closest available facility (e.g., cardiac catheterization laboratory for the patient with an OMI), and on overall patient status. The question for the transport team is whether to divert the ambulance/aircraft or continue to the destination after weighing all these factors.

The third essential issue relates to the service's available resuscitation equipment and medications. This equipment should, at minimum, include oxygen, endotracheal tubes, advanced cardiac life-support medications, fluids, and the battery power on life-support equipment. Given the limited supplies available in a transport vehicle, particularly with long-distance transports, the transport team may need to make a decision based on exhausting all resuscitation supplies or medications.

Finally, the endurance of the personnel on the transport should be considered, especially for transports that also require extended ground times. The transport team may need to contact their medical director or when this is not available, use preexisting protocols to recommend ceasing resuscitation efforts if the patient does not respond to medical therapy on a long transport. Transport teams that regularly perform long-distance transports should strongly consider the feasibility of adding a mechanical CPR device to their vehicles and aircraft.[23]

Do Not Resuscitate or Allow Natural Death Orders

Because various states have different definitions for Do Not Resuscitate (DNR) orders (sometimes called Do Not Attempt Resuscitation [DNAR] or Allow Natural Death [AND]), transport teams must be familiar with the state laws and agency policies governing these directives. A DNR order is not an absolute contraindication to CCT, but goals of care and clarification of the DNR status must be discussed prior to transport. Occasionally, patients or their authorized decision-maker may temporarily suspend an existing DNR in the hopes of correcting a temporary critical event. Other times, transport services may provide palliative care transports for patients with DNR orders in place to repatriate or return to home or a dedicated hospice facility.

Documentation[1,20,23,89]

Copies of any relevant documentation from the referring agency or EMS care providers should accompany the patient. If pictures of the scene of the accident are available, the transport team should bring them as well. Customized charting software for use with laptop computers and handheld devices provides an efficient and thorough way to document the patient assessment and record any changes or care provided during the transport. The documentation can then be downloaded into a centralized database that allows for storing and categorizing collected data. As there is often a delay in completing the final electronic record, programs may consider using a "preliminary" record that conveys critical information to the receiving team in advance of the full, formal record. In general, however, full documentation should be completed and available to the receiving facility as soon as possible, but no later than 24 hours after the transport.[23]

Copies of laboratory results, radiographic and diagnostic studies, and documentation by other healthcare providers should also accompany the patient unless they can be received electronically. Even still, it may be helpful for transport teams to receive a physical copy of any diagnostic test results, medication administration records, and other pertinent portions of the medical record for their own reference during transport. Consent forms, reasons for transport, and any other pertinent papers should be placed in the transport vehicle so that the team does not forget them when the patient arrives at the receiving facility. Remember to maintain patient confidentially when transporting or reviewing patient records.

What is documented and who does the documentation are determined by the transport service and applicable professional standards. Specific documentation elements may be required to maintain compliance with state or local EMS regulations; accreditation bodies, including the Commission on Accreditation of Medical Transport Services (CAMTS)[89] and the Joint Commission; or by professional organizations, including the Air and Surface Transport Nurses Association (ASTNA) and the International College of Advanced Practice Paramedics (ICAPP).[1,20] Box 11.13 outlines commonly recommended documentation elements.

In general, documentation by the transport team should reflect the reason the patient was transported; the interventions performed before, during, and after transport; and the patient's response to those interventions. Documentation of not only what specific intervention was performed but also of how the decision was made and what diagnostic tools were implemented is important. For example, why was the decision made to perform rapid sequence induction to secure the patient's airway? If medications were administered for pain or arrhythmia management, did they influence the patient and what was that effect?

The patient's chart is not only used to document interventions and their indications but also for continuous quality improvement and reimbursement of services. Documentation and data collection are an integral part of tracking and trending of quality metrics that may be used to identify quality practices, patient care, and improved patient outcomes. It must be clear, complete, and readable and allow for data collection and reporting.

Preparation for the Transport of the Bariatric Patient

Obesity is an unhealthy epidemic in the United States that is rapidly spreading to other parts of the world. A patient is considered

> **• BOX 11.13 Recommended Documentation Elements[1,20,23,89]**
>
> - Clinical documentation should consist of the following, within the transport service's scope of care:
>   - Reason for transport or transfer
>   - History of present illness or injury
>   - Pertinent medical/surgical history, medications, and allergies
>   - Physical exam findings
>   - Results of any applicable assessment scales (e.g., stroke scale)
>   - Vital signs, including patient temperature and weight
>   - Waveform capnography values for patients with advanced airway
>   - Pain assessments
>   - Treatments, procedures, and medications administered, including the patient response to these interventions
>   - Intake and output measurements
>   - Ventilator settings and any changes to these settings
>   - Laboratory, imaging, and diagnostic results, including any point-of-care studies performed by the transport team and any pertinent findings reported from a referring facility or EMS agency
>   - Ongoing reassessment of patient condition
>   - The name of the referring agency or facility, destination facility, and the person(s) to whom report was provided
> - Documentation should clearly depict which member of the transport team performed each intervention (e.g., treatment, procedure, or medication administration)
> - Each care provider should sign the documentation
> - Full documentation should be completed and available to the receiving facility as soon as possible, but no later than 24 hours after the transport

overweight when their body mass index (BMI) is greater than 25 and obese when their BMI is 30 or greater. Because of the increase in larger patients, the care of the bariatric patient has become an integral part of preparing a patient for transport. A bariatric patient includes patients who are overweight, obese, and morbidly obese and those who have had some sort of bariatric surgery. The transport team must consider several issues in the care and preparation for the transport of the bariatric patient.

Selection of an Appropriate Vehicle

The mode of transport is influenced by weight and balance of aircraft, as well as the ability to provide safe care given space limitations. Each transport program must have policies and procedures that address the weight and size of the patient that can be safely managed within the aircraft or ground vehicles. For example, a weight restriction may identify one limitation, but the girth of the patient can also impede safe and competent care in some transport vehicles.

It is imperative to comply with weight limitations for a helicopter or fixed-wing transport to maintain aircraft structural integrity and performance. Balance is also critical to address the center-of-gravity deviations in fully loaded helicopters that may change or affect handling characteristics. Operating within the aircraft weight and balance is a Federal Aviation Administration (FAA) requirement. Weight calculations include the weight of everything and everyone on board, and crew weights should be accurate and include any additional gear they carry, such as survival bags. All equipment, both standard on all transports as well as added in for mission-specific transports, need to be included. Aircraft performance is also affected by temperature, altitude, and landing zone location, as discussed in Chapter 3.

The transport team should be aware of and adhere to stretcher and loading ramp weight restrictions. The team must also assess the patient's physical limitations regarding mode of transport. For example, in a fixed-wing aircraft, rules and regulations require that a patient be flat for takeoff and landing and some patients may not be able to tolerate lying in a supine position for any period of time.

Patient Assessment and Intervention Differences in the Bariatric Patient

Given the current obesity epidemic, the transport team should understand the management challenges of the severely and morbidly obese patient in the acute care setting. They should be aware of and prepared for the comorbid conditions that may be exacerbated or emerge during acute illness. These factors and the implications for patient care are summarized in Table 11.7.[100–102]

The most challenging issues that transport members face when caring for an obese patient is the management of the patient's airway, breathing, and circulation. The excess fatty tissue on the breast, neck, thoracic wall, abdomen, and in the mouth, pharynx, and around internal organs affects airway access, airway patency, and pulmonary function. Intubation, surgical airway, and ventilation require proper planning and preparation including positioning, preoxygenation, and intubation pharmacology selection. An obese patient can be difficult to ventilate with a BVM because of reduced pulmonary compliance, increased upper airway resistance, and abnormal diaphragmatic position. The transport program should have developed and practiced difficult airway algorithms so they are prepared for complications and can respond effectively and efficiently. Mechanical abnormalities, increased airway

resistance, and reduced lung compliance can all affect the management of ventilation in the morbidly obese patient.[100,101] Advanced airway interventions and ventilation management of the bariatric patient are discussed in detail in Chapters 12 and 13.

Increased risk of gastroesophageal reflux will increase the risk of vomiting and aspiration with BVM ventilation. Even if a patient does not require intubation or BVM ventilation, the transport team should position the obese patient with the head elevated, as condition allows, for prophylaxis against aspiration and to ease spontaneous ventilatory efforts by reducing the effort needed to initiate a breath.

Several cardiovascular disorders in patients with significant obesity will affect the clinical course and complicate management in the transport setting. The obese patient requires a higher blood volume to meet the perfusion needs of adipose tissue, and the heart compensates by increasing the stroke volume, without necessarily increasing heart rate, and subsequently results in an increase in cardiac output, left ventricular workload, and oxygen consumption. In addition, there is a decrease in the systemic vascular resistance. Pressure overload, increased blood viscosity, and hypertension make these patients more prone to left ventricular hypertrophy, which elevates the risk for systolic and diastolic dysfunction, congestive heart failure, cardiac dysrhythmias, and stroke.[100,101]

Fluid resuscitation and medication administration must be calculated and monitored. The transport team should be aware of whether the medication dosage of drugs they infuse or deliver is based on actual or predicted body weight.

Preparation for Transport

The transport team must be familiar with physical and physiologic changes related to the bariatric patient. Airway, ventilation, and circulation management must be approached with the appropriate training, equipment, and monitoring devices. Preparation is key for preventing complications.

Airway management must include equipment for a potential failed airway such as a laryngeal tracheal mask airway. Failed airway management is discussed in Chapter 12.

Excessive weight makes vascular access difficult. Alternative access, depending on skill and training, includes IO access and central venous cannulation. Catheter length should be considered in all forms of venous access. Ultrasound-guided peripheral or central line access has become more common in the transport setting with the advancement of lightweight, portable ultrasound devices.

Transport of the bariatric patient requires specialized equipment. Stretchers should be rated for the weight of the patient. These weight limits must be posted on the stretcher. In addition to the ability to support the patient's weight, securing devices, such as seatbelt extenders, should be available in all modes of transport to safely secure a patient to the stretcher. The stretcher must support the weight of the torso in the elevated head position. Obese patients are at higher risk of skin breakdown, particularly those with diabetes, and the ability to reposition during transport is often not reasonable. With that in mind, patients should be carefully positioned so the skin integrity is protected. Loading ramp limitations on fixed-wing aircraft must also be observed.

Adequate personnel must be available to get the patient both in and out of the transport vehicle. EMS crews, hospital personnel, or additional transport crews may be called on to assist with loading and unloading in all modes of transport. Consider the total weight of the patient and what that translates to in terms of

TABLE 11.7	Comorbid Factors That May Accompany Obesity
Comorbid Factor	**Implications to Care**
Alveolar hypoventilation	Hypoxia may already be present in these patients
	Sedation and pain medication may increase hypoxia
Obstructive apnea	Patient may not be able to lay flat for loading or transport
	Preexisting hypoxia can be increased as well if the patient must be flat for transport
Gastroesophageal reflux	Patient is at greater risk for vomiting and aspiration
	Can be aggravated if patient must be flat for loading, unloading, and transport
Increased body tissue	Equipment may not obtain accurate readings
	Pulse oximeters may be unreliable because of increased finger thickness and poorly transmitted light waves
	Inappropriately fitting blood pressure cuffs do not provide accurate blood pressure readings
	Low QRS voltage interferes with cardiac monitoring

weight distributed to each person assisting in the lift. Several commercial devices are now available that have been found to ease patient transfer from beds to stretchers. Some transport companies also have specially equipped winch-capable vehicles to transport morbidly obese patients.

The care and transport of the bariatric patient presents unique challenges to the transport team. The primary key to safe and competent transport is identification of the physiologic changes related to obesity, provision of care based on these differences, and preparation for the transport.

Patient Assessment and Reassessment During Transport

Assessment and preparation are the foundations of patient transport. Primary and secondary assessments provide initial information about the patient's current and potential problems. Based on these assessments, the transport team initiates appropriate interventions. The nature of the patient's illness or injuries and the initial interventions performed influence the assessment and management needed during CCT. Each of the clinical chapters in this textbook addresses the specific care needed during transport because of the patient's illness or injury. Some general principles of assessment and management during transport include the following:

- Transport team members should position themselves in the transport vehicle or aircraft so that they can effectively manage the patient's airway, breathing, and circulation (ABCs).
- Airway equipment, including suction equipment, should be easily accessible.
- All IV, central, or IO lines should be accessible and functioning.
- All tubes and drainage systems should be functioning and secured to decrease the risk of dislodgement.
- If any question exists about cervical spine injury, the cervical spine should be immobilized for transport.
- A combative patient should be properly restrained, physically and/or chemically, if indicated. If chemical restraint is chosen, the transport team needs to ensure that the patient receives adequate analgesia, sedation, and environmental control during the transport. This must always be followed with careful investigation for potential medical causes of psychomotor agitation.
- All monitors should be placed within the transport team's field of vision.

Patient preparation includes not only obvious care but also anticipation of what may occur. In the prehospital care environment, resources are limited and anticipatory planning, safety, and prevention are key care interventions.

Ongoing reassessment is important for all patients. It allows the transport team to maintain an ongoing awareness of the patient's condition and response to interventions. The nature and frequency of reassessment will be dictated by the patient's condition and the length of the transport.

Fixed-Wing Patient Transport

In fixed-wing aircraft patient transport, the transport team must pay critical attention to preflight preparation because of long periods of time typically spent on the ground and in flight. Fixed-wing aircraft transports usually entail lengthy periods of patient care; thus detailed preflight information must be obtained so that

air medical personnel can make appropriate preparations for the transport. The aircraft should not depart to pick up the patient until all preflight preparations are complete. In addition to preparation for the medical aspects of the flight, the logistics and itinerary must be worked out, and any other preflight information needed by the pilots must be obtained. The transport team and pilots should collaborate in gathering this preflight information and in coordinating the entire flight to ensure appropriate safe and quality patient care.

In this section of the chapter, issues encountered by care providers in the fixed-wing transport environment are discussed. The following topics are covered: preflight preparation, preparation for patient transport, patient "packaging," in-flight factors that influence patient care, air medical personnel resources, in-flight codes, and safety and emergency procedures. In addition, issues related to international transports and escort flights are highlighted.

Preflight Preparation

Fixed-wing aircraft flight times are usually much longer than rotor-wing aircraft flight times and may vary greatly from service to service. Fixed-wing aircraft flight times may be as brief as 40 minutes within the state or as long as 3 to 6 hours within a particular region, across the country, or across international borders. In addition, transport distances may range from 150 to 500 miles for a propeller or turbopropeller aircraft to more than 500 miles for a jet. Preplanning by air medical personnel and the pilot is necessary if the patient transport is to go smoothly.

Once the patient transfer has been confirmed by a receiving physician and facility, the transport team should begin gathering information such as physicians' names, telephone numbers, and an accurate account of the patient's diagnosis and condition. This information will, it is hoped, ensure that the skills of the air medical personnel and the medical equipment available during transport are appropriate for the anticipated medical needs of the patient. In addition, logistical information such as patient and luggage weights, the number of family members who will ride along and their weights, and the DNR status of the patient must also be obtained.

Preflight preparation also entails coordination of information with the pilot and appropriate authorities (e.g., Transportation Safety Administration, Customs and Immigration, State Department, and Department(s) of Public Health). Issues to be discussed should include the location of airports, refueling and restroom stops, weight and balance issues, in-flight times to and from airports, ground ambulance times to referring and receiving facilities, ground unit resources, nutritional and fluid requirements, notifications needed depending on the patient condition or diagnoses, and disposal of wastes. The transport team must consider in-flight and ground times when calculating the amount of IV fluids, medications, medical supplies, and oxygen that will be needed and when checking to ensure that medical equipment is fully charged.

Preparation for Patient Transport

Transferring and Accepting Physician and Facility

The transport team must ensure that an appropriate referral is arranged for the fixed-wing transport. Because additional time is usually available to preplan for an interfacility fixed-wing transport, the names of both the referring and the accepting physician should be documented for the transfer.

In 1985, Congress enacted COBRA, which was amended in July and November 1990. COBRA protects indigent uninsured patients from being denied access to emergency care by hospitals or from being transferred inappropriately between hospitals based on the patient's ability to pay. This legislation requires that the referring hospital assume liability for the adequacy of stabilization before transfer. COBRA also requires documentation that the receiving hospital and accepting physician have been verified before patient departure. If a transfer is necessary for a patient whose condition is not yet stabilized, COBRA states that various conditions are to be met, including the following: (1) the physician certifies in writing that, in his or her professional opinion, the benefits of the transfer outweigh the risks; (2) the transferring hospital treats the patient within its capacity, which minimizes the risks to the patient; (3) the receiving facility agrees to accept the patient and has available space and qualified personnel to provide appropriate medical treatment; (4) the transferring hospital sends to the receiving facility all medical records (copies) available at the time of transfer; and (5) the transfer is effected through qualified personnel and transportation equipment.[18,19]

The transport team must often validate transfer information from the communication center. This information must be validated because these patients are transferred from towns, cities, and states in which air medical personnel are not necessarily familiar with the hospitals and physicians involved in the transfer.

Oxygen Requirements

Determination of in-flight and ground ambulance times from the referring to the receiving facility assists the transport team in calculating the amount of oxygen needed to meet the needs of the patient. The transport team must ensure sufficient oxygen to deliver 1.0 FiO_2 or to operate a ventilator, if needed, for 1 to 1.3 times the entire length of the patient transport. In some patient transports, more time is spent on the ground than in flight. Time spent on the ground may be 90 minutes or longer. Therefore, all fixed-wing aircraft should carry a portable backup oxygen tank in case the main system fails or the ground ambulance has no oxygen available. Table 11.8 provides a means to calculate oxygen cylinder duration once the tank

TABLE 11.8 **Oxygen Cylinder Duration Calculation**

$$Time = \frac{P \times CF}{V}$$

Cylinder Size	Conversion Factor
D	0.16
Jumbo D	0.25
E	0.28
M	1.56
G	2.41
H	3.14
K	3.14

CF, Conversion factor; P, current pressure in cylinder; V, flow rate in liters per minute.
From Oakes D. *Clinical Practitioner's Pocket Guide to Respiratory Care.* Health Educator Publications; 2006.

size, pressure, and estimated flow are known. Some transport ventilators also have the ability to calculate this information. If refilling oxygen may be required during a ground stop, this must be coordinated well in advance. Additionally, some foreign countries do not carry oxygen in their ambulances.

Patient Medical Equipment Requirements

Air medical services are advancing fixed-wing aircraft standards by providing dedicated aircraft with custom medical configurations, which allows services to hard-mount ventilators, cardiac monitors, and other durable medical equipment. Equipment that is needed may be chosen based on the mission and the scope of care provided by the air medical service. For example, a program that provides critical care services should have appropriate transport equipment readily available, which may include a cardiac monitor capable of electrical therapy and invasive pressure monitoring, a transvenous pacemaker, IV pumps, suction equipment, a transport ventilator, diagnostic devices such as POCUS and point-of-care laboratory equipment, cardiac assist devices (e.g., intraaortic balloon pump), and an isolette for neonatal CCTs.[23,89]

With the improvement of medical transport equipment in recent years, the most critical patients who need the support of several different pieces of medical equipment may now be transported without difficulty. Transport equipment, including IV pumps, ventilators, intraaortic balloon pumps, fetal heart monitors, ECMO equipment, and other devices, has been designed and tested for the transport environment.

Medical equipment that requires battery power should also have auxiliary power capabilities that can connect to the aircraft's inverter. The transport team should verify that the inverter power source on the aircraft and ground ambulance works properly in case batteries fail. Because many ground ambulances outside the United States do not have inverters, the transport team should have enough spare batteries available to complete the transport.

A portable suction unit should also be included in the standard equipment for fixed-wing transports. This unit provides the team with backup equipment should the main suction system fail. The portable suction unit is also valuable during transport once the patient is transitioned from the aircraft to areas or vehicles without functional or compatible power sources.

Finally, transport services must comply with state licensure requirements for air medical aircraft, which include specifications about medical equipment that must be placed on the aircraft. Because these requirements vary from state to state, some aircraft may be required to carry additional equipment per state regulations.

Patient Care Supplies and Medications

The fixed-wing aircraft must be stocked with sufficient medical supplies and medications to deliver necessary patient care for the full duration of transport. The medical bags should include equipment and medications for a wide range of patient conditions and accommodate for anticipated as well as unanticipated events. For example, patient condition may require continuous nebulizer treatments during transport. If this information was available before transport, the medical team should carefully consider the need to add to their medication stock before departure, particularly if the transport period is long. However, the patient condition could deteriorate between receiving patient information before transport and on arrival. As much as reasonably possible, given space constraints, the volume of medications regularly stocked should consider these possibilities. Most referring facilities are very accommodating in providing the team with additional medications needed for transport, but this cannot always be relied on because of smaller hospital medication stock limitations. For long-distance transports, supplies and medication availability (including oxygen) should be carefully calculated.

Bedding and Linens
Because fixed-wing flights involve longer periods of patient care, comfort becomes a major issue. The traditional fixed-wing aircraft stretcher pads are hard, thin, and narrow and have limited flexibility. The transport team can plan ahead and attempt to use bedding, egg crates, or blankets on top of the stretcher to provide extra padding and create a softer surface. If an air mattress is to be used, air must be able to be released to prevent the mattress from rupturing in flight because of gas expansion at higher altitudes.

In addition, the transport team may stock extra pillows and egg crates for use in supporting the head, neck, back, and knees and for positioning between knees and elbows and elevating extremities and feet. On longer flights, the team must pay greater attention to the patient's position. Patients, especially those who are comatose or paralyzed, may need to be turned to prevent skin breakdown. The patient may be placed on a "turn" or "draw sheet" so that air medical personnel can reposition the patient more easily in flight. The transport team should also pay attention to their own immobility on long flights. Stretching exercises and increased fluid intake can help prevent circulatory problems.

Nutrition and Fluid Requirements
Adequate nutrition and fluids should be provided for all persons on board the aircraft. Depending on the transport time and the time of day, food may be catered for the patient, family, pilots, and air medical personnel at planned refueling stops. The team must choose the proper food or provide the specialized diet (e.g., a low-fat or diabetic diet) needed by the patient. Proper storage of food and fluids is necessary. In addition, an adequate stock of fluids, such as juice, and plenty of water for the entire length of the transport should be available. Because of the longer in-flight times, higher altitudes, and stresses of flight, the team should provide sources for replenishing energy and preventing dehydration for all persons on board the aircraft. Emphasis should be placed on taking care of oneself, in addition to the patient and other passengers during the transport.

Disposal of Contaminated Wastes
All air medical personnel must comply with Occupational Safety and Health Administration (OSHA) regulations regarding occupational exposure to blood-borne pathogens.[103] The medical transport service must have an exposure-control plan. Policies, procedures, and equipment must be addressed in the plan to comply with these regulations and protect employees from infectious disease exposure. Transport personnel must follow infection control policies by observing standard precautions and stocking extra PPE, supplies, and cleaning agents for these long flights. Depending on the flight distance and in-flight patient care times, the team must plan for the containment and disposal of contaminated needles, dressings, empty IV fluid bags, and human wastes per OSHA regulations. The team must also plan for providing care and properly disposing of wastes should the patient have a bowel movement. Multiple large red biohazard bags may be used to dispose of wipes, bedpans, and urinals.

Medical transport personnel, pilots, and family members should plan to use restroom facilities before departure and during fuel stops. Some fixed-wing aircraft may have toilet facilities.

Required Ground Ambulance Capabilities
For fixed-wing transports, the transport team can never assume that a ground ambulance unit is available. The team must investigate the capabilities and resources of the ambulance that arrives at the airport to include safety considerations such as available fire extinguishers and access to other safety equipment. If the patient requires multiple medical devices, inverter power should be available in the ambulance to power the equipment. The transport team should also assess the resources of the ambulance service to determine whether it can provide the appropriate BLS or advanced life support (ALS) services. In some countries, no resources may be available in the ambulance, in which case all medical equipment with adequate battery power, medications, and oxygen needed for the patient must be provided by the transport team.

Patient "Packaging" for Transport
Preparation
Preparation of a patient for a fixed-wing transport follows along the same lines as discussed previously regarding a thorough assessment, stabilization, and preparation process. Because of the longer transport times with the associated stressors of flight, the potential to deteriorate over the length of the transport should be assessed. If risk for decompensation is considerable, the transport team should look at risk vs. benefit of intervening before departure. In rare cases, such as in time-dependent conditions or when transfer is on the tarmac, the transport team may expedite loading the patient. Most of the time, however, the team performs an assessment at the referring facility and initiates patient care. Thorough communication before the team's arrival and a preflight plan help minimize the amount of time spent on the ground before departure.

Loading Considerations
After ground transport to the aircraft, air medical personnel must plan to transfer the patient into the aircraft and secure the medical equipment. Because most aircraft doors are relatively narrow, the team must make the patient package as slender as possible. Many air ambulance operators have recognized patient loading and unloading guidelines with predefined team member roles for optimal patient loading. Once on the aircraft, equipment must be secured per FAA regulations and placed in a position that permits continuous assessments while maintaining tubes and catheter patency and accessibility.

Numerous manufacturers provide equipment for loading a patient into fixed-wing aircraft. Because of an increase in fixed-wing transports, these companies have developed and marketed stands, lifts, slides, and sleds to assist with loading and unloading patients through narrow fixed-wing aircraft doors. These loading devices have significantly eased the loading procedure, but more importantly, they assist with preventing excessive movement and potential injury to the patient during loading and unloading and work-related injuries for the pilot and air medical personnel.

Immobilization Equipment
Immobilization devices present unique challenges for loading a patient through a fixed-wing aircraft door and positioning the patient in the aircraft. Some aircraft doors are too narrow to accommodate standard backboards for loading patients into aircraft. For this reason, tapered backboards are suggested if a backboard must be used. The team must also prepare for patients who have other immobilization devices, such as a traction splint, in place. Loading the patient on the aircraft may be difficult because

of the length of the splint. In addition, positioning the patient can present challenges, especially for transports involving greater distances and longer periods of time inside the aircraft.

Bulky dressings, splints, and the need to maintain a position of comfort for an injured extremity may make transfer of the patient smoothly through the aircraft door difficult. In addition, the patient needs to be positioned in the aircraft so that the extremity can be supported while optimal positioning is maintained and access for care is allowed.

As discussed previously, if air-filled splints are used on fixed-wing transports, the transport team must closely monitor distal circulation during flight and must be able to release air from the splint as needed to prevent patient injury because of gas expansion at higher altitudes.

In-Flight Factors That Influence Patient Care

Limited Space

Just as with rotor-wing and some ground transport vehicles, fixed-wing transport team members must consider several issues that may not be the factors in rotor-wing aircraft transport. Space may vary greatly from one aircraft to another. Propeller and turbopropeller aircraft tend to be more spacious than some of the jet models, which can be extremely important when patients need large ALS equipment or immobilization devices or when family members desire to accompany the patient.

Air Conditioner and Heater

In-flight climate-control systems may not meet most caregiver expectations. The thin walls and floor of the fuselage do not allow much space for thermal insulation. Therefore, the air conditioning may not adequately cool the airplane to the desired temperature on extremely hot summer days; in the winter, some aircraft cabins may still feel cool when heaters are performing at maximum capacity. During fuel stops, most aircraft are dependent on the availability of an Auxiliary Power Unit (APU) to maintain comfortable cabin temperatures. Measures should be implemented to monitor and manage temperature extremes to prevent untoward patient outcomes and detrimental effects on medical equipment, pharmaceuticals, and supplies.

Extended Flight Times

Fixed-wing transports may involve longer flight times than generally appreciated with helicopter transfers. The patient should be assessed for risks related to the development of venous thromboembolic (VTE) events and pressure ulcers often experienced with extended flight exposure. The effects of altitude combined with immobility place the patient at a greater risk for these complications. For any flights that involve lengthy flight times, the transport team should initiate measures to prevent the patient's development of these conditions, such as passive range-of-motion exercises, frequent repositioning, and the use of antiembolic stocking. Passive range-of-motion exercises also decrease the risk of blood pooling, VTE, and additional skin injury from immobility. There are patients who may be ill or at great risk of VTE that may require pharmacologic agents for anticoagulation during transport. These decisions should be discussed in the preflight planning of the fixed-wing transport with the medical director or the referring physician.

Diversions

Because fixed-wing transport times are often longer than other types of patient transport, the potential for diversion of the flight is increased. Diversion can be prompted by mechanical problems, weather, or even a significant deterioration in the patient's status. Contingency plans must be in place before transport to address diversion so that patient care is not jeopardized.

Air Medical Personnel Resources

One of the most critical factors for fixed-wing transports is the team's knowledge of available resources and how these resources can be accessed. The transport team must be familiar with medical control policies and procedures. Medical control may be extremely helpful to those involved with political situations, a patient whose condition is deteriorating, cardiac arrests that occur during the flight, interstate transports, and flights outside of the United States. The transport team must ensure that the air medical service has policies and procedures in place and must know how to contact medical control to deal with these situations. In addition, the transport team must be able to access communication center resources to contact the program director, clinical supervisor, or medical director as needed to assist with patient care decisions and coordination of patient transfer in emergency situations.

Medical Control

Most air medical services receive medical control services from the medical director and the designated medical control physicians. As discussed previously, most fixed-wing aircraft flights are interfacility transports. Therefore, a physician referral has been made to transfer the patient to an accepting physician and facility. Before departure from the referring facility, a transport team member may contact a medical control physician via telephone to discuss a patient's medical condition and request further orders as needed. Once the team is in the ground ambulance or in flight, the opportunities for telephone communication may be limited to satellite services, two-way pagers, or less-than-reliable cellular services. Some CCT teams are using advanced practice providers or physicians to transport critically ill patients, which may help ensure patient care orders can be adjusted even when medical control is unreachable.

Communication

The transport team should be familiar with all the communication devices available to them to contact the communication center, hospitals, and EMS agencies. If medical support is needed, the team should be able to contact medical control or the receiving facility while in flight. Use of flight or satellite telephones is legal during flight, whereas use of cellular telephones or two-way pagers is illegal when airborne. Flight telephones are licensed and regulated by the Federal Communication Commission. Satellite telephones use global satellites for connection rather than the traditional cellular sites. When a flight or satellite telephone is available, the transport team can contact medical control during in-flight medical emergencies.

Safety and Emergency Procedures

Safety is the number one priority for any patient transport. In the fixed-wing aircraft transport environment, the transport team should receive initial and annual ongoing education regarding fixed-wing aircraft operations, regulations, and unscheduled aircraft emergencies. Per Federal Aviation Regulations (FARs), Parts 91.505 and 135.331, all flight crew members should receive emergency training for each aircraft type and model. Because air medical personnel are considered passengers and not flight crew, however, an air medical service may not provide all the crew member emergency training requirements. All air medical personnel should receive safety education in potential in-flight emergencies and procedures appropriate for each kind and model of aircraft flown, which allows the air medical personnel to understand and assist the pilot with various procedures. According to ASTNA, the ability to function appropriately in an emergency is dependent on repetitive training and education with equipment and procedures. At a minimum, education should be provided for dealing with the following emergencies: (1) fire during the flight; (2) electrical failure; (3) hydraulic failure; (4) slow or rapid decompression; (5) water ditching, if flying over water; (6) rapid egress procedures; and (7) survival procedures, survival packs, personal survival gear, and other available equipment. For further review of emergency procedures and survival, see Chapter 10.

International Transport Issues[104,105]

Air Medical Service International Transports

The discussion of air medical transport no longer focuses only on domestic transports. International transports continue to expand for patients who need medical transport between countries. Although similarities exist between domestic and international air medical transports, there are many unique differences. This section focuses on some of the issues and obstacles that may be encountered with international transports, such as preflight preparation and logistics, documentation, language barriers, patient locations, ground ambulance times and resources, pilot and air medical personnel duty times, and medical equipment and supplies.

Preflight Preparation and Logistics

Preflight preparation is critical for international air medical transports. As with long-distance fixed-wing transports, extensive logistical planning must be completed by the entire team because of the extensive transport times. Preflight plans must include customs, immigrations, international weather briefings, landing permits, refueling stops, ground handling, international travel risk assessments, oxygen requirements, catering arrangements, medical equipment needs, and rest requirements. Inadequate preparations or failure to notify the appropriate authorities only frustrate the air medical team and create significant delays. In addition, meticulous attention should be given to obtaining as much accurate patient information as possible to prepare for the medical needs of the patient. Because international transports of critically ill and injured patients may not be accomplished on commercial airlines because of patient transport restrictions, some air medical services have expanded their profile to conduct international transports. These programs have dedicated jets that are medically configured, including redundant medical equipment and systems. These jets also offer lavatory facilities and APUs for maintaining a comfortable cabin environment and charging medical equipment during the ground time portion of the transport. Many aviation companies can assist an air medical service in preparation for international transport.

Documentation

Air medical personnel and pilots should always have the appropriate documentation for customs and immigration requirements on their person. This documentation includes passports, entry and exit visas, and immunization records for not only the destination location, but may also be required for locations traversed en route to or from the destination. International guideline charts are available to explain requirements for different countries. The State Department can advise on the specific customs and immigration requirements for a country.

The Centers for Disease Control and Prevention and the World Health Organization publish guidelines for required and recommended immunizations for each country. The patient and all accompanying passengers should also have the required customs and immigration papers. The transport company is held responsible for any fines or citations incurred from the lack of these required documents.

When planning for the flight, the appropriate documentation must also be verified for the patient and any passengers. Frequently the pilot organizes this information when filing the flight plan and making arrangements with customs.

As discussed previously, the team must document all assessment findings, care administered during the transport, and the patient's status throughout the transport as part of the medical record. Documentation must be done in a manner that allows the nurse to leave a copy of the chart with the patient when care is transferred to the receiving facility.

Language Barriers

When attempting to obtain an accurate patient diagnosis and discover the patient's medical condition and care needs, air medical personnel may deal with language barriers from the referring facility, physician, or family members that may require the use of a translator. Many long-distance telephone companies and hospitals now offer translators fluent in multiple languages. The use of a medical professional translator is preferred. Allowing family members to provide translation is less than optimal but may be used if other options are not available. In addition, insurance companies, travel assistance companies, and air ambulance providers that coordinate these international flights often have multilingual professionals available for translating patient information.

The medical director or clinical supervisor and the transport team involved with the flight must use the necessary resources to obtain patient information that is as accurate as possible, even if this delays the transport. This information ensures that the skills of the air medical personnel and the available medical equipment are appropriate for the anticipated medical needs of the patient.

The air medical personnel must also plan for language barriers when arriving at the patient location and during the flight. An interpreter may be needed at the referring hospital or clinic to translate the medical terms, current treatment, and patient care needs. In addition, the air medical personnel on the flight benefit from learning specific medical terms and words related to caring for the patient during the flight (e.g., terms related to current chest pain status and restroom needs).

Patient Location

International air medical transports may involve patients who are located not only in hospitals but also in clinics, private homes, infirmaries, first-aid stations, trailers, hotels, physician offices, cruise ships or docks, and other locations that may never have been encountered. The stability of the patient's condition on arrival may be unpredictable and the initial information provided inaccurate; therefore, the transport team must be prepared for the worst-case scenario. Patients may arrive at the airport via taxi with minimal initial medical treatment. The air medical personnel may be the first ALS providers to assess the patient and should be prepared, with skills and supplies, to initiate a higher level of medical assessment and intervention.

Transport preparations should include a visit to the patient by the medical team at the referring facility before transport. This time should involve a patient evaluation, obtaining medical records, and completing final arrangements. Each team member must always practice professional courtesy and obtain permission before entering the patient care area, examining the patient, and reviewing medical records. The transport team must keep in mind that medical care and local customs may influence their approach to the patient and the referring facility.

Ground Transport Times

Preflight planning must include an accurate calculation of the distance and ground times between the patient's location and the airport and from receiving city airport to the receiving hospital.

Information such as traffic and road conditions may also be sought. This information is extremely important for calculating oxygen requirements; the battery life of equipment; and necessary supplies, such as medication infusions, to safely complete the transport from starting point to end.

Ground Ambulance Resources

Whether the patient is transported to the airport or the team is transported to the patient, the resources of the ground unit may be limited. The ground transport vehicle may be a private car, a taxicab, a suburban vehicle, a travel trailer or camper, a pickup truck with a camper shell, or an ambulance unit. Some ambulances may be stripped to an empty unit with no oxygen source or suction equipment, whereas others may be elaborately stocked with supplies and medical equipment. In addition, the skills of the ambulance personnel that accompany the team and patient may vary widely, from a driver with no medical knowledge to emergency medical personnel, nurses, or physicians with varying degrees of skills.

Finally, one must consider the safety issues of the ground transport to and from the airplane. Road conditions, driving skills and compliance with traffic laws, the inability to secure equipment, and the lack of familiarity with the ground transport unit and local area by the medical team are a few of the concerns that may be faced during the ground transport. These issues contribute additional stresses to the international transport of patients (see Chapter 24 for how to manage the stresses of transport).

Pilot and Air Medical Personnel Duty Times

Duty and rest times must be considered for each international transport for the pilot and air medical personnel. This issue is already addressed for pilots because they must comply with FAR Part 135.267 flight time limitations and rest requirements. Therefore, during the preflight preparation, rest requirements must be calculated into the plan and arrangements made for relief pilots to assume flight duties at appropriate fuel stops or at the destination.

When making preflight preparations, air medical personnel should determine the length of the flight and patient care times and use judgment in scheduling adequate team breaks. Depending on the duty times of the flight and medical crew members, an overnight stay may be necessary to comply with crew rest and FAA requirements. This stay may involve the acquisition of lodging for each team member. Many times these arrangements are easily facilitated with use of a handling agent in the country to which the patient is transferred; this agent can assist with hotel arrangements, aircraft refueling, catering, ground transportation, and any other needs of the team.

Rest for air medical personnel may be accomplished during the flight depending on available rest areas on board the aircraft, with members of the team resting in a rotation in which the transport nurse, paramedic, physician, or other medical team member is always monitoring and managing patient status and needs. For extremely long transports, the air medical service may send a relief team of air medical personnel to a scheduled fuel stop to assume patient care. Programs should have policies that define when rests occur and when relief medical teams are required.[89]

Medical Equipment and Supplies

As with preflight preparations for any fixed-wing aircraft transport, the transport team must ensure that plans are complete for international transports. The transport team must be meticulous in planning and arranging for adequate oxygen, medical equipment, batteries, supplies, pharmaceuticals, bedding and linens, nutrition and fluids, and disposal of contaminated wastes. A greater potential for unexpected delays exists for these transports because of customs coordination, ambulance delays, and refueling stops. In addition, international transports may be of longer duration than other transports and to destinations with no or limited medical supplies or supplies that are incompatible with that of the air medical personnel. Therefore air medical personnel should stock enough medical supplies and medications for twice the predicted time of transport.

Many countries require special permits or have adopted specific requirements for the transport of certain medications. These requirements should be identified before the team's arrival to prevent any delays or confiscation of the medications needed to care for the patient. Medications should be kept in kits or medical packs, identified as medications needed for patient care, and never carried in the team members' personal luggage.

Finally, the compatibility of medical equipment with foreign electrical current may need to be considered. The team may need to obtain several types of foreign adapters to convert the current so that monitors and suction units can be properly charged. The equipment manufacturer should be consulted on the ability to fully charge the equipment on differing hertz, or cycles per second, of foreign electrical currents.

Escort and Medical Assist Transports on Commercial Airliners

One more form of patient transport, called a commercial medical escort flight or medical assist transport, should be discussed. Escorts may be either domestic or international transports. These transports are referred to as commercial medical escorts. A commercial medical escort is defined as the escort of a patient with a stable condition on a contracted aircraft or a commercial airliner with the airline's approval with only one attendant who may be an emergency medical technician (EMT), paramedic, registered nurse, respiratory therapist, or physician.[89] These flights may involve transporting a patient at the BLS level who needs medical assistance, one who needs ALS or extensive nursing care, or a critically ill or injured patient. The number and expertise of the accompanying attendants needed depends on the patient's condition, the ability to ambulate, and the length of the transport. In addition, when determining the medical escort team configuration, the requirements of the commercial airline must also be considered.

Regarding preflight preparation and logistics for this type of transport, the transport professional should ensure that all arrangements are complete and plan to address several unique obstacles.

These issues include not only commercial air carrier regulations, documentation, airline oxygen requirements, oxygen adapters, and electrical power, but also privacy, wheelchair or other assistance as needed for transfers through airports and terminals during plane changes, and accommodations during layovers or delays. Because transport of a patient on a commercial airliner requires approval of the escort by the air carrier's medical desk and coordination that is not under the control of the air medical service, these arrangements may take several days to an entire week to complete.

Commercial Air Carrier Regulations

Regulations for transporting a patient on an airliner vary, depending on the patient's designated level and condition. Many commercial air carriers allow a patient in stable condition who needs limited care to sit in the first-class or business-class section for transport. With these cases, the patient must be able to sit upright during taxi, takeoff, and landing. On the other hand, transfer of a critically ill patient may necessitate the purchase of multiple seats (6–12) in the business-class section or in the rear coach compartment of the airplane so that the litter can be secured and patient can be safely restrained in a supine position during critical times of flight. Many airlines prohibit stretcher-bound patients. Most of the airliners that can accommodate patients that are unable to travel in a seated position have a dedicated patient litter that rests above the folded passenger seats and is bolted to the seat tracks. Special arrangements should be made with each commercial airline because each carrier has a different patient litter, loading and securing procedures, and quantity of medical oxygen available. The transport team should plan for the logistics of these escorts to ensure that the transport is completed smoothly.

In addition, provisions must be made for transporting medical equipment and supplies in such a way that they are readily available for the patient and yet secured per FARs. The equipment should also be organized so that it can be easily transferred and checked by customs and immigration authorities.

Documentation

Air medical personnel must organize all the paperwork necessary for the entire transport, including airline tickets, passports, itinerary, and customs documents. This documentation for the air medical personnel, patient, and family members must be readily available for customs and immigration authorities. Air medical personnel should always keep this paperwork on their person.

As with other transports, patient documentation must be completed, and copies of the medical record must be left with the patient at the receiving facility.

Airline Oxygen Requirements

Each air carrier has a different procedure for obtaining oxygen and securing the oxygen tanks. The oxygen tanks routinely provided by most airlines deliver only 2 to 4 L/min. Therefore, arrangements must be made to have extra oxygen tanks available for patients who require 100% oxygen, a ventilator, or an oxygen concentrator. A minimum of 24 hours of notice is necessary, but frequently several days are needed to make such arrangements. Many airlines charge additional fees to provide medical oxygen and may restrict the amount that can be secured because they have limited capacity to accommodate and secure larger oxygen tanks. In addition to having oxygen provisions during flight, the availability of oxygen within the terminals during layovers and plane changes must be considered. The commercial airline may not have the ability to provide oxygen outside the aircraft and gate area.

Oxygen Adapters

Particular attention should be given to the oxygen adapters and regulators available on each airliner. Most of this equipment is not compatible with air medical transport ventilator fittings. In addition, oxygen flow meters are often irregular.

Electrical Power and Adapters

The commercial air carrier's electrical power sources must be assessed and coordinated to power the medical equipment to include adapters, voltage output, and amperage. A power source may be needed for transport ventilators, heart monitors, IV pumps, and suction equipment. As previously mentioned, the appropriate adapters must be obtained to convert the current in these foreign airplanes.

Privacy

Most commercial airlines have various rules pertaining to patients in critical condition. Their presence may disturb or upset other passengers. Some airlines provide privacy for the patient by installing temporary curtains, but most of the time, they are inadequate. Other airlines may require the patient be transported in a private medical suite. Additional sheets or drapes may be necessary to provide adequate privacy for the patient.

Nonstop Flight or Flight With Minimal Plane Changes

Every attempt should be made to make reservations on a nonstop flight or to minimize the number of plane changes and layovers for the patient transport. Decreasing the number of stops or delays eliminates the frustrations of making additional arrangements to get on and from the airplane, to transfer the patient, and to provide documentation for customs and immigration officials. In addition, plans must be made to organize all the medical equipment, patient and family belongings, and luggage of air medical personnel for each transfer.

Summary

Although many general principles of practice and patient care are identical in the transport environment and process, whether by air or surface, differences do exist. The complex nature of the transport environment provides many challenges. Preparation for transport requires education and training, preplanning, and intuition. All members of the transport team must be able to deliver safe and competent patient care in the transport environment in which they practice.

References

1. Treadwell D, Santiago JP, eds. *Standards for Critical Care and Specialty Transport.* 2nd ed. ASTNA; 2019.
2. Lyng JW, Braithwaite S, Abraham H, et al. Appropriate air medical services utilization and recommendations for integration of air medical services resources into the EMS system of care: A joint position statement and resource document of NAEMSP, ACEP, and AMPA. *Prehosp Emerg Care.* 2021;25(6):854–873. doi:10.1080/10903127.2021.1967534
3. Newgard CD, Fischer PE, Gestring M, et al. National guideline for the field triage of injured patients: Recommendations of the national expert panel on field triage, 2021. *J Trauma Acute Care Surg.* 2022;93(2):e49–e60. doi:10.1097/TA.0000000000003627
4. American Academy of Pediatrics Section on Transport Medicine. *Guidelines for Air and Ground Transport of Neonatal and Pediatric Patients.* 4th ed. AAP; 2016.

5. American Academy of Pediatrics, American College of Obstetrics and Gynecology. *Guidelines for Perinatal Care.* 8th ed. AAP & ACOG; 2017.

6. Warren J, Fromm RE, Orr RA, Rotello LC, Horst HM. Guidelines for the inter- and intrahospital transport of critically ill patients. *Crit Care Med.* 2004;32(1):256–262. doi:10.1097/01.CCM.0000104917.39204.0A

7. American College of Emergency Physicians. Appropriate interfacility transfer. *Ann Emerg Med.* 2022;79(6):e121–e123. doi:10.1016/j.annemergmed.2022.02.022

8. Chen X, Gestring ML, Rosengart MR, et al. Logistics of air medical transport: When and where does helicopter transport reduce prehospital time for trauma? *J Trauma Acute Care Surg.* 2018;85(1):174–181. doi:10.1097/TA.0000000000001935

9. Swickard S, Swickard W, Reimer A, Lindell D, Winkelman C. Adaptation of the AACN synergy model for patient care to critical care transport. *Crit Care Nurse.* 2014;34(1):16–28. doi:10.4037/ccn2014573

10. Sperry JL, Guyette FX, Brown JB, et al. Prehospital plasma during air medical transport in trauma patients at risk for hemorrhagic shock. *N Engl J Med.* 2018;379(4):315–326. doi:10.1056/NEJMoa1802345

11. Guyette FX, Sperry JL, Peitzman AB, et al. Prehospital blood product and crystalloid resuscitation in the severely injured patient: A secondary analysis of the prehospital air medical plasma trial. *Ann Surg.* 2021;273(2):358–364. doi:10.1097/SLA.0000000000003324

12. American College of Surgeons. *Resources for Optimal Care of the Injured Patient: 2022 Standards.* ACS; 2022.

13. O'Gara PT, Kushner FG, Ascheim DD, et al. 2013 ACCF/AHA guideline for the management of ST-elevation myocardial infarction: A report of the American College of Cardiology Foundation/American Heart Association task force on practice guidelines. *Circulation.* 2013;127(4):e362–e425. doi:10.1161/CIR.0b013e3182742cf6

14. Powers WJ, Rabinstein AA, Ackerson T, et al. Guidelines for the early management of patients with acute ischemic stroke: 2019 update to the 2018 guidelines for the early management of acute ischemic stroke: A guideline for healthcare professionals from the American Heart Association/American Stroke Association. *Stroke.* 2019;50(12):e344–e418. doi:10.1161/STR.0000000000000211

15. Hiratzka LF, Bakris GL, Beckman JA, et al. 2010 ACCF/AHA/AATS/ACR/ASA/SCA/SCAI/SIR/STS/SVM guidelines for the diagnosis and management of patients with thoracic aortic disease. A report of the American College of Cardiology Foundation/American Heart Association task force on practice guidelines, American Association for Thoracic Surgery, American College of Radiology, American Stroke Association, Society of Cardiovascular Anesthesiologists, Society for Cardiovascular Angiography and Interventions, Society of Interventional Radiology, Society of Thoracic Surgeons, and Society for Vascular Medicine. *J Am Coll Cardiol.* 2010;55(14):e27–e129. doi:10.1016/j.jacc.2010.02.015

16. Grotta JC, Yamal J, Parker SA, et al. Prospective, multicenter, controlled trial of mobile stroke units. *N Engl J Med.* 2021;385(11):971–981. doi:10.1056/NEJMoa2103879

17. Bartos JA, Frascone RJ, Conterato M, et al. The Minnesota mobile extracorporeal cardiopulmonary resuscitation consortium for treatment of out-of-hospital refractory ventricular fibrillation: Program description, performance, and outcomes. *EClinicalMedicine.* 2020;29–30:100632. doi:10.1016/j.eclinm.2020.100632

18. Examination and treatment for emergency medical conditions and women in labor. 2020;42 U.S.C. § 1395dd.

19. Special responsibilities of Medicare hospitals in emergency cases. 2013;42 CFR § 489.24.

20. Walter R. Professional issues. In: Wolfe AC, Santiago J, Frakes MA, Farmer S, eds. *Critical Care Transport Core Curriculum.* 2nd ed. ASTNA; 2022:85–108.

21. Air & Surface Transport Nurses Association, Emergency Nurses Association, International Association of Flight and Critical Care Paramedics. Responsible "helicopter shopping" through selective resource management. *Air Med J.* 2019;38(3):143–146. doi:10.1016/j.amj.2019.02.007

22. Continenza K, Hill JH. Transport of the critically ill child. In: Blumer J, ed. *A Practical Guide to Pediatric Intensive Care.* 3rd ed. Mosby; 1990:17–27.

23. Association of Critical Care Transport. *Critical Care Transport Standards.* 2nd ed. ACCT; 2019.

24. Air Medical Physician Association. *Safe Handoff of Care in Air/Ground Medical Transport: Position Statement of the Air Medical Physician Association.* AMPA; 2012.

25. Appelbaum R, Martin S, Tinkoff G, Pascual JL, Gandhi RR. Eastern Association for the Surgery of Trauma – quality, patient safety, and outcomes committee – transitions of care: Healthcare handoffs in trauma. *Am J Surg.* 2021;222(3):521–528. doi:10.1016/j.amjsurg.2021.01.034

26. Maddry JK, Simon EM, Reeves LK, et al. Impact of a standardized patient hand-off tool on communication between emergency medical services personnel and emergency department staff. *Prehosp Emerg Care.* 2021;25(4):530–538. doi:10.1080/10903127.2020.1808745

27. Williams AR. Legal issues in air and ground medical transport. In: Blumen IJ, Bolton L, Davidoff JB, et al. eds. *Principles and Direction of Air Medical Transport.* 2nd ed. AMPA; 2015:170–203.

28. Venkat A, Huckestein V, Dhindsa HS. Ethical issues in air medical transport. In: Blumen IJ, Bolton L, Davidoff JB, et al. eds. *Principles and Direction of Air Medical Transport.* 2nd ed. AMPA; 2015:32–39.

29. Bennett KJ, Probst JC, Bullard JC, Crouch E. The importance of rural hospitals: Transfers and 30-day readmissions among rural residents and patients presenting at rural hospitals. *Popul Health Manag.* 2019;22(2):120–126. doi:10.1089/pop.2018.0050

30. Greenwood-Ericksen M, Kamdar N, Lin P, et al. Association of rural and critical access hospital status with patient outcomes after emergency department visits among Medicare beneficiaries. *JAMA Netw Open.* 2021;4(11):e2134980. doi:10.1001/jamanetworkopen.2021.34980

31. George BP, Doyle SJ, Albert GP, et al. Interfacility transfers for US ischemic stroke and TIA, 2006–2014. *Neurology.* 2018;90(18):e1561–e1569. doi:10.1212/WNL.0000000000005419

32. American College of Emergency Physicians. Policy statement: Emergency medical services interfaces with health care systems. *Ann Emerg Med.* 2018;71(6):e119–e120. doi:10.1016/j.annemergmed.2018.03.013

33. National Association of EMS Physicians. Ambulance diversion and emergency department offload delay. *Prehosp Emerg Care.* 2011;15(4):543. doi:10.3109/10903127.2011.598620

34. Cooney DR, Millin MG, Carter A, Lawner BJ, Nable JV, Wallus HJ. Ambulance diversion and emergency department offload delay: Resource document for the National Association of EMS Physicians position statement. *Prehosp Emerg Care.* 2011;15(4):555–561. doi:10.3109/10903127.2011.608871

35. Miller JA. Patient assessment and transport. In: Wolfe AC, Santiago J, Frakes MA, Farmer S, eds. *Critical Care Transport Core Curriculum.* 2nd ed. ASTNA; 2022:109–134.

36. Alson RL, Han KH, Campbell JE, eds. *International Trauma Life Support for Emergency Care Providers.* 9th ed. Pearson; 2021.

37. Federal Aviation Administration. *FAR/AIM 2022: Federal Aviation Regulations and Aeronautical Information Manual.* Aviation Supplies & Academics; 2021.

38. Collopy K, Ender V. Patient assessment. In: McEvoy M, Rabrich JS, Kivlehan SM, Mejia A, eds. *Critical Care Transport.* 3rd ed. Jones & Bartlett; 2023:121–154.

39. Halliwell K, ed. *Transport Professional Advanced Trauma Course Provider Manual.* 7th ed. ASTNA; 2018.

40. Hertel K, Hamill M, Perez-Fernandez J, eds. *Fundamental Critical Care Support.* 7th ed. SCCM; 2021.

41. Committee on Tactical Combat Casualty Care. Tactical Combat Casualty Care (TCCC) guidelines for medical personnel. *J Spec Oper Med.* Spring;22(1):11–17. doi:10.55460/ETZI-SI9T

42. National Association of State EMS Officials. *National Model EMS Clinical Guidelines.* 3rd ed. NASEMSO; 2022.

43. Panchal AR, Bartos JA, Cabañas JG, et al. Part 3: Adult basic and advanced life support: 2020 American Heart Association guidelines for cardiopulmonary resuscitation and emergency cardiovascular care. *Circulation.* 2020;142(16 Suppl 2):S366–S468. doi:10.1161/CIR.0000000000000916

44. Bulger EM, Snyder D, Schoelles K, et al. An evidence-based prehospital guideline for external hemorrhage control: American College of Surgeons Committee on Trauma. *Prehosp Emerg Care.* 2014;18(2):163–173. doi:10.3109/10903127.2014.896962

45. Pfeifer R, Halvachizadeh S, Schick S, et al. Are pre-hospital trauma deaths preventable? A systematic literature review. *World J Surg.* 2019;43(10):2438–2446. doi:10.1007/s00268-019-05056-1

46. Drake SA, Holcomb JB, Yang Y, et al. Establishing a regional trauma preventable/potentially preventable death rate. *Ann Surg.* 2020;271(2):375–382. doi:10.1097/SLA.0000000000002999

47. Devlin JW, Skrobik Y, Gélinas C, et al. Clinical practice guidelines for the prevention and management of pain, agitation/sedation, delirium, immobility, and sleep disruption in adult patients in the ICU. *Crit Care Med.* 2018;46(9):e825–e873. doi:10.1097/CCM.0000000000003299

48. Nakajima M, Aso S, Yasunaga H, et al. Body temperature change and outcomes in patients undergoing long-distance air medical transport. *Am J Emerg Med.* 2019;37(1):89–93. doi:10.1016/j.ajem.2018.04.064

49. Roberts DJ, Leigh-Smith S, Faris PD, et al. Clinical presentation of patients with tension pneumothorax: A systematic review. *Ann Surg.* 2015;261(6):1068–1078. doi:10.1097/SLA.0000000000001073

50. Ron E, Alattar Z, Hoebee S, Kang P, vanSonnenberg E. Current trends in the use of ultrasound over chest x-ray to identify pneumothoraces in ICU, trauma, and ARDS patients. *J Intensive Care Med.* 2022;37(1):5–11. doi:10.1177/0885066620987813

51. Siemieniuk RAC, Chu DK, Kim LH, et al. Oxygen therapy for acutely ill medical patients: A clinical practice guideline. *BMJ.* 2018;363:k4169. doi:10.1136/bmj.k4169

52. Newgard CD, Cheney TP, Chou R, et al. Out-of-hospital circulatory measures to identify patients with serious injury: A systematic review. *Acad Emerg Med.* 2020;27(12):1323–1339. doi:10.1111/acem.14056

53. Heffner AC, Swords DS, Neale MN, Jones AE. Incidence and factors associated with cardiac arrest complicating emergency airway management. *Resuscitation.* 2013;84(11):1500–1504. doi:10.1016/j.resuscitation.2013.07.022

54. Acker SN, Ross JT, Partrick DA, Tong S, Bensard DD. Pediatric specific shock index accurately identifies severely injured children. *J Pediatr Surg.* 2015;50(2):331–334. doi:10.1016/j.jpedsurg.2014.08.009

55. Teasdale G, Jennett B. Assessment of coma and impaired consciousness. A practical scale. *Lancet.* 1974;2(7872):81–84. doi:10.1016/s0140-6736(74)91639-0

56. Teasdale G, Maas A, Lecky F, Manley G, Stocchetti N, Murray G. The Glasgow Coma Scale at 40 years: Standing the test of time. *Lancet Neurol.* 2014;13(8):844–854. doi:10.1016/S1474-4422(14)70120-6

57. Teasdale G. Forty years on: Updating the Glasgow Coma Scale. *Nurs Times.* 2014;110(42):12–16.

58. Borgialli DA, Mahajan P, Hoyle JD, et al. Performance of the pediatric Glasgow Coma Scale score in the evaluation of children with blunt head trauma. *Acad Emerg Med.* 2016;23(8):878–884. doi:10.1111/acem.13014

59. James HE. Neurologic evaluation and support in the child with an acute brain insult. *Pediatr Ann.* 1986;15(1):16–22. doi:10.3928/0090-4481-19860101-05

60. Healey C, Osler TM, Rogers FB, et al. Improving the Glasgow Coma Scale score: Motor score alone is a better predictor. *J Trauma.* 2003;54(4):671–678. doi:10.1097/01.TA.0000058130.30490.5D

61. Wijdicks EFM, Bamlet WR, Maramattom BV, Manno EM, McClelland RL. Validation of a new coma scale: The FOUR score. *Ann Neurol.* 2005;58(4):585–593. doi:10.1002/ana.20611

62. Foo CC, Loan JJM, Brennan PM. The relationship of the FOUR score to patient outcome: A systematic review. *J Neurotrauma.* 2019;36(17):2469–2483. doi:10.1089/neu.2018.6243

63. Sanello A, Gausche-Hill M, Mulkerin W, et al. Altered mental status: Current evidence-based recommendations for prehospital care. *West J Emerg Med.* 2018;19(3):527–541. doi:10.5811/westjem.2018.1.36559

64. Spaite DW, Bobrow BJ, Keim SM, et al. Association of statewide implementation of the prehospital traumatic brain injury treatment guidelines with patient survival following traumatic brain injury: The excellence in prehospital injury care (EPIC) study. *JAMA Surg.* 2019;154(7):e191152. doi:10.1001/jamasurg.2019.1152

65. Spaite DW, Hu C, Bobrow BJ, et al. Optimal out-of-hospital blood pressure in major traumatic brain injury: A challenge to the current understanding of hypotension. *Ann Emerg Med.* 2022;80(1):46–59. doi:10.1016/j.annemergmed.2022.01.045

66. Ratcliff JJ, Morrison C, Tran DS, Ruzas CM. *Emergency Neurological Life Support: Intracranial Hypertension and Herniation Protocol, Version 4.0.* Neurocritical Care Society; 2020. https://www.neurocriticalcare.org/NCS-Learning-Center/ENLS/Protocols

67. Mota MAL, Santos MR, Santos EJF, Henriques C, Matos A, Cunha M. Trauma prehospital hypothermia prevention and treatment: An observational study. *J Trauma Nurs.* 2021;28(3):194–202. doi:10.1097/JTN.0000000000000583

68. Mota M, Cunha M, Santos M, et al. Prehospital interventions to prevent hypothermia in trauma patients: A scoping review. *Aust J Adv Nurs.* 2020;37(3):29–36. doi:10.37464/2020.373.88

69. Bloemen EM, Rosen T, Cline Schiroo JA, et al. Photographing injuries in the acute care setting: Development and evaluation of a standardized protocol for research, forensics, and clinical practice. *Acad Emerg Med.* 2016;23(5):653–659. doi:10.1111/acem.12955

70. Bergrath S, Rossaint R, Lenssen N, Fitzner C, Skorning M. Prehospital digital photography and automated image transmission in an emergency medical service – an ancillary retrospective analysis of a prospective controlled trial. *Scand J Trauma Resusc Emerg Med.* 2013;21:3. doi:10.1186/1757-7241-21-3

71. Smith HAB, Besunder JB, Betters KA, et al. 2022 Society of Critical Care Medicine clinical practice guidelines on prevention and management of pain, agitation, neuromuscular blockade, and delirium in critically ill pediatric patients with consideration of the ICU environment and early mobility. *Pediatr Crit Care Med.* 2022;23(2):e74–e110. doi:10.1097/PCC.0000000000002873

72. Teoh SE, Loh CYL, Chong RIH, et al. A scoping review of qualitative studies on pre-hospital analgesia administration and practice. *Am J Emerg Med.* 2022;57:81–90. doi:10.1016/j.ajem.2022.04.038

73. American Nurses Association Center for Ethics and Human Rights. *Position Statement: The Ethical Responsibility to Manage Pain and the Suffering It Causes.* ANA; 2018.

74. Hartjes TM, ed. *Core Curriculum for High Acuity, Progressive, and Critical Care Nursing.* 7th ed. Elsevier; 2018.

75. Sessler CN, Gosnell MS, Grap MJ, et al. The Richmond Agitation-Sedation Scale: Validity and reliability in adult intensive care unit patients. *Am J Respir Crit Care Med.* 2002;166(10):1338–1344. doi:10.1164/rccm.2107138

76. Brunsveld-Reinders AH, Arbous MS, Kuiper SG, de Jonge E. A comprehensive method to develop a checklist to increase safety of intra-hospital transport of critically ill patients. *Crit Care.* 2015;19:214. doi:10.1186/s13054-015-0938-1

77. Vincent J, Moreno R. Clinical review: Scoring systems in the critically ill. *Crit Care.* 2010;14(2):207. doi:10.1186/cc8204

78. Desai N, Gross J. Scoring systems in the critically ill: Uses, cautions, and future directions. *BJA Educ.* 2019;19(7):212–218. doi:10.1016/j.bjae.2019.03.002

79. Guan G, Lee CMY, Begg S, Crombie A, Mnatzaganian G. The use of early warning system scores in prehospital and emergency department settings to predict clinical deterioration: A systematic review and meta-analysis. *PLoS One.* 2022;17(3):e0265559. doi:10.1371/journal.pone.0265559

80. Riwitis C. *Cultural Diversity and Gender Inclusivity in the Emergency Care Setting.* ENA; 2018.

81. American College of Emergency Physicians. Cultural awareness and emergency care. *Ann Emerg Med.* 2020;76(4):e85. doi:10.1016/j.annemergmed.2020.06.010

82. Greene-Moton E, Minkler M. Cultural competence or cultural humility? Moving beyond the debate. *Health Promot Pract.* 2020;21(1):142–145. doi:10.1177/1524839919884912

83. Pagana KD, Pagana TJ, Pagana TN. *Mosby's Diagnostic & Laboratory Test Reference.* 15th ed. Elsevier; 2020.

84. Mettler FA, ed. *Essentials of Radiology.* 4th ed. Elsevier; 2018.

85. Scott S, Messer B. Critical care chest radiology. *Surgery (Oxford).* 2018;36(12):694–698. doi:10.1016/j.mpsur.2018.09.020

86. Nentwich LM, Veloz W. Neuroimaging in acute stroke. *Emerg Med Clin North Am.* 2012;30(3):659–680. doi:10.1016/j.emc.2012.06.005

87. Air Medical Physician Association. Ultrasound in the air medical environment. *Air Med J.* 2018;37(6):351. doi:10.1016/j.amj.2018.09.003

88. Amaral CB, Ralston DC, Becker TK. Prehospital point-of-care ultrasound: A transformative technology. *SAGE Open Med.* 2020;8:2050312120932706. doi:10.1177/2050312120932706

89. Commission on Accreditation of Medical Transport Systems. *12th Edition Accreditation Standards of the Commission on Accreditation of Medical Transport Systems.* CAMTS; 2022.

90. McEvoy M. Hemodynamic monitoring. In: McEvoy M, Rabrich JS, Kivlehan SM, Mejia A, eds. *Critical Care Transport.* 3rd ed. Jones & Bartlett; 2023:783–839.

91. Weigand DL, ed. *Procedure Manual for High Acuity, Progressive, and Critical Care.* 7th ed. AACN; 2017.

92. Hatfield JL, Poirier G, Thomas SH. Considerations in air medical transport of the critically ill patient. In: Blumen IJ, Bolton L, Davidoff JB, et al. eds. *Principles and Direction of Air Medical Transport.* 2nd ed. AMPA; 2015:433–440.

93. Stoddard K, Vincent K. Mechanical circulatory devices. In: Wolfe AC, Santiago J, Frakes MA, Farmer S, eds. *Critical Care Transport Core Curriculum.* 2nd ed. ASTNA; 2022:523–534.

94. Motov S, Strayer R, Hayes BD, et al. The treatment of acute pain in the emergency department: A white paper position statement prepared for the American Academy of Emergency Medicine. *J Emerg Med.* 2018;54(5):731–736. doi:10.1016/j.jemermed.2018.01.020

95. Hachimi-Idrissi S, Dobias V, Hautz WE, et al. Approaching acute pain in emergency settings; European Society for Emergency Medicine (EUSEM) guidelines-part 2: Management and recommendations. *Intern Emerg Med.* 2020;15(7):1141–1155. doi:10.1007/s11739-020-02411-2

96. Manterola C, Vial M, Moraga J, Astudillo P. Analgesia in patients with acute abdominal pain. *Cochrane Database Syst Rev.* 2011:CD005660. doi:10.1002/14651858.CD005660.pub3

97. Gavriilidis P, de'Angelis N, Tobias A. To use or not to use opioid analgesia for acute abdominal pain before definitive surgical diagnosis? A systematic review and network meta-analysis. *J Clin Med Res.* 2019;11(2):121–126. doi:10.14740/jocmr3690

98. Kupas DF, Wydro GC, Tan DK, Kamin R, Harrell AJ, Wang A. Clinical care and restraint of agitated or combative patients by emergency medical services practitioners. *Prehosp Emerg Care.* 2021;25(5):721–723. doi:10.1080/10903127.2021.1917736

99. Condition of participation: Patient's rights. 2019;42 C.F.R. §482.13.

100. Binks A, Pyke M. Anaesthesia in the obese patient. *Anaesth Intens Care Med.* 2008;9(7):299–302. doi:10.1016/j.mpaic.2008.04.018

101. Schetz M, De Jong A, Deane AM, et al. Obesity in the critically ill: A narrative review. *Intensive Care Med.* 2019;45(6):757–769. doi:10.1007/s00134-019-05594-1

102. Hannibal GB. Interpretation of the low-voltage ECG. *AACN Adv Crit Care.* 2014;25(1):64–68. doi:10.4037/NCI.0000000000000001

103. Bloodborne pathogens. 2019;29 C.F.R. § 1910.1030.

104. Holdefer WF, Diethelm AG, Tolbert JT. International air medical transport. Part I: Methods and logistics. *J Air Med Transp.* 1990;9(7):6–8. doi:10.1016/s1046-9095(05)80401-5

105. Holdefer WF, Diethelm AG, Tolbert JT. International air medical transport. Part II: Results and discussion. *J Air Med Transp.* 1990;9(8):8–11. doi:10.1016/s1046-9095(05)80432-5

12

Airway Management

DAVID J. OLVERA AND MICHAEL A. FRAKES

COMPETENCIES

1. Describe the process of primary and secondary assessment in airway management.
2. Identify the indications for basic and advanced airway management.
3. Describe and use the universal emergency airway algorithm for airway management.
4. Identify the indications and contraindications for specific airway interventions.
5. Formulate a plan to decide on an approach to advanced airway management.
6. Demonstrate the ability to execute alternative airway management.
7. Describe the pharmacology of advanced airway management.

Maintaining a patent airway is the first priority in patient care, and airway management may account for some of the most challenging clinical situations encountered by transport personnel. The most common errors in airway management are failures to anticipate the need for airway management and failure to prepare the patient, provider, and team for the procedure.

Although many skills and a great deal of equipment are needed to control the airway, the essential component of the airway management skill set is critical thinking. The transport team must know when to intervene, when not to intervene, how to intervene, and how to avoid complications. Critical thinking and technical skills are developed through quality education, practice, and repetition, all of which must be developed in concert. It is foolish to practice technical skills without attention to the critical thinking and decision-making criteria that accompany their use.

Technical perspectives are woven into the critical thinking approach defined in this chapter, which will address patient and airway assessment, considerations in planning the approach to airway management, techniques to optimize preparation, strategies to optimize procedural success, and strategies to prevent procedural and physiologic complications.

Patient Assessment

The assessment associated with airway management falls into four broad categories: primary assessment, secondary assessment, indications for management, and evaluation of the patient's anatomy and physiology related to an indicated procedure. The history, mechanism of injury, and illness progression may also provide subjective and objective data and assist the transport team in determining a course of action. Utilizing the combination of these categories will not only assist with appropriate airway management but also opportunities to improve resuscitation outcomes in patient care.

Primary and Secondary Assessment Surveys

All patient care begins with an evaluation of the primary assessment – ensuring that the airway is patent and that the patient is breathing in an adequate manner. If either of these conditions is not met, a basic life support intervention is necessary to help maintain lifesaving measures. Airway patency can almost always be reestablished with basic interventions such as patient positioning unless precluded by injury involving the cervical spine, using a suction device, and using oral and/or nasal airway adjuncts. Patients who have a patent airway, but inadequate or ineffective spontaneous ventilation, should have ventilatory assistance with a bag-valve-mask (BVM) device, such as a self-inflating or a flow-inflating bag. Those who require basic life support interventions for their airway or breathing for more than a few minutes will almost always require more advanced interventions for longer-term management. The circulatory portion of the primary survey can also offer useful information because skin color, temperature, moisture, and heart rate can suggest hypoxia or shock states.

The secondary survey can provide anatomic and physiologic indications that may indicate the need for an intervention, even in the face of a satisfactory primary examination. Look again at color; pallor, rather than cyanosis, is an indicator of shock. Sympathetic nerve stimulation causes blood to shunt from minor to major organs, and the skin is considered a minor organ. Cyanosis does not occur until approximately 5 g of hemoglobin per 100 cc of capillary blood is deoxygenated.[1] This makes cyanosis a late indicator of hypoxia, although an earlier one in patients with profound anemia. Pallor suggests shock from decreased peripheral perfusion, and mental status change suggests decreased oxygen delivery to the brain. Patients with mental status changes and normal blood sugar should be presumed to have a brain oxygenation defect until it is ruled out.

Working caudally, inspect the neck for obvious injuries and for an expanding hematoma, edema, and jugular vein distention. Palpate for subcutaneous emphysema, and look at the patient, the neck, and the chest for the use of accessory muscles, nasal flaring, and the position the patient assumes. Auscultation identifies absent or decreased breath sounds, which suggest pneumothorax, hemothorax, other effusion, obstruction, infection, or consolidation. Auscultation may also reveal grunting, wheezing, or stridor. Upper airway problems usually involve a barking cough or strider, whereas wheezing and grunting breath sounds are associated with lower airway disease or obstruction. Adventitious breath sounds provide indications about pathology in lower airway structures and lung parenchyma.

Palpate the chest wall for tenderness, crepitus, subcutaneous air, and symmetry of movement. Particularly in noisy environments, palpation can help identify equal rise and fall of the chest. Percussion, like palpation, can provide excellent information about the status of the underlying thoracic structures. The normal lung sound is resonant, a hemothorax is dull, and a tension pneumothorax is hyperresonant.

When evaluating the airway, consider the anticipated clinical course of the patient:

- Is the patient maintaining their airway?
- Will the patient be able to maintain it during transport?
- Is there a chance that the mechanism of injury or illness will lead to a need to intervene during transport?

Also, consider the range of resources and expertise available at the present location, at nearby locations, and during transport. At times it may be reasonable to seek assistance with a difficult or potentially difficult airway from the resources at a local hospital before proceeding with airway interventions at the scene or before beginning transport.

Indications for Airway Management

The indications for airway management, whether noninvasive or invasive, can be generally summarized as the "Six Ps":

- Protection of the airway: Indication for patients who do not have adequate protective airway reflexes to manage secretions. Classically, these patients cannot swallow, follow basic commands, or have a Glasgow Coma Score that has dropped below 9 from their original baseline of a normal score.
- Positive pressure: Indication for patients with insufficient ventilatory effort.
- Partial pressure of oxygen (Po_2): Indication for patients who will benefit from a higher Fio_2 or mean airway pressure to maintain a saturation above 93% or, in rare circumstances, whatever higher target is required. Additionally, an imbalance exists between oxygen supply and demand when a patient is in shock: oxygen consumption increases linearly with work of breathing, and respiratory efficiency declines as the work of breathing increases. External ventilator support can reduce that oxygen demand while increasing oxygen delivery, so early intubation may be beneficial in patients with septic or hypovolemic shock.[2]
- Pulmonary toilet: Indicated when it is necessary to access the airway to remove blood, secretions, infection, or foreign bodies.

- Patient progression: Indicated for patients likely to develop difficulties with protection, effort, oxygenation, or ventilation during transport.
- For the transport provider, a sixth "P," protection, may also be a factor. The management of aggressive behavior in the transport environment, particularly the air transport environment, may necessitate the use of sedation to a depth that creates impairment of one of the previously listed factors triggering consideration of invasive airway management.

Physical Examination in Anticipation of a Procedure

When airway management interventions aim to improve the patient's hemodynamic and physiologic status, it is essential not to cause deterioration in oxygenation, ventilation, or vital signs. Accordingly, if the primary and secondary examinations suggest the need for intervention in the airway, the third critical phase of the patient assessment is for factors that suggest the potential for difficulty or complications with the airway management procedure, physiology, or postprocedure management.

Many mnemonics can help remember factors associated with difficulty in performing various basic and advanced procedures.

Difficult Bag-Valve-Mask Ventilation: ROMAN

R: Radiation/restriction. The term *stiff lungs* refer to patients with difficulty and resistance in ventilation requiring high-ventilation pressures. These patients usually have airway obstruction or reactive airway disease. More commonly, it is noted that patients with chronic obstructive pulmonary disease (COPD), acute respiratory distress syndrome, advanced pneumonia, or term pregnant patients are susceptible to stiff lungs. It can also be noted if a patient snores when they sleep or has sleep apnea, which could result in difficulty with ventilation.

O: Obesity/obstruction/obstructive sleep apnea. Patients who are obese (body mass index [BMI] >26 kg/m²) and women in their third trimester of pregnancy have decreased compliance which can make BVM ventilation more challenging. Obstruction caused by angioedema, Ludwig angina, upper airway abscess, epiglottis, and similar conditions will make BVM more difficult.

M: Mask seal/male sex/Mallampati. Consider facial features such as bushy beards, blood, and disruption of the facial anatomy as issues that may cause difficulty providing a proper mask seal. Both male sex and a Mallampati class 3 or 4 airway can also appear to be independent predictors of difficult BVM. The Mallampati score describes the ability to see structures in the oropharynx. Classically, the patient sits up, opens the mouth maximally, and protrudes the tongue maximally without phonating. In a class I airway, the soft palate, uvula, fauces, and tonsillar pillars are visible. In a class II airway, the tonsillar pillars disappear, but the soft palate, uvula, and fauces are visible. In a class III airway, only the base of the uvula and soft palate are visible. In a class IV airway, none of the soft palates is visible. The Mallampati classes are illustrated in Fig. 12.1.

A: Age. Diminishing muscle tone with advancing age, particularly over age 55, can lead to difficulty in bag-mask ventilation. Pediatric patients under 3 can also be problematic because their muscle tone has not yet fully developed.

N: No teeth. It may be challenging to provide a proper seal on edentulous patients because of the diminished structure of the airway. If a patient has dentures, consider leaving the

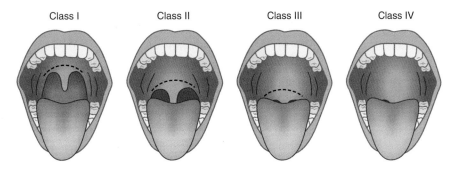

Class I   Class II   Class III   Class IV

• **Figure 12.1** Mallampati classes. (From Karan SB, Bailey PL. *Techniques in Gastrointestinal Endoscopy.* Elsevier; 2004.)

dentures in place during application of BVM and removing them for instrumentation.[3]

Difficult Direct Laryngoscopy: LEMON(S)

L: Look externally. Evaluate normal face and neck anatomy, face and neck pathology, face shape, sunken cheeks, protruding front teeth, and a receding mandible. Include an evaluation for a beard, which reduces the ability to get a seal for mask ventilation and consider neck circumference. Increasing neck circumference is an independent predictor of intubation difficulty, with the risk beginning to increase at about 40 cm. Very high BMI, >50 kg/m², is also associated with risk for difficult laryngoscopy and intubation.[4,5]

E: Evaluate the 3-3-2 rule. Direct laryngoscopy (DL) requires the ability to line up oral, pharyngeal, and laryngeal axes. The 3-3-2 rule identifies patients in whom the ability to achieve that alignment is more likely to be complicated. Patients should be able to place three of their own fingers between the upper and lower incisors of a fully opened mouth, three fingers along the mandible from the tip of the chin posteriorly, and two fingers from the laryngeal prominence to the floor of the mouth.

M: Mallampati score. The Mallampati score describes the ability to see structures in the oropharynx. Intubation is typically not difficult in class I and class II airways. In a class III airway, DL is predicted to be moderately difficult. In a class IV airway, DL is unlikely to be successful (see Fig. 12.1).

O: Obstruction. Evaluate for potential mechanical obstruction from a foreign body, tumor, swelling, expanding hematoma, or abscess.

N: Neck mobility. The neck should flex freely, and the head should extend freely so the patient can assume the classic sniffing position.

S: Saturation. Attempting to preoxygenate or maintain saturations above 93% during intubation attempt.[3]

Difficult Extraglottic Device: RODS

R: Restricted mouth opening. Ensuring the patient can open the mouth enough to allow access of the rescue device.

O: Obstruction/obesity. Assess if it is possible to pass the extraglottic device into the mouth to allow adequate oxygenation or if there is an obstruction caused by increased extraglottic tissue.

D: Disrupted/distorted airway. When placing the extraglottic device, will it be able to be seated correctly, or is the airway disrupted or distorted?

S: Stiff lungs. Is there a resistance to ventilation caused by airway resistance (asthma, COPD) or issues with pulmonary compliance?[3]

Difficult Cricothyrotomy: SMART

S: Surgery (recent or remote). After surgery, it could be noted that the anatomy might not be in correct alignment, and it might be difficult to find landmarks. Another consideration is the scar tissue after surgery; accessing the membrane might be more difficult.

M: Mass. A hematoma or mass over the cricothyroid membrane might make access to the surgical airway more difficult.

A: Access/anatomy. Patients with higher BMI can make identifying landmarks more difficult because of extra tissue. Other challenges might include a patient wearing a C-collar or a short neck.

R: Radiation (and other deformity or scarring). A patient with a history of radiation may have distortion and scarring.

T: Tumor. Access to the airway, either from outside or inside, when a tumor is present can lead to increased bleeding and difficulty identifying landmarks.[3]

These preparation guidelines can be helpful memory aids and triggers. At the same time, the accuracy of any prediction rule for difficult airway management is limited. Even among professional anesthesia providers, 93% of patients with difficult airway were unanticipated, and some of the rules can be difficult to apply in emergency situations. Interestingly, anesthesia providers found technical difficulty in only one-quarter of patients in whom difficult airways were anticipated.[6,7] It is most prudent to approach each patient with the idea that the airway will be difficult.

Physiologic Examination and Considerations Associated With Airway Management

The assessment must include both physical findings associated with technical procedures and factors suggesting peri-intubation physiologic deterioration. Three classic physiologic risk factors should be considered in airway evaluation and preparation: hypoxia, hypotension, and severe metabolic acidosis.[8] Additionally, patients who have complex cardiovascular physiology that affects right ventricular function (such as chronic pulmonary hypertension, massive pulmonary embolism, or right-sided myocardial infarction) or patients with altered cardiac anatomy from repair of congenital heart defects will require particular thought and care in the development of an induction and intubation plan.

Hypoxemia

Hypoxemia is a failure to maintain adequate arterial oxygenation and often represents one of the triggers for both invasive and noninvasive airway management. Intubation, particularly intubation facilitated by medications that suppress spontaneous ventilation, creates a risk for desaturation. The goal is to prolong the duration of the safe period of hypoventilation before desaturation below a peripheral oxygen saturation (SpO_2) of 93%. It is impossible to predict how long the period of desaturation will last, and hypoxia develops more quickly in patients with hyperdynamic conditions, high oxygen demands, or with poor oxygen delivery capabilities. Children normally have twice the metabolic demand of adults, along with a smaller reserve capacity, so they commonly desaturate more quickly than adults. Pregnant women and patients with a higher BMI. Have decreased functional residual capacity (FRC), so can be more difficult to preoxygenate and will desaturate more rapidly.

Pulse oximetry measurement in the setting of emergent intubation is often confounded by loss of signal, and there is a well-known latency period between desaturation and the detection of desaturation on peripheral monitors. Finger pulse oximetry reflects oxygen saturation changes by a mean of about 2 minutes after arterial blood gas samples change in healthy patients. Probe location, physiologic state, and body temperature affect the delay.[9,10] Fig. 12.2 shows the relationship between oxygen saturation and the partial pressure of oxygen.

Patients who are about to have invasive airway management procedures performed on them should have optimal preoxygenation before the procedure begins and should have passive oxygenation throughout the procedure. Raising the head of the bed 30 degrees during ventilation helps with oxygenation, and any patient requiring ventilatory support or being prepared for airway management should have head elevation. Even a trauma patient on a backboard can be placed in reverse Trendelenburg position. Physiologically, head elevation lowers the gastric bubble below the cardiac sphincter, increases FRC, improves dynamic compliance by removing weight from the chest, and increases lung volumes – almost 50% of lung volume is lost when the patient is laid flat.[8,9,11] Raising the head of the bed can also decrease the time to reoxygenation if a patient desaturates during an airway procedure.

With the patient's head elevated, apply high-flow oxygen through a tight-fitting face mask with high-flow oxygen to maximize the oxygen saturation, partial pressure of oxygen, and exchange nitrogen in the residual capacity of the lungs for oxygen. In light of this, preoxygenation should get the SpO_2 as close to 100% as possible and ideally persists for at least 3 minutes. Remember that it is possible to preoxygenate many patients who have reduced ventilation if there is effective tidaling, and positive-pressure ventilation (PPV) may not be required.[8,11]

For patients whose oxygen saturation cannot be raised above 93% with supplemental oxygen, consider using positive pressure through a continuous positive airway pressure (CPAP) or bilevel positive airway pressure (BiPAP) device or with a bag-valve device. If positive pressure is used, there should be at least 5 cm H_2O of positive end-expiratory pressure (PEEP) in the system for any positive-pressure device.[8,11] Some experts suggest using a "delayed-sequence" intubation technique, in which sedation improves the ability to use positive pressure to improve saturation before an airway procedure. In planning such an approach, pay attention to the patient's protective airway reflexes; inadequate airway protection indicates invasive airway management and a contraindication to noninvasive ventilation.[8,11,12]

At the start of the invasive airway procedure, begin passive oxygenation. This technique, first described more than 50 years ago and well known to critical care practitioners in conjunction with brain death examinations, capitalizes on the ability of hemoglobin to take up oxygen by diffusion. Even without lung expansion, oxygen diffuses into the blood at least 12 times as fast as carbon dioxide accumulates in the alveoli. Extension of this concept to emergency intubation can prolong the duration of safe hypoventilation without desaturation. The requirements for oxygen uptake are a patient airway for oxygen delivery and a high oxygen concentration gradient. For emergency intubation, the easiest method is to place a nasal cannula on patients during their preparation for intubation and to begin 15 L/min of oxygen flow through the cannula as the patient becomes obtunded.[11]

Hypotension

Approximately 25% of patients develop transient hypotension after emergent intubation and transition to PPV.[13–15] Sedative and anxiolytic medications, as well as many induction agents, have vasodilatory and negative inotropic qualities, and the conversion from negative pressure (spontaneous) to PPV changes preload and afterload.

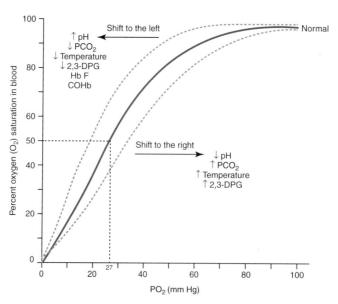

• **Figure 12.2** Oxyhemoglobin dissociation curves: Normal and shifted. (From Schick L, Windle P. *PeriAnesthesia Nursing Core Curriculum: Preprocedure, Phase I and Phase II PACU Nursing.* 3rd ed. Saunders; 2016.)

Patients should be evaluated for current hemodynamic stability and their risk for postprocedure deterioration. Patient age, low systolic blood pressure, lower pulse oximetry value, and elevated shock index are associated with peri-intubation cardiovascular decline.[13,14,16,17] An identified inflection point in the prehospital setting has been evaluated; multiple studies indicate the use of shock index (HR/SBP) greater than 0.9 or the overlap of $EtCO_2$ of 24 mm Hg or below and a systolic blood pressure less than 80 mm Hg.[18]

Conceivably, if the patient has a tenuous blood pressure or cardiac function, it makes sense to have a vasopressor, either as an infusion or in the form of a temporizing "push-dose pressor" available, or volume resuscitation prepared, to help stabilize a patient with these issues. Interestingly, preprocedure volume and vasopressor use has not been shown to eliminate the risk of cardiovascular decline during and immediately after emergent intubation.[13,15,19]

In a practice extrapolating from the operating room (OR), in which most induction agents and vapor anesthetics are vasodilators, some nonanesthesia providers will use so-called push-dose pressors to temporarily stabilize hemodynamics in the peri-intubation patient. There is little doubt that small IV doses of epinephrine, vasopressin, and phenylephrine will most often improve blood pressure, both through vasoconstriction and, for epinephrine, by increasing heart rate and contractility.[20-22] In the transport environment, at least 79% of patients had reversal of hypotension and nearly all had an increase in systolic blood pressure after push-dose administration of either vasopressin or phenylephrine. There was little rebound hypotension.[23]

The practice is well discussed in popular literature, but practice appears to be nonstandardized.[24] The individualized approach, unfamiliar dilutions and doses, and need for providers to dilute the agents themselves create some patient safety risks. Nontrivial rates of both adverse hemodynamic responses and medication errors, up to 100-fold, are reported.[25,26] Teams considering the use of push-dose pressors need to build systems to protect against these risks. Bolus doses of infusion agents are no substitute for adequate preprocedure preparation or for the appropriate use of continuous infusion vasopressor agents.

The most common medications considered for push dose pressors are epinephrine, phenylephrine, and vasopressin. Epinephrine is a potent agonist of alpha-, beta$_1$-, and beta$_2$-adrenergic receptors, which increases inotropy, chronotropy, and mean arterial pressure.[27] The common dose is 10 to 20 µg given every 2 minutes until the desired effect is achieved. Onset is approximately 1 minute, with a duration between 5 and 10 minutes. Adverse events include hypertension, tachydysrhythmias, and increased myocardial oxygen use. Phenylephrine is a pure vasoconstrictor, a strong alpha agonist that allows for an increase of systematic vascular resistance and is noted to be a vasopressor of choice when attempting to raise the mean arterial pressure with a patient with a high cardiac output. Administration of phenylephrine is usually given at 100 to 200 µg, repeated in two minutes, if needed. Adverse events include hypertension, bradycardia, and extravasation risk. For patients with either left or right ventricular dysfunction, an increase in vascular resistance without inotropic support can further reduce cardiac output. Vasopressin is an antidiuretic hormone vasoconstrictor targeting the vasopressin V1 and V2 receptors. It may be particularly beneficial in patients with hemorrhagic or septic shock, as it can directly affect the smooth muscle tone. Vasopressin is usually given at 0.2 to 2 units every 2 to 5 minutes.

Severe Metabolic Acidosis

One of the physiologic compensatory mechanisms for patients with severe metabolic acidosis is hyperventilation. Accordingly, the period of hypoventilation associated with medication-assisted intubation can disrupt that compensatory effort, as can careless postprocedure ventilator management. In these patients, it may be reasonable to avoid intubation, if possible, or to intubate the patient while maintaining spontaneous respiration. Once the patient is intubated, postprocedure management must include a minute ventilation that matches the preintubation ventilation volume.[8]

Intervention

Basic Life Support Airway Interventions

In patients with a history of trauma, all airway interventions must be performed with consideration of the cervical spine. The airway should be opened, all blood or emesis suctioned, and foreign bodies removed. The need for ready access to a working suction machine throughout transport cannot be overemphasized. The tongue may be displaced from the oropharynx through the placement of an airway adjunct, or the use of a modified jaw thrust. If the patient's mandible is not intact, the tongue can be protracted directly.

The addition of a simple mechanical adjunct can maintain the patient's airway. When properly positioned, both oral and nasal airways rest in the lower posterior pharynx and can improve the effectiveness of mask ventilation or free the provider to perform other activities. The appropriate size for an oral airway (OPA) is obtained by measuring the level of the teeth to the angle of the jaw. The proper-sized nasal airway (NPA) is obtained by measuring from the tip of the nose to the tip of the earlobe (Figs. 12.3 and 12.4).

In patients with intact airway reflexes, placement of either device may precipitate vomiting, gagging, or laryngospasm. An incorrectly placed oropharyngeal airway may worsen airflow or create an airway obstruction where none existed that is created by the tongue being pushed posteriorly against the pharyngeal wall or the epiglottis being pushed against the laryngeal opening.

Nasopharyngeal airways may be used in patients with marginal stupor or coma who need assistance in maintaining an open airway and cannot tolerate an OPA, but it should be avoided for any patient with suspected head or facial trauma.[28] Selection of the appropriate size of the NPA is important because traumatic insertion may cause severe epistaxis or adenoid bleeding, especially in children. Lubricant use facilitates insertion, and the airway is initially placed with the beveled edge along the nasal septum. When the left nostril is used, the nasopharyngeal airway must be inserted upside down to maintain the beveled edge against the septum and then rotated once the airway tip is in the posterior pharynx. If significant resistance is met, the other nostril should be tried. In a nonfacial trauma patient, the tip of the nose can be lifted to allow for direct passage of the nasopharyngeal airway.

The proper position for both adjuncts must be confirmed with airflow assessment and ventilation efficacy. Breath sounds must be assessed after placement to ensure airway patency has not been compromised; likewise, a head position must be optimized to ensure obstruction has not occurred. Where indicated, the cervical spine must be protected.

For patients with hypoxia, provide supplemental oxygen to achieve saturations above 93%. Good BVM skills are essential for the transport professional. Ventilatory assistance is indicated for patients with apnea, severe hypoventilation, or patients needing

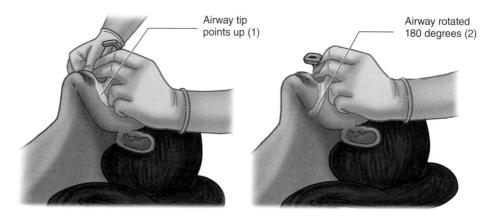

Airway tip points up (1)

Airway rotated 180 degrees (2)

• **Figure 12.3** Insertion of oropharyngeal airway. (From Lynn-McHail D, Carlson K, eds. *AACN Procedure Manual for Critical Care*. 4th ed. Saunders; 2001.)

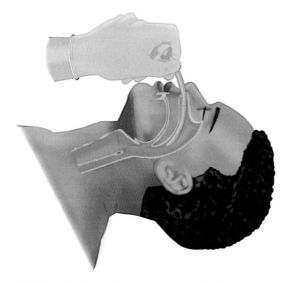

• **Figure 12.4** Correct placement of nasopharyngeal airway. (From Proehl J. *Emergency Nursing Procedures*. 4th ed. Saunders; 2009.)

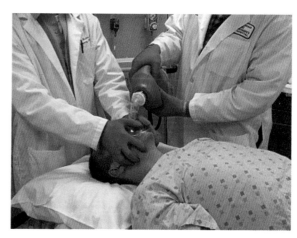

• **Figure 12.5** The two-hand thenar eminence technique of bag-mask ventilation. (From Reardon RF, Mason PE, Clinton JE. *Clinical Procedures in Emergency Medicine*. Elsevier; 2010.)

positive pressure to improve saturation. Delivered tidal volumes vary with bag type, hand size, and patient body characteristics; the transport team must evaluate the effectiveness of BVM ventilations. Optimal technique includes an oxygen flow rate of at least 15 L per minute, PEEP of at least 5 cm H_2O, an oropharyngeal airway, and a two-person technique: one clinician creates a two-handed mask seal with a head-tilt and chin-lift maneuver, while the other provides ventilation of at ten breaths per minute with the smallest volume required to generate a visible chest rise.[29] The thenar eminence technique, achieved by placing the thenar eminence of the hand on the mask, wrapping the mask on the face, and placing the fingers under the prominent line of the jaw and avoiding the submandibular soft tissues, may be helpful (see Fig. 12.5).[30]

Again, raising the head of the bed 30 degrees during ventilation helps with oxygenation and ventilation. Any patient requiring ventilatory support or being prepared for airway management should have head elevation. An integrated pressure manometer can also help with safe ventilation. Pulse oximetry should be available to aid in oxygen desaturation detection, and if end-tidal CO_2 capnography is available, a regular waveform with exhalation should be noted.

The ROMAN mnemonic described earlier identifies patients at risk of being difficult to ventilate with a BVM device. Additionally, in edentulous patients, leaving the teeth in place to give the cheeks structure and removing them just before intubation often aids ventilation. After BVM ventilation is begun in a patient with the head elevated and an oral or nasal airway in place, evaluate for effective chest rise. If there is no effective chest rise, or if there is persistent or new desaturation, the mnemonic MR. SOPA describes interventions to improve the effectiveness of mask ventilation:

M: Mask is tightly applied to the face
R: Reposition the head into the "sniffing" position
S: Suction the nares and the pharynx
O: Open the mouth
P: Pressure of PPV can be increased to a maximum of 40 cm H_2O
A: Alternate airway plan and consideration[31]

Advanced Airway Management Techniques

Although intubation is a life-saving procedure, it is not without the potential for the development of serious complications. These include physical and physiologic adverse events; soft tissue injuries to the mouth, dental injury, vocal cord injury, tracheal injury, endotracheal tube (ETT) misplacement, aspiration, pneumothorax, cardiac dysrhythmias, vital sign deterioration, and hypoxia.

Complications can also occur with the use of neuromuscular blocking agents (NMBAs), anxiolytics, and sedative-hypnotics that are used to facilitate intubation.[32,33]

Using a checklist in high-stakes operations is a well-proven strategy to improve safety. In medicine, checklists have improved safety and reduced complications for various procedures in various settings.[34,35] The risk of an intubation-related complication for patients intubated in the emergency department (ED) is approximately 12%.[36] Particularly in the emergency and transport environments, where ad hoc teams come together at critical times, using a preintubation checklist to aid in team and equipment preparation is intuitively a best practice. In the limited literature, using a checklist improved preparation and reduced patient complications by up to 84% without increasing preparation time or time to intubation.[37,38]

Developing a checklist is a complex venture and will likely need to be individualized for each practice group.[39,40] Generally, factors related to preparing primary and backup equipment, primary and backup medication and procedure plans, preparing the patient physiologically, reviewing team roles, and reviewing critical decision points should be included.

Tracheal Intubation

Anatomy

Intubation of the trachea is considered the gold standard for artificial airway support, providing protection against aspiration, allowing for controlled ventilation, and offering a method of emergency drug administration. In addition, intubation protects the airway in situations of potential upper airway closure from the progression of processes such as epiglottitis, airway burns, soft tissue trauma, or infections. Orotracheal intubation is the most common method of invasive airway management for all age groups. The procedure requires finesse and psychomotor skills.

Few, if any, true contraindications to orotracheal intubation exist in the emergency setting. However, circumstances that create challenges to effective mask ventilation are relative contraindications. Similarly, conditions that will make a surgical airway difficult should give the transport team pause before inducing hypoventilation or apnea in a patient for intubation.

Endotracheal intubation is generally successful, with variability linked to context. The incidence of failed intubation is about 1 per 2000 in elective surgery, 1 per 300 in obstetric anesthesia, and under 1 per 100 in the ED.[36,41] The Ground Air Medical Quality Transport Quality Improvement Collaboration collects information specific to critical care transport and reports intubation, ventilation, and airway management performance data.[42]

The ability to perform advanced airway maneuvers begins with knowledge of normal anatomy. Endotracheal intubation entails manipulating the anatomy to allow the passage of an ETT through the larynx. Understanding the relationship between the cartilage of the larynx and its relative position helps with faster and more confident intubation. This knowledge is especially important when structures are only partially visible or displaced due to injury. Familiarity with the anatomic differences between the adult and pediatric airway is also helpful.

The larynx, or voice box, is an intricate arrangement of nine cartilages, three single and six paired, connected by membranes and ligaments and moved by nine muscles. From above, it attaches to the hyoid bone and opens into the laryngopharynx, and on the inside, it is continuous with the trachea. In an adult, it extends from the level of the fourth to the sixth cervical vertebrae.

The three single cartilages – the epiglottis, the thyroid cartilage, and the cricoid cartilage, form the basic boxlike structure of the larynx and provide the major external landmarks. The epiglottis, a spoon-shaped structure that lies directly over the glottic opening, prevents anything other than air from entering the tracheal inlet. The epiglottis is the primary visual landmark for performing tracheal intubation (Figs. 12.6–12.8).

The thyroid cartilage, commonly known as the Adam's apple, is formed by the fusion of two curving cartilage plates and is typically more prominent in men than in women because of the growth-stimulating influence of male sex hormones during puberty. The ring-shaped cricoid cartilage is sandwiched between the thyroid cartilage above the first tracheal ring and connected to the thyroid cartilage by the cricothyroid membrane. That membrane is the desired location for a cricothyrotomy.

The upper free edge of the cricothyroid membrane forms the vocal cords. Because of the attachment of the vocal cords to the cricoid ring and the cricoid ring to the thyroid cartilage, external laryngeal manipulation (ELM) may help bring the vocal cords into view during intubation. The Sellick maneuver (posterior pressure on the cricoid cartilage designed to occlude the esophagus and prevent aspiration) is a part of medical history. Sellick's original study was a nonrandomized case series of head-down patients.[43] There is no evidence clearly demonstrating a benefit or a harm in the routine use of cricoid pressure to prevent regurgitation or aspiration.[44,45]

The most important paired cartilages of the larynx are the arytenoids. They are pyramid shaped and anchor the vocal cords in the larynx. The remaining two pairs of cartilages, the cuneiform and corniculate, form the posterior wall of the larynx. Committing these structures to memory assists the laryngoscopist in quickly identifying the glottic opening; when the opening is obscured from view, the ETT can be steered into position with the structures in view as reference points.

The vocal cords look pearly white because of their avascular nature but, over time, could lose color and become grey or even black depending on environmental exposure. At rest, the vocal cords lie partially separated or abducted. Excessive secretions or aspiration stimulate the airway and activate the defense reflexes. Laryngospasm, or spasmodic closure of the vocal cords, is the most severe form of airway closure and can totally prevent ventilation and the passage of an ETT. If a tube is forced through the cords with excessive pressure, an arytenoid can be dislocated, and permanent hoarseness can result.

Cormack and Lehane quantified the ability to visualize the glottic opening during laryngoscopy (Fig. 12.9). In the Cormack-Lehane scale, grade I is the visualization of the entire glottic opening, grade II is just the arytenoids cartilages or posterior glottic opening, grade III is only the epiglottis, and only the tongue is visible in grade IV. Grade I and II views are associated with high intubation success rates, and grade III and IV views are linked with lower success rates. Other operators simply describe the percent of glottic opening that is visible during the laryngoscopy.[3]

Potential Complications

Complications of oral and nasal endotracheal intubation can be both significant and disastrous (Box 12.1). The need for first-pass success is imperative because the incidence of airway and hemodynamic adverse events correlates with the number of intubation attempts. Even a second attempt at intubation can increase the complication rate close to 47%, and the rate rises to 63% with a third attempt.[32,33,46] It is interesting that self-reported rates of

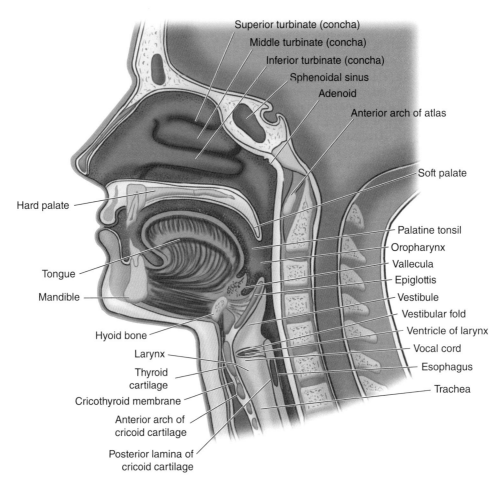

- **Figure 12.6** Sagittal view of airway. (From Rosen P, Ron M. Walls, Robert S. Hockberger et al. *Emergency Medicine: Concepts and Clinical Practice,* vol 1. 2nd ed. Mosby; 1988.)

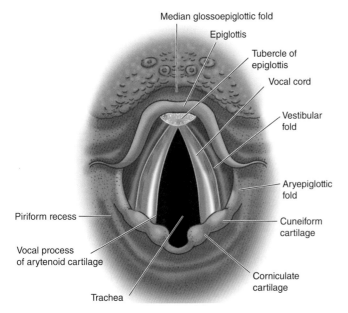

- **Figure 12.7** Laryngoscopic view of airway. (From Rosen P, et al. *Emergency Medicine: Concepts and Clinical Practice,* vol 1. 2nd ed. Mosby; 1988.)

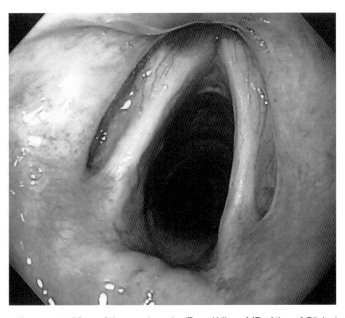

- **Figure 12.8** View of the vocal cords. (From Wilcox MD. *Atlas of Clinical Gastrointestinal Endoscopy.* 3rd ed. Saunders; 2012.)

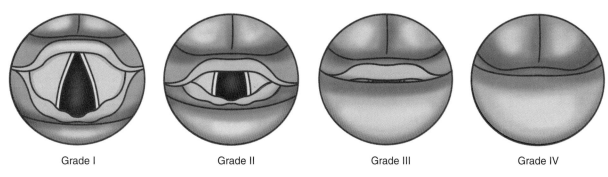

Grade I   Grade II   Grade III   Grade IV

• **Figure 12.9** Cormack Lehane grades. (From Miller RD, Pardo M. *Basics of Anesthesia*. 6th ed. Saunders; 2012.)

Early Complications That Occur During the Intubation Procedure

1. Neck
Cervical strain: subluxation/dislocation, fracture, and neurologic injury

2. Mouth
Soft tissue injury that results in abrasion and hemorrhage involving lips, tongue, buccal mucosa, and pharynx
Temporomandibular joint subluxation/dislocation
Dental injury

3. Airway/respiratory
Arytenoid: dislocation and avulsion
Vocal cord: spasm, avulsion, and laceration
Pyriform sinus perforation that results in pneumothorax and pneumomediastinum
Tracheal and bronchial rupture
Right mainstem bronchus intubation, with atelectasis and respiratory compromise
Bronchospasm

4. Gastrointestinal
Esophageal: intubation and perforation
Vomiting and aspiration

5. Cardiovascular
Hypertension, tachycardia, bradycardia, and dysrhythmias
Cardiac arrest and interruption of CPR

Late Complications That Occur After Tube Is in Place

1. Airway/respiratory
Tube obstruction: secretions, blood, and kinking
Accidental extubation and endobronchial intubation
Vocal cords: ulceration
Trachea: ulceration, ischemic necrosis, and paralysis
Pneumothorax and pneumomediastinum
Aspiration and atelectasis
Cough that results in increased intrathoracic, intracranial, and intraocular pressures

2. Gastrointestinal
Esophageal intubation
Tracheoesophageal fistula

3. Cardiovascular
Tracheoinnominate artery fistula

4. Infections
Sinusitis, pneumonia, tracheobronchitis, mediastinitis, and abscess

5. Tube dislodgment

---

airway management complications underreport those confirmed by direct observation of the procedure.[47]

Trauma to the teeth, soft tissues of the mouth, posterior pharynx, or vocal cords caused by improper use of the laryngoscope blade or by forcing an ETT is a complication of oral intubation. Unrecognized right mainstem bronchus intubation is a complication that may lead to inadequate ventilation and left lung atelectasis.

Unsuccessful intubation or a missed inadvertent esophageal intubation may lead to prolonged hypoxia, hypotension, or cardiac arrest and result in long-term injury or death. Oxygenation must be maintained throughout airway management attempts, and other means of oxygenation and ventilation must be used if a patient cannot be intubated.

Intubation predisposes the patient to several harmful physiologic responses, including laryngospasm, bronchospasm caused by airway irritability or aspirated secretions, hypertension, and dysrhythmias unrelated to hypoxia. The stimuli of DL and endotracheal intubation produce a sympathetic response that increases mean arterial pressure above baseline by up to 44%, heart rate by up to 36%, and intracranial pressure (ICP) by up to 22 mm Hg.[48,49]

The safety of inline immobilization of the trauma patient's cervical spine with a gentle laryngoscopy is well established. Once the patient has adequately become obtunded, have an assistant hold the cervical spine and remove the anterior part of the C-collar during the intubation attempt to maintain spinal motion restriction while still allowing the mandible to be displaced anteriorly, facilitating mouth opening and a satisfactory glottic view. Upon completion of the intubation, replacing the anterior part of the collar is necessary to maintain the correct position.

The ETT cuff pressure should be measured. Although no ideal pressure has been defined, most recommendations are between 20 and 30 cm H_2O. High cuff pressures can cause complications, including tracheal ischemia and fistula formation, and mucosal damage can begin to occur within 14 minutes.[50,51]

Direct Laryngoscopy

When using DL, a direct line of sight is used to perform the intubation. Laryngoscope blades come in curved shapes, such as the MacIntosh, or straight shapes, such as the Miller, Phillips, or Wisconsin. Generally speaking, the wide flange of the curved blade aids in controlling the tongue, considered the primary obstacle to intubation, better than the straight blade. The ability of the flanged curved blade to control the tongue also leaves more room on the right side of the mouth to manipulate the endotracheal blade into place. In addition, the curved blade follows the natural curvature of the anatomy better than the straight blade, which often must be inserted in a stepwise fashion of lifting, relaxing, and advancing.

The straight blade, although more difficult for control of the tongue, has an advantage in viewing the glottic opening of patients who are considered to have an anteriorly positioned larynx. Such is the case in pediatric patients, patients with receding chins, and patients with short, muscular necks. In these patients, the larynx is located more forward, and curved blades often do not provide an adequate view. If the laryngoscopist secures a good view of the cords with a straight blade, but without totally maintaining the tongue to the left of the blade, the tongue may lap over the blade and prevent manipulation of the tube through the cords.

The curved tip of the MacIntosh is inserted into the vallecula, the space between the base of the tongue and the pharyngeal surface of the epiglottis. The tip of the blade must be inserted to engage the hypoepiglottic ligament, then it is possible to indirectly open the epiglottis to expose the larynx (Fig. 12.10). The straight Miller blade is passed so that the tip lies beneath the laryngeal surface of the epiglottis. The epiglottis is then directly lifted to expose the vocal cords (Fig. 12.11). Steps for orotracheal intubation are included in Box 12.2.

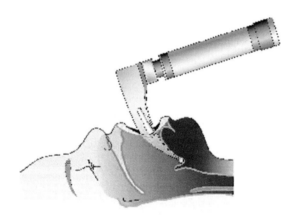

• **Figure 12.10** Use of a curved laryngoscope blade. (From Donoghue AJ, Walls RM. *Pediatric Emergency Medicine.* Elsevier; 2008.)

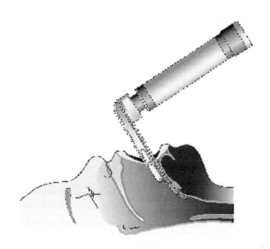

• **Figure 12.11** Use of a straight laryngoscope blade. (From Donoghue AJ, Walls RM. *Pediatric Emergency Medicine.* Elsevier; 2008.)

• BOX 12.2 Steps for Orotracheal Intubation

1. Position the patient. Nontrauma patient: Flex the neck forward and extend the head backward, creating a sniffing position. Trauma patient: Maintain in-line traction.
2. Preoxygenate the patient.
3. Hold the laryngoscope in the left hand and open the patient's mouth with the right hand.
4. Insert the blade into the right side of the mouth, sweep the tongue to the left, and advance to the appropriate landmarks. The Miller (straight) blade tip goes beyond the epiglottis; the MacIntosh (curved) blade tip enters the vallecula.
5. Pull the laryngoscope blade at a 45-degree angle; avoid twisting the laryngoscope handle. Visualize the epiglottis and vocal cords. Apply cricoid pressure.
6. Insert the ETT from the right corner of the mouth and watch the tube pass through the vocal cords. Use the largest tube possible. Remove the stylette.
7. Inflate the tube cuff with 5 to 10 mL of air or to minimal occluding volume. (Minimal occluding volume is determined by placing the hand over the mouth and noting cessation of air leak with ventilation.) Capillary flow pressure in the tracheal mucosa is approximately 25 mm Hg, so cuff pressure should be less than that.
8. Confirm tube placement.
9. Secure the tube in place.

When the laryngoscopist uses a hand to improve laryngeal visualization, the method is also called ELM. ELM from an assistant or with the laryngoscopist's free right hand may also assist the intubator in visualizing the laryngeal inlet. Use caution with pressure directed posteriorly because too much cricoid pressure may worsen the laryngeal view and reduce airway patency.[52]

MacIntosh, the British anesthesiologist who developed the MacIntosh laryngoscope blade, is credited with developing the *endotracheal tube introducer* (ETI) in the 1940s. The ETI is 60 cm long and is curved 35 degrees at the end. The tip permits it to be steered behind the epiglottis and into the glottic opening, even when only the posterior arytenoids or the epiglottis are visualized during the intubation attempt.

To use the introducer, often referred to as a "bougie," perform laryngoscopy in the usual manner. Hold the ETI in the right hand and advance it toward the epiglottis, or where the cords are presumed. As the introducer goes blindly down the trachea, the laryngoscopist receives confirmation by way of feeling "clicks" as the curved tip of the introducer slides over the tracheal rings or "holdup" where the introducer reaches the carina or the right or left mainstem bronchus and cannot be further advanced. If a holdup is noted, which may or may not be accompanied by clicks, it is nearly 100% confirmation that the introducer is in the trachea. Clicks are confirmed in 90% of tracheal intubations with the ETI. Holdup may possibly occur in a patient with esophageal stenosis with a false-positive result or with cricoid pressure. If the introducer is advanced without clicks or holdup, it has likely gone down the esophagus. This route is confirmed when the laryngoscopist realizes that the entire introducer has been inserted with only a few centimeters left in the hand. In this situation, pull back on the introducer until the curved tip is seen again and redirect it.

Once the intubation specialist is confident the ETI has entered the trachea, with positive holdup, click, or both signs, an assistant places an ETT over the introducer. The intubation specialist then advances the tube, similar to the Seldinger technique, over the introducer while holding the laryngoscope in the left hand. Maintaining the laryngoscope in place facilitates sliding the tube over the introducer. The assistant can stabilize the introducer by holding the free end above the ETT as the intubation specialist advances it.

At times, the ETT may resist passing through the cords. If this should occur, back the tube out slightly and rotate the tube 90 degrees to the left (the Murphy eye is now in the upright position), and then advance. If this maneuver is unsuccessful, rotate the tube to the right 90 degrees and advance. In rare situations, the tube may need to be rotated 180 degrees to pass through the cords. Once the ETT passes through the cords, remove the introducer and confirm placement in the usual manner.

Video-Assisted Intubation

With the advancement of video-assisted laryngoscopy, the need for direct visualization is assisted with using a video-transmitting device on the tip of the laryngoscope blade. Using a hybrid videoscopic intubation device with both video and DL is the best practice in advanced airway management. The video transmits an image to a monitor via a camera element located on the laryngoscope blade. The views obtained with the video-assisted laryngoscope can be enhanced via magnification and wide-angle view. The improvement in the ability to visualize the airway is due to both the placement of the video camera and the angulation of the laryngoscope blade.[53]

Video devices often have blades with increased angulation, from traditional MacIntosh curvature to hyperangulated blades with a 60-degree angulation. Hyperangulated blades look around the curvature of the tongue very effectively and can facilitate procedure success when the anatomy is "anterior." However, their perspective (looking upward at the glottic opening from the base of the tongue) can lead to difficulty in tube delivery. If the blade is inserted too deeply, the video-imaging element gets very close to the larynx. In this instance, the view will be great, but the extreme angle of approach will create difficulty passing the tube because of the angle, the shortened delivery area, and the decreased field of view on the screen. Additionally, operators must be careful to look in the mouth while inserting an ETT on a hyperangulated stylette to avoid injury to the soft palate, tonsils, or hypopharynx.[54]

Reported advantages over DL include a better view of the larynx with no need for head extension in patients with limited cervical spine motion, improved ability to visualize the larynx when anatomic disruption is present, and a faster learning curve for inexperienced intubators.[55,56]

The mnemonic HEAVEN can help illuminate the choice between video and DL:

H: Hypoxemia. DL is faster, although video laryngoscopy (VL) may be easier with anatomic difficulty.

E: Extremes of size. VL (out to in) uses a slow, controlled advancement toward the epiglottis. DL (in to out) advances into the airway with the slow removal of the laryngoscope blade until the airway comes into sight. In pediatrics, a straight blade will lead to increased success.

A: Anatomic disruption/obstruction. The process is VL out to in and DL in to out.

V: Vomited blood or fluid in the airway. Use DL if bloody or uncontrollable vomiting.

E: Exsanguination. DL is faster but use VL with anatomic difficulty.

N: Neck mobility. VL is gentler.[57]

The approach to the airway with an indirect tool is slightly different than with DL. The patient should be in a supine, neutral position, compared with the classic sniffing position. Malposition, along with a small mouth opening, are known predictors of difficult VL.[58] Follow the curvature of the specific blade when forming the ETT and stylette. The blade is inserted to the midline or slightly to the left of midline, rather than along the right side. Once an attempt is started slowly, walk the blade down the tongue until exposure of the uvula, then lift to expose the epiglottis. Once the epiglottis is found, position the device, and obtain a glottis view. A Cormack-Lehane grade II view might be more successful than a grade I because it allows the camera to work in a further recessed manner, allowing more room for manipulation of the ETT to pass through the cords. Once the tube is at the entry to the vocal cords, continue to advance the tube through the cords while a partner removes the stylette.

In reality, the distinction between VL and DL is not as concrete. Video-assisted devices permit, and are often used, with a "crossover" technique, in which the operator can use the same tool for either direct or video-assisted laryngoscopy.[53]

Extraglottic Devices

The category of extraglottic covers a spectrum of devices separated into two subclasses: supraglottic devices and retroglottic devices. Extraglottic devices were traditionally thought to be used as "rescue" or "backup devices"; however, they are used as primary or temporizing devices in proper situations, particularly when preprocedural airway assessment suggests that the use of a traditional device might be difficult. Uses for extraglottic devices can be summarized as follows:

- An airway rescue device when intubation has failed.
- A "single-attempt" rescue device performed simultaneously with preparation for cricothyrotomy in the "*can't* intubate, *can't* oxygenate" failed airway.
- An easier and more effective alternative to BVM in the hands of basic life support providers or nonmedical rescue personnel.
- An alternative to endotracheal intubation by advanced life support providers.
- An alternative to endotracheal intubation for elective airway management in the OR for appropriately selected patients.
- A conduit to facilitate endotracheal intubation, such as an intubating laryngeal mask airway (LMA).[3,59]

Two concerns with extraglottic devices are compression of the carotid artery with impaired cerebral blood flow and the stability of the device. There is some disagreement in the literature about whether extraglottic devices impair carotid blood flow in patients, either in cardiac arrest or at all.[60,61] The Combitube is the airway appliance that is most difficult to dislodge, and other common supraglottic devices, the LMA and King airway are removed with force similar to an ETT.[62]

Supraglottic Airway Devices

Supraglottic devices surround the area around and above the glottis. Examples of supraglottic devices are LMAs, or the I-gel.

Laryngeal Mask Airway

The first-generation LMA was developed by the British anesthesiologist Archie Brain and introduced in 1988. The device comes in appropriate sizes for all patients, including neonates to large adults, and LMAs reliably provide rescue ventilation in cases when difficult airways are encountered. The LMA consists of an airway tube, a mask, and a mask inflation tube. It provides ventilation by forming a seal over the larynx above the cords. The tip of the LMA rests in the esophagus, and there are two rubber bars that cross the tube opening at the mask end to prevent herniation of the epiglottis into the LMA tube. Sizing is based on patient weight. Insertion of the LMA is shown in Fig. 12.12. Typical first-time insertion success rates range between 90% and 95%, with insertion times between 30 and 50 seconds.[63]

The LMA is also available in several variations, including versions with the addition of a port to allow for gastric decompression, with a more rigid shape to facilitate insertion, and with an improved seal pressure up to 40 cm H_2O. The intubating LMA allows for ventilation while providing a conduit for blind passage of a specially designed ETT for intubation.

A classic concern about the LMA is that it does not offer a definitive defense against regurgitation and aspiration, leaving the airway less protected than one secured by a cuffed ETT. A meta-analysis of 547 published studies on the LMA, however, concluded that "(p)ulmonary aspiration with the LMA is uncommon and comparable to that for outpatient anesthesia with the face mask and tracheal tube."[64]

All air-filled devices, including cuffed ETTs and the cuffs of supraglottic devices, may expand at altitude, and pressures should be monitored with changes in altitude.

I-Gel

The I-gel is a newer supraglottic airway. Unlike previous devices, it does not use inflatable cuffs to achieve a seal of the esophagus and pharyngeal structures. The I-gel is produced from an entirely synthetic medical-grade thermoplastic, which gives it a gel-like feel and is anatomically designed to fit snugly into the perilaryngeal structures, essentially mirroring the supralaryngeal anatomy. Current available sizes allow use in patients who weigh between 2 and 100 kg. It is easily placed, with 98% success on one or two

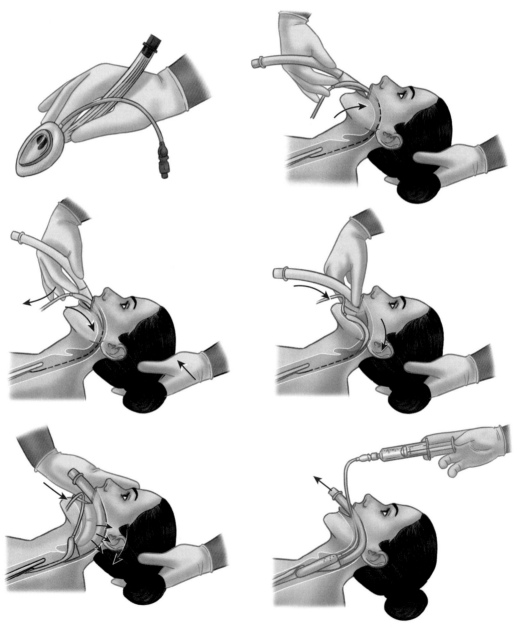

• **Figure 12.12** Insertion of laryngeal mask airway. (Courtesy of LMA North America, Inc.)

attempts, sustains a peak airway pressure of 30 mm Hg, and incorporates into its design a bite block and a gastric channel that allows for the passage of a gastric tube up to 14 French in size.[65]

Retroglottic Devices

Retroglottic, or esophageal tube, airways are blind-insertion devices designed with high-volume, low-pressure cuffs that occlude the esophagus and posterior oropharynx, directing PPVs through the esophagus. The pharyngeal balloon may also tamponade oral bleeding and prevent the aspiration of blood into the trachea. The oropharyngeal balloon does not prevent the aspiration of teeth or other oral debris, and the oropharyngeal balloon can migrate out of the mouth anteriorly, partially dislodging the airway. Retroglottic airways are contraindicated in patients who are awake and semi-obtunded. They cannot be used in patients with known esophageal injury or in situations of caustic ingestion.

Retroglottic devices can be used with blind insertion, but it is recommended to use a laryngoscope blade with insertion to help facilitate smooth insertion and prevent any folding of the distal tip of the device. If an esophageal tube airway is inserted and ventilation is not possible, then it is generally because the placement is too deep, and stepwise withdrawal of the device with attempted ventilation should result in successful ventilation.

For the King LT version, the device will sustain a peak pressure of 60 mm Hg, and pediatric sizes are available. Proper sizing is essential to successful use (Box 12.3).

Surgical Airway

In rare cases, it is necessary to use a percutaneous approach to secure the airway. The procedure is rare across the spectrum of emergency medical service, transport, and hospital care, but it has a high success rate.[66–68] A firm understanding of the anatomy of the neck is needed to facilitate success in these cases (Fig. 12.13).

Needle Cricothyrotomy

Needle cricothyrotomy involves the insertion of an over-the-needle cannula through the cricothyroid membrane into the trachea. Conceptually, the needle cricothyrotomy is quicker and easier to perform than a surgical cricothyrotomy and is an alternative technique for practitioners unable to perform a surgical cricothyrotomy. The procedure is performed infrequently, with reported success rates between 37% and 100% and some papers reporting significant complications.[66–69]

Steps for this procedure are included in Box 12.4. Using a kink-resistant catheter with a 10-gauge, 14-gauge, or 16-gauge

• BOX 12.3	King-LT Sizing Guide				
Size	**2**	**2.5**	**3**	**4**	**5**
Connector color	Green	Orange	Yellow	Red	Purple
Patient criteria	35–45 inches (90–115 cm) Or 12–25 kg	41–51 inches (105–130 cm) or 25–35 kg	4–5 feet (122–155 cm)	5–6 feet (155–180 cm)	Greater than 6 feet (>180 cm)

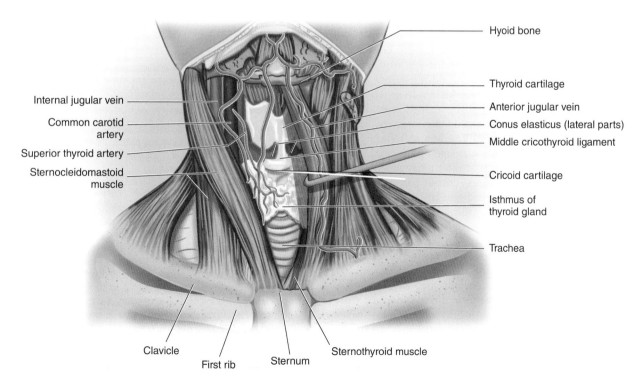

• **Figure 12.13** Anterior aspect of neck with relative anatomic structures. (From Rosen P, et al. *Emergency Medicine: Concepts and Clinical Practice*. Vol. 1. 2nd ed. Mosby; 1988.)

1. Stabilize the patient's head in a neutral position.
2. Identify the cricothyroid membrane and prepare the skin.
3. Stabilize the cricoid and thyroid cartilages with the nondominant hand.
4. Insert a 12-gauge or 14-gauge over-the-needle intravenous catheter into the membrane at a 45-degree angle caudally (toward the feet). On passage into the trachea, the needle is removed, and the cannula is advanced caudally.
5. The hub of the needle is connected, preferably to a jet ventilator capable of delivering oxygen at a pressure of 50 psi. Otherwise, the connector is removed from a 3.0-mm ETT and attached to the intravenous catheter. It is then connected to a bag-valve-mask device. This method is temporary until other means of airway securement can be achieved.

cannula is recommended. The needle is removed, and the cannula is left in place. Commercially available cannulas are designed with side holes in addition to the distal port and incorporate a flange that aids the securement of the catheter. The additional holes decrease pressure-related mucosal damage.

Use in adults has become mostly obsolete with the advancement of retroglottic devices as well as surgical airway approaches. However, when a surgical cricothyrotomy is contraindicated (unable to palpate or identify landmarks), a needle cricothyrotomy can be performed. When used in pediatric patients, a pressure regulator set at a maximal pressure of 20 to 30 psi should be used to decrease the risk of barotrauma. This method of ventilation is known as *translaryngeal jet ventilation.* It provides emergency oxygenation and ventilation by passive recoil of the chest wall and exhalation by way of the upper airway. In situations in which complete upper airway obstruction is suspected, a needle cricothyrotomy does not allow for exhalation and barotrauma results. In such a situation, a cricothyrotomy is the airway of choice.[3]

The ventilatory rate should be from 12 to 20 breaths per minute (bpm) with an insufflation time of about 1 to 2 seconds. In young children under 5 years old, an alternative method to the use of the jet ventilator allows for the connector from a No. 3 ETT to be connected to the cannula, which is then connected to a resuscitation bag. This technique meets oxygen requirements. However, ventilation is minimal at best, and respiratory acidosis quickly results. The respiratory acidosis that results generally limits ventilation in this manner to approximately 30 minutes. The use of a resuscitation bag is at best a temporary measure, whereas jet ventilation is considered a true PPV technique.[3]

Regardless of the circumstances surrounding the need to perform a needle cricothyrotomy, it is at most a temporizing intervention. A definitive airway or surgical cricothyrotomy is needed to allow both proper oxygenation and ventilation.

Surgical Cricothyrotomy

Surgical cricothyroidotomy is performed when other forms of airway management have failed and the patient cannot be adequately ventilated and oxygenated with a bag and mask. The indication for surgical airway is the patient who cannot be ventilated or oxygenated by other means. Airway inaccessibility may be the result of trauma, which can cause abnormal anatomy or profuse bleeding, obscuring visualization of the glottic opening, or the result of a foreign body, mass lesion, or edema. There is no absolute contraindication because the alternative is hypoxic death. Relative contraindications include the inability to locate the correct landmarks, primary laryngeal injury, and coagulopathy. As a

surgical airway is a possibility with every airway management plan that includes suppressing spontaneous ventilation, such an approach should be planned with extreme caution in patients who have relative contraindications.

There are three variations of the surgical cricothyrotomy technique: classic surgical, Seldinger, and rapid four-step (Boxes 12.5–12.7). Generally, a vertical incision over the midline is recommended to minimize bleeding. If the incision is too small, identifying the structures is more difficult. The nondominant hand should be used to grasp and stabilize the larynx from the beginning of the skin incision until the airway is secured. This keeps structures in midline and in place. A 6.0-cuffed ETT or #4 Shiley tracheostomy tube is placed through the incision and into the trachea. The angle and rounded tip of the tracheostomy tube can make inserting that tube more difficult than a standard ETT.

1. Stabilize the patient's head in a neutral position.
2. Identify the cricothyroid membrane and prepare the skin.
3. Stabilize the cricoid and thyroid cartilages with the nondominant hand.
4. Make a vertical incision 5 to 7 cm through the skin.
5. Identify the cricoid membrane and insert the tracheal hook. Use the tracheal hook, now in the nondominant hand, to stabilize the thyroid. Apply upward traction (45-degree angle) on the inferior margin of the thyroid cartilage.
6. Use the tip of a No. 11 blade to create a horizontal incision through the cricoid membrane. Avoid insertion of the blade too deeply and injury of the posterior wall of the trachea or the esophagus.
7. Insert a Trousseau dilator and spread vertically to enlarge the diameter of the cricoid space. Mayo scissors may be used to help enlarge the space in the transverse direction.
8. Remove the tracheal hook.
9. Place a cuffed ETT or tracheostomy tube through the dilator.
10. Remove the dilator. Secure the tube and verify proper position in the usual manner.

1. **Palpation** (Fig. 12.14A). To perform the procedure, one should position oneself at the patient's left shoulder and palpate the cricoid membrane with the index finger of the left hand, allowing the thumb and middle finger to palpate and stabilize the trachea.
2. **Incision** (Fig. 12.14B). With the right hand, a No. 20 scalpel is used to make a horizontal incision into the inferior aspect of the cricothyroid membrane. The scalpel is pushed through the membrane at a 60-degree angle to create a 2.5-cm horizontal incision. The scalpel is *not* removed; it is held in place.
3. **Traction** (Fig. 12.14C). A tracheal hook is held perpendicular to the longitudinal axis of the patient. With the left hand, the tracheal hook is placed flush against the caudal surface of the scalpel blade and slid down along the trachea. The tip of the hook is rotated 90 degrees in the inferior direction, and ventral/caudal traction is applied to the superior margin of the cricoid cartilage. The scalpel is then removed, and traction is maintained on the trachea by placing the left hand on the patient's sternum.
4. **Intubation** (Fig. 12.14D). This step is similar to orotracheal intubation. A cuffed endotracheal tube or tracheostomy tube is placed with the right hand. Tube placement is confirmed, and the hook is removed. If an endotracheal tube is used, the beveled side initially should be facing cephalad during insertion to decrease advancement of the tube superior to the vocal cords.

1. Position the patient and identify appropriate landmarks.
2. Insert a small locator needle into the cricothyroid membrane. Aspirate air to confirm needle placement into the trachea.
3. Pass a soft-tipped wire through the needle and thread it into the trachea. Keep control of the wire at all times to prevent wire aspiration.
4. With a No. 11 blade, cut a small incision adjacent to the needle to facilitate passage of the airway device.
5. Place the airway tube with its internal dilator over the wire through the tissue into the trachea. If resistance is met, extend or deepen the skin incision. A gentle screwing motion may also facilitate passage.
6. Confirm tube placement.

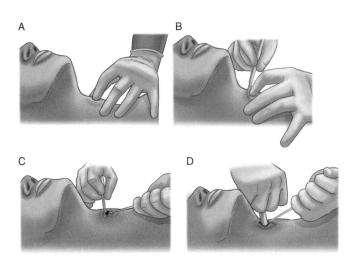

• **Figure 12.14** Four-step cricothyrotomy: **A.** Palpation. **B.** Incision. **C.** Traction. **D.** Intubation. (From Brofeldt BT, Osborn MI, Sakles JC, et al. Evaluation of the rapid four-step cricothyrotomy technique: An interim report. *Air Med J.* 1998;17(3):127.)

For the traditional open technique, a modification is to place a bougie or ETI in the trachea after the incision is made, assisting with securing the airway as well as preventing intubation of a false passage.[35] The rapid four-step cricothyrotomy technique, also known as scalpel finger bougie, was developed for use in the prehospital environment. This technique relies on palpation rather than direct visualization of the cricothyroid membrane, which decreases the need for suction and additional light (Fig. 12.14). Studies suggest the rapid four-step technique aids in establishing an airway quicker than the traditional technique but may be associated with a higher complication rate.

Circumstances in which identification of the anatomy of the surgical airway is difficult to represent a contraindication to inducing apnea for intubation. If the anatomy of the neck is distorted, the trachea can be identified with the slow advancement of a needle connected to a syringe through the skin and attempted aspiration of air. Once the air has been aspirated, signaling entrance into the trachea, the needle and syringe should be left in place, and the tissues cut down over the needle.

Pediatric Management

The pediatric airway differs from the adult until about the age of 8 years, when the larynx resembles that of the adult in structure and position. The most significant differences exist in the child who is 2 years or less, and patients between the years of 2 and 8 represent a transitional period.

An infant's head is much larger in proportion to the rest of the body, resulting in a natural sniffing position. As a result, neck flexion is not necessary to attain the sniffing position and bag-mask ventilations. In infants and some young children, the sniffing position is too pronounced, and the transport team provider may need to place a towel under the infant's shoulders to raise the rest of the body and straighten the airway, improving airflow.

The infant is also an obligate nose breather, and secretions or edema in this area can cause airway compromise more easily than in adults. Infants and small children have tongues that are large in relation to the size of the oropharynges, which makes the tongue, as it is in the adult, the most common cause of airway obstruction. The relatively small size of children's mouths also makes intubation more difficult. Because of the small size of the pediatric airway, minimal edema can create a life-threatening obstruction. An infant's airway, normally 4 mm in diameter, decreases to 2 mm with 1 mm of circumferential edema caused by secretions or trauma caused by intubation. In comparison, the adult airway, normally 8 mm in diameter, decreases to 6 mm with 1 mm of circumferential edema (Fig. 12.15). The result is only a 25% decrease in diameter in the adult compared with a 50% decrease in the infant with an equal amount of swelling.

The vocal cords of a young child are more pliable than those of an adult and are easier to damage, resulting in potential obstruction. The presence of hypertrophied tonsils and adenoid tissues can cause rapid development of upper airway obstruction and is a significant source of bleeding when traumatized. In addition, the larynx is situated higher in relation to the cervical spines than the adult. In the infant, the glottic opening is at C1; as the child ages,

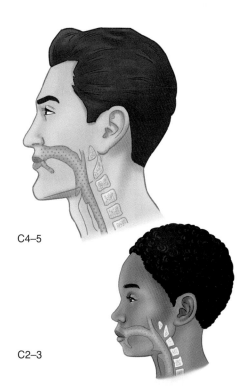

C4–5

C2–3

• **Figure 12.15** Comparative anatomy of adult and infant airways. (From Nichols DG, et al. eds. *Golden Hour: The Handbook of Advanced Pediatric Life Support.* 2nd ed. Mosby; 1996.)

the glottic opening moves down to the level of the adult at C4 to C5. The anterior position of the larynx in the infant and young child leads to more frequent intubations of the esophagus. In a situation where the laryngoscopist recognizes no landmarks, a likely indication is that the laryngoscope blade has been passed too far and needs to be withdrawn until structures are recognized.

The anatomic differences between the pediatric and adult airways are illustrated in Fig. 12.12 and can be summarized as follows:

1. A child's larynx lies more cephalad than an adult's larynx.
2. A child's epiglottis is at an angle of 45 degrees to the anterior pharyngeal wall, whereas an adult's larynx lies parallel to the base of the tongue.
3. A child's epiglottis is large, stiff, and U-shaped, whereas an adult's epiglottis is flattened and more flexible.
4. The larger tongue of infants and children and the position of the hyoid bone depress the epiglottis.
5. The cricoid ring is the narrowest portion of a child's airway.

In addition to the anatomic differences noted, the critical care transport team members must be aware of the physiologic differences between children and adults. Of critical importance is the recognition that infants and children experience oxygen desaturation much quicker than adults. This faster desaturation time after apnea results from the higher metabolic oxygen consumption rate compared with the adult. The infant and child's oxygen consumption rate is twice that of adults, and the FRC is significantly less.

Lungs can easily be overdistended, and barotrauma induced by overzealous PPV can develop. Ventilation should be limited to the amount of air needed to cause the chest to rise. Excessive volumes exacerbate gastric distention and increase the risk of pneumothorax. When possible, a self-inflating bag-valve ventilation system should be used optimally with a pop-off valve. Resuscitation bags are available for neonates (delivering volumes of 500–600 mL) and adults (delivering volumes of 1.0–1.5 L). An oxygen reservoir should be used to enhance the oxygen concentration. Initial respiratory rates for controlled ventilation should approximate normal spontaneous respiratory rates based on age.

The proper ETT size can be determined in several ways. An indispensable tool in assisting with and reducing medication dosing errors is using a colorimetric weight-based measuring device. The original variations were designed to assist in the estimation of weight in cases of pediatric trauma. Since then, information on equipment sizes and medications has been added, significantly reducing caregivers' anxiety who primarily treat adult patients.

Cuffed ETTs are a reasonable choice for infants and children, and may have the advantages of improved capnography accuracy, decreased need for tube changes, and improved pressure and tidal volume delivery. Because cuff pressure can cause mucosal damage, it is particularly important to measure ETT cuff pressure in pediatric patients.[70,71] Tube size can be estimated by age. For neonatal patients, the gestational age (in weeks) divided by 10 and rounded down defines the tube size. For older children, the size of an uncuffed ETT is estimated by (age in years/4) + 4, and a CUFFED tube size is estimated by the formula (age in years/4) + 3.5.[72] The use of length-based tools may improve equipment size estimation, and intubators should prepare tubes a half size larger and smaller than predicted when setting up their kit before the procedure.[70]

The ETT depth is estimated as three times the inside diameter of the tube size. This rule of thumb applies to premature infants and adults when the appropriately sized tube for the patient's age is in place.

A part of airway management for children is placing a gastric tube. A child's stomach is relatively larger than an adult's and may contain food and a significant amount of air. Children tend to swallow air when crying (aerophagia). If full, the stomach may impinge on the diaphragm and decrease vital capacity. If a postintubation chest radiograph is available, the tip of the ETT should be at the T2 to T3 vertebral level or at the level of the lower edge of the medial aspect of the clavicle.

Medication-Assisted Airway Management

Since the 1980s, the use of sedation and NMBAs to facilitate advanced airway management before and during transport has evolved. It is clear that using NMBAs facilitates improved success and patient safety in emergency airway situations.[33] There are two approaches available: rapid and delayed sequence intubation.

RSI of anesthesia was introduced for patients with a full stomach to protect the airway from potential aspiration of the gastric contents. The practice includes preoxygenation, administration of a predetermined induction drug dose, using NMBAs, and then tracheal intubation when relaxation has occurred. In the early 1980s, the technique of rapidly gaining control of the airway with the same drugs as in the OR became known as RSI when done in the ED. The practice is identical in both situations. While the classic performance of RSI avoids the use of positive pressure ventilation until the airway is controlled with an ETT, it is clear that properly performed mask ventilation can be interposed in the process, as needed, to prevent desaturation.[29]

Delayed sequence intubation is a "procedural sedation, where the procedure is preoxygenation," designed to permit activities that improve preoxygenation and subsequently extend the duration time of safe apnea. In contrast to RSI, the technique of delayed sequence intubation temporally separates the administration of the induction agent from the administration of the muscle relaxant to allow adequate preoxygenation, which the patient might not otherwise tolerate. When the desired level of preoxygenation is achieved, the muscle relaxant is given, and the procedure progresses.[11,12,73]

Premedications

The stimuli of laryngoscopy and endotracheal intubation produce a well-documented sympathetic response that increases mean arterial pressure, heart rate, and ICP. This sympathetic response may be particularly detrimental to patients with cardiovascular disease and head injury. While not routinely done in the emergency and transport environments, pretreatment medications can be considered in situations where the sympathetic response to intubation must be controlled.[74,75]

Opioids provide anesthesia and analgesia and decrease sympathetic tone. Compared with morphine, fentanyl has greater lipid solubility and causes less histamine release, which gives it a faster onset, shorter duration, and greater hemodynamic stability. Accordingly, it is preferred for use in induction. Doses of 5 mcg/kg effectively minimize the reflex sympathetic response to laryngoscopy but are at an increased risk of premature apnea. More moderate doses of 2.5 to 3 mcg/kg decrease adverse effects while still blocking roughly half of the sympathetic response. Blood pressure moderation is more effective than heart rate control.[49,74,76–78] Fentanyl can cause chest wall muscle rigidity that makes ventilation impossible. Muscle rigidity appears to be related to dose and administration rate. The likelihood of chest wall rigidity is rare in doses of 5 mcg/kg or less in adults, but the risk, even at traditional doses, is real in neonatal and pediatric patients.[79]

Routine use of atropine is not recommended for preintubation in infants and children; atropine may be considered in situations with a high risk of bradycardia. Atropine is used to counterbalance the cholinergic effects of succinylcholine, which can produce bradycardia.

The use of peri-induction vasopressors, particularly push-dose vasopressors, is discussed earlier in this chapter.

Sedation

Induction agents are given to render the patient unconscious during intubation. Administer an induction agent to all patients, even those with apparent unconsciousness, unless the patient is in full arrest. Common induction agents in use today are etomidate, propofol, and ketamine.

Etomidate is a barbiturate-like derivative without the adverse effects of barbiturates. It acts rapidly, producing hypnosis in less than 30 seconds at a dose of 0.3 mg/kg, and recovery is prompt. Cardiovascular stability is characteristic of patients receiving etomidate, with little or no decreases in mean arterial pressure in normovolemic patients and in patients with limited cardiac reserve. Blood pressure changes are more likely to occur in hypovolemic patients. Etomidate decreases cerebral blood flow, cerebral metabolic oxygen demand, and ICP. Etomidate does not suppress the sympathetic response to laryngoscopy.[3,8,75]

Disadvantages of etomidate administration include pain during injection, involuntary skeletal muscle movements, and adrenocortical suppression. During this time, the adrenal cortex is not responsive to the adrenocorticotrophic hormone. This may be detrimental to patients on long-term steroid replacement therapy, or other forms of adrenal suppression, or patients in septic shock.[3,8,75]

Propofol is a lipid-soluble induction agent that combines rapid onset with rapid awakening. Unconsciousness and excellent amnesia occur within 30 seconds following a dose of 2 to 2.5 mg/kg. The awakening from propofol is more rapid and complete than from any other induction agent. Propofol, however, is a direct myocardial depressant that blunts compensatory tachycardia. Accordingly, in patients with cardiac disease or hypovolemia, propofol may be a suboptimal choice for induction. It may be associated with the development of peri-intubation hypotension.[13]

Ketamine is a phencyclidine derivative that produces dissociative anesthesia. Anesthesia and analgesia come from dissociation between the thalamus and limbic system. Patients appear to be in cataleptic states in which the eyes remain open with a slow nystagmus gaze. Ketamine is unique among induction agents because it is the only induction agent that provides amnesia and analgesia. Induction in 60 seconds is achieved following a dose of 1 to 2 mg/kg IV or within 2 to 4 minutes following an intramuscular dose of 5 to 10 mg/kg.

Ketamine administration triggers the release of centrally mediated catecholamines and inhibits their reuptake, producing an indirect sympathomimetic effect that is believed to preserve hemodynamic stability and which may be beneficial in patients with reactive airway disease. Skeletal muscle tone remains intact, which helps maintain a patent upper airway; however, the presence of protective upper airway reflexes should vomiting or regurgitation occur cannot be assumed.

There are some adverse effects of the drug. Ketamine-induced cardiac stimulation may adversely increase myocardial oxygen demands in patients with ischemic heart disease. Caution should be taken in patients involved in a hypertensive crisis because the administration of ketamine can cause an increase in blood pressure.

Airway secretions are increased by ketamine and may precipitate laryngospasm, which can be attenuated with the use of an anticholinergic agent, such as atropine, as a premedication.

Historically, ketamine was considered to be contraindicated in patients involved in severe head injuries; however, further research shows no evidence that it causes harm in traumatic brain injury patients.[80,81] Awakening from ketamine anesthesia may be associated with unpleasant visual, auditory, and proprioceptive illusions that may progress to delirium. Administration of benzodiazepines can decrease the incidence of emergence reactions associated with ketamine.

Both etomidate and ketamine have been suggested to reduce the incidence of peri-intubation arrest and hemodynamic instability. It is not clear that either agent, or a particular dose of either agent, has universal superiority.[13,82,83] The intubation of patients with undifferentiated critical illness is complex and nuanced. It is probably unlikely that a single agent holds the key to success, particularly in comparison to patient selection and preparation, provider knowledge and preparation, and careful clinical surveillance.

Neuromuscular Blocking Agents

All *NMBAs* work at the level of the neuromuscular end plate, disrupting neurotransmitter (acetylcholine [ACh]) function and preventing effective contraction of skeletal muscle (Fig. 12.16). These agents do not produce analgesia, anesthesia, or amnesia, and reports exist of patients with total recall and pain perception who received NMBAs without sufficient anesthesia during operations and procedures. Therefore, sedation of the patient is essential before and during extended periods of use of NMBAs.

NMBAs can be classified in three ways: type of block produced (depolarizing vs. nondepolarizing), duration of action (ultrashort, short, intermediate, or long), and structure (ACh-like, benzylisoquinoline compound, or aminosteroid compound). Table 12.1 compares common NBAs.

Succinylcholine

Succinylcholine, the only depolarizing NMBA in use, is two joined ACh molecules. When Ach receptors are activated, they open and then close voltage-sensitive sodium channels, which

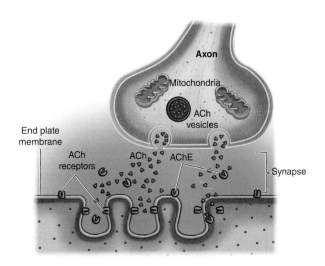

• **Figure 12.16** Neuromuscular junction. (From Clark JB, Queener SF, Karb VB. *Pharmacologic Basis of Nursing Practice.* 4th ed. Mosby; 1993.)

TABLE 12.1	**NMBAs**			

NMBAs	Intravenous Dosage (mg/kg)	Onset (min)	Duration (min)	Comments
Depolarizing				
Succinylcholine	Adult dose: 1.0–1.5 Pediatric dose: 1.5–2.0	1.5–2.0	4–6	Pretreat with atropine in children and adolescents; many adverse effects.
Nondepolarizing				
Pancuronium	00.04–0.01	3–5	60–100	Stimulate heart rate and cardiac output; no histamine release.
Atracurium	0.4–0.5	2–3	20–45	Metabolism independent of kidney or liver function; histamine release.
Rocuronium	0.5–1.0	1–2	20–40	Shortest onset of all nondepolarizing NMBAs; no histamine release.
Vecuronium	0.1	2–3	20–40	Minimal cardiovascular effects; no histamine release.
Mivacurium	0.15–0.25	2–3	12–20	Shortest duration of all nondepolarizing NMBAs; histamine release. No longer available in the United States.

inactivates them. In the interval, until the membrane potential is reset, junctional neuromuscular transmission is blocked, and the muscle is flaccid. The use of succinylcholine produces many side effects and clinical considerations. Because of succinylcholine's structural resemblance to ACh, the primary parasympathetic neurotransmitter, it stimulates cholinergic receptors at other sites in addition to those at the neuromuscular junction. The stimulation of nicotinic receptors in the sympathetic and parasympathetic nervous system and muscarinic receptors in the sinoatrial node of the heart can produce bradycardia and lead to hypotension. Associated bradycardia is more pronounced in children and adults who receive repeated doses and is attenuated by the use of atropine as a pretreatment drug.

Fasciculations signal the onset of paralysis by succinylcholine. They result from uncoordinated motor unit contractions that may be clinically important.[84,85]

Succinylcholine-induced hyperkalemia is rare but continues to be reported in the literature and is associated with cardiovascular instability, hyperkalemic dysrhythmias, and death. Normal muscle releases enough potassium during succinylcholine-induced depolarization to raise serum potassium by 0.5 to 1.0 mEq/L. Pathologic conditions with potential for hyperkalemia with succinylcholine include upper or lower motor neuron defect; prolonged chemical denervation with muscle relaxants or clostridial toxins, direct muscle trauma, tumor, or inflammation; thermal trauma; disuse atrophy; and severe infection.

In denervation injuries, ACh receptors develop outside the neuromuscular junction, which is referred to as upregulation. These extrajunctional receptors allow succinylcholine to affect widespread depolarization and extensive potassium release. The higher the upregulation is, the more profound is the hyperkalemia. The potential for severe hyperkalemia with succinylcholine can occur as early as 4 to 5 days of immobilization and can persist as long as the condition that induced it continues to present. Patients with quadriplegia or paraplegia, therefore, could have the potential for succinylcholine hyperkalemia throughout life.

A common belief is that the use of succinylcholine for induction in patients with open globe injuries is contraindicated. Physiologically, succinylcholine is associated with increased intraocular pressure (IOP). However, when an open globe injury occurs, it is often associated with crying, forceful blinking, and rubbing of the eyes, all of which create a much larger rise in IOP than that associated with the use of succinylcholine. The belief that succinylcholine caused vitreous extrusion has been perpetuated for nearly 50 years and relied on anecdote rather than documented case reports.[86]

Succinylcholine is known to trigger malignant hyperthermia (MH) in susceptible patients. MH is a hypermetabolic disorder of the skeletal muscles. Classic signs include hyperthermia, tachycardia, increased carbon dioxide production, increased oxygen consumption, acidosis, muscle rigidity, and rhabdomyolysis. If untreated, the syndrome is fatal. Early detection is essential and relies on observed increases in end-tidal carbon dioxide and body temperature, followed by laboratory confirmation of acidosis. The incidence of MH in adults is rare; however, children are at higher risk, with more than 50% of all cases of MH appearing in children less than 15 years of age. MH is treated with dantrolene sodium administered in doses of a 2.5 mg/kg bolus followed by additional doses up to 10 mg/kg. Further treatment is aimed at cooling the patient, treatment of arrhythmias (avoid calcium channel blockers), aggressive fluid therapy to maintain urine output, and monitoring for coagulation abnormalities. Patients should be monitored for 48 to 72 hours after the initial event because as many as 25% of patients have a recurrence of symptoms.

Nondepolarizing Agents

The explorers of the new world described the South American arrow poisons known as curares as early as the 16th and 17th centuries. Investigations into these poisons led to the development in 1943 of the first nondepolarizing drug, tubocurarine, which was used as a muscle relaxant during surgical anesthesia.

Unlike succinylcholine, which binds to the muscle receptor and acts as an agonist, nondepolarizing muscle relaxants bind to the receptors and prevent depolarization with ACh. Therefore, nondepolarizing NMBAs are referred to as competitive antagonists. Most nondepolarizing agents have a slower onset of action and maintain neuromuscular blockade longer than succinylcholine.

The search for a nondepolarizing muscle relaxant with an onset of action equal to that of succinylcholine and with minimal side effects led to the development of rocuronium, which is a steroidal nondepolarizing agent with an intermediate duration. When dosed in the range of 1.0 to 1.2 mg/kg, rocuronium produces intubation conditions similar to succinylcholine in a similar time frame.[85,87,88] The agent's onset and duration are dose-dependent, and pediatric patients seem to experience a shorter time of relaxation. There are suggestions in the literature that rocuronium has a favorable hemodynamic profile and may have a beneficial effect on mortality compared with succinylcholine. There is no consensus that a meaningful difference exists or on the potential mechanisms that would contribute to such variability.[85,87–91] There is also a small risk for anaphylaxis from rocuronium, seemingly (but not certainly) higher than from other NMBAs.[92]

Vecuronium is also a steroidal, nondepolarizing NMBA. The usual dose is 0.1 mg/kg. It is not possible to achieve intubating conditions with vecuronium in a time similar to rocuronium or succinylcholine. Even when the vecuronium dose is tripled, the speed of onset is still around 90 seconds.[87,90] With the slow onset of intubation conditions, operators use more of the safe apnea time waiting for the development of good intubating conditions. Because of this, they have less time to do the procedure. There is a greater likelihood of multiple attempts and the need to interpose mask ventilation because of desaturation. Both increase the risk of adverse events.[32,33]

Medications, disease processes, and physiologic conditions may interfere with the effectiveness of NMBAs. Neurologic diseases such as myasthenia gravis can prolong paralysis. Hyperthermia and hypothermia may have an impact on the pharmacology of selected NMBAs. Electrolyte imbalances such as hypermagnesemia may also prolong paralysis.

Sugammadex is a noncompetitive antagonist for the reversal of nondepolarizing neuromuscular blocking agents. It rapidly encapsulates rocuronium or vecuronium by one-to-one molecular binding, providing fast and predictable reversal effects. It is commonly used in anesthesia practice and appears safe for pediatric and adult patients.[93,94]

Monitoring Airway Patency During Transport

There is no single perfect way to ensure that an airway appliance is properly placed. Physical examination alone is insufficient, and even direct visualization of the ETT can be imperfect in the context of an airway that is difficult to visualize. A combination of physical examination and mechanical detection techniques must be used on every patient and reused throughout the episode of care.[95] The rate of undetected ETT misplacement in the out-of-hospital environment is significant.[96]

End-Tidal Carbon Dioxide Detection

End-tidal CO₂ detection is the most accurate and easily available method to monitor correct ETT position and ventilator circuit integrity in patients with adequate tissue perfusion. It is highly reliable in pulseless patients with high-quality cardiopulmonary resuscitation. Continuous end-tidal CO_2 detection is the standard of care for any patient with an airway appliance during transport.[97–99]

Disposable qualitative end-tidal CO_2 detectors evaluate proper ETT placement by incorporating a nontoxic, pH-sensitive, chemically treated indicator that changes color in the presence of carbon dioxide. False-negative results (color remains purple despite correct tracheal placement) can occur during cardiac arrest, severe airway obstruction, and pulmonary edema and in severely hypocarbic infants. In low-perfusion states, such as occur in cardiac arrest, the colorimetric end-tidal CO_2 can produce a detectable color change. In a study of 566 prehospital intubations of patients in cardiac

arrest, a color change occurred in 95.6%, with only one false-positive result.[100] In addition to verification of endotracheal placement after intubation, the device can also be used to monitor tube placement during transport.

Capnometry is the measurement of end-tidal CO_2 values with each breath. The instrument works by emitting an infrared light beam through a gas sample either located immediately distal to the ETT (mainstream capnometry) or by analyzing a gas sample from the breathing circuit (sidestream capnometry). A capnogram is a time-scaled graphic representation of the capnometry values.

Similar to the way that an electrocardiogram adds helpful information about the pulse rate, the waveform of a capnogram adds valuable information about the presence of CO_2 or even the capnometry value. A sudden decrease in CO_2 to zero with no waveform indicates a dislodged ETT, a kinked or obstructed ETT, or a ventilator disconnect. An incremental decrease in CO_2 may indicate sudden and severe hypotension or cardiac arrest. An incremental increase in CO_2 can indicate hypoventilation or partial endotracheal obstruction and can occur with sodium bicarbonate administration or rising body temperature. A sudden and dramatic rise in end-tidal CO_2 is one of the clinical indicators of MH. However, as with any piece of equipment, caution should be exercised when capnography is used to ensure the clinical picture matches the readings: carbon dioxide present in the exhaled gas indicates that alveolar ventilation has transpired but does not necessarily mean that the ETT is in the trachea. A tube positioned in the pharynx also provides normal readings (Figs. 12.17 and 12.18).[18,97]

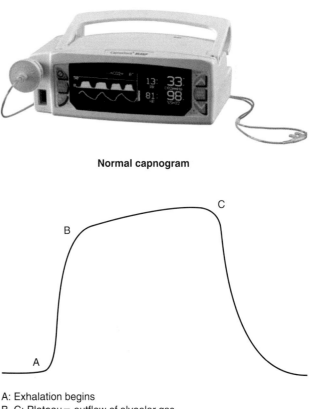

Normal capnogram

A: Exhalation begins
B–C: Plateau = outflow of alveolar gas
C: End-tidal CO_2

• **Figure 12.17** End-tidal carbon dioxide waveform. (From Dean JA, *McDonald and Avery's Dentistry for the Child and Adolescent.* 10th ed. Elsevier; 2016.)

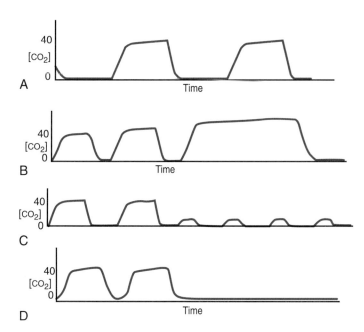

• **Figure 12.18** Normal and abnormal end-tidal carbon dioxide waveforms. **A.** Normal waveform. **B.** Decreasing respiratory rate, preserved tidal volume. **C.** Hypoventilation from decreased tidal volume. **D.** Loss of waveform from apnea or extubation. (From Nagler J, Krauss B. Capnography: A valuable tool for airway management. *Emerg Med Clin North Am.* 2008;26(4):881–897.)

It is important to emphasize that the end-tidal CO_2 value and the arterial partial pressure of CO_2 are not reliably related. The end-tidal value is a function of metabolic rate, minute ventilation, cardiac output, and not just gas exchange. Accordingly, any alteration in metabolism, minute ventilation, or cardiac output affects the end-tidal value, whereas only changes in minute ventilation affect the arterial value. Arterial partial pressure can be higher or lower than the exhaled value, and the difference between the two varies with patient position, disease state, and medication use.[97]

Pulse Oximetry

In the ED or critical care unit, healthcare providers rely on arterial blood gases (ABGs) or, more specifically, the partial pressure of oxygen tension (PaO_2) drawn intermittently to guide therapy. Oxygen in the blood is dissolved in the plasma or is bound to hemoglobin. The oxygen dissolved in the plasma is referred to as the partial pressure of oxygen (PO_2). The normal value ranges from 80 to 100 mm Hg. The PO_2 accounts for only 1% to 2% of the total oxygen content. The vast majority of oxygen is bound to hemoglobin molecules and is reported as oxygen saturation (SaO_2 or SpO_2). Total oxygen-carrying capacity of the blood (CaO_2) is $[(1.39 \times Hb \times SpO_2/100) + (0.003 \times PO_2)]$. In arterial blood, the normal value of oxygen saturation (SaO_2) ranges from 95% to 97.5%.

Pulse oximetry provides a reliable and continuous evaluation of oxygenation. The relationship between the PaO_2 and SaO_2 is displayed in Fig. 12.2 in the oxyhemoglobin dissociation curve. The relationship is not a linear one. The upper portion of the curve shows a compensatory mechanism of the body. In a healthy adult, more oxygen than necessary is carried. A drop in the PaO_2

from 100 to 80 mm Hg shows a minimal change in the SaO_2. The steep portion of the curve shows a rapid decline in SaO_2 with small decreases in PaO_2. When the SaO_2 falls to less than 90%, a rapid decline is seen in the oxygen content.

There is a time lag, referred to as latency, of up to 3 minutes, between a change in arterial oxygen tension and a change in pulse oximetry values. It may make sense to think of pulse oximetry as reporting the history of oxygen saturation and not necessarily the current state.[9,10]

Pulse oximeters use a light source and photo-detector device. Accordingly, successful use depends on good alignment between the light source and detector in the sensor and on the placement of the sensor over a good pulse site. Thus, the accuracy of pulse oximetry may be affected by clinical conditions causing vasoconstriction, such as hypotension, hypothermia, or vasopressor therapy, and oximetry signal reliability is affected by motion, hypothermia, dyshemoglobinemias, and intravenous dye. There are racial and ethnic differences in pulse oximetry measurement that can translate into delayed care delivery for Asian, Black, and Hispanic patients.[101,102]

Postintubation Management

Hypotension is expected in the postintubation period and is often caused by diminished venous blood return due to the increased intrathoracic pressure that attends mechanical ventilation, exacerbated by the hemodynamic effects of the induction agent. If significant hypotension is present, proper management should be considered.

The intubating clinician should pay close attention to postintubation sedation. Up to 7.4% of patients receiving neuromuscular blockade for intubation in the ED are at risk for awareness. Exposure to rocuronium and decreased level of consciousness are factors which may be associated with increased risk for awake paralysis in the ED.[103,104] Immediate postintubation sedation and analgesia must be guided empirically, with understanding of the duration of the various neuromuscular blocking agents, sedatives, and analgesic agents. Transport teams may underestimate the timing and need for sedatives immediately after intubation.[105]

For sedation after muscle relaxation has abated, using a sedation scale, such as the Richmond Agitation Sedation Scale (Table 12.2), helps to optimize patient comfort and to guide decision-making. Optimal sedatiogesia practice is to provide analgesia first, then a sedative. This is particularly important in the context of most classic sedative agents – the benzodiazepines, propofol, and dexmedetomidine, having no analgesia properties at all. Physiologic responses (hypertension, tachycardia, lacrimation) are not completely reliable in indicating the need for sedation or analgesia.[3,105]

Summary

Assessment and management of the patient's airway is the primary role of the transport team. Knowledge of when and how to perform basic and advanced airway management is critical in the transport environment. When in doubt, it is best to use a solid basic technique to help prepare for advanced airway management. Good clinical judgment, skill, and familiarity with the pharmacology of airway management are necessary so that patients receive competent care and complications that can occur in the care of the critically ill or injured patients are prevented.

TABLE 12.2 Richmond Agitation-Sedation Scale (RASS)

Score	Term	Description	
+4	Combative	Overly combative, violent, immediate danger to staff	
+3	Very agitated	Pulls or removes tube(s) or catheter(s), aggressive	
+2	Agitated	Frequent nonpurposeful movement, fights ventilator	
+1	Restless	Anxious but movements not aggressively vigorous	
0	Alert and calm		
−1	Drowsy	Not fully alert but has sustained awakening (eye opening/eye contact) to *voice* (≥10 seconds)	Verbal stimulation
−2	Light sedation	Briefly awakens to *voice* with eye contact (<10 seconds)	
−3	Moderate sedation	Movement or eye opening to *voice* (but no eye contact)	
−4	Deep sedation	No response to voice but movement or eye opening to *physical* stimulation	Physical stimulation
−5	Unarousable	No response to *voice* or *physical* stimulation	

References

1. Martin L, Kahil H. How much reduced hemoglobin is necessary to generate central cyanosis. *Chest.* 1990;97(1):182–185.

2. Medicine SoCC. *Fundamental Critical Care Support.* 7th ed. Society of Critical Care Medicine; 2021.

3. Brown C, Sakles J. *Walls Manual of Emergency Airway Management.* 5th ed. Wolters Kluwer; 2017.

4. Brodsky JB, Lemmens HJ, Brock-Utne JG, Vierra M, Saidman LJ. Morbid obesity and tracheal intubation. *Anesth Analg.* 2002;94(3):732–736; table of contents. doi:10.1097/00000539-200203000-00047

5. Riad W, Vaez MN, Raveendran R, et al. Neck circumference as a predictor of difficult intubation and difficult mask ventilation in morbidly obese patients: A prospective observational study. *Eur J Anaesthesiol.* 2016;33(4):244–249. doi:10.1097/eja.0000000000000324

6. Levitan RM, Everett WW, Ochroch EA. Limitations of difficult airway prediction in patients intubated in the emergency department. *Ann Emerg Med.* 2004;44(4):307–313. doi:10.1016/j.annemergmed.2004.05.006

7. Norskov AK, Rosenstock CV, Wetterslev J, Astrup G, Afshari A, Lundstrom LH. Diagnostic accuracy of anaesthesiologists' prediction of difficult airway management in daily clinical practice: A cohort study of 188 064 patients registered in the Danish Anaesthesia Database. *Anaesthesia.* 2015;70(3):272–281. doi:10.1111/anae.12955

8. Mosier J, Joshi R, Hypes C, Pacheco G, Valenzuela T, Sakles J. The physiologically difficult airway. *West J Emerg Med.* 2015;16(7):1109–1117.

9. Davis DP, Aguilar S, Sonnleitner C, Cohen M, Jennings M. Latency and loss of pulse oximetry signal with the use of digital probes during prehospital rapid-sequence intubation. *Prehosp Emerg Care.* 2011;15(1):18–22. doi:10.3109/10903127.2010.514091

10. MacLeod DB, Cortinez LI, Keifer JC, et al. The desaturation response time of finger pulse oximeters during mild hypothermia. *Anaesthesia.* 2005;60(1):65–71. doi:10.1111/j.1365-2044.2004.04033.x

11. Weingart S, Levitan R. Preoxygenation and prevention of desaturation during emergency airway management. *Ann Emerg Med.* 2012;59(3):165–175.

12. Weingart SD, Trueger NS, Wong N, Scofi J, Singh N, Rudolph SS. Delayed sequence intubation: A prospective observational study. *Ann Emerg Med.* 2015;65(4):349–355. doi:10.1016/j.annemergmed.2014.09.025

13. Russotto V, Tassistro E, Myatra SN, et al. Peri-intubation cardiovascular collapse in patients who are critically Ill: Insights from the INTUBE study. *Am J Respir Crit Care Med.* 2022;206(4):449–458. doi:10.1164/rccm.202111-2575OC

14. Kim WY, Kwak MK, Ko BS, et al. Factors associated with the occurrence of cardiac arrest after emergency tracheal intubation in the emergency department. *PLoS One.* 2014;9(11):e112779. doi:10.1371/journal.pone.0112779

15. Russell DW, Casey JD, Gibbs KW, et al. Effect of fluid bolus administration on cardiovascular collapse among critically Ill patients undergoing tracheal intubation: A randomized clinical trial. *JAMA.* 2022;328(3):270–279. doi:10.1001/jama.2022.9792

16. Heffner AC, Swords DS, Neale MN, Jones AE. Incidence and factors associated with cardiac arrest complicating emergency airway management. *Resuscitation.* 2013;84(11):1500–1504. doi:10.1016/j.resuscitation.2013.07.022

17. Trivedi S, Demirci O, Arteaga G, Kashyap R, Smischney NJ. Evaluation of preintubation shock index and modified shock index as predictors of postintubation hypotension and other short-term outcomes. *J Crit Care.* 2015;30(4):861.e1–e7. doi:10.1016/j.jcrc.2015.04.013

18. Davis JS, Johns JA, Olvera DJ, et al. Vital sign patterns before shock-related cardiopulmonary arrest. *Resuscitation.* 2019;139:337–342. doi:10.1016/j.resuscitation.2019.03.028

19. Guyette FX, Martin-Gill C, Galli G, McQuaid N, Elmer J. Bolus dose epinephrine improves blood pressure but is associated with increased mortality in critical care transport. *Prehosp Emerg Care.* 2019;23(6):764–771. doi:10.1080/10903127.2019.1593564

20. Panchal AR, Satyanarayan A, Bahadir JD, Hays D, Mosier J. Efficacy of bolus-dose phenylephrine for peri-intubation hypotension. *J Emerg Med.* 2015;49(4):488–494. doi:10.1016/j.jemermed.2015.04.033

21. Tilton LJ, Eginger KH. Utility of push-dose vasopressors for temporary treatment of hypotension in the emergency department. *J Emerg Nursing.* 2016;42(3):279–281. doi:10.1016/j.jen.2016.03.007

22. Weingart S. Push-dose pressors for immediate blood pressure control. *Clin Exp Emerg Med*. 2015;2(2):131–132. doi:10.15441/ceem.15.010

23. Davis DP, Olvera D, Selde W, Wilmas J, Stuhlmiller D. Bolus vasopressor use for air medical rapid sequence intubation: The vasopressor intravenous push to enhance resuscitation trial. *Air Med J*. 2022. doi:10.1016/j.amj.2022.09.004

24. Kubena A, Weston S, Alvey H. Push-dose vasopressors in the emergency department: A narrative review. *J Emerg Crit Care Med*. 2022;6. https://jeccm.amegroups.com/article/view/7558

25. Cole JB, Knack SK, Karl ER, Horton GB, Satpathy R, Driver BE. Human errors and adverse hemodynamic events related to "push dose pressors" in the emergency department. *J Med Toxicol*. 2019;15(4):276–286. doi:10.1007/s13181-019-00716-z

26. Rotando A, Picard L, Delibert S, Chase K, Jones CMC, Acquisto NM. Push dose pressors: Experience in critically ill patients outside of the operating room. *Am J Emerg Med*. 2019;37(3):494–498. doi:10.1016/j.ajem.2018.12.001

27. Nawrocki PS, Poremba M, Lawner BJ. Push dose epinephrine use in the management of hypotension during critical care transport. *Prehosp Emerg Care*. 2020;24(2):188–195. doi:10.1080/10903127.2019.1588443

28. Ellis DY, Lambert C, Shirley P. Intracranial placement of nasopharyngeal airways: Is it all that rare? *Emerg Med J*. 2006;23(8):661. doi:10.1136/emj.2006.036541

29. Casey JD, Janz DR, Russell DW, et al. Bag-mask ventilation during tracheal intubation of critically ill adults. *N Engl J Med*. 2019;380(9):811–821. doi:10.1056/NEJMoa1812405

30. Gerstein N, Carey M, Braude D, et al. Efficacy of facemask ventilation techniques in novice providers. *J Clin Anesth*. 2013;25(3):193–197.

31. *Textbook of Neonatal Resuscitation*. 8th ed. American Academy of Pediatrics an American Heart Association; 2021.

32. Mort T. Emergency tracheal intubation: Complications associated with repeated laryngoscopic attempts. *Anesth Analg*. 2004;99(2):607–613.

33. Wilcox SR, Bittner EA, Elmer J, et al. Neuromuscular blocking agent administration for emergent tracheal intubation is associated with decreased prevalence of procedure-related complications. *Crit Care Med*. 2012;40(6):1808–1813. doi:10.1097/CCM.0b013e31824e0e67

34. Gawande A. *The Checklist Manifesto: How to Get Things Right*. Henry Holt and Company; 2010.

35. Hales BM, Pronovost PJ. The checklist – a tool for error management and performance improvement. *J Crit Care*. 2006;21(3):231–235. doi:10.1016/j.jcrc.2006.06.002

36. Brown CA 3rd, Bair AE, Pallin DJ, Walls RM. Techniques, success, and adverse events of emergency department adult intubations. *Ann Emerg Med*. 2015;65(4):363–370.e1. doi:10.1016/j.annemergmed.2014.10.036

37. Smith K, High K, Collins S, Self W. A preprocedural checklist improves the safety of emergency department intubation of trauma patients. *Acad Emerg Med*. 2015;22(8):989–992.

38. Long E, Fitzpatrick P, Cincotta DR, Grindlay J, Barrett MJ. A randomised controlled trial of cognitive aids for emergency airway equipment preparation in a paediatric emergency department. *Scand J Trauma Resusc Emerg Med*. 2016;24:8. doi:10.1186/s13049-016-0201-z

39. Anthes E. Hospital checklists are meant to save lives – so why do they often fail? Nature 2015;523(7562):516–518. doi:10.1038/523516a

40. Brunsveld-Reinders AH, Arbous MS, Kuiper SG, de Jonge E. A comprehensive method to develop a checklist to increase safety of intra-hospital transport of critically ill patients. *Crit Care*. 2015;19:214. doi:10.1186/s13054-015-0938-1

41. Cook TM, MacDougall-Davis SR. Complications and failure of airway management. *Br J Anaesth*. 2012;109(Suppl 1):i68–i85. doi:10.1093/bja/aes393

42. Aspiotes CR, Gothard MQ, Gothard MD, Parrish R, Schwartz HP, Bigham MT. Setting the benchmark for the ground and air medical quality in transport international quality improvement collaborative. *Air Med J*. 2018;37(4):244–248. doi:10.1016/j.amj.2018.03.002

43. Sellick B. Cricoid pressure to control regurgitation of stomach contents during induction of anesthesia. *Lancet*. 1961;2(7199):404–406.

44. Algie CM, Mahar RK, Tan HB, Wilson G, Mahar PD, Wasiak J. Effectiveness and risks of cricoid pressure during rapid sequence induction for endotracheal intubation. *Cochrane Database Syst Rev*. 2015;(11):Cd011656. doi:10.1002/14651858.CD011656.pub2

45. Bhatia N, Bhagat H, Sen I. Cricoid pressure: Where do we stand? *J Anaesthiol Clin Pharmacol*. 2014;30(1):3–6.

46. Sakles J, Chiu S, Mosier J, Walker C, Stolz U. The importance of first pass success when performing orotracheal intubation in the emergency department. *Acad Emerg Med*. 2013;20(1):70–78.

47. Kerrey BT, Rinderknecht AS, Geis GL, Nigrovic LE, Mittiga MR. Rapid sequence intubation for pediatric emergency patients: Higher frequency of failed attempts and adverse effects found by video review. *Ann Emerg Med*. 2012;60(3):251–259. doi:10.1016/j.annemergmed.2012.02.013

48. Wadbrook P. Advances in airway pharmacology. *J Emerg Med Clin North Am*. 2000;18(4):767–788.

49. Frakes M. Esmolol: A unique drug with ED applications. *J Emerg Nurs*. 2001;27(1):47–51.

50. Sengupta P, Sessler D, Maglinger P. Endotracheal tube pressure in three hospitals and the volume required to produce an appropriate cuff pressure. *BMC Anesthesiol*. 2004;4(1):8.

51. Tollefsen WW, Chapman J, Frakes M, Gallagher M, Shear M, Thomas SH. Endotracheal tube cuff pressures in pediatric patients intubated before aeromedical transport. *Pediatr Emerg Care*. 2010;26(5):361-363.

52. Levitan RM, Kinkle WC, Levin WJ, Everett WW. Laryngeal view during laryngoscopy: A randomized trial comparing cricoid pressure, backward-upward-rightward pressure, and bimanual laryngoscopy. *Ann Emerg Med*. 2006;47(6):548–555. doi:10.1016/j.annemergmed.2006.01.013

53. Olvera D, Davis D, Wolfe A, Swearingen C. Implementation of CMAC PM device and focused airway management training to improve first pass success (Abstract). Critical Care Transport Medicine Conference. Charlotte, NC; 2015.

54. Phelan MP, Dhimar J. Techniques for improving video laryngoscopy with a hyperangulated blade. *Acad Emerg Med*. 2016. doi:10.1111/acem.13011

55. Griesdale DE, Liu D, McKinney J, Choi PT. Glidescope® video-laryngoscopy versus direct laryngoscopy for endotracheal intubation: A systematic review and meta-analysis. *Can J Anaesth*. 2012;59(1):41–52. doi:10.1007/s12630-011-9620-5

56. Sakles JC, Mosier J, Patanwala AE, Dicken J. Learning curves for direct laryngoscopy and GlideScope® video laryngoscopy in an emergency medicine residency. *West J Emerg Med*. 2014;15(7):930–937. doi:10.5811/westjem.2014.9.23691

57. Olvera D, Davis D, Wolfe A, Swearingen C. Prospective validation of a novel difficult airway prediction algorithm for emergency airway management (Abstract). World Airway Management Meeting. 2015.

58. Aziz MF, Bayman EO, Van Tienderen MM, Todd MM, Brambrink AM. Predictors of difficult videolaryngoscopy with GlideScope® or C-MAC® with D-blade: Secondary analysis from a large comparative videolaryngoscopy trial. *Br J Anaesth*. 2016;117(1):118–123. doi:10.1093/bja/aew128

59. Frerk C, Mitchell V, McNarry A, et al. Difficult Airway Society 2015 guidelines for management of unanticipated difficult intubation in adults. *Br J Anesth*. 2015;115(6):827–848.

60. Segal N, Yannopoulos D, Mahoney BD, et al. Impairment of carotid artery blood flow by supraglottic airway use in a swine model of cardiac arrest. *Resuscitation*. 2012;83(8):1025–1030. doi:10.1016/j.resuscitation.2012.03.025

61. White JM, Braude DA, Lorenzo G, Hart BL. Radiographic evaluation of carotid artery compression in patients with extraglottic airway devices in place. *Acad Emerg Med*. 2015;22(5):636–638. doi:10.1111/acem.12647

62. Carlson JN, Mayrose J, Wang HE. How much force is required to dislodge an alternate airway? *Prehosp Emerg Care.* 2010;14(1):31–35. doi:10.3109/10903120903349879

63. Flaishon R, Sotman A, Friedman A, Ben-Abraham R, Rudick V, Weinbroum AA. Laryngeal mask airway insertion by anesthetists and nonanesthetists wearing unconventional protective gear: A prospective, randomized, crossover study in humans. *Anesthesiology.* 2004;100(2):267–273.

64. Brimacombe JR, Berry A. The incidence of aspiration associated with the laryngeal mask airway: A meta-analysis of published literature. *J Clin Anesth.* 1995;7(4):297–305.

65. Middleton PM, Simpson PM, Thomas RE, Bendall JC. Higher insertion success with the i-gel supraglottic airway in out-of-hospital cardiac arrest: A randomised controlled trial. *Resuscitation.* 2014; 85(7):893–897. doi:10.1016/j.resuscitation.2014.02.021

66. Marcollini E, Burton J, Bradshaw J, Baumann M. A standing order protocol for cricothyrotomy in prehospital emergency patients. *Prehosp Emerg Care.* 2004;8(1):23–28.

67. McIntosh S, Swanson E, Barton E. Cricothyrotomy in air medical transport. *J Trauma.* 2008;64(6):1543–1547.

68. Hubble MW, Wilfong DA, Brown LH, Hertelendy A, Benner RW. A meta-analysis of prehospital airway control techniques part II: Alternative airway devices and cricothyrotomy success rates. *Prehosp Emerg Care.* 2010;14(4):515–530. doi:10.3109/10903127.20 10.497903

69. Peterson GN, Domino KB, Caplan RA, Posner KL, Lee LA, Cheney FW. Management of the difficult airway: A closed claims analysis. *Anesthesiology.* 2005;103(1):33–39.

70. Topjian AA, Raymond TT, Atkins D, et al. Part 4: Pediatric Basic and advanced life support: 2020 American heart association guidelines for cardiopulmonary resuscitation and emergency cardiovascular care. *Circulation.* 2020;142(16_suppl_2):S469–S523. doi:10.1161/CIR. 0000000000000901

71. Shaffner DH, McCloskey JJ, Schwartz JM. Cuffed endotracheal tube use in children: Times (and minds) are 'A changing. *Pediat Crit Care Med.* 2019;20(8):789–790. doi:10.1097/pcc.0000000000002001

72. Manimalethu R, Krishna S, Shafy SZ, Hakim M, Tobias JD. Choosing endotracheal tube size in children: Which formula is best? *Int J Pediatr Otorhinolaryngol.* 2020;134:110016. https://doi.org/10.1016/j. ijporl.2020.110016

73. Weingart SD. Preoxygenation, reoxygenation, and delayed sequence intubation in the emergency department. *J Emerg Med.* 2011;40(6): 661–667. doi:10.1016/j.jemermed.2010.02.014

74. Feng CK, Chan KH, Liu KN, Or CH, Lee TY. A comparison of lidocaine, fentanyl, and esmolol for attenuation of cardiovascular response to laryngoscopy and tracheal intubation. *Acta Anaesthesiol Sin.* 1996;34(2):61–67.

75. Masoudifar M, Beheshtian E. Comparison of cardiovascular response to laryngoscopy and tracheal intubation after induction of anesthesia by Propofol and Etomidate. *J Res Med Sci.* 2013;18(10):870–874.

76. Gupta S, Tank P. A comparative study of efficacy of esmolol and fentanyl for pressure attenuation during laryngoscopy and endotracheal intubation. *Saudi J Anaesth.* 2011;5(1):2–8. doi:10.4103/1658-354X.76473

77. Miller DR, Martineau RJ, Wynands JE, Hill J. Bolus administration of esmolol for controlling the haemodynamic response to tracheal intubation: The Canadian Multicentre Trial. *Canadian J Anaesth.* [Journal canadien d'anesthesie] 1991;38(7):849–858. doi:10.1007/bf03036959

78. Ugur B, Ogurlu M, Gezer E, Nuri Aydin O, Gursoy F. Effects of esmolol, lidocaine and fentanyl on haemodynamic responses to endotracheal intubation: A comparative study. *Clin Drug Investig.* 2007;27(4):269–277.

79. Dewhirst E, Naguib A, Tobias JD. Chest wall rigidity in two infants after low-dose fentanyl administration. *Pediatr Emerg Care.* 2012;28(5). https://journals.lww.com/pec-online/Fulltext/2012/05000/Chest_Wall_Rigidity_in_Two_Infants_After_Low_Dose.15.aspx

80. Cohen L, Athaide V, Wickham ME, Doyle-Waters MM, Rose NGW, Hohl CM. The effect of ketamine on intracranial and cerebral perfusion pressure and health outcomes: A systematic review. *Ann Emerg Med.* 2014;65(1):43–51.e2. doi:10.1016/j.annemergmed.2014.06.018

81. Miller M, Kruit N, Heldreich C, et al. Hemodynamic response after rapid sequence induction with ketamine in out-of-hospital patients at risk of shock as defined by the shock index. *Ann Emerg Med.* 2016. doi:10.1016/j.annemergmed.2016.03.041

82. April MD, Arana A, Schauer SG, et al. Ketamine versus etomidate and peri-intubation hypotension: A National emergency airway registry study. *Acad Emerg Med.* 2020;27(11):1106–1115. doi:10.1111/acem.14063

83. Foster M, Self M, Gelber A, et al. Ketamine is not associated with more post-intubation hypotension than etomidate in patients undergoing endotracheal intubation. *Am J Emerg Med.* 2022;61:131–136. doi:10.1016/j.ajem.2022.08.054

84. Schreiber JU, Lysakowski C, Fuchs-Buder T, Tramer MR. Prevention of succinylcholine-induced fasciculation and myalgia: A meta-analysis of randomized trials. *Anesthesiology.* 2005;103(4):877–884.

85. Taha SK, El-Khatib MF, Baraka AS, et al. Effect of suxamethonium vs rocuronium on onset of oxygen desaturation during apnoea following rapid sequence induction. *Anaesthesia.* 2010;65(4):358–361. doi:10.1111/j.1365-2044.2010.06243.x

86. Murgatroyd H, Bembridge J. Intraocular pressure. *Contin Educ Anesth Crit Care Pain.* 2008;8(3):100–103.

87. Chatrath V, Singh I, Chatrath R, Arora N. Comparison of intubating conditions of rocuronium bromide and vecuronium bromide with succinylcholine using "timing principle." *J Anaesthesiol Clin Pharmacol.* 2010;26(4):493–497.

88. Perry JJ, Lee JS, Sillberg VA, Wells GA. Rocuronium versus succinylcholine for rapid sequence induction intubation. *Cochrane Database Syst Rev.* 2008;(2):Cd002788. doi:10.1002/14651858.CD002788.pub2

89. Patanwala AE, Erstad BL, Roe DJ, Sakles JC. Succinylcholine is associated with increased mortality when used for rapid sequence intubation of severely brain injured patients in the emergency department. *Pharmacotherapy.* 2016;36(1):57–63. doi:10.1002/phar.1683

90. Magorian T, Flannery KB, Miller RD. Comparison of rocuronium, succinylcholine, and vecuronium for rapid-sequence induction of anesthesia in adult patients. *Anesthesiology.* 1993;79(5):913–918.

91. Lyon RM, Perkins ZB, Chatterjee D, Lockey DJ, Russell MQ. Significant modification of traditional rapid sequence induction improves safety and effectiveness of pre-hospital trauma anaesthesia. *Crit Care.* 2015;19(1):134. doi:10.1186/s13054-015-0872-2

92. Reddy JI, Cooke PJ, van Schalkwyk JM, Hannam JA, Fitzharris P, Mitchell SJ. Anaphylaxis is more common with rocuronium and succinylcholine than with atracurium. *Anesthesiology.* 2015;122(1): 39–45. doi:10.1097/aln.0000000000000512

93. Lang B, Han L, Zeng L, et al. Efficacy and safety of sugammadex for neuromuscular blockade reversal in pediatric patients: An updated meta-analysis of randomized controlled trials with trial sequential analysis. *BMC Pediatrics.* 2022;22(1):295. doi:10.1186/s12887-022-03288-0

94. Honing GHM, Martini CH, Bom A, et al. Safety of sugammadex for reversal of neuromuscular block. *Expert Opinion on Drug Safety.* 2019;18(10):883–891. doi:10.1080/14740338.2019.1649393

95. Rudraraju P, Eisen LA. Confirmation of endotracheal tube position: A narrative review. *J Intensive Care Med.* 2009;24(5):283–292. doi:10.1177/0885066609340501

96. Wang H, Yealy D. Out of hospital endotracheal intubation: Where are we? *Ann Emerg Med.* 2006;47:532–541.

97. Gravenstein JS, Jaffe MB, Gravenstein N, Paulus DA. *Capnography.* Cambridge University Press; 2011.

98. American Society of Anesthesiologists ASo. Standards for Basic Anesthetic Monitoring. http://www.asahq.org/publicationsAndServices/standards/02.pdf

99. Takeda T, Tanigawa K, Tanaka H, Hayashi Y, Goto E, Tanaka K. The assessment of three methods to verify tracheal tube placement in the emergency setting. *Resuscitation.* 2003;56(2):153–157. doi: 10.1016/s0300-9572(02)00345-3

100. Hayden SR, Sciammarella J, Viccellio P, Thode H, Delagi R. Colorimetric end–tidal CO_2 detector for verification of endotracheal tube placement in out–of–hospital cardiac arrest. *Acad Emerg Med.* 1995;2(6):499–502. https://doi.org/10.1111/j.1553-2712.1995.tb03247.x

101. Gottlieb ER, Ziegler J, Morley K, Rush B, Celi LA. Assessment of racial and ethnic differences in oxygen supplementation among patients in the intensive care unit. *JAMA Intern Med.* 2022;182(8):849–858. doi:10.1001/jamainternmed.2022.2587

102. Fawzy A, Wu TD, Wang K, et al. Racial and ethnic discrepancy in pulse oximetry and delayed identification of treatment eligibility among patients with COVID-19. *JAMA Intern Med.* 2022;182(7):730–738. doi:10.1001/jamainternmed.2022.1906

103. Pappal RD, Roberts BW, Mohr NM, et al. The ED-AWARENESS study: A prospective, observational cohort study of awareness with paralysis in mechanically ventilated patients admitted from the emergency department. *Ann Emerg Med.* 2021;77(5):532–544. doi:10.1016/j.annemergmed.2020.10.012

104. Driver BE, Prekker ME, Wagner E, et al. Recall of awareness during paralysis among ED patients undergoing tracheal intubation. *Chest.* 2022. doi:10.1016/j.chest.2022.08.2232

105. Ender V, Leisten D, Zheng H, et al. Postintubation sedation after a formulary change from succinylcholine to rocuronium in a critical care transport organization. *Air Med J.* 2022;41(3):287–291. doi:10.1016/j.amj.2022.02.009

13

Mechanical Ventilation

ERIC BAUER

COMPETENCIES

1. State and describe the different modes of ventilation in transport.
2. Describe the different settings and effects of patient outcomes.
3. Discuss the importance of proper management of patients with adult respiratory distress (ARDS).
4. State the indications for noninvasive ventilation and management of oxygenation and ventilation in this mode.
5. Perform oxygenation calculations.

The air medical and critical care transport community has moved mountains in the past decade in advancing education to meet the rigors of an ever-changing landscape. This landscape would demonstrate a convergence of new evidence-based research, new technologies, new industry-wide accreditation standards, system-wide acceptance of free open-access medical education (FOAMed), and a generation that seeks to think differently. These collective efforts have propelled the critical care transport community forward more in the past 10 years than ever. Gone are the days of ventilating patients in the critical care environment with a bag-valve-mask (BVM). The decision is not based on whether one should use a mechanical ventilator but on how mechanical ventilation will assist in providing the highest quality care for the patient. It is then essential to have an in-depth understanding of transport ventilation and its application in the vast areas of the ever-changing world of critical care (Table 13.1).

Ventilator-Induced Lung Injury

Ventilator-induced lung injury (VILI) is damage inflicted on the lung directly from mechanical ventilation. Patients with acute lung injury (ALI), adult respiratory distress syndrome (ARDS), chronic obstructive pulmonary disease (COPD), and asthma are particularly prone to VILI associated with high transpulmonary pressures, high tidal volume (Vt), and cyclic atelectasis which compounds the difficulty in ventilation management. *Transpulmonary pressure* is the pressure difference across the lung calculated by subtracting the pleural pressure from the alveolar pressure. Alveolar pressure is most closely approximated in ventilated patients by the end-inspiratory plateau pressure (Pplat). The Pplat is believed to be a better indicator of alveolar overdistention than the peak inspiratory pressure (PIP) because it is not influenced by upper airway resistance or ventilator equipment.[1,2] The transport team measures the Pplat by performing an inspiratory hold maneuver. It is essential to point out that the methods for obtaining the Pplat measurement will vary based on the

ventilator manufacturer. Goal Pplat is less than 30 cm H_2O. Pplat can only be measured in volume-cycled modes; Pplat cannot be measured in pressure-limited modes. It is essential to know that the patient's Pplat will always be the lower pressure compared with the PIP. When using a ventilator that only delivers a pressure-limited breath, the provider can use the PIP as a surrogate for Pplat. With that in mind, the provider must use industry standards and current recommendations for upper-limit trending, with a PIP of less than or equal to 35 cm H_2O as a stopping point. As highlighted above, the PIP will always be the higher of the two pressures. Using PIP as a surrogate, the program guidelines can be tailored to limit PIP to less than or equal to 30 cm H_2O for alveolar pressure protection. Keep in mind, a PIP of 30 cm H_2O is conservative, with a normal PIP maximum of 35 cm H_2O being standard. The consideration for a PIP of 30 cm H_2O would only be used as a surrogate of Pplat within a pressure-limited breath type. If using a volume breath, the Pplat should be evaluated once the patient is placed on the mechanical ventilator and trended every 10 to 15 minutes or based on the patient's presentation. Lastly, the patient must be well sedated to get an accurate Pplat. If the patient actively attempts to breathe during the inspiratory hold maneuver, it will result in an erroneous reading.

Barotrauma

Barotrauma is damage to lung tissue that causes alveolar rupture and air migration into the extrapulmonary space. Historically, this has been attributed to high airway pressure. In a retrospective study of patients enrolled in the ARDS Network trial of low Vt ventilation, mean airway pressure (MAP) and Pplat were not predictive indicators of barotrauma.[1,2] However, it has been shown that barotrauma may lead to pneumothorax, tension pneumothorax, pneumomediastinum, pneumopericardium, pneumoperitoneum, subcutaneous emphysema, and air embolus (rare). Whether high PIPs are a direct cause of barotrauma or just a marker of severe lung disease is not clear.[1]

209

TABLE 13.1	Terminology Related to Mechanical Ventilation
Term	**Definition**
ARDS – Berlin definition	Differentiated by a PaO_2/FiO_2 ratio Mild: 200 mm Hg $<$ PaO_2/FiO_2 $\leq$300 mm Hg with PEEP or CPAP $\geq$5 cm H_2O Moderate: 100 mm Hg $<$ PaO_2/FiO_2 $\leq$200 mm Hg with PEEP $\geq$5 cm H_2O Severe: PaO_2/FiO_2 $\leq$100 mm Hg with PEEP $\geq$5 cm H_2O
Asynchrony	Incongruity between patient's respiratory effort and ventilator breath delivery; increases work of breathing
Auto-PEEP	Gas trapped in alveoli at the end of expiration caused by insufficient expiration time, bronchospasm, or mucous plugging; causes dynamic alveolar hyperinflation and increases work of breathing; also referred to as intrinsic PEEP
Barotrauma	Damage to lung tissue from high airway pressures; alveolar rupture may lead to pneumothorax, pulmonary interstitial edema, and pneumomediastinum
Cyclic atelectasis	Repeated opening of alveoli on inspiration and collapsing on expiration
Derecruitment	The collapse of open alveoli
Dynamic alveolar hyperinflation	Increase in lung volume at the end of expiration caused by incomplete exhalation
Extrinsic PEEP	Mechanical application of PEEP (see PEEP)
FiO_2	Fraction of inspired oxygen; ranges from 0.21 (21%) to 1.0 (100%); normal ambient air FiO_2 is 0.21
FRC	The volume of air remaining in the lungs at the end of normal expiration
IBW	Expected weight of person based on gender and height; used to base targeted Vt in the adult population
Male	IBW = 50 kg + 2.3 kg for each inch over 5 feet
Female	IBW = 45.5 kg + 2.3 kg for each inch over 5 feet
I:E ratio	Inspiratory to expiratory ratio. In normal conditions, the expiratory phase is passive and twice as long as the active inspiratory phase (1:2)
Inspiratory flow	The rate at which the breath is delivered on the ventilator, measured in liters per minute; the higher the flow, the faster the breath is delivered; flow is equal to Vt divided by inspiratory time
Intrinsic PEEP	See auto-PEEP
P_{aw}	Average pressure to which lungs are exposed over one inspiratory/expiratory cycle
PaO_2/FiO_2 ratio	The calculation used to quantify the degree of hypoxemia and oxygenation abnormality in patients with acute respiratory failure; PaO_2 derived from arterial blood gas is divided by the fraction of inspired oxygen (normal is 500); patients with ALI are at $<$300, and patients with ARDS are at $<$200; the lower the number, the greater the degree of pulmonary abnormality; for example, a patient on 60% FiO_2 has a PaO_2 of 70 mm Hg (70/0.6 = 116)
PEEP	Positive pressure is maintained at the end of expiration; therapy is used in mechanical ventilation to increase the volume of gas remaining in the lungs at the end of expiration (FRC)
Permissive hypercapnia	Lung-protective ventilation strategy that uses low Vt or lower rates to reduce lung injury associated with high volumes and alveolar overdistension; carbon dioxide is allowed to rise as a consequence
PIP	Measurement in lungs at the peak of inspiration
Plateau pressure	The pressure exerted on small airways and alveoli; measured by holding inspiratory pause during ventilator delivered inspiration; plateau pressures $>$30 mm Hg have been associated with alveolar overdistension lung injury
Recruitment	Refers to the opening of collapsed alveoli; alveolar recruitment maneuvers refer to increasing PEEP for short durations to open collapsed alveoli and improve oxygenation; the level of PEEP, duration, and frequency of this maneuver is determined by the transport team
tI	Time over which Vt is delivered or pressure maintained (depending on mode); set as I:E ratio or inspiratory flow
Tidal volume	The volume of gas inspired or expired in one breath
Trigger – sensitivity	The measure of the amount of negative pressure or inspiratory flow that must be generated by the patient to trigger the mechanical ventilator into the inspiratory phase
VE	The volume of air that moves in and out of the lungs in 1 minute, which is the product of tidal volume and respiratory rate: VE = Vt $\times$ R
Vte	Exhaled tidal volume; measured by the mechanical ventilator after each breath cycle
High V/Q ratio	High V/Q = dead space ventilation; alveoli are ventilated, but perfusion to lungs is impaired; examples are pulmonary embolus and hypotension
Low V/Q ratio	Low V/Q = shunt ventilation; alveoli are perfused, but there is impaired aeration; examples are ARDS and pneumonia
Volutrauma	Volume-related overdistension injury of alveoli inflicted by mechanical ventilation

ALI, Acute lung injury; *ARDS*, acute respiratory distress syndrome; *CXR*, chest x-ray; *FiO₂*, fraction of inspired oxygen; *FRC*, functional residual capacity; *IBW*, ideal body weight; *I:E*, ratio of inspiratory time to expiratory time; *MV*, minute ventilation; *P_aw*, mean airway pressure; *PEEP*, positive end-expiratory pressure; *PIP*, peak inspiratory pressure; *R*, rate; *tI*, inspiratory time; *VE*, minute ventilation; *V/Q*, ventilation/perfusion ratio; *Vt*, tidal volume; *Vte*, exhaled tidal volume.

Volutrauma

In years past, patients were ventilated with Vt ranges between 10 and 15 mL/kg. This was based on the idea that larger Vt would prevent atelectasis. In 1994 a group of researchers came together and established the ARDS Network. Their landmark study, published in May 2000, proved that lower Vt led to a decrease in mortality and established a new norm for mechanical ventilation: Vt of 6 to 8 mL/kg of ideal body weight (IBW). Based on this study and later studies on this subject, we now know that the use of lower Vt strategies (more specifically 6 mL/kg IBW) helps to limit the pulmonary damage during ARDS. The question now is: should we be using this strategy in all mechanically ventilated patients? Anatomically speaking, it makes sense. We know that the standard physiologic Vt for humans is approximately 6 mL/kg IBW. This does not mean that one size fits all, with each patient needing evaluation for the right Vt approach. With that in mind, attention has been placed on ventilator-induced injury caused by high volumes and *alveolar overdistension*, also referred to as *dynamic hyperinflation*. The stretch of alveoli causes microvascular injury, high permeability pulmonary edema, accumulation of fluid in the interstitial and alveolar space, disruption of surfactant function, and alveolar collapse.[3] Ongoing monitoring and controlling the Pplat is one strategy used to prevent or minimize the excessive alveolar stretch associated with VILI. The ARDS Network study demonstrated that maintenance of the Pplat at or less than 30 cm H_2O was associated with a statistically significant decrease in ventilator days and improved mortality rates.[4]

Cyclic Atelectasis

Cyclic atelectasis is the opening of alveoli on inspiration and collapsing on expiration. Animal models have shown that this repeated opening and closing causes the release of cytokines and the development of local and systemic inflammatory response, further extending lung injury.[5] positive end-expiratory pressure (PEEP) should be used to curtail the cyclic open and closing of lung units, particularly in low Vt strategies. It is important to remember that Vt is the key to alveolar recruitment. PEEP is needed to maintain alveolar recruitment during the exhalation process. Alveoli that suffer from repeated cyclic opening and closing will eventually not reinflate, and atelectasis trauma ensues.

Oxygen Toxicity

High levels of oxygen over a prolonged period of time have been shown to produce cytotoxic effects, presumably as the result of free radical production.[1,3] How this relates to the clinical care of patients with acute respiratory failure is still being researched. It is thought that the causes of pulmonary atelectasis stem from three different mechanisms: airway closure resulting from the reduced functional residual capacity (FRC), mechanical lung compression, and absorptive atelectasis, respectively. The pathophysiology behind this phenomenon is related to the high concentrations of oxygen.

Absorptive Atelectasis

During normal breathing, atmospheric air is made up of multiple gases, primarily nitrogen at 78% and oxygen at 21%. Nitrogen and oxygen are both very close in size, with oxygen having a larger molecular size and molecular weight. Nitrogen has a molecular weight of 28, with oxygen having a larger molecular weight of 32. Nitrogen, despite being a larger molecule overall, does not diffuse as well as oxygen. Why? It comes down to the electronic signature of the molecules. Every molecule has a diffuse "cloud" surrounding the nuclei of the atoms in the molecule. The simple fact is that the electron cloud around the oxygen nuclei in the O_2 molecule is smaller and more compact in size due to attractive electrostatic interactions between the electrons and proton in its nucleus. To compare Nitrogen and Oxygen from that standpoint, each oxygen atom has eight protons in its nucleus, while each nitrogen atom has only seven protons in its nucleus. Thus, the overall size and shape of the electron cloud of the O_2 molecule are smaller than that of nitrogen because of the greater positive charge on the nuclei that brings the electron cloud inward. Think of this as a tighter force toward the center, causing the size to be smaller.

As stated above, nitrogen makes up 78% of atmospheric air but is chemically inert in our bodies. It plays no role in breathing. We all have nitrogen gas dissolved in our blood and tissues. Nitrogen has a partial pressure (760 mm Hg) at sea level of 593 mm Hg [(0.78)(760)] = 593 mm Hg. Once we take a breath and equilibrium is reached, there is no net change in the partial pressure of nitrogen in the alveoli of your lungs, 593 mm Hg in, 593 mm Hg out.

Oxygen (O_2) and carbon dioxide (CO_2) have reciprocal roles in gas exchange within the lung: inhaled atmospheric oxygen is partly absorbed into the venous blood, which is deficient in oxygen and has a partial pressure of 40 mm Hg. Meanwhile, carbon dioxide, which is absent from inhaled gas, comes out of venous blood to enter the gas exchange phase inside the lung's alveoli, in an amount that roughly replaces. Oxygen and carbon dioxide gases move along concentration gradients by passive diffusion to move into or out of blood, i.e., gas exchange. In the case of nitrogen, there is no gradient to drive diffusion. The nitrogen stays behind because the partial pressures in a normal environment are equal.[6] The nitrogen creates some pressure (partial pressure based on Dalton's Law) in the alveoli, but we would be wrong to label this as an "intrinsic peep."

When we start administering supplemental oxygen, less nitrogen is inhaled. For example, if we administered 50% oxygen, there is still approximately 50% nitrogen in inhaled air. But, if we increase oxygen concentrations greater than 50%, oxygen replaces nitrogen as the primary gas in the lungs. The term for this is nitrogen washout. The partial pressure of oxygen is now higher than that of nitrogen, thus causing a diffusion gradient.

Administration of 100% oxygen to patients is reasonable during emergencies and resuscitation but should be weaned down during transport if the patient's oxygen saturations allow. Life-threatening hypoxia should always be treated with 100% oxygen delivered via facemask, endotracheal tube (ETT), or tracheotomy. Some patients may be more susceptible to high levels of oxygen; for example, preterm neonates are at risk for long-term retinal damage and bronchopulmonary dysplasia (BPD). Also susceptible are children with congenital cyanotic and partially repaired cyanotic-heart lesions who are at risk of hemodynamic instability as a result of oxygen-induced excess pulmonary blood flow.[7,8] The Neonatal Resuscitation Program (NRP) guidelines have recommended preductal oxygen saturation parameters beginning at 1 minute after birth and going to 10 minutes, with 1-minute preductal oxygen saturation goals of 60% to 65% and a 10-minute goal of 85% to 95%.[9] Treating neonates with supplemental oxygen should only occur if their preductal oxygen saturation is less than the recommended parameters from NRP and should only be treated until their oxygen saturations reach the recommended levels based on minutes since birth. Any neonate with bradycardia (heart rate less than 100 beats per minute) despite the oxygen saturation, will be treated with positive pressure ventilation and 100% supplemental oxygen. During neonatal resuscitation, a neonate having an appropriate heart rate but low oxygen saturation despite oxygen administration at high concentrations, with no correlating increase in oxygen saturation, suggests an undiagnosed congenital heart defect. If that is the case, the standard approach within neonatal guidelines is to reduce oxygen concentrations to 30% and continue resuscitation with the assumption of an undiagnosed congenital heart defect.[8]

Ventilator Settings

Selection of ventilator mode and settings are determined by clinical assessment, degree of alteration in oxygenation or ventilation, disease pathophysiology, institutional or physician preference, and capabilities of the transport ventilator.

Tidal Volume

Tidal volume is set in volume-cycled ventilation modes. To reduce the likelihood of alveolar overdistension and high airway pressures, Vt should be based on IBW rather than actual body weight in adult patients.

In light of the study outcomes, Vt should be initiated at 6 mL/kg IBW in patients with ARDS/ALI.[10] Adjust the respiratory rate to achieve the desired partial pressure of carbon dioxide in arterial blood ($PaCO_2$) or pH. Low Vt ventilation often requires acceptance of a degree of respiratory acidosis (permissive hypercapnia), which is discussed in more depth in the section, "Ventilation Strategies."

Patients with obstructive diseases, such as COPD and asthma, benefit from lower Vt of 6 to 8 mL/kg IBW to reduce lung inflation and extend exhalation time. In most other patients, using a Vt greater than 8 mL/kg is rarely necessary (and may be harmful), and a starting Vt of 6 to 8 mL/kg with subsequent ventilator adjustments to meet the pH and $PaCO_2$ targets are reasonable.[10]

Rate, Breaths per Minute, and Frequency

During the initial selection of the rate, consider the patient's age (newborn, pediatric, and adult), minute ventilation, and Vt. *Minute ventilation*, or minute volume, is equal to the respiratory rate multiplied by the tidal volume (Vt × R), with a normal range of 4 to 8 L/min. In the neonate, VE requirement will be in the range of 0.2 to 0.3 L/min/kg. Adjustments to the rate depend on the clinical goal and disease process to meet the desired pH or $PaCO_2$ range. Historically, when Vt of 10 to 12 mL/kg were used, ventilator rates of 12 breaths/min were common for adults. However, with Vt now appropriately set at 6 to 8 mL/kg of IBW, initial rates of 14 to 16 breaths/min are more appropriate. Pediatric rates often range from 20 to 30 breaths/min, depending on the age of the child. Generally, increasing the rate decreases the $PaCO_2$ and increases the pH. Conversely, decreasing the rate increases the $PaCO_2$ and decreases the pH. With assisted ventilation modes in spontaneously breathing patients, care must be taken to monitor for hyperventilation and auto-PEEP.

The frequency is the total sum of mandatory breaths and patient-triggered breaths combined. Respiratory rate and frequency are often mislabeled or referenced and need to be reflected correctly when evaluating the patient. Looking at an overall frequency can give insight into correct sensitivity (*trigger*) settings, sedation status, metabolic activity, and overall patient comfort. Frequency should also be evaluated to calculate overall minute ventilation, which includes patient-triggered breaths. Overall evaluation of frequency can give the transport team ongoing information that will help guide pharmacologic decisions for ongoing sedation and pain management.

Minute Ventilation

Minute ventilation (VE) can be defined as Vt × RR. For an adult patient, the resting physiologic norm for VE is 4 to 8 L/min, which matches the normal cardiac output requirement range of 4 to 8 L/min. In contrast, neonates have a VE requirement in the range of 0.2 to 0.3 L/min/kg and a higher cardiac output requirement compared to the adult patients.[11] The normal physiological norm for VE requirements can be simplified based on a per person, per minute requirement. The average person produces approximately 60 mL/kg/min of VE, with a patient intubated and being mechanically ventilated needing an increase to approximately 100 mL/kg/min on average. The transport team should maintain consistent assessment to ensure the VE requirements for the patient being mechanically ventilated are met.

Dead Space

Dead space is the amount of volume loss that does not reach the alveolar level during each mechanically delivered breath. It is measured in milliliters (mL) and is lost in multiple areas. Dead space can be separated into two segments, with anatomical dead space being a product of volume lost within the upper airways, chest, bronchioles, and lung units. The second form of dead space is called mechanical dead space and reflects the loss in volume within the ventilator circuit, ETT, viral filters, $EtCO_2$, or suction devices. It is essential to understand the impact of dead space on minute ventilation (VE) and how to account for any reduction in VE resulting from each form. We are reminded that VE requirements are between 4 and 8 L/min for adults and pediatrics. However, we need to understand that when delivering a breath via the ventilator, all that volume does not reach the alveolar-capillary membrane for gas exchange leading to hypoventilation and hypercapnia. The key concept here is identifying actual alveolar minute ventilation and not just overall minute ventilation delivered by the ventilator.

Anatomical dead space is the product of the loss of gas within the upper airways, chest, bronchioles, and lung units. There are two ways to calculate anatomical dead space. The textbook answer is to calculate this by using 1 mL/1 pound of IBW; for an average adult patient, that is approximately 150 mL per breath. However, with anyone under 70 kg or 150 pounds, it is best to use the 1 mL/1 pound of IBW formula. Anatomical dead space impacts alveolar minute ventilation, which is what counts for gas exchange. If the transport team has a preset Vt of 480 mL using 6 mL/kg (80 kg IBW), the VE target would be 8 L/min using 100 mL/kg/min for any intubated patients baseline VE requirement (80 kg × 100 mL).[1] To identify the desired respiratory rate, the transport team divides the VE requirement for the patient by the calculated Vt. The target VE is 8 L/min. Convert 8 liters per minute to 8000 milliliters per minute (8 L to 8000 mL), to have like terms. Take the VE requirement and divide it by Vt (8000 mL/480 mL), which will give you a respiratory rate of 16 breaths per minute.

Now do the same thing to identify the impact of anatomical dead space and alveolar minute ventilation. Once the anatomical dead space (150 mL) is removed from the Vt of 480 mL using 6 mL/kg (80 kg IBW), Vt would be approximately 330 mL. The 330 mL must be the focus of your calculation for VE. What impact, positive or negative, will the reduced Vt have on overall VE? Using the same formula above but using reduced Vt as a result of the anatomical dead space loss, there is an increased need for respiratory rate. Using the target VE of 8 L or 8000 mL and Vt of 330 mL (8000 mL/330 mL), the respiratory rate requirement increased. Use clinical judgment and evaluate the exhaled tidal volume (Vte) to see what the loss is breath by breath. In most adult ventilation scenarios, the reduction in Vt seen breath to breath is not going to impact the patient negatively. However, each patient is different and should be evaluated as such. The math formula used above is the foundational way of breaking down minute ventilation and alveolar minute ventilation to identify the Vt and respiratory rate requirements to meet the patient's physiological requirements at a minimum. Keep in mind that the physiological requirements may be altered based on the underlying pathophysiology of the disease process, with higher VE requirements needed. Patients suffering from chronic COPD and acute pulmonary embolism will have a much greater anatomical dead space loss within each of the disease processes. Patients in severe acidemia with partially compensated metabolic acidosis at the core will require careful consideration for VE requirements that can be impacted negatively by anatomical dead space.

In the pediatric population, anatomical and mechanical dead space can have a huge impact on VE as well; with the smaller VE and Vt requirement, pediatric patients can see a larger impact on delivered Vt and VE overall. Mechanical dead space is the core area of focus with the pediatric population specifically. Adult patients notwithstanding, pediatrics have a smaller Vt and VE delivery requirement, and the margin for error is much smaller.

Mechanical dead space is the loss of volume in the ventilator circuit, ETT, viral filters, $EtCO_2$, or suction devices. Breaking each of these areas down is essential because of how each impacts the VE differently. First, mechanical dead space loss within the ventilator circuit is only a factor within volume ventilation scenarios. Compliance loss within the ventilator circuit because of PIP will impact the volume moving down the circuit. If higher PIP exists, the expansion within the circuit increases resulting in lost volume that doesn't reach the patient's ETT. The higher the PIP, the more mechanical dead space loss realized, which is one reason it is recommended to use pressure-limited ventilation in pediatrics. If a pediatric patient has a Vt requirement of 60 mL, hypothetically, the transport team could ventilate the child with volume ventilation. If the transport team's ventilator is both volume-cycled and pressure-limited (Vyaire ReVel®, Vyaire LTV 1200®, and Zoll EMV+®), it will deliver a volume down to 50 mL. It is often tempting to use volume on most patients because of the added simplicity of this manner of delivery. However, the transport team should use caution and understand the impacts of not only anatomical dead space but, most importantly, mechanical dead space. The transport team must not be late in recognizing the reduction in Vt from the preset Vt secondary to the mechanical dead space loss in the ventilator circuit and any ancillary devices put between the circuit and ETT. For interfacility pediatric transports, the transport team must also be aware of differences in mechanical dead space loss when switching from the hospital ventilator to the transport ventilator.

The rule of thumb to calculate mechanical dead space loss in the circuit while using volume-cycled ventilation is (2 mL × PIP) for adult ventilator circuits and (1 mL × PIP) for pediatric ventilator circuits. If a pediatric patient had a Vt requirement of 60 mL and a current PIP of 25 cm H_2O, the mechanical dead space loss is approximately 25 mL.[1] Meaning the delivered Vt secondary to the 25 mL mechanical dead space loss is only 35 mL. Consideration for additional mechanical dead space loss with the ancillary devices such as viral filters (90 mL/min), heat moisture exchange devices (HME) (30 mL/min), and $EtCO_2$ (50 mL/min), to name a few, can impact Vt and overall VE even more. The devices listed are not all-encompassing and do not reflect each specific manufacturer or patient demographic. Some will have a larger loss, and some will have smaller losses. It is important to know your equipment and plan accordingly.

Mechanical dead space loss is significantly reduced when the transport team uses pressure-limited ventilation methods. The difference is seen in how the mechanical ventilator measures the breath or target pressure. In pressure-limited ventilation, the ventilator targets a preset inspiratory pressure and measures the target pressure at the flow sensor. This means that any compliance loss prior to the flow sensor is accounted for and not a factor because pressure-limited ventilation is based on a compliance-volume relationship. Adjustments in the inspiratory pressure up or down impact Vt up or down. This, however, does not impact mechanical dead space within the circuit because of where the target pressure is measured. The only impact on the patient while using pressure-limited ventilation will be the ancillary devices placed after the flow sensor and between the distal end of the ventilator circuit and ETT. In the case example from above, this would reduce mechanical dead space in the pediatric patient by 25 mL at a minimum if using pressure-limited versus volume-control ventilation.

Exhaled Tidal Volume

Exhaled tidal volume is a monitored parameter on any ventilator that gives you a second-by-second account of chest wall compliance and volume delivered compared to the volume received. Standard teaching says a +/− 50 mL variation from the delivered Vt and measured Vte may exist. Verify the patient has adequate chest wall compliance; poor Vte compared to Vt suggests impending poor compliance or possible leak. As highlighted in the section on dead space, any difference in the delivered Vt and Vte should be evaluated for mechanical and anatomical dead space loss. Additional assessment advantages with Vte surround evaluation of leak, specifically ETT cuff leak.

During pressure-limited ventilation, the Vte will be used to identify whether the delivered volume meets the physiological needs of the patient as per initial calculations using IBW, gender, and disease presentation. The Vte will be used as a surrogate because there is no preset Vt when using pressure-limited ventilation. Because pressure-limited ventilation is compliance-based and each breath will have a variation, the Vte is the only parameter the transport team can use to see if the preset inspiratory pressure is generating the Vt that is required.

Peak Inspiratory Pressure

PIP is set in pressure-targeted modes. When initiating pressure-control ventilation, the target pressure should initially be set to give the patient a measured exhaled Vt of 6 to 8 mL/kg IBW, with peak pressures of 16 to 24 cm H_2O commonly required. As stated previously, Vt and minute ventilation are not static, but they change dynamically with lung compliance, which warrants ongoing monitoring.

In volume-cycled modes, PIP is a dynamic value reflective of a combination of patient and ventilator variables. Vt, PEEP, and inspiratory time are ventilator settings that contribute to inspiratory pressures. On some ventilators, inspiratory time is not a set parameter but is determined by the set respiratory rate and the ratio of inspiratory time to expiratory time (I:E ratio). PIP increases or decreases as lung compliance worsens or improves.

Plateau Pressure

Plateau pressure (Pplat) is a pressure that is reflective of the pressure applied to the small airways and alveoli at the end of inspiration. The Pplat represents the alveolar pressure based on the elastic recoil of the respiratory system. The transport team can only measure the Pplat in a volume breath; it cannot be measured in pressure-targeted modes. The Pplat will always be measured at the end of the inspiratory phase by performing an inspiratory hold for 0.5/sec.

As discussed in the Vt section, controlling the Pplat is one strategy to prevent or minimize the excessive alveolar stretch associated with VILI. The ARDS Network study demonstrated that maintenance of the Pplat at or less than 30 cm H_2O was associated with a statistically significant decrease in ventilator days and improved mortality rates.[4] The ARDS Network ventilation protocols set a goal Pplat of less than 30 cm H_2O and recommend it be checked after each change in PEEP or Vt. Some controversy exists regarding the need to reduce Vt if the Pplat is greater than 30 cm H_2O; however, a secondary analysis of the ARDS Network trial suggested that a beneficial effect was seen in Vt reduction from 12 mL/kg IBW to 6 mL/kg, regardless of the Pplat before Vt was reduced.[3] In the case of a high Pplat greater than 30 cm H_2O, the transport team needs to take steps to reduce the Pplat to less than 30 cm H_2O. Pplat management strategies include:

1. Identify the pathophysiology behind the potential high Pplat. Attempt to correct problems, i.e., pneumothorax, tension pneumothorax, gastric distension (via orogastric/nasogastric tube placement).
2. Reduce the patient's Vt to the lower levels of the lung-protective strategy. The volume will cause transiently high alveolar pressures. Lowering the Vt in 1-mL/kg increments until the Pplat is less than 30 cm H_2O or 4 mL/kg is reached is the ultimate goal. At this point, the provider starts sacrificing volume and overall minute ventilation. In addition, while lowering the Vt to achieve the desired Pplat of less than 30 cm H_2O, the same minute ventilation needs to be maintained. This requires increasing the respiratory rate to match the starting minute ventilation if possible. Always keep in mind the impact of increasing the respiratory rate will have on anatomical dead space loss, which could impact hemodynamic status. It comes down to which will cause more harm and how we can overcome one versus the other. Alveolar damage can be profound, and hemodynamic status and treating the patient can easily be accomplished with pharmacological intervention. Additionally, a certain degree of elevation in the arterial $PaCO_2$ level is acceptable while attempting to maintain a pH greater than 7.30. Refer to the ARDS.net protocol card that shows the recommendations from the May 2000 study (Fig. 13.1).

Driving Pressure

Driving pressure is the difference between Vt and static compliance. Driving pressure equals the (Pplat – PEEP). This takes our Pplat goal of <30 cm H_2O and really throws it out the window. Example: Your patient has a current Pplat 25 cm H_2O and PEEP 5 cm H_2O. This would be a driving pressure of 20 cm H_2O. This is significant in ALI or ARDS patients. We need to either lower our Pplat or increase our PEEP. To lower our Pplat, we lower our Vt. We can lower our Vt down to 4 mL/kg and evaluate our Pplat with each 1 mL/kg drop in Vt. We can also bring down our driving pressure by increasing our PEEP. In the end, this theory is only applicable to those ALI and ARDS patients. In a normal healthy lung, there is no set driving pressure. We all have different driving pressures and shouldn't worry about this for other nonlung-injured patients.

Fractional Concentration of Oxygen in Inspired Gas

The fractional concentration of oxygen in inspired gas (FiO_2) is the percentage of oxygen given through different devices within patient care. If the partial pressure of oxygen in arterial blood (PaO_2) is unknown, the (FiO_2) is typically set at 100% on initiation of mechanical ventilation but should be reduced as soon as possible and as tolerated by PaO_2 or pulse oximetry. FiO_2 is used in combination with PEEP to maintain the PaO_2 or peripheral oxygen saturation (SpO_2) above the minimum threshold. The oxygenation goals set by the ARDS Network for patients with ALI/ARDS are PaO_2 of 55 to 80 mm Hg or SpO_2 of 88% to 95%.[4,12] The Brain Trauma Foundation recommends that PaO_2 be maintained at more than 60 mm Hg or SpO_2 at more than 90% in patients with TBIs.[2,12] The American Heart Association recommends supplemental oxygen to maintain SpO_2 greater than 90%.[3] If high levels of FiO_2 do not reverse hypoxia, then PEEP can be added incrementally to achieve oxygenation goals. The FiO_2 selections may be limited by the transport ventilator's blending or air entrainment capabilities.

Positive End-Expiratory Pressure

PEEP exerts pressure in the patient's airway above the atmospheric level throughout the respiratory cycle, increasing the FRC by opening collapsed alveoli. The FRC is the air that remains in the lungs at the end of passive expiration; it is reduced with the loss of chest wall mobility (obesity) or lung compliance.[1,13] The increase in FRC through the addition of PEEP is referred to as *recruitment* and decreases intrapulmonary shunting of blood through lung regions with collapsed alveoli, improving ventilation-to-perfusion ratio matching. The ideal PEEP setting prevents cyclic atelectasis and overdistension injury while optimizing oxygenation. When possible, the overall goal should be to use the lowest PEEP setting necessary to acquire an acceptable PaO_2 with an FiO_2 of less than 0.60. Most patients benefit from the addition of 5 cm H_2O PEEP to overcome the decrease in FRC as a result of the airway resistance caused by the ETT. Unless otherwise indicated, initial ventilator settings should include a PEEP of 5 cm H_2O.

In several circumstances, PEEP should be used with caution because it increases intrathoracic pressure, reducing venous return and preload. However, it has been shown that it may be better to apply more PEEP and reduce FiO_2 in an attempt to optimize oxygenation and, at the same time, limit the oxygen toxicity potential.[1,10,13] In addition, many patients may suffer from refractory hypoxia and require the added PEEP. In these cases, it may be necessary to augment the additional PEEP with vasopressors in order to ensure optimal oxygenation and mean arterial pressure can be achieved.

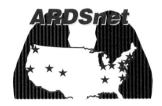

NIH NHLBI ARDS Clinical Network
Mechanical Ventilation Protocol Summary

INCLUSION CRITERIA: Acute onset of
1. PaO_2/FiO_2 ≤300 (corrected for altitude)
2. Bilateral (patchy, diffuse, or homogeneous) infiltrates consistent with pulmonary edema
3. No clinical evidence of left atrial hypertension

PART I: VENTILATOR SETUP AND ADJUSTMENT
1. Calculate predicted body weight (PBW)
   Males = 50 + 2.3 [height (inches) - 60]
   Females = 45.5 + 2.3 [height (inches) -60]
2. Select any ventilator mode
3. Set ventilator settings to achieve initial V_T = 8 ml/kg PBW
4. Reduce V_T by 1 ml/kg at intervals ≤2 hours until V_T = 6ml/kg PBW.
5. Set initial rate to approximate baseline minute ventilation (not >35 bpm).
6. Adjust V_T and RR to achieve pH and plateau pressure goals below.

pH GOAL: 7.30–7.45
Acidosis Management: (pH <7.30)
If pH 7.15–7.30: Increase RR until pH >7.30 or $PaCO_2$ <25 (Maximum set RR = 35).

If pH <7.15: Increase RR to 35.
If pH remains <7.15, V_T may be increased in 1 ml/kg steps until pH >7.15 (Pplat target of 30 may be exceeded).
May give $NaHCO_3$
Alkalosis Management: (pH >7.45) Decrease vent rate if possible.

I: E RATIO GOAL: Recommend that duration of inspiration be ≤ duration of expiration.

PART II: WEANING
A. **Conduct a SPONTANEOUS BREATHING TRIAL daily when:**
   1. FiO_2 ≤0.40 and PEEP ≤8 OR FiO_2 ≤0.50 and PEEP ≤5.
   2. PEEP and FiO_2 ≤ values of previous day.
   3. Patient has acceptable spontaneous breathing efforts. (May decrease vent rate by 50% for 5 minutes to detect effort.)
   4. Systolic BP ≥90 mmHg without vasopressor support.
   5. No neuromuscular blocking agents or blockade.

OXYGENATION GOAL: PaO_2 55–80 mmHg or SpO_2 88–95%
Use a minimum PEEP of 5 cm H_2O. Consider use of incremental FiO_2/PEEP combinations such as shown below (not required) to achieve goal.

Lower PEEP/higher FiO2

FiO2	0.3	0.4	0.4	0.5	0.5	0.6	0.7	0.7
PEEP	5	5	8	8	10	10	10	12

FiO2	0.7	0.8	0.9	0.9	0.9	1.0
PEEP	14	14	14	16	18	18–24

Higher PEEP/lower FiO2

FiO2	0.3	0.3	0.3	0.3	0.3	0.4	0.4	0.5
PEEP	5	8	10	12	14	14	16	16

FiO2	0.5	0.5–0.8	0.8	0.9	1.0	1.0
PEEP	18	20	22	22	22	24

PLATEAU PRESSURE GOAL: ≤30 cm H_2O
Check Pplat (0.5 second inspiratory pause), at least q 4h and after each change in PEEP or V_T.
If Pplat >30 cm H_2O: decrease V_T by 1ml/kg steps (minimum = 4 ml/kg).
If Pplat <25 cm H_2O and V_T <6 ml/kg, increase V_T by 1 ml/kg until Pplat >25 cm H_2O or V_T = 6 ml/kg.
If Pplat <30 and breath stacking or dys-synchrony occurs: may increase V_T in 1ml/kg increments to 7 or 8 ml/kg if Pplat remains ≤30 cm H_2O.

B. **SPONTANEOUS BREATHING TRIAL (SBT):**
If all above criteria are met and subject has been in the study for at least 12 hours, initiate a trial of UP TO 120 minutes of spontaneous breathing with FiO_2 ≤0.5 and PEEP ≤5:
   1. Place on T-piece, trach collar, or CPAP ≤5 cm H_2O with PS ≤5
   2. Assess for tolerance as below for up to two hours.
      a. SpO_2 ≥90: and/or PaO_2 ≥60 mmHg
      b. Spontaneous V_T ≥4 ml/kg PBW
      c. RR ≤35/min
      d. pH ≥7.3
      e. No respiratory distress (distress = 2 or more)
         ➤ HR >120% of baseline
         ➤ Marked accessory muscle use
         ➤ Abdominal paradox
         ➤ Diaphoresis
         ➤ Marked dyspnea
   3. If tolerated for at least 30 minutes, consider extubation.
   4. If not tolerated resume pre-weaning settings.

Definition of <u>UNASSISTED BREATHING</u>
(different from the spontaneous breathing criteria as PS is not allowed)

1. Extubated with face mask, nasal prong oxygen, or room air, OR
2. T-tube breathing, OR
3. Tracheostomy mask breathing, OR
4. CPAP less than or equal to 5 cm H_2O **without pressure support or IMV assistance.**

• **Figure 13.1** Mechanical ventilator protocol card. (From NIH-NHLBI ARDS Network.)

In patients with unilateral lung disease, preferential distribution of minute ventilation and PEEP may be directed to areas of healthy lung (least resistance) and do minimal for the injured or diseased lung. This can cause alveolar overdistension injury of healthy alveoli and compress the vasculature surrounding the alveoli, worsening the shunt.

Auto-PEEP

Auto-PEEP refers to air trapped in the alveoli at the end of expiration. Causes include high minute ventilation, mechanical expiratory flow limitation (foreign body obstruction and mucous plug), and physiological expiratory resistance (asthma and COPD).

Large Vt or high respiratory rates increase the minute ventilation and reduce exhalation time. A new breath is delivered before full exhalation occurs and traps air in the alveoli. Similarly, patient-generated rapid respiratory rates in assisted ventilator modes (Assist Control) caused by agitation, patient-ventilator asynchrony, or low sensitivity thresholds can lead to subsequent incomplete exhalation and auto-PEEP. Patients with obstructive lung disease are particularly vulnerable to air-trapping because of airway collapse or narrowing. Auto-PEEP can lead to hypotension, barotrauma, and increasing ventilator-patient asynchrony. Modern transport ventilators can measure auto-PEEP with an expiratory hold maneuver, so it should be monitored, and efforts made to minimize the occurrence, especially in asthma and COPD patients. If the patient develops clinically significant auto-PEEP or has lung hyperinflation to the point of potential decompensation, the transport provider needs to immediately disconnect the ventilator circuit from the patient's ETT and allow time for exhalation. Axial compression is also beneficial in aiding in complete exhalation. Once the exhalation has been completed (30–45 seconds), reapply the ventilator circuit and evaluate settings to optimize the time for exhalation.

Inspiratory Time

Inspiratory time is the time over which the Vt is delivered (volume delivery) or the pressure is maintained (pressure delivery), depending on the mode of delivery. By changing the I-time, the I:E ratio will change accordingly.

Inspiratory-to-Expiratory Time Ratio

Inspiratory-to-Expiratory Time Ratio (I:E Ratio) is the ratio between the inspiratory and expiratory time within a respiratory cycle. A respiratory cycle is the amount of time needed to fully inhale and exhale. We can calculate the respiratory cycle by dividing the respiratory rate into 60 seconds. Using a respiratory rate example of 14 breaths per minute (60/14) equals a respiratory cycle time of ~4.25 seconds. The normal I:E ratio is 1:2 or 1:3, depending on adult versus pediatric physiologic requirements. An increase in the flow rate, or how fast a breath is given, causes a decrease in the inspiratory time, which allows for a longer period of expiration. The I:E ratio may be adjusted for disease pathology. The inspiratory time can be adjusted directly on most transport ventilators. If there is no inspiratory time adjustment, the inspiratory flow rate, Vt, and respiratory rate can be used to affect the I:E ratio. Patients with reactive airway disease, or asthma, benefit from a longer expiratory time of 1:4 to 1:5 in many cases. However, have caution in putting all patients into silos: some reactive airway patients may benefit from a 1:1 I:E ratio as well. Patients with hypoxia may benefit from a longer inspiratory time, reflective of an inverse I:E ratio.

Flow Rate

For most adults, flow rates of 50 to 60 L/min are usually adequate, although a higher flow may be needed to produce adequate ventilation, particularly in patients with obstructive lung disease.[1,2] Some transport ventilators are not equipped with the ability to adjust the flow, and longer expiratory times are adjusted through the I:E ratio or inspiratory time settings. The flow limitations of some transport ventilators limit extension of the expiration time and shortening of the inspiration time. In this situation, an inadequate time for expiration in patients with obstructive disease may lead to auto-PEEP, high plateau pressures, overdistension, and barotrauma. Transport teams can overcome this to some extent by decreasing the Vt or respiratory rate. This decrease may require some degree of respiratory acidosis to prevent lung overdistension from air trapping. However, patients tend to do better being in a state of hypercapnia compared with hypocapnia, and the maintenance of mild respiratory acidosis may be warranted at times.

Flow Pattern

Some transport ventilators allow the transport team to select flow patterns, which dictate how an inspiratory flow is delivered. Flow pattern advantage depends on the patient's lung compliance, chest wall elasticity, airway resistance, and transport ventilator capability. Determination of which pattern optimizes ventilation-perfusion is not always predictable and is often an exercise of trial and error.[13,14]

Trigger Sensitivity

An assisted breath (assist-control ventilation, pressure-controlled ventilation (PCV), or pressure support ventilation) can be triggered by either pressure or flow. Most transport ventilators use a flow trigger as the primary trigger source. However, each ventilator is different, and every user should consult their manufacturer's guide for correct understanding and application of the trigger. *Flow triggering* detects a change in the flow of gas with spontaneous effort. A base (or bias) flow of gas continuously moves past the patient. When the patient makes an inspiratory effort, the ventilator detects a deviation in the flow, which triggers the ventilator to deliver a supported breath. A bias flow of 3 to 10 L/min is often used with a trigger sensitivity threshold of 2 L/min.[4] When the trigger is set at a specific level, it is setting a trigger in liters per minute (L/min) of the total bias flow. This total L/min can be reduced to its simplest form to understand how the ventilator uses this technology for triggering. If, for example, the trigger setting was set to a level of 5, the bias flow available for the flow trigger is 5 L/min. Converting 5 L/min to the lowest form means milliliters per second (mL/sec). First, convert 5 L to 5000 mL and 1 minute to 60 seconds. This allows simplification into a smaller number that makes sense; dividing 5000 mL/60s equals 83 mL/sec. This means that the patient's effort must change the speed of the flow by 83 mL. Essentially, a flow change is being recognized. This doesn't necessarily mean the patient is taking a breath of 83 mL. Can you drive 83 MPH without driving 83 miles? The answer is yes. The flow trigger is doing the same; the flow change is a speed change that allows the ventilator the ability to recognize the need for a mandatory breath (*AC*) or patient-triggered breath (synchronized intermittent mandatory ventilation [*SIMV*]). This same method also can be applied to any other sensitivity settings within the parameters of the manufacturer's capabilities. One negative to the transport ventilators being primarily flow-triggered stems from the low threshold for auto-triggering.[4] As the previous example illustrated, a sensitivity level of 5 allows a triggered breath with the patient producing a minimum effort of 83 mL/sec. By simply grabbing the ventilator circuit, the transport team can easily simulate this and cause an auto-triggered breath to be given if the ventilator is in the AC mode, for example. It is for this reason that the transport team should always start at a higher sensitivity level than in a normal stationary patient environment, with 5 being a good starting point.

Pressure triggering requires a demand valve that senses a negative airway pressure generated by the patient during the initiation of a spontaneous respiratory effort. The demand valve sensitivity is set at a level that allows the patient to easily take a breath but is not so sensitive that it interprets artifacts, such as patient movement, air leak, or water in the ventilator circuit, as an attempted breath. This could cause unintended hyperventilation, respiratory alkalosis, and auto-PEEP. If the sensitivity is set too high, the ventilator does not trigger a breath when the patient makes a spontaneous effort and increases the patient's work of breathing. The usual threshold is set at –2 to –3 cm H_2O in the transport environment. For example, the ReVel ventilator has a feature that allows transport team members to move from the standard default flow trigger to a pressure trigger by turning the trigger setting knob counterclockwise until "P" is seen. The ventilator is then in a pressure trigger mode, with a default trigger of –3 cm H_2O for an adult patient. This is a great feature and useful if difficulties arise in transport with auto-triggering in the standard flow trigger setting.[4] The Zoll EMV+® uses a pressure trigger as the only triggering source, with the same threshold of -0.5 to -6 cm H_2O available in the default settings for patient triggering. In contrast, the Hamilton T-1 ventilator is a 100% flow-triggered ventilator and has a wide flow trigger range of 0.5 to 20 L/min for adult patient settings. Within the neonatal software available on the Hamilton T-1, a range of 0.1 to 5 L/min is used. As you can see, the range is wide and specific to the age demographic.

Changing one ventilator parameter may affect other ventilator variables and should be reassessed after adjustments are made. For example, inspiratory time (tI) is equal to Vt divided by flow (tI = Vt/flow). Changing these parameters changes the other parameters. Likewise, on some ventilators, alteration in the FiO_2 may change the flow enough to alter the delivered Vt. Transport teams should be familiar with ventilator capabilities and limitations. Be aware of the parameters that are automatically adjusted by the ventilator to compensate for changes made by the user.

Rise Time

Rise time determines the rate at which the ventilator reaches a set target pressure while in pressure control, pressure support, pressure-regulated volume control, or even bilevel positive airway pressure (BiPAP) applications. Each ventilator has a different form of rise time and applies this function a little differently. Rise time is one of the least utilized adjustments made by respiratory therapists and physicians alike.

Rise time determines the rate at which the ventilator reaches a set target pressure during inspiration. The ventilator may provide rise time based on a percentage of the breath cycle or in fractions of a second. It does this by adjusting the inspiratory flow rate. While *inspiratory time* is the total time of inspiration, the *rise time* is the segment of inspiration from initiation to peak inspiratory flow. Once peak inspiratory flow is reached, flow is tapered during the remaining inspiratory time to maintain the set target pressure. Prolonged rise time causes the inspiratory flow to be decreased, resulting in a decreased Vt during pressure control ventilation and slower alveolar recruitment. The end result will be increased work of breathing and decreased patient comfort. Prolonged rise time would benefit patients with small ETT diameters because these patients need longer rise times (filling time) to allow for adequate tidal volumes. Additionally, obstructive lung patients requiring high flow rates and peak airway pressures (PIP) to generate enough volume will benefit by prolonging the rise time; this will

result in a reduction of inspiratory flow rates, which will reduce PIP. This is simply based on the compliance-volume relationship.

In contrast, faster rise times are often used in noninvasive positive pressure ventilation (NiPPV) patients, hypoxic air-starved patients, and patients requiring faster inspiratory times. It is important to point out that any rise time setting will need to fall inside the inspiratory time you have set. An example would be a patient with an inspiratory time of 0.5 seconds and a rise time that is lengthened to greater than 0.5/sec. This makes no sense and will not benefit the patient.

Classification of Positive Pressure Ventilation

No universal consensus exists on the classification of ventilators or ventilation modes, and descriptions vary within the literature. Understand your specific ventilator and the manufacturer-specific language that exists. The elements in classification that are most pertinent to transport teams are volume control ventilation, pressure control ventilation, NiPPV/BiPAP, and continuous positive airway pressure (CPAP). No research exists to suggest improved outcomes between volume-cycled and PCV strategies. Within these categories, ventilation modes can be described as mandatory, assisted, or spontaneous, depending on the dynamic necessary to initiate an inspiratory breath.

- *Mandatory:* Mandatory breaths are initiated, controlled (volume or pressure), and terminated by the ventilator. No synchronizing of the ventilator breaths occurs with patient-initiated breaths. Example: continuous mandatory ventilation (CMV).
- *Assisted:* Spontaneous breaths are initiated by the patient but controlled and ended (assisted) by the ventilator. Example: assist-control (AC).
- *Spontaneous:* Spontaneous breaths are initiated, controlled, and terminated by the patient. Example: CPAP.

In the sections below, we will discuss volume, pressure, pressure regulation, and modes of ventilation, with a focus on differentiating the manufacturer-specific differences. In an attempt to be thorough but target the most widely used ventilators on the market today, we will focus on the following ventilators: Hamilton T-1®, Vyaire ReVel®, Vyaire LTV 1200®, and Zoll Impact EMV+®. Keep in mind this list is not all-inclusive.

Volume Ventilation (Vyaire ReVel®, Vyaire LTV 1200®, and Zoll Impact EMV+®)

Volume-cycled pressure-variable ventilation (VC) is the most common mode of ventilation used on transport ventilators. The Vt is preset and delivered during the set inspiratory time of the ventilatory cycle. Once that Vt is reached, inspiration ends and exhalation begins. The inspiratory pressure varies depending on the compliance and resistance of the lungs, with higher pressures associated with greater lung resistance or low compliance. The advantage of this form of ventilation is the guarantee of minute ventilation (respiratory rate multiplied by the tidal volume, Vt × R). On the other hand, the potential for lung injury exists when high pressures are required to deliver the set Vt in patients with low lung compliance. To mitigate against ventilator-induced barotrauma or lung injury, pressure limits are set. If the high-pressure limit is reached during the delivery of the set Vt, the inspiration is terminated, even if the targeted Vt has not been achieved. This is an important parameter to understand within the realm of ventilation, but also with the specific manufacturing differences seen in the industry. Volume ventilation can be delivered using various modes of ventilation, with or without pressure support (PS), depending on the brand of the ventilator.

Ventilator-specific differences are important to point out. The manufacturer differences will dictate if the ventilator has the capability of delivering a true volume breath. The Vyaire ReVel®, Vyaire LTV 1200®, and Zoll Impact EMV+® can deliver a volume breath or a pressure breath, depending on the transport team's settings. In contrast, the Hamilton T-1 does not deliver a "true" volume breath but instead uses the terminology of volume-targeted, adaptive pressure control. This is not volume ventilation despite the transport team putting a target Vt into the ventilator. It uses adaptive pressure control to reach the preset targeted Vt. One important key capability within any ventilator that delivers a volume breath is the ability to measure a Pplat using an inspiratory hold maneuver.

Pressure Ventilation (Hamilton T-1®, Vyaire ReVel®, Vyaire LTV 1200®, and Zoll Impact EMV+®)

Pressure-controlled ventilation (PCV) delivers an inspiratory breath at a preset pressure limit. The inspiratory cycle is terminated when the rise time interval is met and the inspiratory time, set on the ventilator by the transport team, has been reached. The transport team sets the base ventilatory rate, the inspiratory pressure, the inspiratory time, and inspiratory rise time. The Vt delivered varies depending on the compliance and resistance of the lung. For example, smaller volumes are delivered in patients with low pulmonary compliance or high airway resistance. The advantage of this method of delivery is that it limits the distending pressure of the lung, reducing the risk of VILI. The disadvantage of this method of delivery is the absence of guaranteed minute ventilation with the potential for hypoventilation and hypercapnia. Most modern ventilators can deliver pressure ventilation using AC, SIMV, or variations of each mode based on the manufacturer.

As discussed in the volume ventilation section, each ventilator has specific capabilities. It is important to note that the Hamilton T-1 delivers each breath using pressure-limited or adaptive controlled methods.

Pressure-Regulated Volume-Cycled Ventilation (Vyaire ReVel®)

Pressure-Regulated Volume-Cycled Ventilation (PRVC) is a relatively new mode of ventilation that attempts to blend the best of volume and pressure ventilation modes. The transport team sets a Vt and a high-pressure limit. After a test breath, the ventilator software will adjust the inspiratory flow wave pattern to attempt to deliver the set Vt within the pressure parameter that has been set. If it is unable to do so, inspiration continues (until the set inspiratory time has been reached), but the ventilator will begin to limit the Vt once the PIP has reached 5 cm H_2O below the set high-pressure limit. In pure pressure ventilation, the Vt can increase significantly when resistance and compliance fall, but in PRVC, if a patient's airway resistance or lung compliance improves, the Vt will not exceed what has been set. This helps protect against over-inflation and maintains consistent minute ventilation.

Modes of Ventilation

There are many different perspectives regarding which mode of ventilation is better for the highly critical patients transported in the critical care environment. In a hospital setting with quiet environments, little patient movement, and more sophisticated ventilators that can stop auto-triggering, AC may be a great mode of ventilation. In contrast, the transport environment brings many different dynamics that may cause transport ventilator auto-triggering if used incorrectly. Considering the standard dynamics that transport teams encounter, including patient movement, ambulance and aircraft vibrations, and the new industry standard of attempting to maintain patients on pain management and sedation only while withholding long-acting paralytics, some transport teams feel that SIMV may offer added benefits during transport. Others, however, feel that in the early stages of acute illness, AC is the preferred mode because it provides the most support for the patient. There is no clinical evidence proving one mode is superior to another, so many transport programs follow the preferences of their medical directors or pulmonologists at the receiving tertiary care facility in their region.

Continuous Mandatory Ventilation

CMV is a volume-initiated or pressure-initiated mode of ventilation in which the Vt and ventilatory rate are set. Any spontaneous respiratory effort by the patient is ignored, and no patient triggering is possible. This method of ventilation is uncomfortable and is not used much anymore. If used, the patient would need to be deeply sedated, chemically paralyzed, and treated for pain. This mode may be used for patients who have no spontaneous respiratory effort but shows no advantage compared to AC. *CMV-assist* is a term used by some ventilator manufacturers to refer to AC ventilation; however, the primary transport ventilators used in the critical care environment do not use this language. CMV is assumed by using AC and turning any patient trigger off. The only ventilators that may use this terminology are the simplified ventilators like the AutoVent 3000.

Assist-Control Ventilation (Vyaire ReVel®, Vyaire LTV 1200®, and Zoll EMV+®)

In Assist-Control (AC) ventilation, the transport team will set a base ventilatory rate; however, the patient is allowed to breathe faster than the set rate. Every breath, whether patient or ventilator initiated, receives the full set Vt. This mode of ventilation requires minimal work from the patient and is often used during the early hours and days after intubation to allow the patient to rest while the underlying cause of respiratory failure is addressed.

AC can be either volume-cycled or pressure-controlled. In volume mode AC, both the ventilatory rate and Vt are set parameters. Parameters also set by the transport team on more sophisticated transport ventilators include either inspiratory flow rate or inspiratory time, waveform, and trigger sensitivity. Patient hyperventilation may occur in this mode; therefore, minute ventilation should be monitored. Historically, AC has been the primary mode seen in the hospital setting, but in the transport environment, this mode can cause additional issues with ventilation. Ambulance and aircraft vibration as well as simple movements by the transport crew, can cause auto-triggering to occur. This can cause added discomfort, air trapping, and subsequent auto-PEEP. Patients need to be monitored closely for these potential problems during transport.

Pressure-Control Plus (Hamilton T-1®)

Pressure-Control Plus (PCV+) ventilation is a Hamilton T-1 specific mode in which all breaths, whether triggered by the patient or ventilator, are pressure-controlled and mandatory. The transport team sets a starting inspiratory pressure and ventilatory rate; however, the patient can trigger the ventilator, with all breaths being ventilator delivered.

Synchronized Continuous Mandatory Ventilation Plus (Hamilton T-1®)

Synchronized Continuous Mandatory Ventilation Plus (S)CMV+ is a specific mode for this ventilator using volume-targeted, adaptive pressure control. The terminology, volume-targeted, adaptive pressure control is the same thing as *PRVC Ventilation*. It is not a true volume breath, but volume targeted with pressure regulation to achieve the preset Vt. Despite the terminology of CMV, this is how AC is labeled in this brand. The transport team sets a base ventilatory rate; however, the patient is allowed to breathe faster than the set rate. Every breath, whether patient or ventilator triggered, receives the full set Vt. The difference as discussed previously, is the pressure regulation to achieve this desired preset Vt.

Synchronized Intermittent Mandatory Ventilation (Vyaire ReVel®, Vyaire LTV 1200®, and Zoll EMV+®)

Synchronized Intermittent Mandatory Ventilation (SIMV) can be used in either volume or pressure ventilation modes. The primary distinction between SIMV and AC ventilation is how the ventilator contributes to spontaneous respiratory effort. Similar to AC, SIMV mode provides breaths at a set rate and set Vt (or pressure), which will give a guaranteed minimum minute ventilation. However, unlike AC, spontaneous respiratory efforts do not receive an assisted Vt at the set mandatory Vt level. During the respiratory time interval, the ventilator will deliver a mandatory breath or allow a spontaneously triggered breath by the patient. During the next respiratory time interval, if the patient has not triggered another spontaneous breath, the ventilator will then give a mandatory breath. As noted earlier, the patient's spontaneous breath can be augmented with the addition of PS. The main goal of PS is to reduce the work of breathing only during spontaneous breaths initiated by the patient. The patient can initiate spontaneous breaths based on the sensitivity (trigger setting) level set by the transport team, and positive pressure is delivered through the ventilator circuit to help overcome the resistance of the ETT and ventilator circuit. PS levels are commonly set at 5 to 10 cm H_2O over PEEP.

Pressure-Synchronized Intermittent Mandatory Ventilation Plus (Hamilton T-1®)

Pressure-Synchronized Intermittent Mandatory Ventilation Plus (PSIMV+) is a specific mode of pressure control ventilation for the Hamilton T-1. PSIMV+ provides breaths at a set rate and set Vt via pressure control. However, unlike PCV+, spontaneous respiratory efforts do not receive an assisted Vt. During the respiratory time interval, the ventilator will deliver a mandatory breath or allow a spontaneously triggered breath by the patient. During the next respiratory time interval, if the patient has not triggered another spontaneous breath, the ventilator will then give a mandatory breath.

Synchronized Intermittent Mandatory Ventilation Plus (Hamilton T-1®)

Synchronized Intermittent Mandatory Ventilation Plus (SIMV+) is a specific mode of volume-targeted, adaptive pressure control

ventilation for the Hamilton T-1. SIMV+ provides breaths at a set rate and set Vt via volume-targeted, adaptive pressure control. However, unlike (S)CMV+, spontaneous respiratory efforts do not receive an assisted Vt. During the respiratory time interval, the ventilator will deliver a mandatory breath or allow a spontaneously triggered breath by the patient. During the next respiratory time interval, if the patient has not triggered another spontaneous breath, the ventilator will then give a mandatory breath. As noted earlier, the patients' spontaneous breath can be augmented with the addition of PS, which is only available in a SIMV or SIMV+ mode and not available in AC or (S)CMV+.

Adaptive Support Ventilation (Hamilton T-1®)

Adaptive Support Ventilation (ASV) is a mode of ventilation found specifically on the Hamilton-T1 ventilator. This mode of ventilation is a microprocessor-controlled mode of mechanical ventilation that provides an automatic selection of continuous breath-by-breath adaptation of the RR and Vt. The transport team inputs whether the patient is male or female and an estimated height. The ventilator then identifies the desired VE for that patient based on IBW. The target breathing pattern is calculated by the ventilator to optimize breathing patterns, which results in the least work of breathing. By adjusting inspiratory pressure and mandatory rate on a breath-by-breath basis, the ventilator identifies changing lung characteristics such as resistance and compliance in an effort to apply lung protective strategies to meet the patient's targets based on IBW and gender. It is important to note that the transport team does not have any control over the set RR or Vt while using this mode because ASV uses a concept called the "Otis" least work of breathing formula to determine the RR and Vt. Therefore, the rationale for why it is called "adaptive."

Noninvasive Positive Pressure Ventilation

Noninvasive positive pressure ventilation (NiPPV) refers to mechanical ventilatory support provided without an endotracheal or tracheostomy tube. It is applied with a face or nasal mask, mouthpiece, high-flow nasal cannula, or nasal prongs, although generally, it is used with a snug-fitting facial or nasal mask.[5] This method is useful in both chronic and acute disorders and is discussed here as it relates to acute respiratory failure or acute exacerbation of a chronic respiratory condition.

When successful, NiPPV can eliminate the need for intubation and its associated complications while preserving the ability to speak, cough, and swallow. It decreases the work of breathing, increases alveolar ventilation, allows rest for respiratory musculature, and improves gas exchange. The strongest evidence supporting NiPPV is in patients with acute exacerbation of COPD and in patients with acute cardiogenic pulmonary edema.[1,5] It may also be used in patients who refuse intubation. NiPPV is contraindicated for patients who need emergent intubation because of cardiac or respiratory arrest and for patients with hemodynamic instability, inability to protect the airway (high risk for aspiration), upper airway obstruction, facial trauma or deformity, unstable arrhythmias, or organ failure unrelated to respiratory failure (Box 13.1). Patients who have difficulty breathing in the supine position, especially when related to obesity, should be carefully considered before transport via NiPPV.

NiPPV can be delivered via CPAP and volume-cycled or pressure-limited modes. CPAP delivers a constant positive pressure during inspiration and expiration. Volume-cycled ventilators

---

• BOX 13.1 **Indications for Endotracheal Intubation**
Problem: Failure or Anticipated Failure to Protect the Airway

Obtunded or comatose with loss of gag reflex
- Traumatic brain injury
- Overdose
- Anoxia
- Cerebral insults (cerebrovascular accident, aneurysms, etc.)

Obstruction
- Edema related to trauma
- Inhalation injury
- Foreign body aspiration
- Congenital anomaly

Pharmacological therapy: Profound sedation or analgesia used to treat or diagnose certain conditions, such as:
- Status epilepticus
- Increased intracranial pressure
- Diagnostic procedures in combative patients
- Elective procedures

Problem: Failure to Oxygenate
Shunt ventilation: Alveoli are perfused but not ventilated
- Pneumonia
- Acute lung injury
- Pulmonary hemorrhage or contusion
- Atelectasis
- Congenital cardiac disease

Dead space ventilation: Alveoli are ventilated but not perfused
- Pulmonary embolus
- Hypotension
- Low cardiac output states

Diffusion abnormalities: Obstruction or restriction of gas exchange across the alveolar-capillary membrane
- Pulmonary edema
- Pulmonary fibrosis

Oxygen extraction: Inability to extract oxygen
- Sepsis
- Carbon monoxide poisoning
- Cyanide poisoning

Problem: Failure to Ventilate
Neurological
- Spinal cord injury or disease
- Brain injury or disease
- Overdose
- Guillain-Barré syndrome

Muscular
- Myopathies
- Myasthenia gravis

Anatomical
- Pleural effusions
- Hemothorax or pneumothorax
- Abdominal compartment syndrome
- Bronchospasm, reactive airway disease
- Congenital anomalies

Infectious
- Botulism
- Respiratory syncytial virus
- Pertussis

---

are often not well tolerated because masks cause a loss of Vt, leading to constant alarms set off by the ventilator. Pressure-limited modes include PS, pressure-control, and BiPAP. BiPAP ventilation delivers both inspiratory positive airway pressure (IPAP) and expiratory positive airway pressure (similar to CPAP and PEEP). The patient triggers each breath. In the event of apnea, alarms and backup rates should be set.

The success of NiPPV is associated with user expertise, familiarity with equipment, and patient selection.[1,5] NiPPV, more than any other method of ventilation, requires a clinician skilled in the art of mechanical ventilation because the patient is awake, alert, hemodynamically stable, and lightly sedated (or not sedated at all). Patient comfort and cooperation are the keys to success, and it is important that the transport team understand the advanced ventilator adjustments that can potentially increase patient comfort and ventilator synchrony. When initiating NiPPV, a properly fitting mask must be selected. Applying the mask gently (or allowing the patient to hold the mask if they are able) until the patient is comfortable and in sync with the ventilator before securing the straps improves patient comfort.

CPAP, as opposed to PSV or BiPAP, may be selected when hypoxemia from cardiogenic pulmonary edema or upper airway obstruction from underlying obstructive sleep apnea is contributing to respiratory failure. CPAP can be delivered effectively using widely available lower-tech products with no mechanical ventilator required. CPAP devices consist of a tightly fitting facemask and a flow and CPAP generator or PEEP valve. PSV or BiPAP modes are chosen when ventilatory failure is a component and positive pressure ventilation is needed to support failing respiratory muscles, such as in COPD exacerbation or neuromuscular disease. BiPAP

requires a mechanical ventilator designed for noninvasive ventilation (NIV) and transport team members trained in its use.

The efficacy of NiPPV in the transport setting has not been clearly defined. Programs should develop specific criteria that involve not only proper patient selection but also the practicality of use in the medical transport environment. The use of NiPPV in acute hospital and home settings is steadily increasing. Requests to transport patients already successfully managed on NiPPV are on the rise. Transport team members need to be aware that patients being successfully managed in a hospital on sophisticated hospital noninvasive ventilators may not always tolerate the change to the transport ventilator. Transport ventilators often cannot match the inspiratory flow capabilities of the hospital ventilators and may increase the work of breathing on a patient already on the brink of needing intubation. NIV requires high oxygen flow rates and will deplete a portable ventilator's battery faster than conventional ventilation, so transport team members also need to be aware of their vehicle's oxygen capacity and have a power source readily available. Compliance with the aviation provider's protocols regarding electromagnetic interference must be maintained when considering the use of a patient's personal NiPPV device in an aircraft.

Continuous Positive Airway Pressure (Hamilton T-1®, Vyaire ReVel®, Vyaire LTV 1200®, and Zoll EMV+®)

Continuous Positive Airway Pressure (CPAP) is neither volume-cycled nor PCV. Patients breathe spontaneously at their own rate and Vt via an artificial airway with a continuous level of elevated baseline pressure called expiratory positive airway pressure (EPAP). This has the same effect as PEEP in opening collapsed alveoli and increasing FRC. This mode is primarily used to augment the patient's ability to oxygenate. This mode should be used with caution in patients who have the potential to decompensate neurologically or hemodynamically. For this reason, in the setting of the critical care transport environment, CPAP is rarely used for acutely ill patients.

Bi-Level Positive Airway Pressure (Hamilton T-1®, Vyaire ReVel®, Vyaire LTV 1200®, and Zoll EMV+®)

BiPAP can be described as a CPAP system with a time-cycled or flow-cycled change of the applied CPAP level by using PEEP. It delivers a preset IPAP by applying PS and EPAP by applying PEEP. Before we dive into these concepts, we need to define additive versus absolute.

Additive

Additive ventilators are also called "PEEP Compensated." This means that the PS is in addition to the PEEP, or IPAP is in addition to EPAP. If the transport team had a set PEEP of 5 cm H_2O and the goal is an IPAP of 15 cm H_2O, subtract the EPAP setting from the desired IPAP setting of 15 cm H_2O. The result in this example would require the transport team to set the PS (IPAP) at 10 cm H_2O, with an overall goal of IPAP of 15 cm H_2O (PIP would be 15 cm H_2O) and EPAP of 5 cm H_2O.

Absolute

Absolute ventilators are older technology, with some stand-alone hospital systems using this method. This means that the IPAP and EPAP are separate and not in addition to each other. This means the system is not PEEP compensated. The PS (IPAP) is separate from the PEEP (EPAP). If we have a set PEEP of 5 cm H_2O and desire an IPAP of 15 cm H_2O, we would set the desired IPAP setting at 15 cm H_2O. The result in this example would be to set the PS (IPAP) at 15 cm H_2O, ending with an IPAP of 15 cm H_2O (PIP would be 15 cm H_2O) and EPAP of 5 cm H_2O.

Patients with predominantly hypoxemic respiratory failure start with the recommended initial BiPAP settings. If the expected response (increase in oxygenation) is not achieved, increase the EPAP in increments of 2 cm H_2O with each adjustment.[1] But keep the gradient between IPAP and EPAP the same, such that the IPAP will be increased by the same increments as the EPAP. In situations of predominately hypercapnic respiratory failure, the goal is to improve the overall expiratory phase and promote consistent minute ventilation by setting a wider gradient between IPAP and EPAP. If the expected response (a decrease in carbon dioxide) is not achieved, increase the gradient between IPAP and EPAP. The key is to lower the EPAP to a level that allows the patient comfort while in the exhalation phase. Often times it's uncomfortable for a healthy individual attempting to exhale over an EPAP of 5 cm H_2O. Imagine a patient with respiratory failure secondary to asthma or COPD.

Oxygen Consumption in NiPPV

Monitoring oxygen consumption during NiPPV must be at the forefront for every transport team. Some transport ventilators give

the clinician the ability to change settings to conserve oxygen. Many programs have established recommendations and guidelines that guide NiPPV transports, with most establishing low-pressure oxygen sources use instead of using the high-flow (green) supply hose. The key element in evaluating oxygen consumption is to plan ahead. All the guidelines and protocols set forth do not replace critical thinking. Transport teams must be aware of how much oxygen duration their ambulance or aircraft has available prior to each shift. This should be evaluated throughout the shift and before any potential mechanical ventilation transport, whether using NiPPV or not. Oxygen consumption can be calculated by the following, taking the current pressure per square inch (PSI) from the oxygen tank and subtracting 200 PSI. By subtracting 200 PSI, which, provides a safety factor. Then multiply by the tank constant (factor), then divide by the flow in liters per minute (L/min). Examples:

Oxygen Tank Duration

$$([PSI - 200] \times constant) / flow$$

For example, using an M tank with an anticipated flow of 50 L/min.
The M tank has a factor of 1.56.

$$([1800 - 200] \times 1.56)/50$$
$$([1600] \times 1.56)/50$$
$$2496/50$$
$$= 49 \text{ minutes}$$

Common Oxygen Tank Size Constants

D cylinder: 0.16

E cylinder: 0.28

M cylinder: 1.56

H cylinder: 3.14

High-Flow Nasal Cannula

High-flow nasal cannula (HFNC) has slowly become the preferred method of NiPPV for hypoxemic respiratory failure patients. It is important to point out that no existing studies directly looking at HFNC versus noninvasive mask oxygenation, such as nonrebreather mask (NRB) masks. However, evaluation has been conducted through a metaanalysis review of 8 trials with 1084 patients. The metareview showed a reduction in the rate of intubation, ICU-free days, and overall intubation rates compared to patients treated with conventional oxygen therapy.[15] More focused randomized controlled trials are needed to evaluate long-term benefits and future treatment guidelines.

The transport team should have the proper equipment needed to transition the patient to HFNC devices. Stand-alone HFNC devices exist but can be large, cumbersome, difficult to move safely, and difficult to secure in an ambulance or aircraft. HFNC provides a small amount of PEEP. HFNC is excellent in reducing anatomical dead space, leading to a reduction in inspiratory effort. HFNC also "washes out" nitrogen and carbon dioxide in the upper airways, providing 100% oxygen for inhalation. Patients needing higher PEEP settings that exceed 8 to 10 cm H_2O may need to be transitioned to mask or helmet-based NIPPV methods.

One transport ventilator known to have HFNC capabilities is the Hamilton T-1. If transporting a patient with suspected or confirmed COVID-19, the use of a viral or bacterial filter is required. Because HFNC requires much higher inspiratory flow requirements that can be as high as 60 L/min, the transport team must evaluate oxygen consumption prior to transport to ensure adequate oxygen is available during all phases of patient transport. HFNC typically requires a specific HFNC delivery device and a heated-humidified oxygen delivery device that keeps the temperature between a specific range. HFNC will continue to grow in popularity and must be a consideration for guideline development, training initiatives, and overall budget requirements.

Helmet-Based Ventilation NiPPV

Helmet-based ventilation is a form of NiPPV ventilation that uses a technology first invented for hyperbaric oxygen therapy purposes. The Sea Long helmet was redesigned to be used for NIV purposes, with deployment in the critical care transport industry at the start of the Novel Coronavirus (SARS-CoV-2) pandemic. Early in the coronavirus pandemic, it was determined that airway procedures were associated with a high exposure risk potential, with transmission through respiratory droplets and aerosols. Helmet-based ventilation maintains an enclosed environment and significantly reduces droplets and aerosols to be emitted into the environment.

Helmet-based ventilation was first deployed in the hospital setting with success. However, before the coronavirus pandemic, helmet-based NIV had not been deployed in the critical care transport setting. Clinical trials have compared HFNC to high PEEP helmet NIV and showed improved oxygenation, reduced dyspnea, improved inspiratory effort, and a reduction in respiratory rate.[15] Helmet-based ventilation is not without limitations. When used with high-flow NIV delivery methods, these devices require constant flow and will not increase during any patient's inhalation phase. In light of this, the pressure within the helmet drops during any patient inhalation phase, which may make the patient feel like they cannot take an adequate breath. Patients that are significantly air hungry may benefit from standard NiPPV through the helmet.[16]

Helmet-based ventilation can be deployed using standard-flow or high-flow oxygen delivery devices. High-flow oxygen delivery devices with a flow generator capable of flow rates greater than or equal to 60 L/min are essential. The transport team provider should be able to manage the amount of delivered oxygen percentage. The requirement for high flow rates may be a limitation for some programs. The high flow rates that may exceed 60 L/min are necessary to optimize CO_2 elimination and prevent CO_2 rebreathing.[16] In contrast, standard NiPPV delivery through helmet-based ventilation increases the flow during inhalation, which can be much more comfortable for "air hungry" patients. As described above, flow rates must be greater than or equal to 60 L/min. If the transport team does not have a ventilator capable of these high flow rates during NiPPV ventilation or cannot compensate for high leak, then it is not advisable to use this form of NiPPV.

When using standard NiPPV with helmet ventilation, the ventilator circuit is attached to the inflow port on the base of the helmet. The outflow port is used to cause an intentional leak. This is one reason a ventilator with a high leak compensation is needed to function correctly. Regulating the flow within the helmet is not through the inflow port as the name suggests but instead through the outflow port via an external PEEP valve. When the transport team provider wants to increase the flow to the patient, they will lower the delivered external PEEP. This will increase flow. If the flow is too high, then reduce the external PEEP and titrate for patient comfort. In most cases, PEEP levels between 5 and 10 cm H_2O are the most comfortable. If external PEEP levels exceed 10 cm H_2O, it has been shown to cause high pressures within the helmet and to be uncomfortable for the patient. The key is to maintain the required flow rates of at least 60 L/min to eliminate CO_2 buildup within the helmet and the possibility of hypercapnia as a result. The transport provider can apply side-stream nasal cannula $EtCO_2$ while deploying the helmet, which will allow for added monitoring capabilities. If the transport team has point-of-care lab capability, it is encouraged to check ABGs based on ongoing assessment periods or changes in patient status.

As discussed in other NiPPV sections, oxygen consumption is a key element in initial and ongoing decision-making. Because of the high flow rates required, intentional leak, and length of transport, the transport provider must assess oxygen consumption and the capabilities of their equipment. Patients that require higher FiO_2 levels will add even more stress on oxygen usage. Helmet-based ventilation is a great option for programs looking for new NIV methods that allow for safe transport of patients in hypoxemic respiratory failure secondary to chronic respiratory disease or COVID-19.[17] It is recommended that each transport program ensure they have the proper equipment, clear transport guidelines, and proper training on the implementation and use of helmet-based NIV delivery.

Advanced Modes of Ventilation

Airway Pressure Release Ventilation (Hamilton T-1®)

Airway Pressure Release Ventilation (APRV) was designed to be an effective, safe alternative for difficult-to-oxygenate patients with ALI or ARDS. During APRV, the ventilator applies a relatively high level of CPAP for a prolonged time to maintain alveolar recruitment with intermittent timed releases, which help to eliminate CO_2. The high, prolonged CPAP level is referred to as P-high. P-low is the pressure level during the release phase (usually 0–5 cm H_2O). The time spent at P-high is called T-high, and the short time spent at P-low is called T-low. The P-high is usually set at a level between 20 and 30 cm H_2O, whereas P-low is set between 0 and 5 cm H_2O. APRV has been referred to by some as a form of inverse ratio ventilation because inspiration (T-high) is usually 4 to 6 seconds, whereas expiration (T-low) is just 0.2 to 0.8 seconds long.[18] The difference between the P-high and P-Low will serve as your expiratory ramp and one of the primary ways to optimize the release of CO_2. The other difference between inverse ratio ventilation and APRV is that APRV allows the patient brief periods to breathe spontaneously during the P-high phase, which allows for the release of CO_2 and better patient comfort.

When making the decision to switch to APRV, the transport team should evaluate and document the current MAP. It is recommended to use the MAP as your initial P-high. Transport teams should avoid chemical paralytics when using APRV. As outlined above, the T-high should be set at 4 to 6 seconds, which will yield a frequency release between 8 and 12 per minute. A P-Low of zero allows a larger pressure gradient over a shorter amount of time. The goal is to set the T-Low short enough to prevent de-recruitment but long enough to maintain an adequate Vt (4–6 mL/kg).

High-Frequency Ventilation

High-frequency ventilation (HFV) modes provide alveolar ventilation with Vt that is less than or equal to dead space volume by delivering breaths at supraphysiologic frequency. The goal of HFV therapy is to produce adequate alveolar ventilation at low Vt with preservation of end-expiratory lung volume to minimize volu-trauma and barotrauma.[4,10,19] This form of ventilation is more commonly used for newborn and pediatric patients than for adults. In practice, the high-frequency devices most often used are high-frequency oscillatory ventilation (HFOV) and high-frequency jet ventilation (HFJV).

Indications for HFV include disease states such as bronchopleural fistulas and airway injuries, patients at risk for pulmonary barotrauma (i.e., those with mean airway pressures [P_{aw}] greater than 18–20 cm H_2O or plateau pressures >35 cm H_2O), and patients with diffuse alveolar disease (i.e., ALI, ARDS), in which a major therapeutic goal is to preserve end-expiratory lung volume while limiting end-inspiratory lung overdistension.

HFV requires complicated, specialized equipment, and it is strongly recommended that trained respiratory therapists with experience using these devices be part of the transport team if patients are being transported on HFV.

High-Frequency Jet Ventilation

High-frequency jet ventilation (HFJV) delivers inspiratory gas through a jet injector, near the carina, at high velocity. This is accomplished with a specific ETT with a jet injector or an in-line jet injector adapter that is added to the existing ETT. HFJV is most often used simultaneously with a conventional ventilator that is able to provide PEEP and Vt breaths to the patient to preserve end-expiratory lung volume.
- Rates of 100 to 600 breaths/min are delivered with a Vt of 3 to 5 mL/kg.
- Risks include airway injury from the jet flow of gas positioned near the carina and air trapping.
- Expiration is passive.
- HFJV is generally limited to patients less than 8 years of age because of limitations in minute ventilation support.

High-Frequency Oscillatory Ventilation

HFOV is the most widely used HFV technique in clinical practice today. High-frequency oscillatory ventilators maintain lung recruitment by delivering a relatively high distending pressure (i.e., P_{aw}) while providing ventilation through superimposed, piston-generated, sinusoidal pressure oscillations (delta P [ΔP]) at a frequency of 3 to 15 Hz (180–900 oscillations per minute). Adequate oscillatory pressure (ΔP) generally produces visible chest vibration ("wiggle") from the clavicles to the lower abdomen or pelvis.

HFOV uses a relatively high P_{aw} to improve oxygenation. When transitioning to HFOV, the initial P_{aw} is generally set 3 to 5 cm H_2O above the P_{aw} on conventional ventilation immediately before transition. After the transition, the transport team should titrate the P_{aw} in 1- to 2-cm H_2O increments until oxygenation improves enough to allow a reduction in FiO_2 below 0.6. Ideally, chest x-ray will show global lung recruitment with both hemidiaphragms extending to the level of the 8th to 10th posterior ribs.[4,10,19]
- Ventilation is primarily determined by oscillatory pressure amplitude (ΔP). Increase the ΔP in 2- to 3-cm H_2O increments to improve CO_2 clearance. The chest wiggle is attained by adjusting the ΔP on the ventilator.
- Ventilation is also influenced by the oscillation frequency because the frequency is inversely related to delivered Vt in HFOV. At higher frequencies, HFOV generally delivers Vt of 1 to 3 mL/kg; physiological Vt that approaches those used in typical conventional ventilation strategies can be produced at the low end of the frequency spectrum.[10,19]

- HFOV is the only mode of mechanical ventilation in which expiration is active rather than passive.

Gases Used in Mechanical Ventilation

Inhaled Nitric Oxide

Inhaled nitric oxide (iNO) is a naturally occurring vasodilator administered as an inhaled gas for selective pulmonary vasodilation without associated systemic hypotension. As iNO diffuses across the alveolar-capillary membrane, the smooth muscle cells in the adjacent pulmonary vasculature relaxes, therefore decreasing pulmonary vascular resistance (PVR). Oxygenation improves as the vessels that perfuse ventilated alveoli are dilated, redistributing blood flow and reducing intrapulmonary shunting. iNO in the bloodstream is bound to hemoglobin and is rapidly deactivated, causing little effect on systemic vascular resistance and blood pressure.

Therapy indications include pulmonary hypertension and isolated right heart failure. iNO can be administered through a nasal cannula or ventilator circuit at a dose of 5 to 40 parts per million (ppm), with a typical starting point of 20 ppm. Once therapy is started, do not abruptly discontinue or disconnect a patient from iNO without specific medical orders from a physician. PVR could significantly increase and cause acute hypoxia and right ventricular dysfunction.

The most common patient population placed on iNO therapy are newborns with meconium aspiration and pulmonary hypertension. It has also been used with mixed results on adult patients with severe ARDS.

Methemoglobinemia and alveolar cytotoxicity are rare adverse reactions reported with iNO therapy. Monitor methemoglobin levels with blood gas samples if available.

Helium-Oxygen Mixture

Helium-oxygen mixture (Heliox) is a biologically inert gas with a much lower density than oxygen-nitrogen. With inhalation, resistance to airflow is reduced, and areas of turbulent flow through obstructions may be converted to a streamlined, nonturbulent (laminar) flow, improving the work of breathing.

Clinical indications for Heliox include upper airway obstruction associated with edema (postextubation stridor or croup), obstruction from compression, respiratory processes with high airway resistance, obstructive pathology (bronchiolitis or status asthmaticus), or respiratory distress syndrome. Additional indications include children with BPD (to decrease the work of breathing), augmenting the delivery of nebulized bronchodilators to obstructed lower airways, and allowing time for the onset of therapeutic medications or the resolution of the primary disease process. If successful, it may negate the need for intubation. The benefits are usually evident in several minutes. Administration considerations include the following:
- Usually administered with 30% oxygen through a tight-fitting mask.
- Commercially available in helium: oxygen concentrations of 80:20 or 70:30.
- Avoid administration of pure helium; administer with oxygen. If manually blending helium and oxygen, place an in-line oxygen concentration device to ensure adequate oxygen mix.

Positive improvement has been reported in the adult population in patients treated for upper airway obstructions as a result of thyroid masses, radiation injury, lymphoma, cancer, or angioedema.[1,14]

Ventilation Strategies

Obstructive Lung Disease

A measured approach should be taken in patients intubated for severe asthma and acute exacerbations of COPD to minimize air trapping, auto-PEEP, and overventilation. As such, arterial CO_2 levels of greater than 100 mm Hg are common and can be alarming in these patients. However, attempting to quickly lower those CO_2 levels with high set ventilator rates can lead to catastrophic consequences, such as pneumothoraces. The goal for these patients is to provide adequate oxygenation and ventilation support while allowing the other treatment modalities to take effect. The CO_2 level will gradually improve. Vt of 6 to 8 mL/kg with slower rates than normal (10–12 breaths/min in adults), higher inspiratory flow rates, and shorter inspiratory times all allow for the longer exhalation times required in these patients. I:E ratios of 1:4, 1:6, or even 1:8 may be necessary to minimize air trapping.[4]

Management of the Asthmatic Patient

Severe asthma exacerbation is a common patient in the critical care transport environment. Severe asthma can easily progress to status asthmaticus. This defines a patient who does not respond to initial airway and pharmacological therapy, progressing to acute respiratory failure. It has been shown that most patients that have near-fatal or fatal asthma exacerbations have a large allergen exposure and associated emotional distress.[20] Studies have defined two different asthma exacerbation pathways that are either eosinophilic or neutrophilic in nature.[20] Patients that suffer from the eosinophilic form of asthma usually have a more gradual onset and a slower response to the therapy provided. Eosinophils are a type of white blood cell that reacts to parasitic infections or allergic reactions. Within the differential of a standard CBC, the eosinophils will have a normal range of 0% to 7%. Anything >7% would be considered suspicious for parasitic or allergic etiology. In contrast, neutrophilic asthma exacerbations will have a more immediate onset and will also respond quicker to therapies. Neutrophils are white blood cells that destroy and ingest bacteria. They will arrive first at the site of inflammation. Therefore, their numbers increase greatly immediately after an injury or during an inflammatory process. The normal neutrophil range is 45% to 75%.

Asthmatic patients in exacerbation will not only suffer from exhalation failure but will progressively move into inspiratory failure. As the airway caliber narrows and progressive bronchial constriction ensues, the patient will progressively have more and more difficulty taking in the breath. Once the patient is mechanically ventilated, the need for constant evaluation of both inspiratory and expiratory phases is paramount. Considering both phases, the transport team must understand the standard starting recommendation of an I:E ratio of 1:4 is just a starting parameter that must be evaluated and changed if warranted. The goal must be to optimize the I:E ratio setting for both the inspiratory and expiratory phases. In doing so, the clinician may want to use an I:E ratio of 1:1. This will give equal emphasis on both phases and allow for the needed time to fill the lungs during the inhalation phase. Ultimately, an I:E ratio of 1:4 will not only give lengthened time during exhalation but also a short inspiratory time that may not be enough to allow for full lung filling.

To compare both approaches, we will use a respiratory rate of 10. Using the I:E ratio of 1:4 in the first example, we can ascertain the inspiratory phase to be 1.2/sec and the expiratory phase to be 4.8/sec, which equals a 6-second respiratory cycle. As you can see, a 1:4 ratio gives much more emphasis to the exhalation phase. This is true but also a misguided teaching approach that gives such importance to an I:E ratio of 1:4 as the standard. In contrast, using the same respiratory rate of 10 but an I:E ratio of 1:1 as our second example, we can ascertain the inspiratory phase to be 3/sec and the expiratory phase to be 3/sec, which equals a 6-second respiratory cycle. As seen in the second example, a 1:1 ratio provides equal emphasis on the inspiratory and expiratory phases. Ongoing assessment should focus on consistent identification of auto-PEEP levels, with a focus on Pplat evaluation if using a volume breath. If auto-PEEP levels are increasing, determine if the I:E ratio is giving enough time to fill the lungs, while providing an adequate exhalation phase. Further consideration should be focused on proper analgesia/sedation and long-term paralytics to prevent over-breathing, auto-triggering, and increased work of breathing that could interfere with I:E ratio decision-making.

Permissive Hypercapnia

Ventilating with slower rates for obstructive lung disease patients and lower Vt for ARDS patients can result in hypercapnia. *Permissive hypercapnia* is a lung-protective strategy aimed at decreasing alveolar ventilation to prevent lung injury. The use of small Vt or lower rates produces higher $PaCO_2$ and lower pH levels. In permissive hypercapnia strategies, acidemia is tolerated to a pH of ≥7.10. Hypercapnia and acidemia are not the goals of this approach but rather the tolerated consequence. Acidosis at this level is generally well tolerated when achieved gradually. The small Vt and/or slower respiratory rates associated with permissive hypercapnia may be uncomfortable and will require sedation and sometimes paralysis to offset the increased respiratory drive and agitation associated with discomfort. The high $PaCO_2$ in permissive hypercapnia causes cerebral vasodilation and increased intracranial pressure (ICP), so this approach should be avoided in patients with head injuries or cerebral hemorrhage.

The transport team must be aware that increasing $PaCO_2$ and $EtCO_2$ levels should not entice them to increase the respiratory rate in an attempt to drive down the $PaCO_2$. This strategy, although part of basic teaching, is not correct in treating an obstructive lung patient. The foundations built on why increasing the respiratory rate in this scenario is not correct reside in how the change will impact the respiratory cycle and the ratio between the time given for inhalation and exhalation.

Management of the ARDS Patient

The transport team will most certainly encounter an ARDS patient at some point. ARDS is thought to start secondary to a multilayer inflammatory response. This inflammatory response in the early stages causes increased permeability of the alveolar-capillary barrier. This barrier is a thin layer called the endothelial glycocalyx that is made from tiny hair-like follicles that line the endothelial layer. The inflammatory mediators promote neutrophil accumulation in the microcirculation, which in turn causes vascular permeability and gaps in the alveolar endothelial glycocalyx. This endothelial breakdown causes interstitial fluid build-up and can cause the alveoli to separate from the capillary, thus lengthening the alveolar-capillary gradient.

The differential diagnosis protocol for ARDS has always been based on the Berlin Definition criteria that focused on the PaO_2/FiO_2 ratio. Secondary assessment revolved around chest x-ray evaluation, which would show bilateral lung involvement and a ground-glass appearance. Many patients will also suffer from pleural effusions, with the onset of symptoms being acute in nature. With that in mind, it is now thought that ARDS is much more uncommon and involves diffuse alveolar damage throughout the lung units. The newest argument revolves around iatrogenic causes related to the approach taken in the initial resuscitation phase, with volume overload, inadequate lung recruitment, and cyclic opening and closing of alveoli resulting in atelectotrauma.

The ventilation strategy for ARDS patients focuses on lower Vt (4–6 mL/kg) and higher respiratory rates. Vt is decreased to maintain Pplat less than 30 cm H_2O. Oxygenation is usually the primary problem for these patients, so high FiO_2 and high PEEP levels are commonly required. The PaO_2/FiO_2 ratio is used as an ultimate benchmark for diagnosis. If the PaO_2/FiO_2 ratio is <200, the diagnosis is ARDS with the other associated differential diagnosis components present. The key with the pseudo-ARDS argument is all about using a more aggressive approach in lung recruitment. This means these patients need more aggressive initial interventions that attempt to recruit alveolar lung units more quickly. This can be accomplished by early BiPAP intervention or mechanical ventilation using APRV.

Novel Coronavirus (SARS-CoV-2)

The novel coronavirus (SARS-CoV-2, COVID-19) took the medical community by surprise in 2020 and has fundamentally reshaped healthcare. Treatment guidelines during the early phase of the coronavirus pandemic were scarce. Severe illness and secondary decompensation occur in most patients within 1 week after the onset of symptoms. Most often, patients will seek medical care after cough, dyspnea, and fatigue progresses to severe hypoxemia.

As with many patients with respiratory failure, attempting to improve oxygenation with NiPPV techniques is thought to be the best approach. Targeting an SpO_2 greater than or equal to 92% is the recommended goal. Potential harm in maintaining SpO_2 of less than 92% is well documented in ARDS patients without COVID-19. The target of 92% or greater, not exceeding 96%, is backed by the current surviving sepsis 2021 guidelines for COVID-19.[21,22] Careful consideration by the transport team should guide decisions on NiPPV versus transitioning to mechanical ventilation. Adult patients with COVID-19 and accompanying acute hypoxemic respiratory failure may not respond to conventional oxygen therapy. It is safe to say that current and past evidence within any hypoxemic respiratory failure patient has shown that an escalation of correcting hypoxemia is the best approach.

Options now exist for providing enhanced delivery of oxygen through NiPPV methods, consisting of HFNC and BiPAP ventilation, which may be the initial treatment focus. However, the transport team must consistently monitor the patient for worsening respiratory failure despite NiPPV therapy and make the decision for an escalation to intubation and mechanical ventilation support.

Current therapy guidelines exist and are similar to those of standard ARDS treatment recommendations. Lung protective tidal volumes with 4 to 8 mL/kg of IBW, Pplat targets of less than 30 cm H_2O, and SpO_2 titration to 92% to 96% should be the immediate goal. These broad, open-ended management strategies for COVID may be safer, considering how much could change with COVID over the coming year(s). However, the sat goal is slightly different for ARDS versus COVID.

Proning

Prone positioning has been part of the treatment paradigm in hypoxemic respiratory failure patients suffering from ARDS for years. It is thought that proning improves V/Q mismatch, although it is not fully understood.[1] Prone positioning traditionally has not been deployed as a standard of care in the transport environment; however, isolated programs or situations may have existed in the past. The COVID-19 pandemic changed this mindset and forced transport programs to establish proning guidelines and add focused training on how to transport these patients safely and effectively to definitive care. Prior to the COVID-19 pandemic, any research available on proning in the transport setting was minimal at best, so any program attempting to gain insight on any evidence-based practice standards within proning and transport was unsuccessful. Fast-forward a few years and we now have a small amount of data on best practice recommendations secondary to a retrospective study completed by Boston MedFlight, which consisted of a 25-patient sample size.[13]

Safety is key, and each program must establish guidelines around their specific mode of transport, equipment capabilities, transport team dynamics, and overall length of transport. It is important to be able to assess the patient continuously with an unobstructed view. Recommendations exist to always have a 360° view of the patient. This often requires ground transport, as in this study done at Boston MedFlight. There is no existing study showing any data on air medical transport or if there is a benefit with air transport over ground transport in the prone patient. If air transport is the decision by the program, the aircraft should allow for unobstructed 360° views of the patient. It is strongly recommended to have long-acting paralysis in place with consistent pharmacologic intervention with sedation and pain management medications. $EtCO_2$ waveform capnography and SpO_2 monitoring are essential, with reassessment based on your program guidelines. In addition, physically securing the patient within the transport vehicle and preventing dislodgment of invasive lines and tubes require the transport team's constant vigilance. A prediscussed plan for cardiac or respiratory emergencies or arrest should be established.

Proning is a needed and often effective method in the refractory hypoxemic respiratory failure patient that is being mechanically ventilated. It is not without problems and is a much more complex addition to patient transport. In a continual effort to always improve, each program should have a commitment to training and ongoing evaluation of each patient transport, especially transports of proned patients. This will give the program real-time insight into strengths and weaknesses within their program and allow them to make necessary changes that will ultimately impact patients in a positive manner.

Metabolic Acidosis

Metabolic acidemia is one of five possible metabolic derangements that transport teams will face. When making a clinical decision within mechanical ventilation, pH can be a dangerous silent killer that can be easily missed. Within metabolic acidosis lies the *partially compensated metabolic acidosis*. This patient will have increased respiratory compensation and higher metabolic demands, with the need to increase the VE to a level that allows for matched compensation. Some transport teams may have point-of-care lab capability that will give immediate feedback secondary to any mechanical ventilation changes. However, most of the industry does not have point-of-care lab capability and must rely on clinical gestalt and a thorough assessment to make decisions.

The question exists on how to set up minute ventilation (VE), which protects the pH and does not allow the metabolic acidosis to worsen. There has been a long debate on how to correctly accomplish this goal, with high VE formulas (240 mL/kg/min) to (160 mL/kg/min) used to establish the correct respiratory rate.[1] Instead, maybe the transport team should target a pre or postintubation $EtCO_2$ in an attempt to minimize any rise in $PaCO_2$. In many cases, transport teams only have $EtCO_2$ as a surrogate to $PaCO_2$ and can only use $EtCO_2$ to guide decision-making if the patient's hemodynamic status is within normal limits. If there is any hemodynamic instability, then $EtCO_2$ levels will be low because of the low perfusion state. This will give the transport team provider a false sense of hypocapnia if used to guide resuscitation and clinical decision-making in an attempt to match respiratory compensation. The accepted approach is to be conservative with VE targets and to set respiratory rates that are in the range of 26 breaths per minute, with the understanding that most patients are being ventilated with lung-protective Vt ranges. If in doubt, it is best not to correct any identified hypocapnia through $EtCO_2$ assessment but to maintain $EtCO_2$ at the hypocapnic level, allowing the receiving facility to make ventilator adjustments based on ABG results.

Troubleshooting

Monitoring

Patients on mechanical ventilation need vigilant and continuous monitoring of ventilator parameters and clinical assessment. Oxygen saturations and $EtCO_2$ should be monitored, and their limitations in clinical use should be well understood. Pulse oximetry does not detect saturations below 83% with the same degree of precision or accuracy as it does at higher saturations, nor does it perform well in low perfusion states. Many errors made in pulse oximetry readings are related to artifact. The pulse oximetry waveform should be compared with the patient's heart rate to ascertain accurate readings.

Continuous waveform capnography is the gold standard for peri and post prehospital intubation monitoring, ETT placement confirmation, and continuous assessment. Capnography is the standard of care in intubation confirmation, despite a patient having a low flow state. Clinical research using $EtCO_2$ waveform capnography in human cadavers illustrated that ETT placement and continuous confirmation had 100% sensitivity and specificity.[20] As described above, an abrupt loss in $EtCO_2$ is a critical finding and requires immediate recognition and airway reassessment. Outside of cardiac arrest or profound hypoperfusion, an abrupt loss of $EtCO_2$ values can also be caused by ET tube dislodgement or a complication with the $EtCO_2$ line.[23]

$EtCO_2$ monitors have been shown to be accurate in both prehospital and hospital settings. In normal conditions, the $EtCO_2$ reads 3 to 5 mm Hg lower than the $PaCO_2$.[1,5] However, it is important to understand that $EtCO_2$ in hypoperfusion states (hypovolemia, hypotension, and reduced cardiac output) or in patients with ventilation-perfusion abnormalities will be significantly (and unpredictably) lower than the patient's arterial CO_2. $EtCO_2$ reflects a patient's perfusion status as well as ventilation, and a sudden profound drop in the $EtCO_2$ reading may be one of the first indicators that a patient is going into pulseless electrical activity. Additionally, it is important to recognize the $EtCO_2$ will never be higher than the patient's $PaCO_2$. In cases in which transport

teams do not have access to the most recent ABG, $EtCO_2$ can be used to predict $PaCO_2$. One must understand there is a gradient, as stated earlier, and this gradient is not 100% accurate. In patients with increasing dead space or hypoperfusion states related to treatment or worsening conditions, the gradient between $PaCO_2$ and $EtCO_2$ will widen. Although $EtCO_2$ monitoring is an excellent tool for transport and is the standard of practice for determining proper ETT placement, decisions regarding adjusting mechanical ventilator settings should take the entire clinical picture into account, not just the $EtCO_2$ values.

Furthermore, $EtCO_2$ helps identify hypoventilation following pain management or sedation medication administration. $EtCO_2$ will begin showing hypoventilation (Fig. 13.2) and CO_2 retention before a pulse oximeter indicates hypoxemia in patients being managed with positive-pressure ventilation.

Continuous monitoring capabilities extend past ETT confirmation or ongoing perfusion assessment. $EtCO_2$ can assist the transport provider in early identification of breath stacking during mechanical ventilation. As shown below in Fig. 13.3, the $EtCO_2$ waveform will begin to show hypercapnia, with a morphology that does not return to the respiratory baseline. This complication may arise from a reduction in expiratory time where a complete exhalation does not occur. This can be due to incorrect trigger setting, improper I-time, or inadequate sedation status.

Additionally, if a patient has incomplete paralysis or air leak, the patient's $EtCO_2$ waveform will likely show a curare cleft type waveform (Fig. 13.4). The curare cleft waveform will help you detect breakthrough breathing or a leak from the ETT cuff or ventilator circuit.

COPD and Asthma are difficult disease processes that transport providers must manage. $EtCO_2$ can help provide information to

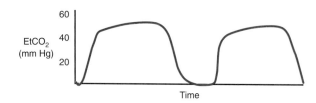

• **Figure 13.2** Hypoventilation.

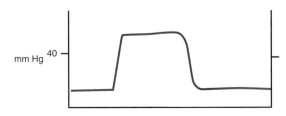

• **Figure 13.3** $EtCO_2$ waveform beginning to show hypercapnia.

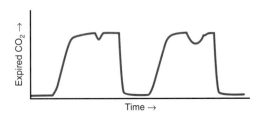

• **Figure 13.4** $EtCO_2$ waveform showing a curare cleft type waveform.

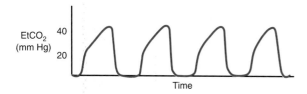

• **Figure 13.5** A shark-fin morphology. (From Karbing DS, Perchiazzi G, Rees SE, Jaffe MB. Journal of Clinical Monitoring and Computing 2018-2019 end of year summary: respiration. *J Clin Monit Comput.* 2020;34(2):197-205.)

support specific pathologies during COPD or asthma exacerbation, which will frequently be illustrated by a shark-fin morphology secondary to poor alveolar emptying (Fig. 13.5). As a result of incomplete exhalation, these patients will begin to retain CO_2 and commonly show signs of hypercapnia. The $EtCO_2$ morphology can be used to assess the effectiveness of these medications over time. As bronchodilation occurs, one can expect less profound shark-fin morphology and a reduction in $EtCO_2$ values.

Ventilator Alarms

Alarms should not replace your critical thinking or the need to constantly evaluate the patient, especially since the source of alarms could be either benign or catastrophic. Alarm limits should be set to warn transport crews of mechanical and physiological problems. Silencing alarms or changing limits without carefully considering the cause can be deleterious to the patient. Additionally, setting alarms should not give the transport team a false sense that the ventilator will warn of potential adverse situations. Continuous

monitoring of the patient and the ventilator should take place throughout the patient interaction.

Because peak inspiratory and plateau pressures are associated with VILI, high-pressure alarm limits should particularly be tightly controlled and assessed. Increased PIP without changes in the Pplat is indicative of increased airway resistance, such as a kinked ETT, secretions, bronchospasm, or obstruction. Elevated peak *and* plateau pressures are associated with decreased compliance, such as pulmonary edema, pneumothorax, pleural effusions, abdominal distension, or auto-PEEP.

Ventilator alarms are difficult to hear in the transport setting. They should be set to maximum volume, and the machine should be positioned so that flashing alarm lights can be visualized. Airway status should be evaluated immediately with any patient deterioration. The DOPE acronym (D, displaced ETT; O, obstructed ETT; P, pneumothorax; E, equipment [ventilator] failure) is a useful tool for remembering possible causes of airway compromise. If any question exists as to the cause of deterioration, the patient should be disconnected from the ventilator and manually ventilated until all possibilities are considered. Common ventilator alarms are listed in Table 13.2.

High-Pressure Alarm

PIP is measured at the peak of inspiration and is a representation of many factors. It includes the volume of each breath, compliance of the lungs, airway resistance, and the force needed to deliver the breath. The ventilator uses the pressure limit to notify the transport team of high pressure. It is important to point out that each ventilator manufacturer has different pressure limit settings. Meaning if we set a high-pressure alarm setting at 35 cm H_2O,

TABLE 13.2 Troubleshooting Ventilator Alarms

Initial assessment:
Airway: Is the ETT in the correct position? Check ETT insertion depth, check $EtCO_2$, and check bilateral breath sounds.
Breathing: Check bilateral breath sounds, look for chest excursion, check pulse oximetry, and check patient skin color.
Circulation: Check the pulse, ECG, and blood pressure.

Remove the patient from the ventilator and manually use a resuscitation bag if any compromise is found; consider adding a PEEP valve.

Alarm	Cause	Management
Apnea	Insufficient spontaneous breathing by the patient in CPAP or pressure support mode	Switch ventilator mode to one that provides a set rate
High airway pressure	ETT obstruction: sputum, kinked, biting Decreased compliance or increased resistance Circumferential burns Bronchospasm, lung collapse, pneumothorax, endobronchial intubation, worsening of lung process Anxiety/fear/pain/fighting the ventilator	Suction airway Treat the cause of resistance Adjust mode or settings Rule out hypoxia before treating agitation CXR analysis Change ventilator mode to one that is better tolerated. Provide sedation/analgesia, consider paralytics
Low airway pressure	Ventilator disconnect Leak in the ventilator system Cuff leak Inadvertent extubation	Ensure that all connections are intact and tight Troubleshoot ETT cuff BVM if ETT was dislodged
Oxygen pressure low	The oxygen cylinder is empty; the cylinder valve is closed; the unit is not connected to the wall terminal Aircraft/ambulance oxygen flow in off position	Switch to a functional oxygen source

BVM, Bag-valve-mask; *CPAP,* continuous positive airway pressure; *CXR,* chest x-ray; *ECG,* electrocardiogram; *EtCO2,* end-tidal CO_2; *ETT,* endotracheal tube.

the ventilator will terminate the breath at a limit below the set high-pressure alarm. The Hamilton-T1, for example, uses Plimit setting that is minus 10 cm H_2O as a safety boundary for its inspiratory pressure adjustment and does not exceed this value. If you set the high-pressure alarm on the Hamilton T-1 at 35 cm H_2O, the Plimit will terminate the breath (even if the target Vt isn't reached) at 25 cm H_2O. A variation of this is with the ReVel or LTV1200, for example, which has a P-limit minus 5 cm H_2O of the high-pressure alarm setting. As you can see, this is an important factor to consider and an alarm parameter that you must take seriously and evaluate within ongoing assessment periods.

Low-Pressure Alarm

The low-pressure alarm is also an important alarm to monitor. The alarm is used to inform the transport team of any disconnections. Use the DOPE (Displaced, Obstruction, Pneumothorax, Equipment) pneumonic (Box 13.2) anytime you have a low-pressure alarm. Most often, this will be due to a circuit disconnection at either the ETT or ventilator connection. This can be more common in some ventilators, with the ReVeL and LTV1200 ventilators also showing a "disc/sense error" within the settings screen. You can also have a low-pressure alarm if an O_2 source disconnection has occurred.

Low Minute Ventilation Alarm

The low minute ventilation alarm is also an excellent warning system for disconnections but it will be a more specific alarm used when using pressure-limited delivery. Because of the potential changes seen in the patient's chest wall compliance, Vt often will vary from breath to breath. The low minute ventilation alarm will inform you of a minute ventilation below the level you set on the alarm screen. Our minute ventilation requirements need to be between 4 and 8 L/min, and an alarm setting at or below this point will give the transport team the ability to identify minute ventilation changes below the required level.

Ventilator Asynchrony

Ventilator asynchrony occurs when disparity is found between patient respiratory effort and ventilator delivery, often described as "fighting the ventilator." Ideally, to decrease the work of breathing and reduce respiratory distress, the ventilator should cycle with the patient's intrinsic respiratory rhythm.[1,2,14] Anxiety and discomfort are often associated with mechanical ventilation. Sedation and pain should be evaluated, treated, and reassessed for adequacy. Initial ventilator settings can be adjusted after connecting the patient to the ventilator and assessing the patient's breathing pattern and demand.

The patient's respiratory effort and trigger sensitivity should be assessed in assisted and spontaneous modes of ventilation, whether volume limited or pressure limited. If the sensitivity threshold is set too high, the patient's respiratory efforts are not recognized, and the ventilator is not triggered to provide a breath. Alternatively, if the trigger is set too low, the ventilator auto-triggers or delivers breaths in response to extrinsic stimuli (ambulance or aircraft vibrations and movement) or water in the circuit.

One problem related to volume-limited ventilators is the inadequate flow of gas, which causes patients to feel like they are not getting enough air and attempt to extract more gas out of the ventilator.[2,14] This situation is uncomfortable for patients, and many transport ventilators only have the option of adjusting inspiratory time, or I:E ratio, and not flow directly. However, some ventilators allow the user to adjust flow via the *Rise Time* profiles found in the extended features menus. By adjusting to a quicker *Rise Time (0.1 seconds)*, you then allow for more flow and a corresponding increase in Vt. Patients with poor lung compliance or obstructive disease need high inspiratory flow rates to receive full Vt support during the set inspiratory time. Lengthening the inspiratory time compromises the long expiratory time needed by these patients who are already prone to air trapping and auto-PEEP.

Patient oxygenation and ventilation requirements may exceed the capabilities of some transport ventilators and may require deep sedation or neuromuscular blockade to complete some patient transports. This is not the absolute norm, and each patient should be given continuous aliquots of pain and sedation medications while attempting to limit long-acting paralytics, if at all possible. This strategy should be undertaken after careful consideration of the cause of asynchrony, the ventilator capabilities, and alternative means of transport. More sophisticated transport ventilators and ventilation strategies often require the skill and knowledge of a respiratory therapist and transport via a larger ambulance or fixed-wing aircraft.

Summary

This chapter provided an overview of mechanical ventilation in the transport environment. The topic of mechanical ventilation and the application of ventilation strategies will be one of the most challenging learning aspects for critical care providers. The transport team must be familiar with indications for mechanical ventilation, pulmonary physiology, and the equipment that is used during patient transport. It is essential to continually broaden your understanding of mechanical ventilation to be prepared for the highly critical patients you will be asked to transport. The learning doesn't stop there; a broad understanding of laboratory values, acid-base balance, and ventilator manufacturer-specific technology must be a constant focus for each transport provider, increasing the ability to make clinical decisions for each patient transported.

References

1. Bauer E. *Ventilator Management: A Pre-Hospital Perspective.* 2nd ed. FlightBridgeED; 2015.
2. Daoud EG. Airway pressure release ventilation: Annals of thoracic medicine. *Ann Thorac Med.* 2007;2(4):176–179.
3. Carlson JN, Colella MR, Daya MR, et al. Prehospital cardiac arrest airway management: An NAEMSP position statement and Resource Document. *Prehosp Emerg Care.* 2022;26(sup1):54-63.
4. COVID-19 Treatment Guidelines Panel. Coronavirus Disease 2019 (COVID-19) Treatment Guidelines. National Institutes of Health. Accessed August 15, 2022. https://www.covid19treatmentguidelines.nih.gov/

• BOX 13.2 DOPE

D: Displaced endotracheal tube
O: Obstructed endotracheal tube
P: Pneumothorax
E: Equipment (ventilator) failure

5. Cairo J. *Pilbeam's Mechanical Ventilation: Physiological and Clinical Applications*. 6th ed. Mosby; 2015.
6. O'Brien J. Absorption atelectasis: Incidence and clinical implications. *ANA J*. June 2013;81:205–208.
7. Remensberger P. *Pediatric and Neonatal Mechanical Ventilation*. Springer; 2015.
8. Walsh B. *Neonatal and Pediatric Respiratory Care*. 4th ed. Elsevier; 2015.
9. Weiner GM. *Textbook of Neonatal Resuscitation*. 8th ed. American Academy of Pediatrics; 2021.
10. Davies JD, Senussi MH, Mireles-Cabodevila E. Should a tidal volume of 6 mL/kg be used in all patients? *Respir Care*. 2016;61(6): 774–790. doi:10.4187/respcare.04651
11. Nourbakhsh E, Nugent K. *A Bedside Guide to Mechanical Ventilation*. Texas Tech University Health; 2011.
12. Elie M, Carden D. *Acute Respiratory Distress Syndrome*. Morgan and Claypool Life Sciences; 2013.
13. Farkas J. ARDS vs. pseudoARDS – Failure of the Berlin definition. January 2018. http://emcrit.org/pulmcrit/pseudoards
14. Esquinas A. *Noninvasive Mechanical Ventilation: Theory, Equipment, and Clinical Application*. 2nd ed. Springer; 2016.
15. Patel BK, Wolfe KS, Pohlman AS, Hall JB, Kress JP. Effect of noninvasive ventilation delivered by helmet vs face mask on the rate of endotracheal intubation in patients with acute respiratory distress syndrome: A randomized clinical trial. *JAMA*. 2016;315:2435–2441.
16. Beckl R. Use of Helmet-Based Noninvasive Ventilation in Air Medical Transport of Coronavirus Disease 2019 Patients. *Air Med J*. 2021;40:16–19.
17. Menga LS, Berardi C, Ruggiero E, Grieco DL, Antonelli M. Noninvasive respiratory support for acute respiratory failure due to COVID-19. *Curr Opin Crit Care*. 2022;28(1):25–50. doi:10.1097/MCC.0000000000000902
18. Commission on Accreditation of Medical Transport Systems – camts. org. *CAMTS 12th Edition Standards*. CAMTS. 2023. Accessed November 24, 2022. https://www.camts.org/wp-content/uploads/2022/10/12th-Edition-Final-with-highlights-for-website.pdf
19. Davis D, Aguilar S, Smith K, et al. Preliminary report of a mathematical model of ventilation and intrathoracic pressure applied to pre-hospital patients with severe traumatic brain injury. *Prehosp Emerg Care*. 2014;19(2):328–325.
20. Marik, Paul. *Evidence-Based Critical Care*. 3rd ed. Springer Cham Heidelberg; 2016. doi:10.1007/978-3-319-11020-2
21. Surviving sepsis campaign guidelines on the management of adults with Coronavirus disease 2019 (COVID-19) in the ICU 1/202. *Society of Crit Care Med*. https://www.sccm.org/sccm/media/ssc/SSC-COVID19GuidelinesRecTable-FirstUpdate.pdf
22. Silvestri S, Ladde JG, Brown JF, Roa JV, Hunter C, Ralls GA. Endotracheal tube placement confirmation: 100% sensitivity and specificity with sustained four-phase capnographic waveforms in a cadaveric experimental model. *Resuscitation*. 2017;115:192–198. doi.org:10.1016/j.resuscitation.2017.01.002
23. Hess D, Kacmarek R. *Essentials of Mechanical Ventilation*. 3rd ed. McGraw-Hill; 2014.

Manuals
Hamilton-T1 Operator's Manual. 2021. Retrieved November 29, 2022. HAMILTON-T1-ops-manual-SW3.0.x-en-USA-10103179.01.pdf

14
Shock

MICHAEL A. FRAKES

Shock, the "rude unhinging of the machinery of life," is a cellular-level imbalance between oxygen supply and demand. It is common in critical care, affecting about one-third of critical care patients.[1] The oxygen utilization defect comes from one or more of four potential, but not necessarily exclusive, mechanisms: hypovolemia, structural or functional cardiac failure, obstruction to cardiac filling or return, and abnormal intravascular volume distribution. Septic shock, a form of distributive and hypovolemic shock, is the most common.[2–4] In one report of intensive care unit (ICU) patients with pressor-dependent shock, septic shock occurred in 62% of patients, cardiogenic shock in 16%, hypovolemic shock in 16%, other types of distributive shock in 4%, and obstructive shock in 2%.[2]

Physiology

When oxygen demand exceeds oxygen supply, no matter the mechanism, cellular respiration shifts to anaerobic metabolism, with decreased energy availability, increased carbon dioxide production, and the accumulation of lactic acid and other toxic byproducts. An understanding of shock, therefore, requires an understanding of both cellular respiration and oxygen delivery.

Cellular Respiration

The processes of cellular respiration break down one glucose molecule into carbon dioxide and water. The final results of the three processes (glycolysis, the Krebs cycle, and oxidative phosphorylation) also generate adenosine triphosphate (ATP; Fig. 14.1).

In glycolysis, glucose is ultimately converted into two molecules of pyruvate, and a small amount of ATP is created. A transition reaction in the mitochondrial matrix, pyruvate oxidation, converts the pyruvate to acetyl coenzyme A. The Krebs, or citric acid cycle, is an eight-reaction series that will occur only in the presence of oxygen. In the cycle, glucose is oxidized to carbon dioxide, carbon dioxide is released, and two molecules of ATP and both NADH and $FADH_2$ are produced.[5]

It is in the process of oxidative phosphorylation that the majority of ATP is produced. Electrons are released from NADH and $FADH_2$ as they are passed along a series of enzymes. The ions then flow back through special pores in the mitochondrial membrane, driving ATP synthesis with a net yield of 34 ATP molecules and 6 water molecules per glucose molecule.[5]

In the absence of oxygen, there is a significant reduction in ATP creation. The absence of this cellular energy source impairs normal processes including active transport, muscle contraction, and protein synthesis. It also decreases energy available for energy-dependent functions, including carbohydrate, lipid, and protein metabolism.

Oxygen-Carrying Capacity and Delivery

Oxygen delivery (DO_2) is the total amount of oxygen delivered to the tissues per minute, irrespective of blood flow distribution. Oxygen delivery can be calculated as $DO_2 = CaO_2 \times CO$, where the oxygen content is $CaO_2 = (1.39 \times Hb \times SpO_2/100) + (0.003 \times PO_2)$. In the context of shock, this emphasizes that decreased oxygen delivery is a function of one or more out of anemia, hemoglobin (Hb) desaturation, or low cardiac output. Cardiac output is $CO = Stroke\ Volume \times Heart\ Rate$, and stroke volume is determined by preload, afterload, and contractility, which essentially leaves six variables for oxygen delivery: Hb, Hb saturation, preload, afterload, heart rate, and contractility (Fig. 14.2).[3,5,6]

In the oxygen delivery equation, it is worth noting that oxygen-carrying capacity is over 450 times more dependent on oxygen saturation than on partial pressure. The S-shaped oxyhemoglobin dissociation curve allows blood to unload oxygen where it is needed most: small changes in PaO_2 lead to large changes in the saturation, which benefits peripheral tissues. Shifts of the oxyhemoglobin dissociation curve result from changes in pH, temperature, 2,3-diphosphoglycerate, and type of Hb (Fig. 14.3). Except in cases of profound anemia, there is essentially no gain, and there may be physiologic harm, in increasing the PaO_2 above the level at which the Hb saturation is 99%. An oxygen saturation of 94% may be sufficient for most patients.[6–8]

Global oxygen consumption (VO_2) measures the total amount of oxygen consumed by the tissues per minute. Body oxygen consumption is the difference between oxygen delivery and consumption: $DO_2 - VO_2$. It can be measured directly or derived from the Fick equation using cardiac output and arterial and venous oxygen measures: $VO_2 = CO \times (CaO_2 - CvO_2)$. Measures of oxygen saturation in the pulmonary artery or superior vena cava provide objective data on the balance between oxygen supply and consumption. The normal range is 60% to 80%.[5,6]

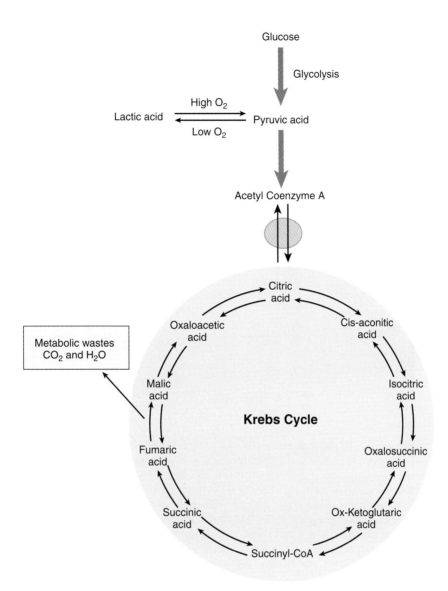

• **Figure 14.1** Krebs Cycle. (Modified from Sanders M. *Mosby's Paramedic Textbook*. 3rd ed. Mosby; 2007.)

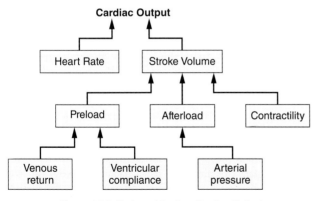

• **Figure 14.2** Factors Affecting Cardiac Output.

Physiologic Response to Shock

The physiologic response to shock also describes the body's compensatory mechanisms for the underperfused or underoxygenated states. The vasomotor centers in the pons and medulla control the immediate response, which are triggered when baroreceptors in the carotid bodies and aortic arch detect falling pressure. Those inhibitory centers normally maintain systolic blood pressures at an individual's physiologic set point somewhere between systolic pressures of about 50 and 180 mm Hg. Chemoreceptors, also located in the carotid sinus and aortic arch, sense decreased oxygenation from decreased carrying capacity or delivery, and hypoxia triggers the same vasomotor center activity that hypotension does.[3,6]

The sympathetic response to hypoperfusion is the release of norepinephrine and epinephrine, which increases heart rate and myocardial contractility; constricts peripheral vasculature, particularly in the arterioles and venules; and increases minute ventilation. In the lungs, hypoxic vasoconstriction shunts blood away from even underventilated areas of the lung to improve gas exchange. The aim of these hemodynamic changes is to maintain perfusion to essential organs. Interestingly, other areas in the brain, including the hypothalamus and cerebral cortex, can also trigger the same vasomotor center activity in response to psychological and physical stimuli such as strong emotions, pain, or cold.[3,6]

Fluids within the body are located in the vascular, interstitial, and intracellular spaces. Movement of fluid between spaces is regulated

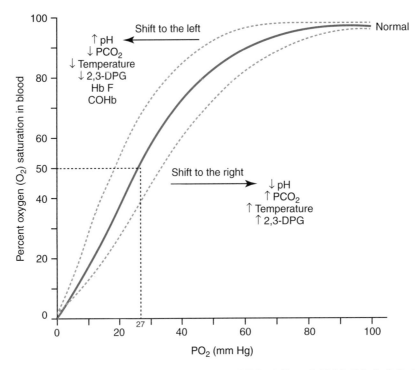

• **Figure 14.3** Oxyhemoglobin Dissociation Curves: Normal and Shifted. (From Schick L, Windle P. *PeriAnesthesia Nursing Core Curriculum: Preprocedure, Phase I and Phase II PACU Nursing.* 3rd ed. Saunders; 2016.)

by solute concentrations and pressure gradients. Neurohormonal changes in response to decreased perfusion states redistribute fluid to the intravascular spaces. Low atrial filling pressures trigger increased arginine vasopressin levels, reaching a maximal antidiuretic effect in about 2 hours. At the same time, renal detection of low circulating blood volume causes the release of renin, triggering the release of angiotensin I, subsequently converted to angiotensin II and stimulating aldosterone release. Aldosterone increases renal sodium retention, decreasing urinary water losses. This takes 12 to 24 hours to reach full effect. There is also an increase in serum blood glucose through a combination of gluconeogenesis, glycogenolysis, and inhibition of glucose uptake by the tissues. This relative hyperglycemia shifts the osmotic gradient within the vascular space in an effort to pull fluid from the other two compartments. Early in shock, the vasculature is primed for increased calcium sensitivity and reactivity (Figs. 14.4 and 14.5).[3,5,6]

Shock becomes decompensated when natural mechanisms fail to maintain perfusion, and hypotension develops. Normally, sodium and potassium are moved against concentration gradients to maintain a slightly negative intracellular charge. Moving these ions against a concentration gradient requires energy. With depleted energy sources, the energy-dependent sodium-potassium pump begins to fail. Normal cell membrane potential also fails, and sodium and water move into the cells, further decreasing microvascular perfusion. Cellular edema causes cell membrane disruption, which releases lysosomal enzymes, injuring surrounding cells. As shock progresses, vascular reactivity and calcium sensitivity begin to decline. Endothelial dysfunction associated with decreased nitric oxide formation and release will also develop, creating an inability for endothelium and smooth muscle to counteract increased sympathetic tone, creating areas of persistent hypoperfusion. This may be one of the links in the progression from inflammation to tissue infarction. An example of this dysfunction is observed in an extremity mottled from shock-induced vasoconstriction, which does not display the

normal blanching and reflow, or "reactive hyperemia," seen when pressure is put on a capillary bed (Figs. 14.6 and 14.7).[3,5,6]

In shock states in which there is vascular endothelial damage or a trigger to the immune system, the linked inflammatory and coagulation cascades are activated. Prolonged cellular hypoxia can also trigger inflammation. The localized inflammatory response is designed to facilitate leukocyte and monocyte migration toward the trigger, augmented by chemotaxis, lymphocyte and macrophage function, lysosome activity, reactive oxygen species (ROS), and superoxide anions. Inflammation generates ROS that, along with other inflammatory mediators, alters the microcirculation. Neutrophil apoptosis may be inhibited, enhancing the release of inflammatory mediators. In other cells, apoptosis may be augmented, increasing cell death, thus worsening organ function. Permeability changes in an underperfused gastrointestinal tract can permit translocation of enteric bacteria, potentially contributing to systemic infection. Septic shock may be more proinflammatory than other forms of shock because of the actions of bacterial endotoxins.[3,5,6]

Coagulopathy always accompanies bleeding or inflammation. Normally, local inflammation and coagulation are protective. With systemic inflammation and decreased microvascular circulation, widespread platelet aggregation and fibrin deposition create distributed microthrombi and simultaneously consume platelets and fibrinogen. This alters the usual balance between procoagulant and anticoagulant processes and stimulates a widespread procoagulant imbalance (Fig. 14.8).[3,5,6]

Diagnosis

A diagnosis of shock is based on clinical, hemodynamic, and biochemical signs, which can broadly be summarized into three components: physical examination findings, vital signs, and laboratory values. Physical signs of shock reflect the compensatory

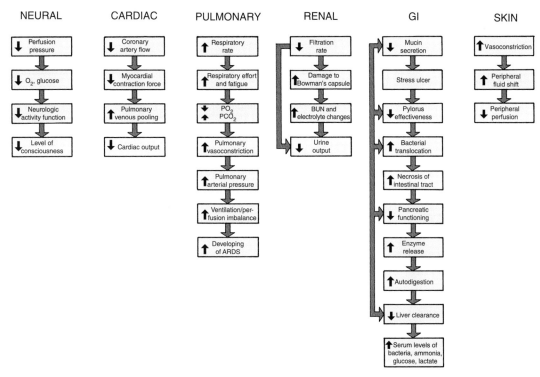

• **Figure 14.4** Major Organ System Changes Associated With Hypoxia and Shock. (Modified from Kitt S, Selfridge-Thomas J, Proehl J, and Kaiser J. *Emergency Nursing: A Physiologic and Clinical Perspective.* Saunders; 1995.)

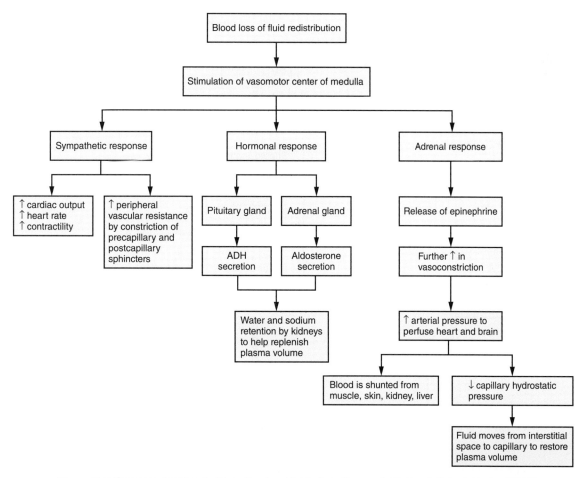

• **Figure 14.5** Compensated Shock. (From Sanders M. *Mosby's Paramedic Textbook.* 3rd ed. Mosby; 2007.)

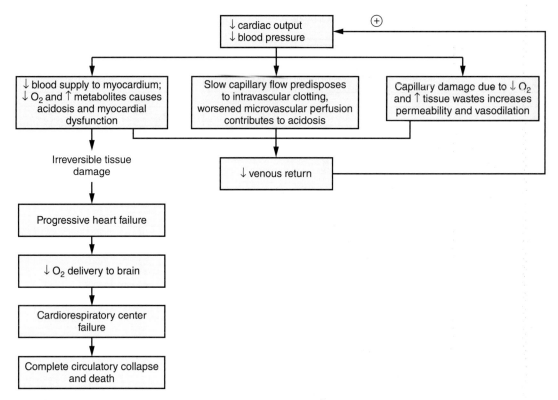

• **Figure 14.6** Uncompensated Shock.

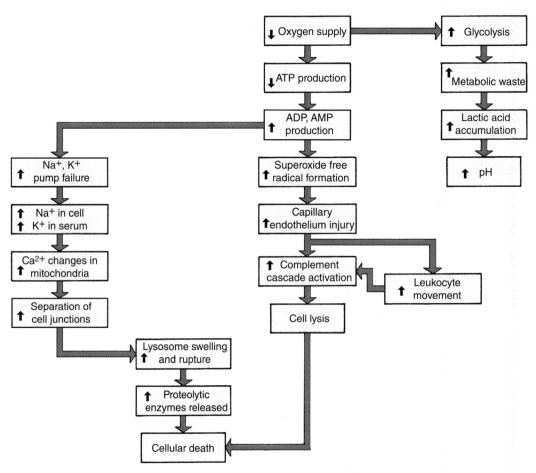

• **Figure 14.7** Micropathophysiologic Changes That Occur During Cellular Ischemia. (Modified from Kitt S, et al. *Emergency Nursing.* Saunders; 1995.)

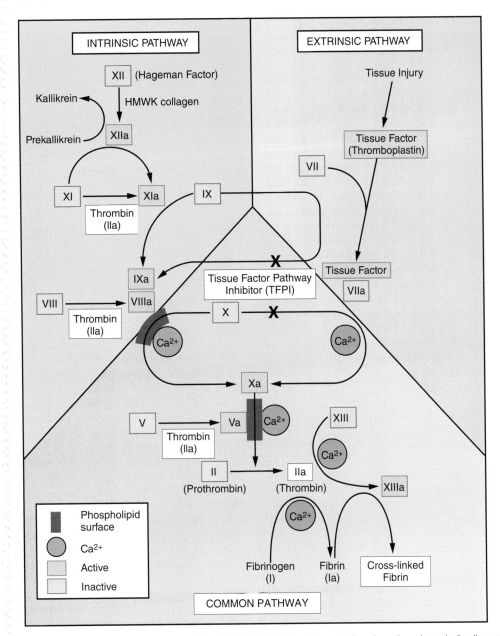

• **Figure 14.8** The Coagulation Cascade. (From Mitchell RN. Hemodynamic disorders, thromboembolic disease, and shock. In Urden LD, Stacy KM, Lough ME, eds. *Critical Care Nursing*. 7th ed. Mosby; 2014.)

mechanisms for shock and the effects of hypoxia. Organs with high metabolic demands will demonstrate altered function most rapidly with the onset of ischemia, whereas those with lower demand will show altered function only if ischemic time is prolonged. Accordingly, three organ systems are most affected: cutaneous (skin that is cold and clammy, with vasoconstriction and cyanosis), renal (urine output of less than 0.5 mL/kg of body weight per hour), and neurologic (altered mental state, which typically includes obtundation, disorientation, and confusion).[3]

The type and cause of shock may seem obvious from the medical history and physical examination. This should not preclude a full physical examination to avoid premature diagnostic closure and missed clinical information.

Vital sign changes also reflect attempts to compensate: heart rate and respiratory rate will increase, as well, unless precluded by other factors, including medications and other physiologic insults.

Blood pressure will ultimately decrease if the shock state is untreated. This decline in blood pressure is considered the point at which compensatory mechanisms have failed and the shock becomes "uncompensated."

All vital signs must be considered in the context of expected values for age. Additionally, the appearance of hypotension can also be masked in patients with chronic hypertension who can be markedly underperfused at arterial pressures that are not hypotensive for those with normal autoregulation.

The shock index (SI) is defined as heart rate divided by systolic blood pressure, with a normal range of 0.5 to 0.7 in healthy adults. First introduced in 1967 to measure hypovolemia in patients with hemorrhagic or septic shock, it appears to be an earlier and more helpful indicator of shock than the vital sign measures in isolation. Physiologically, the SI is inversely related to cardiac index, stroke volume, and mean arterial pressure (MAP). Values over 0.9 or 1.0 are associated with worsened outcomes in patients with circulatory failure, trauma, and septic shock, and increasing SI is also associated with increasing transfusion requirement in traumatic shock.[9–13]

Serum lactate or base deficit measures can help identify patients in shock and assess their response to resuscitation. The lactate produced as a product of anaerobic metabolism is an indirect marker of oxygen debt, and the base deficit values derived from arterial blood gas measures are similarly sensitive and specific. A normal serum lactate is under 2 mmol/L and a normal base deficit is between +2 and –2 mEq/L.[2] Either measure can be used to improve clinical decision-making in any shock state. In an example from trauma patients, the addition of a cellular marker of perfusion to vital sign measures nearly doubles the sensitivity in predicting major injury. Normotensive trauma patients with hyperlactatemia from cellular hypoperfusion have a 4.2 times greater chance of death than normotensive patients with a normal serum lactate. In patients with shock, the degree of lactate or base deficit derangement correlates closely with mortality, and the progression toward normal demonstrates resuscitation success as reliably as trending improvements in mixed or central venous oxygen saturation.[14–20]

It is important to note that there are causes for hyperlactatemia other than shock, particularly excessive muscle activity, including seizures, metformin ingestion, thiamine deficiency, malignancy, liver failure, and mitochondrial disease.[14,21]

Management

Early detection of shock states and early intervention is necessary to prevent worsening organ dysfunction. The cellular effects of an oxygen supply and demand imbalance are consistent across all etiologies of shock, so it is not necessary to clarify the diagnosis before resuscitation begins: initial management is problem oriented. Generally, the "three Vs" (volume resuscitation, attention to ventilation, and consideration of vasopressors) identify the triad of early interventions.

Volume

Where oxygen delivery is a function of oxygen-carrying capacity and cardiac output, cardiac output is related to preload and contractility, and volume status can affect preload and contractility; properly timed and properly balanced intravascular volume expansion is an essential part of the treatment for any form of shock. Even patients with cardiogenic shock may benefit from carefully monitored and titrated fluid boluses.

Properly controlled and timed fluid administration improves outcomes, whereas excess fluid administration can increase shock morbidity and mortality.[22,23] The goal is to reach the plateau portion of the Frank–Starling curve where cardiac output is independent of preload, although this is difficult to assess clinically. The technique used for most patients is administering between a fixed volume of 250 mL up to a weight-based volume up to 10 mL/kg over 15 to 30 minutes while evaluating for a favorable physiologic response (heart rate, blood pressure, pulse pressure, or perfusion signs) and for the absence of adverse effects such as a change in heart or lung sounds.[4]

The "passive leg raise" (PLR) may be beneficial in identifying patients who will benefit from volume administration. Beginning with the patient semirecumbent (head elevated 45 degrees), then lowering the upper body flat and passively raising the legs 45 degrees, about 300 mL of venous blood is relocated from the lower body to the right heart. An increase in cardiac output or a derivative,

such as end-tidal carbon dioxide ($EtCO_2$), indicates a patient who will have a beneficial cardiac output effect from fluid administration.[24] A PLR-induced increase in $EtCO_2$ greater than or equal to 5% predicted a fluid-induced cardiac index change over 15% with 71% sensitivity (95% confidence interval: 48%–89%) and 100% specificity.[25]

Ventilation

Administer supplemental oxygen to achieve a peripheral saturation of at least 93%. Remember that the oxygen-carrying capacity equation demonstrates almost no benefit from supplemental oxygen once the saturation is at 99%, and the literature suggests a possibility of harm from hyperoxemia.[6–8] In addition to improving oxygen delivery, mechanical ventilation reduces the oxygen demand from respiratory muscle work, and the increased intrathoracic pressure decreases left ventricular (LV) afterload. Accordingly, endotracheal intubation is helpful in resuscitation for patients with persistent hypoxemia, persistent or worsening acidemia, and markedly increased work of breathing. The salutary benefits of the LV can be counterbalanced by adverse effects of decreased preload and increased afterload on a failing right ventricle.[26] Patients with shock are not good candidates for noninvasive ventilation.[3]

A clinical pearl linking volume resuscitation and mechanical ventilation is that an abrupt decrease in blood pressure following either the initiation of positive pressure ventilation or an increase in positive end-expiratory pressure suggests that the increased intrathoracic pressure is decreasing preload. Clinicians should include an evaluation for hypovolemia and possibly a thoughtful fluid challenge, along with ventilator causes such as autoPEEP and tension pneumothorax, in the differential diagnosis for the blood pressure decline.[3,27]

Vasopressors

If hypotension persists despite fluid administration, the use of a vasopressor is indicated. Adrenergic agonists are the first-line vasopressors because of their rapid onset of action, high potency, and short half-life, which allows easy dose adjustment. Stimulation of each type of adrenergic receptor has potentially beneficial and harmful effects that must be considered when choosing an agent.[4] The administration of vasopressor agents through peripheral intravenous lines, particularly in short-term, early resuscitation situations, is safe.[28,29]

Norepinephrine is an excellent initial choice for most adult patients. It has mixed α- and β-adrenergic properties that benefit both peripheral vasomotor tone and cardiac output. Dopamine also has both α and β properties but is associated with worse outcomes in many patients. In patients with cardiogenic shock, dopamine induced more arrhythmias and was associated with worsened mortality. It is also associated with worsened outcomes in patients with septic shock.[2,30–33] Unless the adult patient is bradycardic, dopamine is probably not a good first-line vasopressor agent.

Epinephrine has predominantly β effects at low doses and α effects with increasing doses. It can be effective as an added agent for refractory shock states.[34] The addition of low-dose vasopressin to a catecholamine infusion may be associated with a survival benefit for some shock patients requiring a second agent. It should not be used at doses higher than 0.04 U/min, and it should be administered only in patients with a high level of cardiac output.[4,35]

So-called "renal-dose" dopamine, doses under 3 μg/kg/min, may selectively dilate the hepatosplanchnic and renal vasculature and has long been thought to be beneficial for renal protection. Controlled trials have shown no benefit and have suggested the possibility of harm. Dopaminergic stimulation may also have undesired endocrine effects on the hypothalamic-pituitary system, resulting in immunosuppression, primarily through a reduction in the release of prolactin. The concept of renal-dose dopamine in critical care has been relegated to folklore.[2,30–33]

Hypovolemic Shock

Hypovolemic shock can be hemorrhagic or nonhemorrhagic. *Hemorrhage,* loss of plasma and red cell mass from the vascular system, can be either internal or external. Normal blood volume is approximately 7% of the ideal adult body weight (approximately 70 mL/kg) and up to 90 mL/kg in children.[35] Physiologic response varies with volume loss. Changes in blood pressure at times may not be seen until 30% to 40% of the total blood volume is lost, so attention to physical examination findings and other vital signs is important in detecting impending shock.[3,36,37] Remember that an elevated SI is associated with a need for transfusion in hemorrhagic shock.

Hemorrhage is the leading cause of trauma death and of preventable trauma death.[38] Intrathoracic and intraabdominal bleeding are well recognized as causes of hypovolemia in trauma. Significant losses from noncavitary causes (pelvic fracture, skin laceration, and multiple long bone fractures) may also cause a severe shock state. For example, an isolated closed femur fracture can result in a blood loss of up to 2 L. The mortality rate for pelvic fracture is up to 15%, and up to 70% of those deaths are attributed to blood loss.[37]

Not all hemorrhagic shock patients have traumatic hemorrhage. Obstetric hemorrhage is the leading cause of maternal mortality worldwide, and patients with gastrointestinal bleeding and large vessel disruption are also common triggers for large-volume resuscitation.

When available, blood products are optimal for patients with hemorrhagic shock. There is little value to prehospital crystalloid resuscitation for trauma patients. In a large US registry study, unadjusted mortality was significantly higher in patients who received prehospital IV fluids, an outcome reproduced in subgroups of penetrating trauma, hypotensive patients, patients with severe brain injury, and patients undergoing immediate surgery.[39] A large European trial similarly found that increasing prehospital intravenous fluid volumes in trauma patients increased the risk of mortality, particularly in patients without severe brain injury.[40] Massive crystalloid resuscitation is clearly associated with coagulopathy, increased hemorrhage, and the development of the abdominal compartment syndrome.[41,42] When crystalloid is administered, balanced solutions appear to offer a beneficial reduction in coagulopathy, hyperchloremic acidosis, and renal dysfunction compared with normal saline solution.[43]

For trauma patients who need more than two units of packed red blood cells, evidence supports resuscitation strategies with early administration of platelets, fresh frozen plasma, and platelets. There may be an advantage to approximating a 1:1:1 ratio between packed red blood cells, plasma, and platelets in the context of trauma transfusion resuscitation.[44–47] Early plasma and platelet transfusion in nontrauma patients with hemorrhagic shock is common, although the clinical outcome benefits are less clear.[48,49]

Specifically in the out-of-hospital arena, transfusion of both plasma and red cells generates an overall mortality reduction and

is economically advantageous. The clinical benefits are more proven in blunt trauma patients or in those with longer transport times.[50–53] For transfused patients, there is a dose-dependent increase in mortality with coadministered crystalloid volume.[50] Transport providers with immediate access to blood products should use a low/no crystalloid resuscitation strategy for trauma patients. The role of unfractionated donor blood (whole blood) offers logistical advantages and earlier access to mixed-component resuscitation; however, there is currently limited evidence to show a significant benefit compared with component therapy.[54,55]

Transfusion must be approached thoughtfully. Severe anemia is associated with worsened outcomes in critical care patients, but evidence dating back to the last century demonstrates that a liberal transfusion strategy to reverse anemia is not beneficial. Transfusion to a Hb of 7 g/dL in adult patients improves outcomes, or is at least not inferior, compared with transfusion to a higher target in critical care patients, both overall and in the subgroups of patients with cardiovascular disease, traumatic head injury, and mechanical ventilation.[56] The administration of blood products carries real risk to the patient, which should factor into the decision to transfuse (Box 14.1).[57–61]

Patients with hemorrhagic shock and associated resuscitation are at risk for falling into the synergistic and self-perpetuating "bloody vicious cycle" or "triad of death" of acidosis, coagulopathy, and hypothermia (Fig. 14.9). This phenomenon and a thoughtful approach to management have been described for decades.[77–80] As described earlier, metabolic acidosis is a key physiologic derangement in shock. Systemic adverse effects seem to occur when the pH declines below 7.1 and include impaired cardiac output, contractility, ability to maintain vasomotor tone, and impaired platelet function.[42,81]

Hypothermia in shock is multifactorial, with contributors including exposure for resuscitation, administration of relatively cold fluids, medications that reduce normal thermoregulatory mechanisms, reduced metabolic substrate to power heat generation, and the loss of intrinsic adaptive mechanisms such as shivering. A core body temperature below 34°C has deleterious effects on clot formation, especially affecting platelet function, and is independently associated with an 80% increase in mortality.[82,83] Nearly 30% of trauma patients arrive at trauma centers with a temperature below 35°C.[84]

Coagulopathy is a function of the loss of coagulation factors through direct loss and consumption, factor dilution, and the release of anticoagulant factors. There also appear to be genetic differences in susceptibility to coagulopathy, perhaps manifested by an increased coagulopathy from hypoperfusion.[42]

The risk for life-threatening coagulopathy increases with injury severity, hypotension, hypothermia, and severe acidosis and demonstrates the synergistic effects of the triangle. While patients with moderate injury are unlikely to become coagulopathic, about 40% of patients with Injury Severity Score (ISS) over 25 and hypotension develop coagulopathy. Acidosis increases the likelihood of shock by another 50%, and virtually all patients with ISS > 25, pH < 7.1, T < 34°C, and systolic blood pressure < 70 mm Hg have life-threatening coagulopathy.[85]

Shock resuscitation, then, involves attention not only to appropriate efforts to restore hemodynamic function appropriately but also to preventing hypothermia and to the possibility of developing coagulopathy. In trauma, the idea that "damage control surgery," in which hemostasis is achieved through temporizing measures, such as intraabdominal packing and definitive repair, is delayed until temperature, vital signs, and coagulation are managed is a classic

• BOX 14.1 Adverse Effects of Blood Transfusion

Acute Reactions

Acute Hemolytic Transfusion Reactions
A hemolytic transfusion reaction is one in which red cell destruction follows transfusion. Symptoms appear within minutes. The interaction of recipient antibodies with donor red cell antigens results in destruction of transfused cells. Rarely, transfusion of ABO-incompatible plasma or platelets also can cause red cell hemolysis. The incidence of acute hemolytic reaction is about 1 per 76,000 transfusions, with a mortality of 1 per 1.8 million transfused units.[57,58]

Febrile Nonhemolytic Transfusion Reactions
Febrile nonhemolytic transfusion reactions are characterized by an otherwise unexplained rise in temperature of at least 1°C during or shortly after transfusion. Antipyretic premedication may mask the fever, but it does not prevent the cytokine-mediated chills and rigors. Other causes of fever should be excluded before making a diagnosis. These reactions are seen more often after a transfusion of platelets (up to 30% of platelet transfusions) than red blood cells, because platelets are stored at room temperature, which promotes leukocyte activation and cytokine accumulation.[62]

Allergic Reactions
Urticaria is the mildest form of an allergic reaction, with an incidence of 1% to 3%.[58,63] Anaphylaxis occurs in 1 per 20,000 to 50,000 transfusions.[59] The identification and management of anaphylactic shock are discussed elsewhere in this chapter.

Transfusion-Related Acute Lung Injury
Transfusion-related acute lung injury (TRALI) is an important cause of transfusion-associated morbidity and mortality, with a reported incidence between 0.41 and 1 case per 5000 component units transfused. TRALI is the new (within 6 hours) onset or worsening of hypoxemia (PaO_2/FiO_2 <300 mm Hg), with a chest X-ray consistent with pulmonary edema. Lung injury is most often transient: approximately 80% of patients will improve within 96 hours.[57,64] The pulmonary edema in TRALI is noncardiogenic and is not improved by diuretic therapy.[65,66]

TRALI is believed to be an antigen–antibody-mediated reaction. Antibodies can be formed after exposure to foreign antigens by pregnancy, transfusion, or transplantation, and transfusion may lead to neutrophil activation and resultant pulmonary endothelial damage, capillary leakage, and pulmonary edema.[64]

All plasma-containing components have been implicated in TRALI, with the risk greatest for platelets, followed by plasma, then packed red blood cells. Products donated by females, particularly by multiparous females, appear to be more likely to trigger reactions. It may also be that products donated by younger donors carry a greater risk for adverse outcomes. Other risk reduction strategies include using packed red blood cells with storage times under 2 weeks and platelet products with storage times under 2 days, because reactive compounds may accumulate during storage.[61,64–66]

Transfusion-Associated Circulatory Overload
Transfusion-associated circulatory overload may precipitate acute pulmonary edema within 6 hours of transfusion. Management is consistent with the management of other pulmonary edema patients; fluid restriction, diuresis, and consideration for positive pressure ventilation.[67,68]

Citrate Toxicity
When large volumes of blood components containing citrate are transfused rapidly, the increased plasma citrate chelates calcium and magnesium ions, resulting in hypocalcemia and hypomagnesemia. The transfusion rate must be high: over 6 units per hour (35 mL/min) of blood must be transfused to precipitate a reduction in ionized calcium levels. Citrate toxicity/hypocalcemia is more likely in patients with hypothermia, hepatic failure, alkalosis, and pediatric patients.[69,70]

Disorders of Potassium
Extracellular potassium in transfused blood rarely causes problems because of rapid dilution, redistribution into cells, and excretion.[71] An infusion rate of about 120 mL/min is probably required.[70] Irradiated cells have greater potassium leakage. Interestingly, hypokalemia is more common than posttransfusion hyperkalemia because donor cells reaccumulate potassium intracellularly, and citrate metabolism causes further intracellular movement. Catecholamine release and aldosterone urinary loss can also trigger hypokalemia in the setting of massive transfusion.[58]

Delayed Reactions: Occurring After 24 Hours

Alloimmunization
Antibodies are produced in response to immunization by antigen-positive red cells following transfusion, organ transplantation, or fetal–maternal hemorrhage during pregnancy. Up to 3% of patients exposed to foreign red cells will form ABO antibodies, with more in some patient groups: up to 40% of sickle cell anemia patients and 9% of thalassemia major patients have ABO antibodies. An acute life-threatening hemolytic anemia, described earlier, can occur in alloimmunized patients when they are transfused.[72,73]

Transfusion-Associated Immunomodulation
Transfusion-associated immunomodulation (TRIM) is the downregulation of a recipient's cellular immune response as a result of allogenic blood transfusion. This downregulation increases the chances of postoperative infections, hospital-acquired infection, cancer recurrence, and possibly a transfusion-related multiple organ dysfunction syndrome. It is believed to be leukocyte mediated. The use of autologous blood or leukocyte-reduced blood can mitigate the adverse effects of TRIM.[74–76]

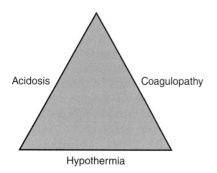

• **Figure 14.9** The "Triad of Death."

and effective demonstration of this.[86] The concepts extend to all states of shock.

It is fairly easy to measure vital signs and temperature. Measurements of pH and perfusion measures such as lactate are also fairly straightforward and can even be completed at the bedside.

Clotting factor function evaluation typically requires some delay for laboratory measurement and is limited: it does not show platelet dysfunction or hyperfibrinolysis. Because laboratory studies are processed at normal body temperature, the results do not reflect the impact of hypothermia.[87]

Tranexamic acid inhibits intrinsic hyperfibrinolysis. It is used extensively in orthopedic and obstetric care and is now ubiquitous in emergency trauma care. For trauma patients, the therapeutic benefit appears to require administration within 3 hours of injury, possibly within the first hour, and it seems to be greatest in patients with severe shock.[88–91]

Thromboelastography (TEG) provides rapid, real-time, and more specific measures of coagulation system function than do traditional laboratory tests. Very simply, TEG measures the strength of fibrin–platelet bonds in whole blood. A small (0.36-mL) whole-blood sample in a heated cup is rotated six times per minute to mimic venous circulation and activate coagulation. The cup has a central pin and connecting torsion wire that measure the speed and strength of fibrin formation and fibrin–platelet binding, which then convert that information to numeric values and a graphical representation of the complete hemostatic process including coagulation, platelet function, and fibrinolysis.[92]

Nonhemorrhagic volume loss usually arises from vomiting, diarrhea, excessive sweating (such as from heat emergency), polyuria, and loss of denuded skin from the body surface area. Patients can also translocate fluid into the "third space" or extravascular space, particularly with sepsis or intraabdominal injury. The shift is caused by direct vessel injury, mediator-driven increases in capillary permeability, and osmotic shifts as plasma proteins move into the interstitial space. Significant edema may be noted either in the affected areas or systemically as these fluid shifts occur. Patients with this third spacing–induced hypovolemia may particularly benefit from the addition of large molecule-containing fluids, such as proteins or starches, to their volume repletion to improve the intravascular osmotic tone.[3]

Distributive Shock

Vasomotor dysfunction results in either high/normal arterial resistance with expanded venous capacitance or low arterial resistance. This dysfunction causes a relative hypovolemia as blood is sequestered in either the arterial or venous beds. The absolute blood volume does not change, but an increase in vascular space results in a decrease in effective blood volume and tissue perfusion. Septic shock and neurogenic shock are classic forms of distributive shock.

Septic Shock

Septic shock is a subset of sepsis in which underlying circulatory and cellular/metabolic abnormalities are profound enough to substantially increase mortality. As described earlier, sepsis involves organ dysfunction, indicating a pathobiology more complex than infection plus an accompanying inflammatory response alone.

Even a modest degree of organ dysfunction when infection is first suspected is associated with an in-hospital mortality in excess of 10%. Patients with suspected infection who are likely to have a prolonged ICU stay or to die in the hospital can be promptly identified at the bedside with a validated scoring tool called Quick Sequential Organ Failure Assessment (qSOFA). These high-risk adult patients have two or more of the following: alteration in mental status (Glasgow Coma Scale <15), systolic blood pressure less than or equal to 100 mm Hg, or respiratory rate greater than or equal to 22 breaths per minute. Positive qSOFA criteria should also prompt consideration of possible infection in patients not previously recognized as infected. Patients with septic shock can be identified with a clinical construct of sepsis with persisting hypotension requiring vasopressors to maintain a mean MAP greater than or equal to 65 mm Hg and having a serum lactate level greater than 2 mmol/L (18 mg/dL) despite adequate volume resuscitation. With these criteria, hospital mortality is in excess of 40%.[93]

For the management of septic shock, a protocolized approach with a goal of effective resuscitation in the first 6 hours is well known to improve results. Care is addressed at volume resuscitation to euvolemia; early support of the MAP to at least 65 mm Hg using vasopressors, if needed; and early appropriate antimicrobial therapy.[3] Norepinephrine is the most commonly used vasopressor and is the better initial choice in most patients.[2] Early use of vasopressin in the face of escalating norepinephrine doses may be a useful approach, and the use of epinephrine as an initial or second-line vasopressor agent is reasonable.[35] Although the role

of steroids in the care of patients with septic shock is unclear, the administration of a single dose of a mineralocorticoid steroid for septic shock patients who require a second vasopressor for blood pressure support is also a reasonable intervention.[94,95]

Lactate or base deficit levels are useful in identifying patients with shock and are helpful in trending the success (or failure) of resuscitative measures.[14,17,18,20]

Neurogenic Shock

A patient with acute spinal cord injury may present with or develop neurogenic shock, suggested by hypotension and a variable heart rate response. This occurs secondary to sympathetic denervation, resulting in arteriolar dilation and pooling of blood in the venous compartment and interruption of cardiac sympathetic innervation, particularly above the T6 level. Loss of supraspinal control of the sympathetic nervous system leads to unopposed vagal tone with relaxation of vascular smooth muscles below the level of the cord injury, resulting in decreased venous return, decreased cardiac output, hypotension, loss of diurnal fluctuations of blood pressure, reflex bradycardia, and peripheral adrenoreceptor hyperresponsiveness.[96–99]

The same physiologic disruption contributes to the autonomic dysreflexia sometimes seen in postacute patients with spinal cord lesions, in which sympathetic-mediated vasoconstriction is induced by afferent peripheral stimulation below the level of the lesion. For example, stimuli such as urinary catheterization, dressing changes, or surgical stimulation can lead to severe blood pressure spikes out of proportion to the stimulus.

Management is first aimed at ensuring euvolemia. Subsequently, vasomotor tone is restored, using an agent that minimizes bradycardia. The appropriate resuscitation end point and optimal mean arterial blood pressure for maintaining spinal cord perfusion is not known; there may be a benefit to maintaining MAP at a minimum of 85 mm Hg for the first 7 days following injury.[96,100] There is no role for steroids in the treatment of neurogenic shock caused by spinal cord injury.[101]

Anaphylaxis

Anaphylaxis is an acute systemic allergic reaction that results from the release of chemical mediators after an antigen–antibody reaction. The reaction is mediated by immunoglobulin E (IgE), which rests on the surface of mast cells and basophils in the body, especially in respiratory and gastrointestinal system cells. A reaction results in the release of mediators including histamine, kinins, and the slow reactive substance of anaphylaxis, which cause three major effects: (1) vasodilation, (2) smooth muscle spasm, and (3) increased vascular permeability with edema formation (Fig. 14.10).[102]

Anaphylactoid reactions are clinically indistinguishable from anaphylactic reactions but are not IgE mediated and do not require prior sensitization; rather, they occur via direct stimulation of mast cells or by complement activation. They are caused most often by drugs, such as iodinated radiograph contrast, nonsteroidal antiinflammatory agents, blood transfusion, some antibiotics, and opiates.[102]

Symptoms of anaphylaxis are usually sudden in onset and can progress in severity over minutes to hours. Patients at risk of severe anaphylaxis include those with peanut and tree nut allergy, preexisting respiratory or cardiovascular disease, previous biphasic anaphylactic reactions, and advanced age. Interestingly, most patients with fatal or near-fatal anaphylaxis do not have a history of severe reactions.[102]

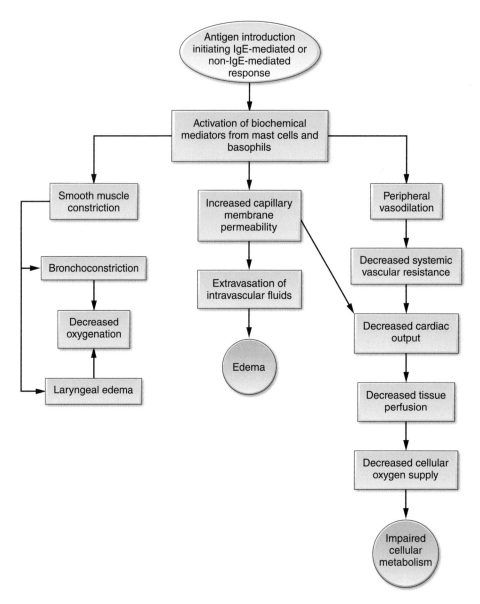

• **Figure 14.10** Allergic Reaction. (From Monahan F, Sands J, Neighbors M, et al. *Phipps' Medical-Surgical Nursing*. 8th ed. Elsevier; 2008.)

The broad spectrum of anaphylaxis presentations requires an index of suspicion and good clinical judgment, because early recognition prevents progression to a more serious outcome. Typically, at least two of the four organ systems are involved: cardiovascular, respiratory, gastrointestinal, or skin. Although most cases of anaphylaxis include cutaneous manifestations, their absence does not exclude the diagnosis. Similarly, anaphylaxis frequently presents without hypotension.

The life-saving therapy in anaphylactic shock is epinephrine, administered initially as an intramuscular (IM) injection in the anterolateral thigh. There are no randomized controlled studies of epinephrine during anaphylaxis; there is agreement on a recommended dose of 0.01 mg/kg (maximum dose, 0.5 mg) IM, repeated every 5 to 15 minutes, as needed. For patients who do not respond to IM epinephrine injections, administer intravenous or intraosseous epinephrine. Crystalloid volume resuscitation and other vasopressors, as adjuncts to epinephrine administration, may be helpful. There is no substitute for epinephrine in

the treatment of anaphylaxis. Administration of H_1 and/or H_2 antihistamines and corticosteroids should be considered adjunctive therapy.[102]

Cardiogenic Shock

Cardiogenic shock is hypoperfusion caused by cardiac failure. The classical diagnostic factors include hypotension, reduced cardiac index (8 L/min/m² without support or under 2.2 L/min/m² with cardiovascular support), and elevated ventricular filling pressures. Myocardial infarction (MI) with LV failure is the most common cause, affecting 5% to 8% of hospitalized ST elevation MI (STEMI) patients and up to 2.5% of non-STEMI patients. Although LV failure is the most common physiologic cause, about 5% of cardiogenic shock patients have right ventricular (RV) failure. Mechanical complications such as ventricular wall rupture, papillary muscle rupture, and valve failure are potential causes of, or contributors to, cardiogenic shock, as are infectious sources (endocarditis and myocarditis), structural cardiomyopathies, and blunt or penetrating cardiac injury.[4,103]

Treatment is aimed in two directions: resolution of the cause and supportive therapy. For patients with STEMI, time-sensitive recanalization is clearly associated with improved outcomes: each 15-minute time reduction saves 6.3 lives per 1000 treated patients.[104] Support until revascularization and recovery from the damage caused before revascularization or the resolution of other causes is permitted by supportive therapies, including pharmacologic and mechanical support. For cardiogenic shock, even more so than for other forms of shock, norepinephrine favors improved outcomes over dopamine.[2,103] The intraaortic balloon pump is a common mechanical aid in cardiogenic shock, putatively improving coronary artery perfusion and reducing afterload. Interestingly, there is still some room for debate on the efficacy of the balloon pump. A series of individual trials and several meta-analyses suggest that it is equivocal or perhaps helpful in most patient groups; most agree that it does not worsen outcomes.[105–109] Other devices to decompress and support the left ventricle exist, as do more robust circulatory support devices. All of these increasingly common approaches are covered elsewhere in this book.

Obstructive Shock

Obstructive shock is an obstruction to cardiovascular flow resulting in impaired diastolic filling or significantly increased afterload. The mechanisms for this are pulmonary embolism (PE), pericardial tamponade, tension pneumothorax, and, in pediatric patients, a structural lesion.

Pulmonary Embolism

Acute PE interferes with both the circulation and gas exchange. Pulmonary artery pressure increases only if more than 50% of the total cross-sectional area of the pulmonary arterial bed is occluded, and RV failure caused by pressure overload is considered the primary cause of death in severe PE. A PE is considered massive when accompanied by shock or hypotension (either relative or absolute).[110]

The patient history is important in making the diagnosis. Major trauma, surgery, lower limb fractures, joint replacements, spinal cord injury, and cancer are common predisposing factors for PE. Oral contraceptive use is the most frequent predisposing factor in women of childbearing age, and PE is a major cause of maternal morbidity and mortality, particularly in the third trimester and extending out to three postpartum months after delivery. Infection and blood transfusion are also associated with PE.[110]

Because PE is the "great masquerader," the diagnosis should be considered in patients with shock and elevated central venous pressure not readily explained by another diagnosis, such as MI, arrhythmia, or other forms of obstructive shock. Symptoms are vague (dyspnea, pleuritic chest pain, and cough are the three most common) but still occur in 50% or fewer patients.[110]

The electrocardiogram (ECG) has low sensitivity and specificity, but it can be helpful. Up to a quarter of patients with PE have a normal EKG, including those with significant clot burden. The most common ECG abnormality in patients with PE is sinus tachycardia, in 28% of patients. Sensitivity for particular EKG findings is low, so they cannot be used to rule out pulmonary embolism. Specificity is high for the RV strain pattern (simultaneous T-wave inversion in the inferior and precordial leads), p-pulmonale, and S1Q3T3, but the prevalence of each is low (11.1%, 0.5%, and 3.7%, respectively).[111]

D-Dimer testing can be useful in excluding the diagnosis of PE. The use of an age-adjusted threshold of 500 μg/L or 10 times the patient age in years, whichever is higher, is safe and improves accuracy.[112]

Acute RV failure is the leading cause of death in patients with massive PE, so management of the patient with massive PE is first directed at supporting the right ventricle. Gentle volume resuscitation in fluid-responsive patients is reasonable; aggressive volume resuscitation without hemodynamic response is of no benefit. It is best to err on the side of withholding volume in these patients, as the right ventricle is poorly responsive to volume loading. Vasopressor support to maintain coronary artery perfusion, particularly with norepinephrine, is indicated in hypotensive patients. Vasopressin is a useful secondary agent, beneficial as a noncatecholamine and likely having some sparing effect on pulmonary vascular resistance compared with adrenergic agents. Inhaled pulmonary vasodilators can be useful.[26] Patients with suspected PE should be rapidly anticoagulated. For those with hemodynamic instability, use of systemic fibrinolysis is associated with a mortality reduction.[113]

Cardiac Tamponade

Cardiac tamponade occurs when blood or effusion accumulates in the closed and relatively noncompliant pericardial sac. The heart is unable to fill, which leads to decreased cardiac output. Acute changes usually become symptomatic rapidly, and surprisingly large chronic accumulations can be well tolerated. The most common causes of larger pericardial effusions are neoplastic, uremic, and idiopathic. Effusions as a complication of MI, coagulopathy, chest radiation, and instrumentation are also common. The treatment is decompression of the pericardial space. Optimization of preload and support of the right ventricle can help temporize the patient until invasive management is possible.[114]

Tension Pneumothorax

Tension pneumothorax results in a complete collapse of one or both lungs with compression on mediastinal vessels and organs. This impairs venous return to the heart and increases afterload. A tension pneumothorax can sometimes be managed with needle decompression; however, the usual intravenous catheter is too short to reach the pleural space in up to a third of trauma patients. A catheter of at least 3.25 inches in length optimizes success rates.[115] The out-of-hospital use of "simple" or "finger" thoracostomy is increasingly accepted as a way to ensure pleural decompression for tension pneumothorax. Physicians and properly trained ground and flight paramedics have demonstrated procedural success, safety, and acceptably low complication rates with this procedure.[116–119] An open pneumothorax can be covered with a three-sided dressing and the patient monitored carefully for the accumulation of air and subsequent development of a tension pneumothorax.

Conclusion

The physiology, presentation, and management of shock is simultaneously complex and simple. Transport teams should be vigilant for the development of the oxygen supply and demand imbalance common to all shock states and should be prepared to intervene before significant vital sign changes are present. The oxygen utilization defect comes from one or more of four, not necessarily exclusive, mechanisms: hypovolemia, cardiac failure, obstruction to cardiac filling or return, and abnormal intravascular volume distribution, and the cellular effects are consistent across all etiologies of shock. For initial resuscitation, it is not necessary to clarify the diagnosis, and the initial problem-oriented management generally follows the triad of volume resuscitation, attention to ventilation, and consideration of vasopressors.

References

1. Cairns CB. Rude unhinging of the machinery of life: Metabolic approaches to hemorrhagic shock. *Curr Opin Crit Care.* 2001;7(6):437–443. (In Eng).
2. De Backer D, Biston P, Devriendt J. Comparison of dopamine and norepinephrine in the treatment of shock. *N Engl J Med.* 2010;362:779–789.
3. Medicine SoCC. *Fundamental Critical Care Support.* 7th ed. Society of Critical Care Medicine; 2021.
4. Vincent J-L, De Backer D. Circulatory shock. *New Engl J Med.* 2013;369(18):1726–1734. doi: 10.1056/NEJMra1208943
5. Hall J, Hall M. *Guyton and Hall Textbook of Medical Physiology.* 14th ed. Elsevier; 2020.
6. Bonanno FG. Physiopathology of shock. *J Emerg Trauma Shock.* 2011;4(2):222–232. doi: 10.4103/0974-2700.82210
7. Singer M, Young PJ, Laffey JG, et al. Dangers of hyperoxia. *Crit Care.* 2021;25(1):440. doi: 10.1186/s13054-021-03815-y
8. Helmerhorst HJ, Roos-Blom MJ, van Westerloo DJ, de Jonge E. Association between arterial hyperoxia and outcome in subsets of critical illness: A systematic review, meta-analysis, and meta-regression of cohort studies. *Crit Care Med.* 2015;43(7):1508–1519. (In Eng). doi: 10.1097/ccm.0000000000000998
9. Koch E, Lovett S, Nghiem T, Riggs RA, Rech MA. Shock index in the emergency department: Utility and limitations. *Open Access Emerg Med.* 2019;11:179–199. (In Eng). doi: 10.2147/oaem.S178358
10. Berger T, Green J, Horeczko T, et al. Shock index and early recognition of sepsis. *West J Emerg Med.* 2013;14(2):168–174.
11. Marenco CW, Lammers DT, Morte KR, Bingham JR, Martin MJ, Eckert MJ. Shock index as a predictor of massive transfusion and emergency surgery on the modern battlefield. *J Surg Res.* 2020;256:112–118. (In Eng). doi: 10.1016/j.jss.2020.06.024
12. Montory K, Charry J, Calle-Toro J, Nunez L, Poveda G. Shock index as a mortality predictor in patients with acute polytrauma. *J Acute Dis* 2015;4(3):202–204.
13. Mutschler M, Nienaber U, Munzbert M, et al. The shock index revisited – a fast guide to transfusion requirement? A retrospective analysis on 21,853 patients derived from the TraumaRegister DGU. *Crit Care.* 2013;17:1–9.
14. Andersen L, Mackenhauer J, Roberts J, Bert K, Cocchi M, Donnino M. Etiology and therapeutic approach to elevated lactate levels. *Mayo Clin Proc.* 2013;88(10):1127–1140.
15. Callaway D, Shapiro N, Donnino M, Baker C, Rosen C. Serum lactate and base deficit as predictors of mortality in normotensive elderly blunt trauma patients. *J Trauma.* 2009;66(4):1040–1044.
16. Donnino M, Andersen L, Giberson T, et al. Initial lactate and lactate change in post-cardiac arrest: A multicenter validation study. *Crit Care Med.* 2014;42(8):1804–1811.
17. Jansen T, van Bommel J, Schoonderbeek F. Early lactate-guided therapy in intensive care unit patients: A multi-center, open-label, randomized controlled trial. *Am J Respir Crit Care Med.* 2010;182(6):752–761.
18. Jones A, Shapiro N, Trzeciak S, Arnold RC, Claremont H, Kline J. Lactate clearance vs central venous oxygen saturation as goals of early sepsis therapy: A randomized clinical trial. *JAMA.* 2010;303(8):739–746.
19. Jones AE. Lactate clearance for assessing response to resuscitation in severe sepsis. *Acad Emerg Med.* 2013;20(8):844–847. (In Eng). doi: 10.1111/acem.12179
20. Liu VX, Morehouse JW, Marelich GP, et al. Multicenter implementation of a treatment bundle for patients with sepsis and intermediate lactate values. *Am J Respir Crit Care Med.* 2016;193(11):1264–1270. (In Eng). doi: 10.1164/rccm.201507-1489OC
21. Hernandez G, Bellomo R, Bakker J. The ten pitfalls of lactate clearance in sepsis. *Intensive Care Med.* 2019;45(1):82–85. doi: 10.1007/s00134-018-5213-x
22. Boyd J, Forbes J, Nakada T. Fluid resuscitation in septic shock. A positive fluid balance and elevated central venous pressure are associated with increased mortality. *Crit Care Med.* 2011;39:259–265.
23. Silversides JA, Fitzgerald E, Manickavasagam US, et al. Deresuscitation of patients with iatrogenic fluid overload is associated with reduced mortality in critical illness. *Crit Care Med.* 2018;46(10):1600–1607. (In Eng). doi: 10.1097/ccm.0000000000003276
24. Cherpanath T, Hirsch A, Geerts B, et al. Predicting fluid responsiveness by passive leg raising: A systematic review and meta-analysis of 23 clinical trials. *Crit Care Med.* 2016;44(5):981–991.
25. Monnet X, Batallie A, Magalhaes E, et al. End-tidal carbon dioxide is better than arterial pressure for predicting volume responsiveness by passive leg raising. *Intensive Care Med.* 2013;39(1):93–100.
26. Wilcox SR, Kabrhel C, Channick RN. Pulmonary hypertension and right ventricular failure in emergency medicine. *Ann Emerg Med.* 2015;66(6):619–628. (In Eng). doi: 10.1016/j.annemergmed.2015.07.525
27. Wilcox SR, Aydin A, Marcolini EG. *Mechanical Ventilation in Emergency Medicine.* Springer International Publishing; 2021.
28. Cardenas-Garcia J, Schaub K, Belchikov Y, Narasimhan M, Koenig S, Mayo P. Safety of peripheral intravenous administration of vasoactive medication. *J Hosp Med.* 2015;10(9):581–585.
29. Ricard J, Salomon L, Boxer A, et al. Central or peripheral catheters for initial venous access of ICU patients. *Crit Care Med.* 2013;41(9):2108–2115.
30. Bellomo R, Chapman M, Finfer S, Hickling K, Myburgh J. Low-dose dopamine in patients with early renal dysfunction. *Lancet.* 2000;356:2139–2143.
31. Jones D, Bellomo R. Renal-dose dopamine: From hypothesis to paradigm to dogma to myth and, finally, superstition? *J Intensive Care Med.* 2005;20(4):199–211. (In Eng). doi: 10.1177/0885066605276963
32. Lauschke A, Teichgraber UK, Frei U, Eckardt KU. "Low-dose" dopamine worsens renal perfusion in patients with acute renal failure. *Kidney Int.* 2006;69(9):1669–1674. (In Eng). doi: 10.1038/sj.ki.5000310
33. Sakr Y, Reinhart K, Vincent L. Does dopamine administration in shock influence outcomes? *Crit Care Med.* 2006;34:589–597.
34. Levy E, Perez P, Perny J, Thivilier C, Gerard A. Comparison of norepinephrine-dobutamine to epinephrine for hemodynamics, lactate metabolism, and organ function variables in cardiogenic shock. *Crit Care Med.* 2011;39:450–455.
35. Demiselle J, Fage N, Radermacher P, Asfar P. Vasopressin and its analogues in shock states: A review. *Ann Intensive Care.* 2020;10(1):9. doi: 10.1186/s13613-020-0628-2
36. Bonanno FG. Hemorrhagic shock: The "physiology approach." *J Emerg Trauma Shock.* 2012;5(4):285–295. doi: 10.4103/0974-2700.102357
37. Trauma ACoSCo. *Advanced Trauma Life Support for Doctors Student Course Manual.* 10th ed. American College of Surgeons; 2018.
38. Koh EY, Oyeniyi BT, Fox EE, et al. Trends in potentially preventable trauma deaths between 2005–2006 and 2012–2013. *Am J Surg.* 2019;218(3):501–506. doi:10.1016/j.amjsurg.2018.12.022
39. Haut ER, Kalish BT, Cotton BA, et al. Prehospital intravenous fluid administration is associated with higher mortality in trauma patients: a National Trauma Data Bank analysis. *Ann Surg.* 2011;253(2):371-377.
40. Hussemann B, Heuer M, Lefering R, et al. Prehospital volume therapy as an independent risk factor after trauma. *BioMed Res Int.* 2015;2015:1–9.
41. Madigan M, Kemp C, Johnson J, Cotton B. Secondary abdominal compartment syndrome after severe extremity injury. *J Trauma* 2008;64(2):280–285.
42. Maegele M, Spinella PC, Schöchl H. The acute coagulopathy of trauma: Mechanisms and tools for risk stratification. *Shock.* 2012;38(5):450–458. doi: 10.1097/SHK.0b013e31826dbd23
43. Hammond NE, Zampieri FG, Tanna GLD, et al. Balanced crystalloids versus saline in critically ill adults – a systematic review

with meta-analysis. *NEJM Evid.* 2022;1(2):EVIDoa2100010. doi: 10.1056/EVIDoa2100010

44. Borgman MA, Spinella PC, Perkins JG, et al. The ratio of blood products transfused affects mortality in patients receiving massive transfusions at a combat support hospital. *J Trauma.* 2007;63(4):805–813. (In Eng). doi: 10.1097/TA.0b013e3181271ba3

45. Holcomb JB, del Junco DJ, Fox EE, et al. The Prospective, Observational, Multicenter, Major Trauma Transfusion (PROMMTT) study: Comparative effectiveness of a time-varying treatment with competing risks. *JAMA Surg.* 2013;148(2):127–136. doi: 10.1001/2013.jamasurg.387

46. Holcomb JB, Tilley BC, Baraniuk S, et al. Transfusion of plasma, platelets, and red blood cells in a 1:1:1 vs a 1:1:2 ratio and mortality in patients with severe trauma: The PROPPR randomized clinical trial. *JAMA.* 2015;313(5):471–482. (In Eng). doi: 10.1001/jama.2015.12

47. Holcomb JB, Wade CE, Michalek JE, et al. Increased plasma and platelet to red blood cell ratios improves outcome in 466 massively transfused civilian trauma patients. *Ann Surg.* 2008;248(3):447–458. (In Eng). doi: 10.1097/SLA.0b013e318185a9ad

48. Etchill EW, Myers SP, McDaniel LM, et al. Should all massively transfused patients be treated equally? An analysis of massive transfusion ratios in the nontrauma setting. *Crit Care Med.* 2017;45(8):1311–1316. (In Eng). doi: 10.1097/ccm.0000000000002498

49. Sommer N, Schnüriger B, Candinas D, Haltmeier T. Massive transfusion protocols in nontrauma patients: A systematic review and meta-analysis. *J Trauma Acute Care Surg.* 2019;86(3):493–504. (In Eng). doi: 10.1097/ta.0000000000002101

50. Pusateri AE, Moore EE, Moore HB, et al. Association of prehospital plasma transfusion with survival in trauma patients with hemorrhagic shock when transport times are longer than 20 minutes: A post hoc analysis of the PAMPer and COMBAT clinical trials. *JAMA Surg.* 2020;155(2):e195085. (In Eng). doi: 10.1001/jamasurg.2019.5085

51. Reitz KM, Moore HB, Guyette FX, et al. Prehospital plasma in injured patients is associated with survival principally in blunt injury: Results from two randomized prehospital plasma trials. *J Trauma Acute Care Surg.* 2020;88(1):33–41. doi: 10.1097/ta.0000000000002485

52. Moore HB, Moore EE, Chapman MP, et al. Plasma-first resuscitation to treat haemorrhagic shock during emergency ground transportation in an urban area: A randomised trial. *Lancet.* 2018;392(10144):283–291. doi: 10.1016/S0140-6736(18)31553-8

53. Hrebinko KA, Sperry JL, Guyette FX, et al. Evaluating the cost-effectiveness of prehospital plasma transfusion in unstable trauma patients: A secondary analysis of the PAMPer trial. *JAMA Surg.* 2021;156(12):1131–1139. (In Eng). doi: 10.1001/jamasurg.2021.4529

54. Jackson B, Murphy C, Fontaine MJ. Current state of whole blood transfusion for civilian trauma resuscitation. *Transfusion.* 2020;60(Suppl 3):S45–S52. (In Eng). doi:10.1111/trf.15703

55. Walsh M, Fries D, Moore E, et al. Whole blood for civilian urban trauma resuscitation: Historical, present, and future considerations. *Semin Thromb Hemost.* 2020;46(2):221–234. (In Eng). doi: 10.1055/s-0040-1702174

56. Cable CA, Razavi SA, Roback JD, Murphy DJ. RBC transfusion strategies in the ICU: a concise review. *Crit Care Med.* 2019;47(11):1637–1644. (In Eng). doi: 10.1097/ccm.0000000000003985

57. Mazzei C, Popovsky M, Kopko P. Noninfectious complications of blood transfusion. In: Roback J, Combs M, Grossman B, eds. *Technical Manual.* 16th ed. American Association of Blood Banks; 2008:715–749.

58. Sahu S, Hemlata, Verma A. Adverse events related to blood transfusion. *Indian J Anaesth.* 2014;58(5):543–551. doi:10.4103/0019-5049.144650

59. Domen R, Hoeltge G. Allergic transfusion reactions. *Arch Pathol Lab Med.* 2003;127:316–320.

60. Goldberg A, Kor D. State of the art management of transfusion related lung injury. *Curr Pharm Dis.* 2012;18:3273–3284.

61. Chassé M, Tinmouth A, English SW, et al. Association of blood donor age and sex with recipient survival after red blood cell transfusion. *JAMA Internal Med.* 2016. doi: 10.1001/jamainternmed.2016.3324

62. Hebert P, Yetisir E, Martin C. Is a low transfusion threshold safe in critically ill patients with cardiovascular disease? *Crit Care Med.* 2001;29:227–234.

63. Hennino A, Berard F, Guillot I, Saad N, Rozieres A, Nicolas JF. Pathophysiology of urticaria. *Clin Rev Allergy Immunol.* 2006;30(1):3–11. (In Eng). doi: 10.1385/criai:30:1:003

64. Toy P, Gajic O, Bacchetti P, et al. Transfusion-related acute lung injury: Incidence and risk factors. *Blood.* 2012;119(7):1757–1767. (In Eng). doi: 10.1182/blood-2011-08-370932

65. Goldberg AD, Kor DJ. State of the art management of transfusion-related acute lung injury (TRALI). *Curr Pharm Des.* 2012;18(22):3273–3284. (In Eng).

66. Kim J, Na S. Transfusion-related acute lung injury; clinical perspectives. *Korean J Anesthesiol.* 2015;68(2):101–105. doi: 10.4097/kjae.2015.68.2.101

67. Agnihotri N, Agnihotri A. Transfusion associated circulatory overload. *Indian J Critical Care Med.* 2014;18(6):396–398. doi: 10.4103/0972-5229.133938

68. Clifford L, Jia Q, Yadav H, et al. Characterizing the epidemiology of perioperative transfusion-associated circulatory overload. *Anesthesiology.* 2015;122(1):21–28. doi: 10.1097/ALN.0000000000000513

69. Dzik WH, Kirkley SA. Citrate toxicity during massive blood transfusion. *Transfus Med Rev.* 1988;2(2):76–94. (In Eng).

70. Sheridan R, Lhowe L, Brown B, et al. *The Trauma Handbook of the Massachusetts General Hospital.* Lippincott, Williams, & Wilkins; 2004.

71. Heddle NM, Klama L, Meyer R, et al. A randomized controlled trial comparing plasma removal with white cell reduction to prevent reactions to platelets. *Transfusion.* 1999;39(3):231–238. (In Eng).

72. Alves VM, Martins PRJ, Soares S, et al. Alloimmunization screening after transfusion of red blood cells in a prospective study. *Rev Bras Hematol Hemoter.* 2012;34(3):206–211. doi: 10.5581/1516-8484.20120051

73. Yazdanbakhsh K, Ware RE, Noizat-Pirenne F. Red blood cell alloimmunization in sickle cell disease: Pathophysiology, risk factors, and transfusion management. *Blood.* 2012;120(3):528–537. doi: 10.1182/blood-2011-11-327361

74. Blajchman MA. Transfusion immunomodulation or TRIM: What does it mean clinically? *Hematology (Amsterdam, Netherlands).* 2005;10 (Suppl 1):208–214. (In Eng). doi: 10.1080/10245330512331390447

75. Sparrow RL. Red blood cell storage and transfusion-related immunomodulation. *Blood Transfus.* 2010;8(Suppl 3):s26–s30. doi: 10.2450/2010.005S

76. Vamvakas EC, Blajchman MA. Transfusion-related immunomodulation (TRIM): An update. *Blood Rev.* 2007;21(6):327–348. (In Eng). doi: 10.1016/j.blre.2007.07.003

77. Duchesne J, McSwain N, Cotton B, et al. Damage control resuscitation: The new face of damage control. *J Trauma Acute Care Surg.* 2010;69(4):976–990.

78. Mikhail J. The trauma triad of death: Hypothermia, acidosis, and coagulopathy. *AACN Clin Issues.* 1999;10(1):85–94.

79. Kashuk J, Moore E, Millikan J, Moore J. Major abdominal vascular trauma: A unified approach. *J Trauma Acute Care Surg.* 1982;22:672–679.

80. Moore E. Staged laparotomy for the hypothermia, acidosis, and coagulopathy syndrome. *Am J Surg.* 1996;172:405–410.

81. Dunn E, Moore E, Breslich D. Acidosis induced coagulopathy. *Surg Forum.* 1979;30:471–478.

82. Reynolds BR, Forsythe RM, Harbrecht BG, et al. Hypothermia in massive transfusion: Have we been paying enough attention to it? *J Trauma Acute Care Surg.* 2012;73(2):486–491. doi: 10.1097/TA.0b013e31825c163b

83. Polderman KH. Hypothermia and coagulation. *Crit Care.* 2012;16(Suppl 2):A20. (In Eng). doi: 10.1186/cc11278

84. Lapostolle F, Couvreur J, Koch FX, et al. Hypothermia in trauma victims at first arrival of ambulance personnel: An observational study with assessment of risk factors. *Scand J Trauma Resusc Emerg Med.* 2017;25(1):43. doi: 10.1186/s13049-017-0349-1

85. Cosgriff N, Moore EE, Sauaia A, Kenny-Moynihan M, Burch JM, Galloway B. Predicting life-threatening coagulopathy in the massively transfused trauma patient: Hypothermia and acidoses revisited. *J Trauma Acute Care Surg.* 1997;42(5):857–862. https://journals.lww.com/jtrauma/Fulltext/1997/05000/Predicting_Life_threatening_Coagulopathy_in_the.16.aspx

86. Rotondo M, Zonies D. The damage control sequence and underlying logic. *Surg Clin North Am.* 1999;77:761–777.

87. Holcomb J, Watts S, Hodgets T. Damage control resuscitation: Directly addressing the early coagulopathy of trauma. *J Trauma Acute Care Surg.* 2008;62:307–310.

88. Guyette FX, Brown JB, Zenati MS, et al. Tranexamic acid during prehospital transport in patients at risk for hemorrhage after injury: A double-blind, placebo-controlled, randomized clinical trial. *JAMA Surg.* 2020;156(1):11–20. (In Eng). doi: 10.1001/jamasurg.2020.4350

89. Boutonnet M, Abback P, Le Saché F, et al. Tranexamic acid in severe trauma patients managed in a mature trauma care system. *J Trauma Acute Care Surg.* 2018;84(6S):S54–S62. doi: 10.1097/ta.0000000000001880

90. Stansfield R, Morris D, Jesulola E. The use of tranexamic acid (TXA) for the management of hemorrhage in trauma patients in the prehospital environment: Literature review and descriptive analysis of principal themes. *Shock.* 2020;53(3):277–283. doi: 10.1097/shk.0000000000001389

91. Karl V, Thorn S, Mathes T, Hess S, Maegele M. Association of tranexamic acid administration with mortality and thromboembolic events in patients with traumatic injury: A systematic review and meta-analysis. *JAMA Netw Open.* 2022;5(3):e220625. doi: 10.1001/jamanetworkopen.2022.0625

92. Schmidt AE, Israel AK, Refaai MA. The utility of thromboelastography to guide blood product transfusion: An ACLPS critical review. *Am J Clin. Pathol.* 2019;152(4):407–422. doi: 10.1093/ajcp/aqz074

93. Singer M, Deutschman C, Seymour C, et al. The third international consensus definitions for sepsis and septic shock. *JAMA.* 2016;315(8):801–810.

94. Cohen J, Venkatesh B. Adjunctive corticosteroid treatment in septic shock. *Anesthesiology.* 2019;131(2):410–419. doi: 10.1097/aln.0000000000002604

95. Nedel W, Lisboa T, Salluh JIF. What is the role of steroids for septic shock in 2021? *Semin Respir Crit Care Med.* 2021;42(5):726–734. (In Eng). doi: 10.1055/s-0041-1733900

96. Consortium for Spinal Cord Medicine. Early acute management in adults with spinal cord injury: a clinical practice guideline for health-care professionals. *J Spinal Cord Med.* 2008;31(4):403-479.

97. Gondim F, Lopes A, Oliveira G, et al. Cardiovascular control after spinal cord surgery. *Curr Vasc Pharmacol.* 2004;2(1):71–79.

98. Guly H, Bouamra O, Lecky F. The incidence of neurogenic shock in patients with isolated spinal cord injury in the emergency department. *Resuscitation.* 2008;76:57–62.

99. Krassioukov A, Claydon V. The clinical problems in cardiovascular control following spinal cord injury: An overview. *Prog Brain Res.* 2006;15:223–229.

100. Ryken TC, Hurlbert RJ, Hadley MN, et al. The acute cardiopulmonary management of patients with cervical spinal cord injuries. *Neurosurgery.* 2013;72:84–92. doi: 10.1227/NEU.0b013e318276ee16

101. Hurlbert RJ, Hadley MN, Walters BC, et al. Pharmacological therapy for acute spinal cord injury. *Neurosurgery.* 2013;72:93–105. doi: 10.1227/NEU.0b013e31827765c6

102. McHugh K, Repanshek Z. Anaphylaxis: Emergency department treatment. *Emerg Med Clin North Am.* 2022;40(1):19–32. (In Eng). doi: 10.1016/j.emc.2021.08.004

103. Tehrani BN, Truesdell AG, Psotka MA, et al. A standardized and comprehensive approach to the management of cardiogenic shock. *JACC Heart Fail.* 2020;8(11):879–891. doi: 10.1016/j.jchf.2020.09.005

104. Nallamothu B, Bradley E, Krumholz H. Time to treatment in primary percutaneous coronary intervention. *N Engl J Med.* 2007;357(16):1631–1638.

105. Fan ZG, Gao XF, Chen LW, et al. The outcomes of intra-aortic balloon pump usage in patients with acute myocardial infarction: A comprehensive meta-analysis of 33 clinical trials and 18,889 patients. *Patient Prefer Adher.* 2016;10:297–312. (In Eng). doi: 10.2147/ppa.s101945

106. Porier Y, Volsine P, Piourde G, et al. Efficacy and safety of preoperative intra-aortic balloon pump use in patients undergoing cardiac surgery: A systematic review and meta-analysis. *Int J Cardiol.* 2016;15(207):67–79.

107. Romeo F, Acconcia MC, Sergi D, et al. The outcome of intra-aortic balloon pump support in acute myocardial infarction complicated by cardiogenic shock according to the type of revascularization: A comprehensive meta-analysis. *Am Heart J.* 2013;165(5):679–692. (In Eng). doi: 10.1016/j.ahj.2013.02.020

108. Thiele H, Zeymer U, Neumann F-J, et al. Intraaortic balloon support for myocardial infarction with cardiogenic shock. *N Engl J Med.* 2012;367(14):1287–1296. doi: doi:10.1056/NEJMoa1208410

109. Zhang J, Lang Y, Guo L, et al. Preventive use of intra-aortic balloon pump in patients undergoing high-risk coronary artery bypass grafting: A retrospective study. *Med Sci Monit.* 2015;21:855–860. doi: 10.12659/MSM.893021

110. Konstantinides SV, Torbicki A, Agnelli G, et al. 2014 ESC guidelines on the diagnosis and management of acute pulmonary embolism [published correction appears in Eur Heart J. 2015 Oct 14;36(39):2666] [published correction appears in Eur Heart J. 2015 Oct 14;36(39):2642]. *Eur Heart J.* 2014;35(43):3033-3069k. doi:10.1093/eurheartj/ehu283

111. Thomson D, Kourounis G, Trenear R, et al. ECG in suspected pulmonary embolism. *Postgrad Med J.* 2019;95(1119):12–17. doi: 10.1136/postgradmedj-2018-136178

112. Righini M, Van Es J, Den Exter PL, et al. Age-adjusted d-dimer cutoff levels to rule out pulmonary embolism: The adjust-pe study. *JAMA.* 2014;311(11):1117–1124. doi: 10.1001/jama.2014.2135

113. Stewart LK, Kline JA. Fibrinolytics for the treatment of pulmonary embolism. *Transl Res* 2020;225:82–94. (In Eng). doi: 10.1016/j.trsl.2020.05.003

114. Sagrista-Sauleda J, Merce AS, Soler-Soler J. Diagnosis and management of pericardial effusion. *World J Cardiol.* 2011;3(5):135–143. (In Eng). doi: 10.4330/wjc.v3.i5.135

115. Wernick B, Hon H, Mumbag R. Complications of needle thoracostomy. *Int J Crit Illn Inj Sci.* 2015;5(3):632–639.

116. Dickson RL, Gleisberg G, Aiken M, et al. Emergency medical services simple thoracostomy for traumatic cardiac arrest: Postimplementation experience in a ground-based suburban/rural emergency medical services agency. *J Emerg Med.* 2018;55(3):366–371. (In Eng). doi: 10.1016/j.jemermed.2018.05.027

117. Hannon L, St Clair T, Smith K, et al. Finger thoracostomy in patients with chest trauma performed by paramedics on a helicopter emergency medical service. *Emerg Med Australas.* 2020;32(4):650–656. doi: 10.1111/1742-6723.13549

118. Mohrsen S, McMahon N, Corfield A, McKee S. Complications associated with pre-hospital open thoracostomies: A rapid review. *Scand J Trauma Resusc Emerg Med.* 2021;29(1):166. doi: 10.1186/s13049-021-00976-1

119. Peters J, Ketelaars R, van Wageningen B, Biert J, Hoogerwerf N. Prehospital thoracostomy in patients with traumatic circulatory arrest: Results from a physician-staffed Helicopter Emergency Medical Service. *Eur J Emerg Med.* 2017;24(2):96–100. (In Eng). doi: 10.1097/mej.0000000000000337

15

General Principles of Trauma Management

ROBERT L. GRABOWSKI

COMPETENCIES

1. Demonstrate the ability to perform scene safety and trauma triage.
2. Perform a primary and secondary assessment of the injured patient.
3. Initiate critical interventions for the injured patient before and during transport.
4. Predict injury patterns based on the mechanism of injury.

*T*rauma is defined as injury to tissue and organs caused by the transfer of energy from an external source. Injuries are caused by the transfer of energy beyond a tissue's resilience to tolerate, resulting in deformation of tissues and cellular damage.[1] Regardless of gender, race, or economic status, unintentional injury is the fourth leading cause of death for all ages in the United States,[2] surpassing stroke in the last few years, and the leading cause of death for those aged 1 to 44 years.[3] In 2020, the National Center for Health Statistics reported 200,955 deaths as the result of trauma.[2] Traumatic events are rarely accidental, and most are preventable.[4] Thus, the term *accident* is replaced by *unintentional*, or the descriptor is omitted entirely. In the United States, unintentional injuries are a major source of morbidity and mortality, having a significant impact on healthcare spending. The cost of trauma-related injuries in the United States exceeds $400 billion annually.[5] These costs include treatment, both medical and psychological; lost wages; benefits; and other productivity losses.[5] For these reasons, injury prevention has become a focus for public health.[6]

Injury Dynamics

The time elapsed from the initial injury to definitive care is a key factor in patient morbidity and mortality. One of the key factors that have historically reduced morbidity and mortality rates in trauma patients is rapid transport. However, the addition of highly trained clinicians has brought critical care management outside the trauma center to the rural hospital or the scene of the trauma, further reducing the patient's time to meaningful intervention.

The transport of the patient with multiple injuries requires in-depth knowledge and skills as well as expert prioritization and organizational skills. A thorough understanding of the mechanisms of injury and the kinematics of trauma is essential for any transport team member caring for injured patients. Knowledge of these principles helps guide appropriate assessment and treatment to ensure the best possible outcome.

History

One of the first steps in caring for a patient with multiple injuries is obtaining a history of events, both preceding and following the trauma. With interfacility transfers, this information is most commonly obtained from other nurses, physicians, and family members. The history at a scene response generally comes from many individuals, including law enforcement, firefighters, other emergency medical services (EMS) personnel, and bystanders.

When responding via rotor-wing aircraft to the scene of a trauma, an aerial view of the situation helps the transport team begin data collection about the patient, mechanism of injury, and other potential circumstances (Fig. 15.1). The transport team has the advantage of evaluating the entire scene, to include damage sustained to vehicles or buildings, extent of impact, and objects thrown or blown out of the central area of impact.

A thorough history is key to direct patient care. Because time is a critical factor for survivability, the history should be obtained while gaining access to the patient or while simultaneously performing the primary assessment. At the scene, life-threatening injuries are always top priority, and a detailed history may be impractical initially, in certain cases. If the patient has an altered

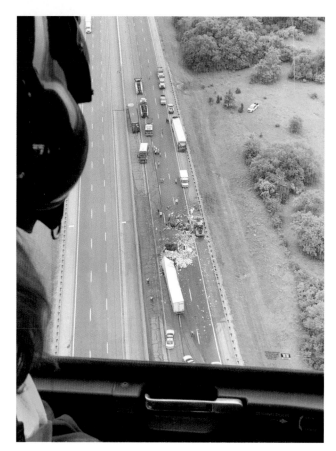

• **Figure 15.1** When approaching a scene from the air, the transport team begins collecting information about the incident.

level of consciousness, the only history available may be from the referring hospital or the emergency personnel present at the scene. Therefore, the history should be elicited during concurrent patient assessment since the team may not get another chance to obtain this critical information. One method of obtaining this critical information is through MIST reporting:

M: Mechanism of injury
 I: Injuries
 S: Symptoms
 T: Treatment

Additional important information includes the time of injury, any force multipliers for the mechanism of injury (i.e., speed of impact, weight of assaulting object, duration of crush, etc.), use of safety devices, alteration in the patient's level of consciousness, as well as the time treatments were provided and the patient's response to the treatment.

The mnemonic AMPLE may be used to help elicit a history from the patient:

A: Allergies
M: Medications currently used
 P: Past illness or Pregnancy
 L: Last oral intake (including food, alcohol, drug use, etc.)
 E: Events leading up to, or Environment factors related to the injury

A more detailed history may be obtained from the patient during the secondary survey as time and patient condition allow, and can be routinely performed in the transport vehicle.

Mechanism of Injury

Injuries occur when external energy is transferred to the body. The type, amount, and duration of energy applied and the tissues' response to that energy determine the extent of injury. When the body's tissue cannot withstand the additional energy, tissue disruption and cellular destruction occurs. This tissue damage is seen in common forms of injuries, such as fractures, lacerations, ruptured internal organs, etc. An understanding of the external energy and the way it is applied is necessary to predict potential injuries and adequately care for the injured patient.

Newton's first law of motion states that a body at rest tends to remain at rest, and a body in motion tends to remain in motion, until acted on by an outside force. When the body contacts an object, energy is transferred, and damage occurs (Fig. 15.2).

Force is a result of energy transference, which can be explained by the laws of physics:

1. Energy can be neither created nor destroyed; it can only change form.
2. Kinetic energy = (Mass × Velocity^2)/2
3. Force = Mass × Acceleration

Because energy is neither created nor destroyed, only transferred, its transference is dependent on the mass of the object multiplied by its speed squared, divided by a common denominator of two.

This same force is applied to destruction of the body. Energy is transferred from the automobile to the human occupant(s) in the vehicle. Several factors determine the amount of energy the human absorbs, including the following:

1. The amount of energy absorbed by the objects that initially collide (e.g., the telephone pole and the automobile).
2. The amount absorbed by protective factors, such as seat belts, helmets, padded steering wheels, dashboards, and air bags.

The forces involved in the impact cause varying degrees of destruction. The slower the mass is applied, the less energy transference and thus the lower the degree of destruction. The extent of injury is also dependent on which body part(s) receive the impact[7]; for example, the skull can take more force before damage occurs, compared to the abdomen.

Force can be delivered via compression, acceleration, deceleration, or shearing.[7]

Compression: Direct pressure on a structure is the most common type of force applied. The amount of injury sustained is dependent on the amount of force, length of time of compression, and the area compressed.[7]

Acceleration/deceleration: Acceleration is the increase in the velocity of a moving object. Deceleration is the decrease in velocity of an object.[7] In an automobile crash, the body is thrown forward (accelerates) by the impact and decelerates as it comes into contact with the steering wheel, seat belt, or dashboard. The internal organs also experience this deceleration as they come into contact with internal structures such as ribs, which causes injury to the tissues and vasculature.

Shearing: Shearing forces occur when tissues, organs, or both are pushed ahead of underlying or overlying structures. This commonly occurs at sites of junction between differently weighed, or affixed versus nonaffixed structures. An example of this is in acceleration/declaration trauma when a nonaffixed portion of the aorta is forced anteriorly while the affixed portion is more or less stable. These opposing forces can then cause a tear in the intima of the vessel.

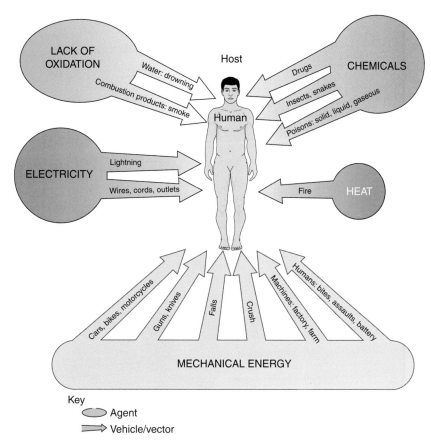

• **Figure 15.2** Energy forces that can affect the human body.

The viscoelastic properties of tissues in the body help absorb and distribute energy. When the energy delivered is below the limit of injury, the energy is absorbed and causes no damage. When the force applied delivers more energy than the body can absorb, strains occur.[7] Strains may be classified as tensile, shearing, or compressive. A tensile strain is a stretching mechanism that typically causes fractures or aortic tears. A shearing strain is movement of tissues in opposite directions causing injuries such as lacerations and avulsions as well as brain injuries. Compressive strain is a crushing force that causes contusions and tissue damage.

Kinematics of Trauma

Injury patterns can be predicted by evaluating the mechanism of injury that has occurred and the estimated amount of force generated. Although all patients should be evaluated individually, certain injuries are common to specific forces and mechanisms of injury. Prediction of these injuries is referred to as *kinematics.* Age, buffers (preventive measures taken), and velocity are factors in the alteration of injury patterns, and the caregiver should consider these factors when evaluating a patient.[8]

Blunt Injuries

Motor Vehicle Crashes

Motor vehicle crashes are the leading cause of injuries and traumatic deaths worldwide, accounting for over 1 million deaths per year and an estimated 20 to 50 million significant injuries (Fig. 15.3).[9]

Head-on Collisions

As an automobile collides with an object head-on, energy is transferred to the vehicle and subsequently, its occupants. The front of the vehicle routinely stops less than one-half second after impact. The rear of the automobile continues to move forward until all the energy is dispersed. Although the front end of the car is destroyed, the rear of the vehicle causes the destruction by its continued forward movement. The same principle of injury occurs with the body during a head-on collision. The initial impact occurs in the front of the vehicle. The unrestrained driver hits the steering wheel with the thorax, the head may hit the windshield, and the knees contact the dashboard (Fig. 15.4). Predictable injuries from initial impact are fractured ribs, pneumothorax, or hemopneumothorax; concussion/traumatic brain injury, skull fractures, patella, and femur fractures; dislocated hips; and acetabular fractures. The progression of injury continues, as does the automobile, and the person's internal organs are thrown forward from the rear until all energy is dispersed. Common internal injuries include ruptured spleen (direct compression from the steering wheel), lacerated liver (stretching of hilum until the tensile strength is exceeded), and ruptured thoracic aortas (heart and aorta are forcibly thrown forward and opposing sections stretch and tear).

The restrained driver in a head-on collision has much of the energy absorbed by the seat belt and air bag, if present. The seat belt may impose a load 20 to 50 times as great as the body weight. The only part of the human body capable of incurring this load is the pelvis. Unless the patient has the belt properly applied securely over the pelvis, direct compression of the abdomen may occur. The first indicator of these injuries is often the presence of abrasions

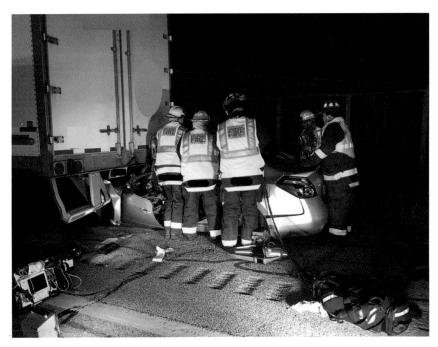

• **Figure 15.3** Motor vehicle crash.

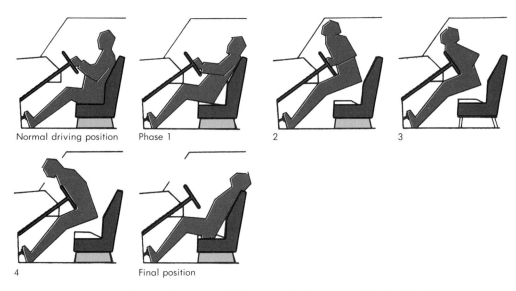

Normal driving position   Phase 1   2   3

4   Final position

• **Figure 15.4** Phases of movement of the unrestrained occupant during frontal collision.

over the abdomen from the seat belt. Other injuries associated with seat belt use include sternal fractures, breast injuries, and lumbar vertebral body fractures. As seen with abdominal seat belt injuries, overlying abrasions, ecchymosis, or both are important indicators. Lap belts should be worn with a diagonal shoulder strap to stop forward movement of the upper body. Diagonal straps worn alone can cause severe neck injuries, including decapitation. Air bags cushion forward motion only. They are effective in a first collision, but because they deflate immediately, they are not effective in multiple-impact collisions. Additionally, when the air bag deploys, it can directly injure the patient. The most common injuries seen are abrasions of the arms, chest, and face, which can include injuries caused by the patient's eyeglasses.[7,10]

Rear-End Collisions

An automobile that sustains a rear impact rapidly accelerates, causing the car to move forward under the patient. Predictable injuries are to the back (T12-L1 is the most common area of injury), legs (femur, tibia/fibula, and ankle fractures), and neck (cervical strain and cervical fractures caused by hyperextension), if the head restraint is not in the proper position.[10] If the automobile undergoes a second collision by striking a car in front of it, the predictable head-on injuries also need to be evaluated.

Side Impact

An automobile struck on the side routinely causes lateral injuries to the patient. An unrestrained occupant sitting on the same side that sustained most of the impact may have initial injuries to the side of the body that received the impact; these may include the clavicle, ribs, femur, and tibia/fibula. Abdominal injuries (such as a ruptured spleen) are seen in these crashes, usually because of the fractured lower lateral ribs, but also because of direct compression on the abdomen.[10] Secondary injuries occur when the patient is propelled to the other side of the car, which causes injuries to the opposite side.

Rollovers

Predictable injuries caused by vehicle rollovers are more difficult to define (Fig. 15.5). The unrestrained patient tumbles inside the vehicle, and injury occurs to the impacted areas of the body. In these circumstances, the caregiver must recognize the potential for multiple-system injuries.

Extrication

Depending on the severity of damage to the vehicle and the response time of the transport team, first responders may still be extricating the patient from the vehicle upon the transport team's arrival. In these situations, transport teams are often not trained in extrication or do not have the proper protective gear to safely provide care in the vehicle during active extrication. Transport team members will need to communicate with the incident commander to establish when it is safe for them to enter the vehicle or to perform quick, episodic assessments. Pauses in extrication can be performed so transport team members can provide supportive interventions, such as placing an intravenous line, applying patient monitors, or providing analgesia. This can be ideal for a stable patient with limited suspicion of injury; however, for unstable patients or those with high suspicion of injury, delays in extrication and on-scene time should be minimized. If life-saving interventions are required (i.e., the patient suffers a cardiac or respiratory arrest), then extrication attempts may be stopped to allow for rapid extrication or to allow interventions to be attempted with the patient in place (Fig. 15.6). After interventions are complete, the transport team should observe the patient from a safe distance and allow extrication to continue; acting as safety

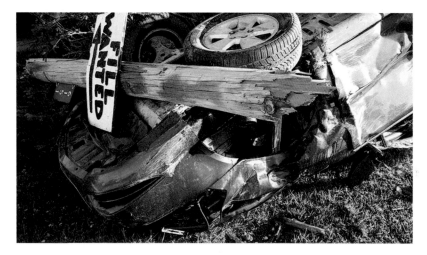

• **Figure 15.5** Rollover motor vehicle crash.

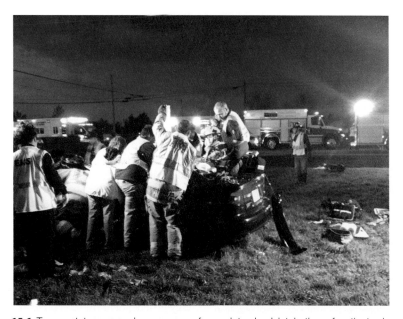

• **Figure 15.6** Transport team member prepares for endotracheal intubation of patient who remains entrapped in motor vehicle rear seat.

officers, watching for patient condition changes requiring intervention, and assuring life support and monitoring equipment are not damaged during extrication. Transport teams should utilize extrication time to prepare all necessary equipment and interventions, to ensure the team is ready to accept and care for the patient as soon as extrication is completed.

Motorcycle Crashes

Because motorcycles offer minimal or no initial energy transference, energy is directly absorbed by the rider, and injuries can be substantially more severe than with other motor vehicle crashes. The predicted injuries during a motorcycle crash, like those during other motor vehicle crashes, depend on the type of collision that occurs.

Head-on Collisions

For accurate prediction of injuries that involve the motorcycle rider, an understanding of the design of a motorcycle is helpful (Fig. 15.7). The center of gravity is located in front of the driver's seat. As the motorcycle strikes an object head-on, the rear (lighter) portion lifts upward, pivoting around the weight under the handlebars. The driver is subsequently propelled forward over the handlebars. Associated injuries with this type of crash are lower extremity fractures (from impact with the handlebars); chest and abdominal injuries (from direct compression against the handlebars or tire); and head and neck injuries (from impact with the tire or any object in front of the cycle). Any motorcycle crash can cause the rider to be ejected, however, ejection is most common during head-on collisions. Suspicion of, and intervention for, major head and cervical spine injuries are imperative with any ejected patient.

Side Impact

Injuries associated with side-impact motorcycle crashes are related to the body parts crushed between the motorcycle and the second object. Most commonly seen injuries involve the leg and foot on the impact side. Open fractures of the femur, tibia/fibula, and malleolus are predictable.

Laying Down the Motorcycle

Motorcycle riders may use the technique of laying down the motorcycle and sliding off to the side before colliding with another object. The energy transference is a result of sliding away from the bike. Injuries commonly seen are abrasions on the affected side. Fractures may occur if the operator hits the road hard or comes in contact with another object. Protective clothing and gear can help absorb more energy than average clothing, preventing abrasions and more serious injuries.

Falls

Falls from heights greater than 15 to 20 feet are associated with severe injuries. In predicting injuries associated with falls, caregivers should keep the following facts in mind.
- The average roof of a one-story house is approximately 15 feet off the ground; a two-story roof is approximately 30 feet off the ground.
- With a fall greater than 15 feet, adults usually land on their feet. At less than 15 feet, adults land in the manner in which they fell (i.e., fall headfirst, strike the ground headfirst).
- Because small children have proportionally larger heads, no matter what the distance, they tend to fall headfirst.

The caregiver must estimate the distance fallen and determine the surface on which the patient landed. A soft-landing surface, such as dirt or sand, absorbs much more energy than a hard surface, such as concrete. Identifying loss of consciousness following a fall can also add to the prognostication for potential head injury.

Three predictable injuries are seen in falls. The forces involved are deceleration and compression. The first injury, calcaneus fractures, is caused by compression of the feet on impact. Second, the energy dissipates after impact and the top of the body pushes down toward the point of impact, and this increased axial pressure load can lead to compression fractures to the thoracolumbar spine, most commonly T12-L1. Finally, as the body moves forward and the patient puts out both arms to complete the fall, bilateral wrist fractures may occur.

Penetrating Trauma

All objects that cause injury from penetration apply the same two types of force: *crushing* and *stretching*.[11–13] Depending on the velocity and size of the penetrating object, the resulting wound can be small or massive.

Stab Wounds

Stab wounds are considered low velocity and produce damage by crushing tissues as the penetrating object enters. An object that is narrow at the beginning and thicker at the end crushes the tissues as it enters and stretches them apart as the thicker part is inserted. The area of injury inflicted by stab wounds is typically localized to the area of direct insult. The penetrating object may still be embedded in the patient. If this is the case, embedded objects should be stabilized with bandages, towel rolls, or other materials for transport and not removed (Fig. 15.8).

Firearm Injuries

Bullet wounds are caused by four different mechanisms: (1) direct contact by the bullet, (2) crushing force in the immediate vicinity of the bullet, (3) temporary cavity formation, and (4) collapse of the temporary cavity.[12,14]

The severity of the wound depends on the amount of energy transferred from the bullet to the body. This transference of energy is dependent on several factors: the type of weapon, the type of bullet or shell, the distance from which the weapon was fired, and the body part penetrated.

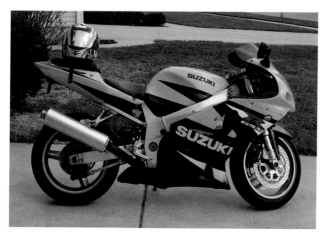

• **Figure 15.7** Construction of a motorcycle places the center of gravity in front of the driver's seat. Head-on collision causes the cycle to tip up and throw the occupant over the front.

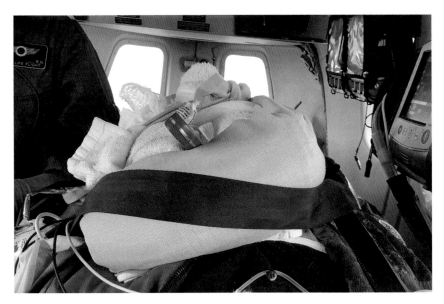

• **Figure 15.8** Kitchen knife impaled in a patient's chest. Knife was stabilized with gauze, towel rolls, and tape.

Firearms can be handguns, rifles, or shotguns. Handguns and some rifles are considered medium energy, while assault rifles and hunting rifles are high energy. The greater the amount of gunpowder in the cartridge, the greater the kinetic energy of the projectile.[7] The degree of damage caused by the projectile is influenced by:

• *Yaw and tumbling:* Yaw is deviation of the leading edge of the projectile up to 90 degrees from its original orientation, and tumbling is rotation of the projectile 360 degrees. Both causes increased crushing and stretching of tissue, resulting in greater damage.

• *Deformation of a* projectile *when striking tissue:* Certain projectiles are constructed of soft lead and flatten on impact. Others have hollow points that cause a mushrooming effect on impact. Hollow-point projectiles are also known as expanding projectiles. The increased diameter of these bullets increases tissue destruction.

• *Fragmentation:* Each fragmented part of the projectile causes damage in its path. Increased velocity increases the potential of fragmentation.

• *Explosive effect:* Explosive projectiles are intended to cause massive damage with a single shot. The projectile is composed of black powder and a metallic shot (traditionally lead). On impact, detonation of the powder causes explosion and disintegration of the projectile casing, which further propels the shot.[7]

The closer to the target the projectile was when fired, the greater the amount of kinetic energy transferred to the tissues, causing more widespread destruction. For this reason, firing distance is important to ascertain during the history taking.

Cavitation occurs with all penetrating objects. The permanent cavity is formed from the crushed tissue caused by the object. Temporary cavity formation occurs from transfer of kinetic energy from the projectile to the tissue (Fig. 15.9). The velocity, size, shape, and ballistic behavior of the projectile and the biophysical properties of the tissue determine the extent of the temporary cavity.[15] As a projectile strikes tissue, temporary cavitation occurs forward of and lateral to the projectile. Relatively elastic tissues, such as lung, bowel wall, and muscle, tolerate the stretch of the temporary cavity much better than the solid nonelastic organs, such as the liver and spleen.[8] It is important to recall that factors

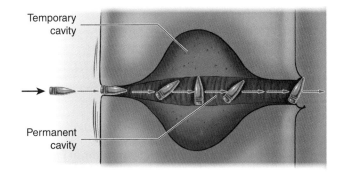

• **Figure 15.9** Effects of yaw and temporary and permanent cavitation from a bullet. Permanent cavity is caused by necrotic muscle tissue. Temporary cavity is caused by stretching of soft tissue. (From Weiner SL, Barrett J. *Trauma Management for Civilian and Military Positions.* Saunders; 1986.)

such as temporary cavitation, projectile fragmentation, and tumbling to lower resistance tissues can cause injury to bodily structures far from the point of entry.[16] Maintaining a high suspicion for serious, diffuse, internal injury is prudent during initial care and transport.

Pathophysiologic Factors

Trauma causes severe stress to the human body and is associated with a flux of hormones and physiologic reactions (Table 15.1). The degree of metabolic and hormonal changes depends on the severity of injury, the effectiveness of resuscitation, and the preinjury condition of the patient. Generally, metabolic response to shock from injury in the early stage differs from that in the late stage (Table 15.2). Review Chapter 13 for a more in-depth discussion of shock physiology.

A critical concept to understand when caring for the bleeding trauma patient is the triad of hypothermia, acidosis, and coagulopathy. Hypothermia may be caused by the environment or by caregiver interventions. When patients are disrobed for assessment, cared for in cold or room-temperature environments, or infused

TABLE 15.1 Major Pathophysiologic Changes in Shock

Change	Effect
Early Stage (Compensatory/Nonprogressive)	
Increased epinephrine and norepinephrine	Increased cardiac output to increase blood flow to tissues
α-Adrenergic receptors stimulated (skin and most viscera)	Vasoconstriction and decreased blood supply
β-Adrenergic receptors stimulated (heart and skeletal muscle)	Vasodilation and increased blood supply and heart rate
Renin–angiotensin response	Vasoconstriction and secretion of aldosterone; sodium and water retention, which supports intravascular volume; potassium loss
Increased glucocorticoids and mineralocorticoids	Sodium and water retention to increase intravascular volume; potassium loss
Hypoxemia	Hyperventilation and bronchodilation; provides more oxygen to tissues; may cause respiratory alkalosis
Decreased hydrostatic fluid pressure	Fluid shifts from interstitial space to intravascular space to increase vascular volume
Late Stage (Noncompensatory/Progressive)	
Decreased blood flow to heart	Impaired cardiac pumping ability (decreased cardiac output); blood pressure decreases
Anaerobic metabolism	Acidosis; decreased adenosine triphosphate; failure of cellular sodium-potassium pump (potassium leaves cell, sodium, and water enter cell); cellular damage
Arteriolar dilation and venule constriction	Fluid shift from intravascular to interstitial space, reducing blood pressure
Decreased blood flow to kidneys with acute tubular necrosis	Decreased kidney function (oliguria or anuria, retention of nitrogenous waste products and potassium)
Decreased blood flow to pancreas	Production of myocardial depressant factor

From Phipps WJ, Sands JK, Marek JF. *Medical-Surgical Nursing: Concepts and Clinical Practice.* 6th ed. Mosby; 1999.

TABLE 15.2 Comparison of Signs and Symptoms in Early and Late Shock by Body System

System	Early Shock	Late Shock
Respiratory system	• Hyperventilation • ↑ Minute volume • ↓ $PaCO_2$ • Normal PaO_2 • Bronchodilation	• Respirations shallow • Breath sounds may sound congested • ≠↑ $PaCO_2$ • ↓ PaO_2 • Pulmonary edema • ↓ Pulse oximetry
Cardiovascular system	• Blood pressure normal to slightly lowered • ↑ Diastolic pressure • Narrowed pulse pressure • Tachycardia • Cardiac output normal in hypovolemic shock, slightly decreased in cardiogenic shock, and increased in septic shock • Mild vasoconstriction in hypovolemic and cardiogenic shock • Vasodilation in septic shock	• ↓ Blood pressure • ↓ Cardiac output • Tachycardia continues • Vasoconstriction worsens in hypovolemic, cardiogenic, and septic shock
Renal system	• Decreased urine output • ↑ Urine osmolarity • ↓ Urine sodium concentration • Hypokalemia	• Oliguria or complete renal shutdown • Hyperkalemia • Buildup of waste products
Acid–base balance	• Respiratory alkalosis	• Metabolic acidosis • Respiratory acidosis
Vascular compartment	• Fluid shift from interstitial space to intravascular compartment • Thirst	• Fluid shift from intravascular to interstitial and intracellular spaces, causing edema

TABLE 15.2 Comparison of Signs and Symptoms in Early and Late Shock by Body System—cont'd

System	Early Shock	Late Shock
Skin	• Minimal to no changes in hypovolemic and cardiogenic shock • Warm flushed skin in septic shock	• Cool clammy skin in hypovolemic, cardiogenic, and septic shock • Cool mottled skin in neurogenic and vasogenic shock
Hematologic system	• Release of RBCs from bone marrow to increase vascular volume • Platelet aggregation	• DIC • ↓ Hematopoiesis, leading to: • ↓ white blood cells • ↓ hemoglobin • ↓ hematocrit • ↓ platelets
Mental-neurologic system	• Restless • Alert • Confused	• Lethargy • Unconsciousness
GI-hepatic system	• No obvious changes	• Perfusion decreases • Bowel sounds diminished • Gastric distention • Nausea, vomiting

DIC, Disseminated intravascular coagulation; *GI*, gastrointestinal; *PaCO₂*, arterial carbon dioxide pressure; *PaO₂*, arterial oxygen pressure; *RBC*, red blood cell.
From Phipps WJ, Sands JK, Marek JF. *Medical-Surgical Nursing: Concepts and Clinical Practice.* 6th ed. Mosby; 1999.

with room-temperature intravenous fluids or refrigerated blood products, a significant drop in core temperature will follow. However, measures can be taken to prevent this occurrence, such as using warmed intravenous fluids, administering blood using a heated transfuser, keeping the transport vehicle or resuscitation bay at a warm temperature, and covering the patient when not actively assessing them. Autoregulation of body temperature requires a much greater than normal amount of oxygen and energy in the already hypermetabolic state of the ill and injured. Not only does hypothermia result in increased energy and oxygen use but it also worsens bleeding. Many reactions within the coagulation cascade are temperature dependent; therefore, a drop in temperature will lead to platelet dysfunction and prolonged coagulation.

Acidosis in the injured patient is most commonly caused by hypoperfusion of the tissues, production of lactic acid as a result of anaerobic metabolism, and hypoventilation, caused by a myriad of reasons, such as traumatic brain injury. Severe acidosis can lead to myocardial dysfunction, worsening hypoperfusion, and worsening coagulopathy (reactions within the coagulation cascade decrease significantly in an acidotic environment).

Coagulopathies, or bleeding disorders, can be caused by hypothermia and/or acidosis. Other cases such as genetic bleeding disorder, massive hemorrhage (loss of clotting factors), dilution (massive intravenous fluid administration and diluting circulating clotting factors), and/or prior medication use (i.e., antiplatelets such as aspirin; vitamin K antagonists such as warfarin; herbal supplements such as garlic, ginger, and ginkgo biloba) can exacerbate coagulopathy for the trauma patient. All three factors of the triad affect each other and should each be considered in concert whenever caring for the hemorrhaging trauma patient.

Recent evidence in trauma literature supports the importance of calcium levels in trauma resuscitation. Some have even proposed adding hypocalcemia as a fourth leg to the lethal triad, creating the "diamond of death."[17] This association of hypocalcemia and mortality has been demonstrated in multiple studies.[18] Calcium performs numerous vital functions, including directly impacting the efficacy of clotting cascade mechanisms. Patients who have

sustained severe traumatic injuries often present to emergency services with hypocalcemia.[18] This hypocalcemia can be further exacerbated by necessary blood transfusions, due to the citrate preservative found in stored blood and its action of binding to a patient's endogenous calcium, rendering it inactive.[19] In order to mitigate the effects of the citrate and to reverse this trauma-induced hypocalcemia, clinicians should consider administering intravenous calcium preemptively and/or concurrently with blood transfusions.

Primary and Secondary Assessment

In development of a systematic approach for assessment of trauma, caregivers must intervene in life-threatening injuries, discover occult injuries, and prioritize care. For the traumatically injured patient, some anticipated interventions could include endotracheal intubation, needle or tube thoracostomy, hemorrhage control with commercial tourniquets, application of a pelvic binder, and/or administration of blood products and tranexamic acid (TXA). In the prehospital setting, scene evaluation is important and includes an assessment of safety. Every transport team member is responsible for recognizing all possible dangers and ensuring that none still exist. No caregiver should become a victim. The scene should be evaluated first for safety and, if necessary, move the patient to a safe area before initiation of treatment. The transport team is challenged by many factors while performing a detailed assessment. Three of the most common factors are time, noise level, and the inability to fully disrobe a patient. The transport team is responsible for evaluating each patient's situation individually to determine the best approach for conducting an assessment. For example, transport of a patient via helicopter from the scene of the accident may routinely require that the team perform the primary assessment on the scene, load the patient, and perform the secondary assessment in the aircraft or ground vehicle, avoiding delay of definitive care. Adjuncts to the assessment, such as the Extended Focused Assessment with Sonography in Trauma (eFAST), and supportive interventions can also be performed during transport to minimize delay. However, the auscultation of breath sounds and bowel sounds is not possible during rotor-wing transport and should be performed before liftoff. For review of the primary and secondary assessment, review Chapter 12, *Patient Assessment*.

Scoring of Trauma Patients

Numeric scoring for determination of the severity of injuries is common practice. Scoring provides a potential outcome classification for trauma patients, through single-system injuries, multisystem injuries, or the patient's physiologic condition. A variety of injury-severity scores exist, but none are 100% accurate, and their reliability should be considered with their use. Common prehospital scoring systems and accepted retrospective scores are discussed in the following subsections.

Prospective Scoring

A goal of emergency response personnel has long been to develop a numeric score to determine the severity of a patient's injuries at the incident scene. Use of such a score would mean rapid verification of trauma patients and appropriate triage to a trauma center; thus, appropriate resources could be used, and morbidity and mortality rates could be significantly decreased. Numerous prehospital scoring indexes have been developed, though few have gained national support.

Trauma Score

The *Trauma Score* is a physiologic index composed of five categories: systolic blood pressure (SBP), respiratory rate, respiratory expansion, capillary refill, and score on the Glasgow Coma Scale (GCS) (Fig. 15.10).[20] The score is a number between 1 and 15. Associated with each score is a probability of survival for that score. The lower scores are associated with higher mortality rates. To increase the reliability of the outcome predictions, the *Revised Trauma Score* was developed. It includes the GCS, SBP, and respiratory rate (Table 15.3), but both capillary refill rate and respiratory expansion have been removed because of subjectivity.[21] The major limitation of the Trauma Score is that it measures physiologic response. As

		Rate	Codes	Score
A.	Respiratory rate	10–24	4	
	Number of respirations in 15	25–35	3	
	seconds: Multiply by 4	>35	2	
		<10	1	
		0	0	A. _____
B.	Respiratory effort	Normal	1	
	Retroactive: Use of accessory	Retractive	0	
	muscles or intercostal retraction			B. _____
C.	Systolic blood pressure	≥90	4	
	Systolic cuff pressure: Either arm,	70–89	3	
	auscultate or palpate	50–69	2	
		>50	1	
	No carotid pulse	0	0	C. _____
D.	Capillary refill			
	Normal: Forehead or lip mucosa			
	color refill in 2 seconds	Normal	2	
	Delayed: More than 2 seconds			
	capillary refill	Delayed	1	
	None: No capillary refill	None	0	D. _____
E.	Glasgow Coma Scale	Total GSC points	Score	
	1. Eye opening			
	Spontaneous _____ 4	14–15	5	
	To voice _____ 3	11–13	4	
	To pain _____ 2	8–10	3	
	None _____ 1	5–7	2	
		3–4	1	E. _____
	2. Verbal response			
	Oriented _____ 5			
	Confused _____ 4			
	Inappropriate words _____ 3			
	Incomprehensible			
	sounds _____ 2			
	None _____ 1			
	3. Motor response			
	Obeys commands _____ 6			
	Purposeful move-			
	ments (pain) _____ 5			
	Withdraw (pain) _____ 4			
	Flexion (pain) _____ 3			
	Extension (pain) _____ 2			
	None _____ 1			
Total GCS points (1 + 2 + 3) _____			Trauma Score _____	

(Total points A + B + C + D + E)

• **Figure 15.10** Components of the trauma score.

TABLE 15.3 Revised Trauma Score Variable Break Points

Glasgow Coma Scale Score	Systolic Blood Pressure (mm Hg)	Respiratory Rate (breaths/min)	Coded Value
13–15	>89	10–29	4
9–12	76–89	>29	3
6–8	50–75	6–9	2
4–5	1–49	1–5	1
3	0	0	0

TABLE 15.4 Mechanism, Glasgow Coma Scale, Age, and Arterial Pressure

Mechanism	Measured Score
Blunt trauma	+4
Penetrating trauma	0
Glasgow Coma Scale	
+ (GCS Score)	
Age	
<60 years	+5
>60 years	0
Systolic Blood Pressure	
>120 mm Hg	+5
60–120 mm Hg	+3
<60 mm Hg	0

long as the patient compensates, or is supported by mechanical ventilation, the score does not accurately reflect condition.

Mechanism, Glasgow, Age, and Arterial Pressure (MGAP)

The mechanism, Glasgow, age, and arterial pressure (MGAP) is a scoring system similar to the Revised Trauma Score; however, MGAP integrates mechanism of injury and age and removes the respiratory component. The score (out of 29) is determined by totaling values for: GCS, SBP, mechanism, and age (Table 15.4). Initial studies for this scoring system identified three groups: low risk (23–29 points), intermediate risk (18–22 points), and high risk (<18 points). Suggested mortality rates for these groups were 2.8%, 15%, and 48%, respectively.[21]

Shock Index

The shock index (SI) is a simple physiologic score derived from the ratio of a patient's heart rate (HR) and SBP ($SI = HR/SBP$).[22] SI has proven useful in identifying patients with higher severity of injury, mortality, and need for massive blood transfusion.[22–24] Initially, an SI greater than or equal to 0.9 was used as the cutoff for these severe findings.[22] However, an agreed-upon cutoff has yet to be established, as clinicians have recently investigated the efficacy of greater than 1.0 as the SI cutoff with similar findings.[23] Given the expected exceptional tachycardic response of pediatric patients in the setting of trauma, researchers identified a need for

an age-adjusted SI. The shock index, pediatric age-adjusted (SIPA) was studied and found to be more effective at identifying a need for endotracheal intubation, emergency surgery, or blood transfusion than age-adjusted hypotension.[24] The values identified for SIPA were: >1.22 (for ages 4–6), >1.0 (for ages 7–12), and >0.9 (for ages 13–16).[24]

Retrospective Scoring

Retrospective scoring is the concept of attaching a numeric score to each diagnosed injury.

Abbreviated Injury Scale

The *Abbreviated Injury Scale* (AIS), published by the American Association for Automotive Medicine, categorizes injuries into six body regions (head, neck, thorax, abdomen, spine, and extremity and external) and assigns an individual score to each injury (Box 15.1).[25] The lower the score is, the less severe the injury. The AIS method was designed to determine the severity of motor vehicle injuries. In the 1985 revision of the AIS, penetrating injuries were addressed in all body regions, but the scale is still considered more sensitive to blunt injuries. The AIS allows determination of individual injury severity but does not take into account multisystem injuries.

Injury Severity Score

The *Injury Severity Score* (ISS) quantifies multisystem injury by use of the AIS scores. The ISS is determined by adding the squares of the highest AIS scores in the three most severely injured body systems (Table 15.5). The ISS is a number between 1 and 75, with 1 being a minor injury and 75 being largely nonsurvivable. A patient who receives a score of 6 in any AIS category is automatically

• BOX 15.1 Abbreviated Injury Scale

0 = No injury
1 = Minor
2 = Moderate
3 = Severe
4 = Serious
5 = Critical
6 = Maximum; virtually nonsurvivable

TABLE 15.5 Injury Severity Score

Region	Injury Description	Abbreviated Injury Scale	Squared Top 3 Scores
Head and neck	Hemorrhagic contusion	3	9
Face	No injuries	0	
Chest	Multiple rib fractures	4	16
Abdomen	Grade V splenic laceration	5	25
Extremity	Bilateral femur fractures	3	—
External	No injuries	0	—
		Injury Severity Score =	50

scored as having an ISS of 75. Any patient with an ISS greater than 15 is widely considered to be a major trauma patient.

Trauma and Injury Severity Score

The *Trauma and Injury Severity Score* method is a statistical equation that ties together the revised trauma score, ISS, age, and type of injury to determine the probability of survival for the patient.[26]

With the focus on percentage of mortality, the injury scoring systems have yet to address the probable morbidity associated with physiologic response and actual injuries. Despite years of experience and research, none of these scoring systems have been found to be significantly superior to the others.[27] However, a recent study has suggested the MGAP scale to be more accurate in predicting mortality than the revised trauma scale.[28]

Field Triage

Use of field triage to determine whether to take a patient to a trauma center is a necessary skill for caregivers in many parts of the United States. Proper identification of patients who meet trauma center criteria is routinely based on physiologic criteria, anatomic criteria, and a field triage score.[1] Fig. 15.11 displays the standard field triage criteria for delivery of a patient to a trauma center.

Mass Casualty Incidents

Mass casualty incidents (MCIs) are situations where the number of patients exceeds the resources, capabilities, or personnel available

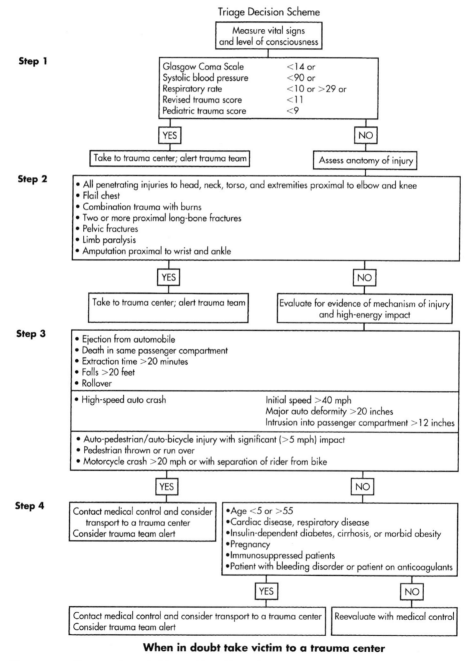

• **Figure 15.11** Trauma triage decision-making. (From Committee on Trauma, American College of Surgeons. *Resources for Optimal Care of the Injured Patient.* American College of Surgeons; 1993.)

to treat them. EMS personnel, particularly in the United States, are responding to MCIs with increasing frequency. Whether the situation involves 4 severely injured patients presenting to 2 EMS personnel, or 30 patients presenting to a rural emergency department, the result is one where normal interventions or timely care will not be available for every patient. Use of triage assessment skills and MCI triage algorithms should be employed to provide the greatest benefit for the greatest number of patients. Many different MCI triage algorithms are used throughout the world. One of the most common systems in the United States is the START (Simple Triage and Rapid Treatment) Triage System (Fig. 15.12).[29] The assessment components within this algorithm are designed for rapid evaluation, so the user may quickly triage several patients with an objective, reliable metric. The triaging clinician uses the

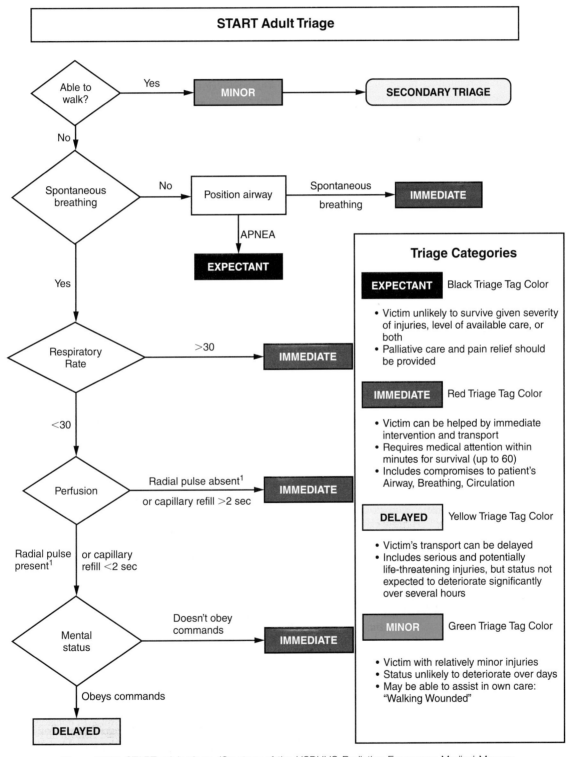

• **Figure 15.12** START adult triage. (Courtesy of the USDHHS Radiation Emergency Medical Management. *Source:* https://chemm.hhs.gov.)

assessment of a patient's ability to walk, presence of breathing, respiratory rate, perfusion, and mental status in order to assign them to one of four color-coded triage categories.[29] Using the color-coded system, patients are treated in the specific order of: red (immediate), yellow (delayed), green (minor), and black (expectant). Of note, patients that may be normally identified as immediate may be identified as expectant in MCIs due to limited resources and the need to treat as many viable patients as possible. The only interventions allowed within the START system are to manually open the airway to assess for spontaneous breathing and to provide hemorrhage control.[29] There is a pediatric version of START, named Jump START, for patients younger than the age of 8. The primary differences for Jump START are the addition of five rescue breaths for patients with apnea but still have a palpable pulse. Additionally, age-appropriate respiratory ranges are provided and Alert, Verbal, Painful, Unresponsive (AVPU) is used in lieu of the adult mental status.[29] As a critical care transport clinician, it is imperative that the clinician is familiar with local MCI systems, triage models, and how to integrate into an active MCI.

Triage Patient Transport

Care during transport of patients with multiple injuries is aimed at maintaining adequate airway; breathing; and circulation, continued resuscitation, and constant monitoring of the patient. The outcome of the patient often depends on the caregiver's ability to anticipate the patient's progression and recognize changes in the patient's condition (Fig. 15.13).

Trends in Trauma Care

Over the last several years, prehospital and tertiary trauma care have undergone significant changes and advancements. Once-new prehospital advances, such as increased use of hemostatic

agents, tourniquets, prehospital ultrasound, and prehospital blood product administration, are now considered mainstays of trauma care in many areas of the world. The concept of "damage control resuscitation" has seen continued support and development.

Damage control resuscitation is the concept of treating hemorrhagic shock in which the provider performs early transfusion of packed red blood cells (PRBC), plasma, and platelets in a 1:1:1 ratio (or whole blood), while restricting crystalloid fluids, to achieve an SPB goal of 90 to 100 mm Hg in adults; while also preventing/correcting hypothermia and coagulopathy (with TXA and thromboelastography guidance).[30] A complimentary component of this concept is immediate damage control surgery, which is the strategy of performing exploratory or hemorrhage control surgery with the aim of stopping internal bleeding and restoring physiologic function, but not anatomic normality. An example of this would be the multisystem trauma patient: the surgeon would perform an open laparotomy to control all sources of bleeding, then pack the abdomen, covering it with a temporary dressing, and admit the patient to the intensive care unit (ICU). Once the patient was stabilized in the ICU, the surgeon would then take the patient back to the operating room for definitive repair of the remaining injuries and surgical wound closure. This generally occurs 1 to 2 days after the initial surgery. It should be noted that there is currently no literature to support the use of damage-control resuscitation in pediatric patients.[31] Additionally, permissive hypotension should be avoided in the pediatric or traumatic brain injury patient populations. Hypotension in these populations can lead to significant worsening of morbidity and mortality.

Another trending treatment strategy is adoption of nonoperative strategies, such as those performed in interventional radiology: balloon occlusion of bleeding vessels, transarterial embolization (purposeful clotting off of a given artery), and stent grafts. Nonoperative management strategies have become the standard of care in the hemodynamically stable patient with blunt abdominal trauma

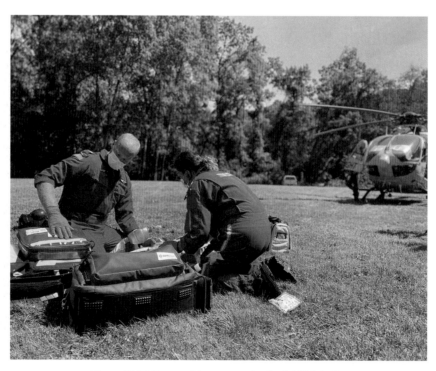

• **Figure 15.13** Transport team preparing for field intubation.

and some vascular injuries. Recent studies have demonstrated the beneficial outcomes of using a nonoperative strategy in select hemodynamically stable patients with penetrating injuries.[32,33]

Resuscitative endovascular balloon occlusion of the aorta (REBOA) is another nonsurgical procedure, which is used for hemorrhagic shock patients. REBOA involves percutaneously placing an endovascular balloon through the femoral artery and threading it up into the aorta. The balloon is inflated in the aorta to augment afterload and decreasing flow to the hemorrhage site, while increasing pressure and flow to proximal vital organs such as the heart and brain. Although generally performed in the emergency department or operating room, REBOA is being further investigated and slowly moving into the prehospital environment.[34,35]

Summary

The members of the transport team provide a critical level of knowledge and expertise of care for the patient with multiple injuries in the prehospital setting. By understanding the kinematics of trauma, performing a thorough assessment, and delivering care in an organized manner, the transport team has a positive effect on decreasing morbidity and mortality rates of these patients.

CASE STUDY

Multiple Trauma

The transport team was dispatched to a multiple-victim scene in a rural area 30 minutes from the hospital. Reports were that two victims were dead, and one other was severely injured. Initial responders performed basic care. On arrival, the flight crew's aerial view of the scene revealed a single car that had been split in half. Rescuers were attending to the victim, and two bodies lying near the wreckage were covered with sheets.

The patient had been thrown from the vehicle over the guardrail, approximately 15 feet. The patient was a 19-year-old girl whose left leg had been amputated above the knee. Bleeding was not being controlled despite application of a pressure dressing before arrival. She had multiple abrasions and lacerations on her face and chest. Her GCS score was 7 (eyes, 1; verbal, 1; motor, 5). She was pale and diaphoretic. She had a palpable femoral pulse of 130 beats/min and a respiratory rate of 8 beats/min. She was immobilized on a backboard, with cervical collar and head blocks in place. She had one intravenous line in place.

The transport team quickly applied a tourniquet to the patient's thigh. Hemorrhage control was obtained. An empiric pelvic binder was placed due to the patient's mechanism of injury and kinematics. The transport team elected to intubate the patient because of her low GCS score, her advanced level of shock, and her anticipated clinical course. While gathering equipment for intubation, a member of the rescue squad placed a second intravenous line. A palpable systolic blood pressure (SBP) of 70 mm Hg was also obtained. One liter of 0.9% sodium chloride had already been infused by the rescue squad team. The transport team carried PRBCs and rapidly began transfusing the patient. The patient's SBP increased to 110 mm Hg. Appropriate rapid sequence induction medications were given, with shock-appropriate dosing, and the patient was intubated without difficulty. The patient was loaded into the aircraft and secured. En route to the hospital, the crew initiated a slow bolus of 1 g of TXA and provided appropriate postintubation sedation and analgesia with respect to hemodynamics. The patient was also placed on the transport ventilator. The transport team kept their remaining blood products and calcium gluconate available in case need for continued transfusion arose en route.

During the 15-minute transport to the trauma center, the patient's SBP remained between 90 and 110 mm Hg and she was tachycardic (100–115 beats/min). No additional neuromuscular blocking agent was administered. The patient was admitted to the shock resuscitation unit, and a report was given to the resuscitation team.

References

1. Marr AB, Stuke LE, Greiffenstein P. Kinematics. In: Moore EE, Feliciano DV, Mattox KL, eds. *Trauma*. 8th ed. McGraw Hill; 2017.
2. National Center for Health Statistics. *Health, United States, 2019: Table 006*. Hyattsville, MD; 2021. https://www.cdc.gov/nchs/hus/contents2019.htm
3. Centers for Disease Control and Prevention, National Center for Injury Prevention and Control. *Web-Based Injury Statistics Query and Reporting System: Leading Causes of Death Reports, 1981–2020*. Atlanta, GA. https://wisqars.cdc.gov/fatal-leading
4. Bonilla-Escobar FJ, Gutierrez Martinez MI. Injuries are not accidents: Towards a culture of prevention. *Colombia Medica*. 2014:132–135. doi:10.25100/cm.v45i3.1462
5. Bergen G, Chen L, Warner M, Fingerhut L. *Injury in the United States: 2007 Chartbook*. Hyattsville, MD: National Center for Health Statistics; 2008.
6. Office of Disease Prevention and Health Promotion, U.S. Department of Health and Human Services. *Injury prevention. Injury Prevention – Healthy People 2030*. Published 2020. https://health.gov/healthypeople/objectives-and-data/browse-objectives/injury-prevention
7. National Association of Emergency Medical Technicians. *PHTLS: Prehospital Trauma Life Support*. Jones & Bartlett Learning; 2020.
8. Emergency Nurses Association. *TNCC: Trauma Nursing Core Course: Provider Manual*. 8th ed. Jones & Bartlett Learning; 2020.
9. World Health Organization. *Road Traffic Injuries*. World Health Organization. Published June 20, 2022. Accessed July 12, 2022. https://www.who.int/news-room/fact-sheets/detail/road-traffic-injuries
10. Klinich KD, Bowman P, Flannagan CAC, Rupp JD. *Injury Patterns in Motor-Vehicle Crashes in the United States: 1998–2014*. University of Michigan Transportation Research Institute; 2016. UMTRI-2016-16.
11. Stefanopoulos PK, Pinialidis DE, Hadjigeorgiou GF, Filippakis KN. Wound ballistics 101: The mechanisms of soft tissue wounding by bullets. *Eur J Trauma Emerg Surg*. 2017;43(5):579–586. doi:10.1007/s00068-015-0581-1
12. Cone DC, Brice JH, Delbridge TR, Myers JB. *Penetrating Trauma in Emergency Medical Services: Clinical Practice and Systems Oversight*. John Wiley & Sons; 2015.
13. Kuhajda I, Zarogoulidis K, Kougioumtzi I, et al. Penetrating trauma. *J Thorac Dis*. 2014;6(Suppl 4):S461–S465.
14. Copes W. *Major Trauma Outcome Study: Letter to MTOS Participants*. American College of Surgeons; 1988.
15. Stefanopoulos PK, Hadjigeorgiou GF, Filippakis K, Gyftokostas D. Gunshot wounds: A review of ballistics related to penetrating trauma. *J Acute Dis*. 2014;3(3):178–185. doi:10.1016/s2221-6189(14)60041-x

16. Stefanopoulos PK, Mikros G, Pinialidis DE, Oikonomakis IN, Tsiatis NE, Janzon B. Wound ballistics of military rifle bullets: An update on controversial issues and associated misconceptions. *J Trauma Acute Care Surg.* 2019;87(3):690–698. doi:10.1097/ta.0000000000002290

17. Wray JP, Bridwell RE, Schauer SG, et al. The diamond of death: Hypocalcemia in trauma and resuscitation. *Am J Emerg Med.* 2021;41:104–109. doi:10.1016/j.ajem.2020.12.065

18. Vasudeva M, Mathew JK, Groombridge C, et al. Hypocalcemia in trauma patients: A systematic review. *J Trauma Acute Care Surg.* 2021;90(2):396–402. doi:10.1097/TA.0000000000003027

19. DiFrancesco NR, Gaffney TP, Lashley JL, Hickerson KA. Hypocalcemia and massive blood transfusions: A pilot study in a level I trauma center. *J Trauma Nurs.* 2019;26(4):186–192. doi:10.1097/JTN.0000000000000447

20. Champion HR, Sacco WJ, Carnazzo AJ, Copes W, Fouty WJ. Trauma score. *Crit Care Med.* 1981;9(9):672–676.

21. Bouzat P, Legrand R, Gillois P, et al. Prediction of intra-hospital mortality after severe trauma: Which pre-hospital score is the most accurate? *Injury.* 2016;47(1):14–18.

22. Montoya KF, Charry JD, Calle-Toro JS, Núñez LR, Poveda G. Shock index as a mortality predictor in patients with acute polytrauma. *J Acute Dis.* 2015;4(3):202–204. doi:10.1016/j.joad.2015.04.006

23. Kheirbek T, Martin TJ, Cao J, Hall BM, Lueckel S, Adams CA. Prehospital shock index outperforms hypotension alone in predicting significant injury in trauma patients. *Trauma Surg Acute Care Open.* 2021;6(1). doi:10.1136/tsaco-2021-000712

24. Acker SN, Bredbeck B, Partrick DA, Kulungowski AM, Barnett CC, Bensard DD. Shock index, pediatric age-adjusted (SIPA) is more accurate than age-adjusted hypotension for trauma team activation. *Surgery.* 2017;161(3):803–807. doi:10.1016/j.surg.2016.08.050

25. Copes WS, Champion HR, Sacco WJ, Lawnick MM, Keast SL, Bain LW. The injury severity score revisited. *J Trauma.* 1988;28(1):69–77.

26. Alam A, Gupta A, Gupta N, Yelamanchi R, Bansal L, Durga C. Evaluation of ISS, RTS, CASS and TRISS scoring systems for predicting outcomes of blunt trauma abdomen. *Pol Przegl Chir.* 2021;93(2):9–15. doi:10.5604/01.3001.0014.7394

27. Farzan N, Foroghi Ghomi SY, Mohammadi AR. A retrospective study on evaluating GAP, MGAP, RTS and ISS trauma scoring system for the prediction of mortality among multiple trauma patients. *Ann Med Surg (Lond).* Mar 28, 2022;76:103536. doi:10.1016/j.amsu.2022.103536

28. Galvagno SM Jr, Massey M, Bouzat P, et al. Correlation between the revised trauma score and injury severity score: Implications for pre-hospital trauma triage. *Prehosp Emerg Care.* 2019;23(2):263–270. doi:10.1080/10903127.2018.1489019

29. Bazyar J, Farrokhi M, Khankeh H. Triage systems in mass casualty incidents and disasters: A review study with a worldwide approach. *Open Access Maced J Med Sci.* Feb 12, 2019;7(3):482–494. doi:10.3889/oamjms.2019.119

30. Leibner E, Andreae M, Galvagno SM, Scalea T. Damage control resuscitation. *Clin Exp Emerg Med.* Mar 2020;7(1):5–13. doi:10.15441/ceem.19.089. Epub 2020 Mar 31.

31. Hughes NT, Burd RS, Teach SL. Damage control resuscitation: Permissive hypotension and massive transfusion protocols. *Pediatr Emerg Care.* 2014;30(9):651–656.

32. Singh A, Kumar A, Kumar P, Kumar S, Gamanagatti S. "Beyond saving lives": Current perspectives of interventional radiology in trauma. *World J Radiol.* 2017;9(4):155. doi:10.4329/wjr.v9.i4.155

33. Matsumoto J, Lohman BD, Morimoto K, Ichinose Y, Hattori T, Taira Y. Damage control interventional radiology (DCIR) in prompt and rapid endovascular strategies in trauma occasions (PRESTO): A new paradigm. *Diagn Interv Imaging.* 2015;96(7–8):687–691. doi:10.1016/j.diii.2015.06.001

34. Tsurukiri J, Akamine I, Sato T, et al. Resuscitative endovascular balloon occlusion of the aorta for uncontrolled haemorrhagic shock as an adjunct to haemostatic procedures in the acute care setting. *Scand J Trauma Resusc Emerg Med.* 2016;24(1):13.

35. Thrailkill MA, Gladin KH, Thorpe CR, et al. Resuscitative endovascular balloon occlusion of the aorta (REBOA): Update and insights into current practices and future directions for research and implementation. *Scand J Trauma, Resusc Emerg Med.* 2021;29(1). doi:10.1186/s13049-020-00807-9

16

Neurologic Trauma

ROBERT L. GRABOWSKI

COMPETENCIES

1. Perform primary and secondary neurologic assessment.
2. Investigate current guidelines for the management of traumatic neurologic injury.
3. Initiate/continue critical interventions during transport for traumatic neurologic injury to reduce morbidity and mortality.

Introduction

Traumatic neurologic emergencies are defined as injury to either the central and/or the peripheral nervous systems. The central nervous system encompasses the brain and spinal cord. The peripheral nervous system includes the cranial nerves, spinal nerves, and peripheral nerves. The risk of morbidity and mortality from neurologic trauma is high. Rapid recognition of neurologic trauma by the transport team and immediate initiation of evidence-based treatment guidelines can dramatically reduce patient mortality and lessen the sequelae of neurologic trauma.

Traumatic Brain Injury

Traumatic brain injury (TBI) statistics are staggering. TBIs are the leading cause of death related to trauma. Estimates are that TBIs lead to over 220,000 hospital admission a year and result in over 64,000 deaths a year in the United States.[1] Seventy-four percent of all TBIs occur in patients 25 years old or younger; however, those 65 years of age and older were most likely to die of TBI, at a rate of 45%.[2] Falls and motor vehicle collisions are the leading causes of fatal TBIs.[1] The cost of care for people who survive neurologic injuries is in the millions of dollars.[1] The primary solution to the death and devastation caused by neurologic trauma is injury prevention.

TBI has a bimodal pathological process. The first is the initial injury which can be blunt or penetrating, mild to severe. The second stage begins immediately after the injury. In this stage, tissue injury, vascular disruption, and cerebral swelling alter the homeostatic processes. The outcome of the second stage is referred to as secondary brain injury. In the transport environment, there is nothing that can be done to change the initial injury. However, rapid injury recognition and intervention can eliminate or reduce secondary brain injury, improving patient outcomes.

Blunt Head Injuries

In general, blunt head injury occurs when the head strikes an object (such as the ground) or an object s strikes the head (such as a baseball bat). Blunt TBI can also occur from rapid acceleration or deceleration as the soft brain bounces around inside the hard skull. The force of impact contributes to the severity of the closed head injury, delineated as mild, moderate, or severe. If forces are severe enough, the skull can be fractured and/or sections of the skull can be depressed, creating an open head injury. Open head injuries are always treated as severe since the force required can translate to significant intracranial injury patterns, and the opening of the skull/dura places the patient at risk for brain and/or meningeal infection.

The hair, skin, and subcutaneous tissues provide some dampening of blunt head trauma. The force remaining is then transferred to the skull, which can flatten, indent, fracture, or dislocate. Maximal depression occurs instantly and is immediately followed by several oscillations. A severe blow to the skull will cause a flattening of the skull in the direction of the impact, which is then extended at right angles to the impact line.[3]

The skull travels faster under impact than does the brain. When the head is impacted, the brain slams into the rigid skull. Rough edges inside the skull, such as the sphenoid wings, can contuse or lacerated brain tissue. The temporal and occipital lobes are particularly vulnerable to shearing impact. Following significant impact, the brain will contact the impacting side of the skull, recoil, and propel backward, striking the opposing side of the skull, causing a "coup-countercoup injury."[4]

Damage may result from direct injury or from compression, tension, or shearing forces created by the injury. In addition, secondary complications result from the TBI. Cerebral edema and subsequent ischemia may ensue. An immediate increase in intracranial pressure (ICP) seems to occur on impact; however, a secondary increase also occurs several minutes after the injury. The increase in ICP at the time of impact results from acceleration and deceleration of the head and deformation of the skull, the former being more significant than the latter.[3]

During impact, cerebrospinal fluid (CSF) may offer some protection to the brain. However, this protective layer is often insufficient in the subarachnoid space, particularly around the frontal and temporal lobes, which are the frequent sites of contusion.

TBI may exist in isolation; however, various combinations of injuries usually occur. Each component of concurrent injuries contributes in a different degree to the overall severity and outcome of the injury.

Types of Traumatic Injuries: Pathologic and Clinical Considerations

Skull Fracture

The skull is composed of three layers: an outer layer, a middle cancellous layer, and an inner layer that is half as thick as the outer layer and contains grooves for large vessels. Whether a fracture occurs in the area of impact depends on the amount of energy and how it is delivered. The more concentrated and focused the impact tends to be, the greater the likelihood of a fracture.

Most skull fractures are linear. A *linear skull fracture* produces a line that usually extends toward the base of the skull. Impact can produce a single linear fracture or multiple fractures, referred to as linear stellate fractures, which radiate outward from the compressed area. Although linear fractures may look benign, they can cause serious complications. Linear fractures may also lead to epidural hematoma formation if the fracture line crosses a groove in the layer of the skull that houses the middle meningeal artery, such as seen with temporal bone fractures. Skull fractures in this area also hold a high risk of inner ear and vestibular complications. Another complication occurs when the dura, which is strongly attached to the skull, tears at the fracture site.

Diastatic and Basilar Skull Fractures

Diastatic fracture involves a separation of bones at a suture line or a marked separation of bone fragments; both are usually visible on computed tomographic (CT) scans. Facial fractures may also play a role in head injuries. A blow to the lower jaw when the jaw is closed can cause the mandibular condyles to displace upward and backward against the base of the skull, leading to a concussion or a basilar skull fracture. Another type of facial fracture, which may or may not involve the cranium, is an orbital blowout fracture, which usually involves the floor of the orbit and is caused by blunt impact to the orbit and its contents.

Basilar skull fractures can occur from direct injury to the base of the skull but most often result from extension of fractures of the calvaria. Basilar fractures are most often associated with temporal bone fractures but can be seen with sphenoid, ethmoid, frontal, or occipital fractures as well. Unique clinical exam findings can lead the clinician to maintain a high index of suspicion for basilar skull fractures, such as Battle's sign (an oval-shaped bruise over the mastoid), hemotympanum, leaking of CSF from the nose or ears, or raccoon eyes (periorbital ecchymosis) within 1 to 3 days of injury.

Depressed Skull Fracture

The presence of depressed elements of a fracture may warrant specific diagnostic and therapeutic measures. If the depressed fracture is closed, the rationale for surgical correction is to evacuate any local mass if present, repair any dural lacerations to prevent cerebral herniation through the defect, and correct any cosmetic disfigurement caused by the depression. Generally, if the depression on the tangential view of the skull is greater than the thickness of the skull, the dura is probably lacerated, and surgery is recommended. A compound depressed skull fracture usually requires surgical debridement, whereas depressions of a lesser degree (e.g., less than 1 cm), unless over the forehead, may not necessitate surgical exploration.

Skull fractures can be the source of various complications, including intracranial infections, hematomas, and pneumocephalus (air within the cranium), as well as meningeal and brain tissue damage. If the skull is fractured open, debris such as hair, dirt, and glass may travel into the cranial vault. This foreign material can cause significant intracranial infection and can complicate patient recovery/outcomes. Traumatic pneumocephalus may occur from a variety of fracture types that allow air to communicate within the cranial vault (e.g., facial bone/sinus fractures or cranial fractures). Air is then able to enter the skull collecting in the epidural, subdural, subarachnoid, interventricular, or intracerebral space. Pneumocephalus seldom produces symptoms unless it is under tension, producing compression of the underlying brain tissue. Without a clear route for the air to escape, Boyle's law demonstrates that bringing a patient to high altitudes will expand that gas volume and increase its compressive effect on surrounding tissues. Therefore, the transport clinician should maintain a high index of suspicion with corresponding injury patterns and should instruct the pilot that the patient has a condition that requires flying at a low altitude. The pilot will determine the safe altitude.

Generally, temporal bone fractures can cause pneumocephalus if dural tearing occurs in conjunction with injury to the eustachian tube, the middle ear, or the mastoid process. The patient may have sensory neurologic hearing loss, otorrhagia, or CSF rhinorrhea in the presence of a temporal bone fracture.[5]

Intracranial Hemorrhage

Subdural Hematoma

A subdural hematoma is a collection of blood in the potential space between the arachnoid mater and the dura mater. It may occur as a result of a contusion or laceration of the brain with bleeding into the subdural space, tearing of the veins that bridge the subdural space, or an extension of an intracerebral hematoma through the brain surface into the subdural space. Subdural hematomas tend to be crescent shaped in appearance on radiologic examination because they follow the layer of the dura and are not affected by the suture lines of the skull (Fig. 16.1). They may or may not be associated with skull fractures.[3]

Subdural hematomas are classified as acute, subacute, or chronic, depending on the time elapsed between the injury. If dysfunction occurs within 24 hours, the hematoma is acute; if it occurs between 2 and 10 days, it is subacute; and if it occurs after 2 weeks, or if the patient remains asymptomatic, the hematoma is chronic. The location of the hematoma, time to develop, and the amount of mass effect play important roles in determination of the timing of surgical intervention.

Elderly patients, alcoholics, and patients with a history of neurologic conditions such as a stroke are at higher risk of sustaining a subdural hematoma. They may also experience larger subdural hematomas, with slower developing symptoms, because they have larger potential subdural spaces to fill as a result of cerebral atrophy. In contrast, symptoms may develop rapidly, along with a marked increase in ICP, in younger patients with smaller subdural hematomas.

Subdural hematomas that occur in children under the age of 2 years may have signs and symptoms that include a bulging fontanel, a large head (because of separation of the sutures), as well as retinal hemorrhages (due to increased ICP or shearing of retinal vessels). The presence of retinal hemorrhages with subdural hemorrhage in the infant should trigger the clinician to be

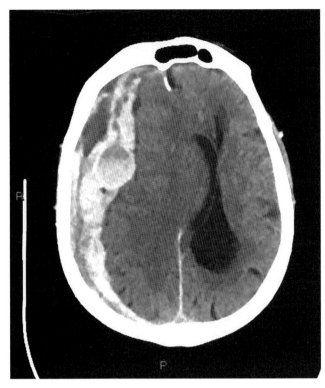

• **Figure 16.1** Subdural hematoma on computed tomographic scan. (From Dr. Derek Smith, Radiopaedia.org.)

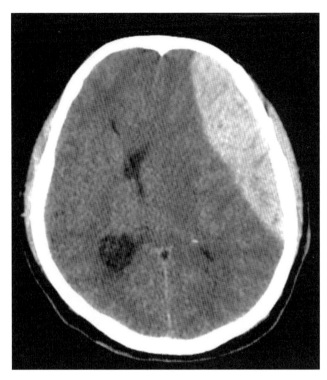

• **Figure 16.2** Epidural hematoma on computed tomographic scan. (From Dr. David Cuete, Radiopaedia.org.)

mindful of nonaccidental trauma, particularly when injury information does not correlate with injury severity. Additionally, the infant patient is at risk for hemorrhagic shock in the presence of subdural hemorrhage (and other intracranial hemorrhages) because of the relatively large blood volume that may be lost in the subdural space, and because of the decreased opposition forces of the skull when sutures have yet to fuse.

Acute subdural hematomas are usually associated with high morbidity and mortality rates. Morbidity is high, with only a quarter of patients returning to functional baseline, though poor outcomes can potentially be mitigated by decreasing time from injury to intervention. Mortality rates can be estimated by the patient's presenting Glasgow Coma Scale (GCS) score; however, this is greatly confounded by patient factors such as age and comorbidities. A GCS score of less than 8 has an associated mortality of 6% to 75%. Patients with a GCS score of 9 to 12 have associated 2% to 32% mortality, and those with a score greater than or equal to 13 have a mortality rate reported as low as 0.3% to 14%.[6] The extremes of age can greatly skew the average mortality, with teenagers demonstrating exceptionally low mortality and geriatrics experiencing near-double the median mortality.[6] The higher mortality rate is generally reflective of the severe nature of the associated injuries and rapidly rising ICP resulting from the mass effect and cerebral edema.

Cerebral contusion and edema are separate yet related pathophysiologic findings common with the presence of blood in the subdural space. The CT scan is valuable in the determination of intracranial processes and whether surgical intervention may be indicated. If the major problem contributing to poor neurologic status is the mass effect, then surgical intervention may be necessary. If the major problem is the cerebral injury, then corrective treatment should be directed toward ICP management.

Epidural Hematoma

An epidural hematoma is the collection of blood between the skull and the outer layer of the dura. Most epidural hematomas are caused by a disruption to a branch of the middle meningeal artery. Epidural hematomas are classified as acute or subacute. An acute epidural hematoma is a life-threatening emergency. A secondary rise in ICP occurs and there is displacement of the brain with mass effect. Once compensatory mechanisms of the inner cranial space have been exhausted, the patient's neurologic status will rapidly deteriorate. On radiologic examination, acute epidural hematomas follow the outer layer of the dura, are usually limited by the suture lines of the skull and take on a lenticular shape (Fig. 16.2). Subacute epidural hematomas are generally venous in origin and may take 2 to 4 days to be recognized. The blood in a subacute epidural hematoma will coagulate into a solid mass. These hematomas are associated with linear skull fractures in many patients. The classic symptoms displayed with epidural hematoma are transient loss of consciousness, recovery with a lucid interval during which neurologic status returns to normal, and the secondary onset of headache and a decreasing level of consciousness (LOC). The classic history and clinical progression, however, are only seen in one-third of patients with epidural hematomas. Another third are unconscious from the time of injury, and the final third are never unconscious. In children, bradycardia and early papilledema may be the only warning signs.

The patient with an acute subdural hemorrhage experiences a downhill course, usually with dilation of the ipsilateral pupil because of third cranial nerve compression by the herniating temporal structures; progressive unconsciousness with weakness or decerebration of either the contralateral extremities or the ipsilateral extremities; Cheyne–Stokes respirations; and, if no treatment is initiated, loss of pupillary reflexes, caloric responses, bradycardia, and death. Thus, on identification of the epidural hematoma

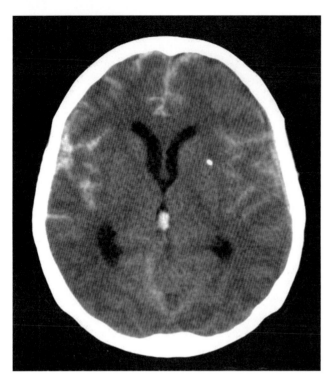

• **Figure 16.3** Subarachnoid hemorrhage on computed tomographic scan. (From Dr. David Cuete, Radiopaedia.org.)

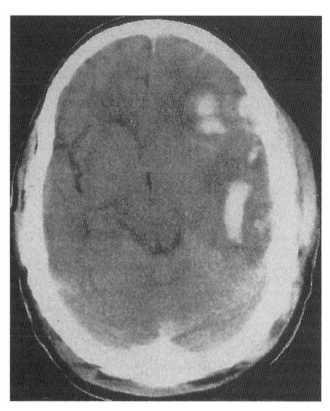

• **Figure 16.4** Intracerebral hematoma (intraparenchymal hematoma). (From Ellenbogen RG, Abdulrauf SI, Sekhar LN. *Principles of Neurological Surgery*. Saunders; 2012.)

in the earliest possible stage, transfer of the patient for immediate neurosurgical intervention is extremely important.[7]

Subarachnoid Hemorrhage

A subarachnoid hemorrhage (SAH) refers to blood collecting between the arachnoid membrane and the pia mater. SAH is identified in 30% to 40% of moderate to severe TBIs (Fig. 16.3).[8] The subarachnoid space is normally occupied by connecting tissue and CSF. CSF circulates through the subarachnoid space and the cerebral ventricles. CSF is reabsorbed into the venous system via arachnoid granulations. Blood from the SAH can clot and block the granulations resulting in a communicating hydrocephalus. In addition to the risk for hydrocephalus, SAH may also increase ICP secondary to the space-occupying hemorrhage or edema. SAH also yields an increased risk for seizures and cerebral vasospasm. Vasospasm is caused by vascular irritation in response to the degradation of the blood in the SAH.[7,9] Generally, traumatic SAH has a better prognostic outcome than does spontaneous SAH. However, it is important to consider if the SAH is a result of the trauma, or if the SAH was the *cause* of the trauma.

Intracerebral Hematoma

Movement of one section of brain tissue over or against another section causes tears in blood vessels, which leads to contusions or intracerebral hematomas, also known as intraparenchymal hematomas. Most intracerebral hematomas are found in the frontal and temporal lobes, are usually very deep, and are associated with necrosis and hemorrhage. The anatomic relationship between these areas and irregularities of the skull has already been discussed. Intracerebral hematomas are readily identified on CT scan (Fig. 16.4). The clinical picture may vary from no neurologic defect to deep coma, depending on the location and severity.

Cerebellar Hematoma

Traumatic cerebellar hematomas are rare, though they may occur in certain injury patters. More commonly, cerebellar hematomas are the result of uncontrolled hypertension. Nestled in the posterior fossa, expanding hematomas of the cerebellum can quickly induce mass effect on the adjacent structures of the brainstem and fourth ventricle. The collapse of the fourth ventricle can lead to increased ICP from hydrocephalus. Herniation of the cerebellum and mass effect onto the brainstem will begin with symptoms of headache, nausea, vomiting, and dizziness. If left untreated, compression of the brainstem will lead to dysregulation of cardiovascular and respiratory function, and ultimately, cardiac arrest. Cerebellar hematomas can be medically managed if small, but lesions greater than about 3 cm will likely require surgical decompression.

Cerebral Contusion

Cerebral contusions frequently occur in patients after TBI. Of the patients who die of TBI, 75% have contusions found on autopsy. Hemorrhagic contusions are infrequently seen in children, but areas of localized decreased density on a CT scan may represent nonhemorrhagic contusions, or possibly local ischemia.[4]

Generally, no surgical intervention is recommended in the treatment of cerebral contusions because brain tissue cannot be removed from areas of the brain that control motor, sensory, or visual functioning. If diffuse, refractory cerebral edema and elevated ICP is present, a decompressive craniectomy may be warranted. However, if the contusion occurs over the frontal or temporal lobes, with significant edema and shift, craniotomy with evacuation of contused portions of the brain is feasible. When a temporal lobe contusion is present, with refractory intracranial hypertension, herniation, and/or diffuse parenchymal damage, surgical excision of the temporal lobe may be performed. Patients with cerebral contusions are most often treated with medical management of elevated ICP; surgical intervention is an uncommon treatment path.

Diffuse Axonal Injuries

Diffuse axonal injury (DAI) occurs when the delicate axons of the brain are stretched and damaged as a result of rapid movement of the brain. Rotational and deceleration forces, like those that occur with high-speed motor vehicle crashes or ejection from a vehicle, can separate the axon from the neuron. When DAI is observed in small children, similar to subdural hematomas with retinal hemorrhages, nonaccidental trauma should be considered.[10] Because axons have been damaged, neuronal transmission is impaired, leading to multiple neurologic deficits ranging from headache and amnesia to severe deficits that include deep coma, posturing, and respiratory compromise. Severe DAI is associated with a high mortality rate. Although there are several treatment strategies currently under investigation, there is no curative treatment for DAI; current goals are aimed at supportive care.

Concussion

A mild form for TBI, concussions are an extremely common finding in patients with head trauma, particularly from contact sports, motor vehicle collisions, and assaults. After the patient suffers a transfer of energy to the head, diffuse dysfunction occurs in the metabolic function of the brain. Functions such as glucose metabolism, neurotransmitter dysfunction, and cerebral blood flow are impaired after a concussion. These changes can affect the patient's cognition, mood, and sleep; and cause a wide range of symptoms, such as headache, dizziness, nausea, and visual disturbances. Treatment of a concussion focuses on supportive interventions for symptom management, physical and cognitive rest, and prevention of reinjury.

Penetrating Injuries

Gunshot Wounds

When a person is shot at close range, evidence of soot or gunpowder may be visible on the skin. When the muzzle of the gun is somewhat farther from the scalp but still close, evidence of powder burns may exist. A bullet striking the skull can cause great destruction of the underlying brain tissue.

Although some of the bullet's kinetic energy may be dissipated on impact by transfer to the bone and soft tissues, the impact on the brain after a bullet penetrates the skull is great. The bullet's ability to destroy tissues is directly related to its kinetic energy at the moment of impact. The degree of damage to the brain depends primarily on the size and velocity of the bullet and the distance between the firearm and its target, as previously discussed in Chapter 15.

A bullet that passes through the head produces a larger defect on the inner table of the skull than that produced on the outer table. Multiple linear fractures that radiate from either the entrance or exit wound are common. Some fractures may be far away from the trajectory of the bullet, particularly in thin bones. The transport team should describe the wounds but not attempt to determine whether they are entrance or exit wounds; variation in size and placement of wounds can be affected by several factors.

Cerebral injuries cause an immediate, but transitory, increase in ICP. The eventual ICP depends on the degree of intracranial bleeding, which may be profuse even in the absence of injury to major vessels. Secondary cerebral edema causes a delayed increase in ICP. Openings in the skull caused by bullets are areas of decreased resistance in which brain tissue may attempt to herniate. Though holes in the skull may act as a means of ICP relief, this does not equate to an effective form of ICP reduction. Damage to the hemisphere causes loss of cerebral autoregulation, decreased cerebral blood flow, an increase in cerebral blood volume and ICP, and eventually brain death.

Intracranial hematomas are frequently associated with penetrating wounds to the brain. If the bullet passes close to or transverses the ventricle, an intraventricular hematoma may result.

Most stab wounds are caused by assaults with sharp instruments such as knives, scissors, and screwdrivers or when the patient (often a child) falls on a stick or sharp toy. If the object is still impaled, leave it in place and immobilize it in order to avoid movement during transport.

If the penetrating object has been removed, determination of exactly where penetration of the skull occurred may be difficult, particularly if entry occurred at the eyelid or sclera. When the patient arrives at the hospital, the area of injury is explored and debrided, as with an open injury.

Blast-Related Traumatic Brain Injury

An explosion triggers a series of potential injury pathways for injury to the body. Following a blast, there are primary, secondary, tertiary, and quaternary mechanisms. Primary injury occurs from direct contact with the blast wave. Secondary injury is caused by the flying debris and shrapnel of the explosive. Tertiary injury occurs from displacement of the body via blast winds that cause the body to strike fixed objects, like walls or cars. Quaternary injuries encompass all other mechanisms for trauma, such as burns and inhalation injuries. The range of injury mechanisms from blast trauma can inflict a myriad of forms of TBI: any severity of concussion from primary injury, penetrating skull injuries from secondary injuries, or skull fractures and intracranial hemorrhage from tertiary injury. The type and severity of injury sustained will depend on the type of explosive, the body's distance from the device, shielding, as well as the type of debris and surroundings.

Traumatic Brain Injury Complications

In addition to the direct effects of hemorrhage, edema, and tissue damage from the trauma, the TBI patient is at risk for a list of complications. The clinician should be alert for posttraumatic seizures, endocrinopathies, and physiologic derangements contributing to secondary brain injury. Posttraumatic seizures can increase ICP, increase oxygen and energy demands of the injured brain, and potentially cause renewed bleeding at the site of injury. Posttraumatic endocrinopathies (i.e., diabetes insipidus, syndrome of inappropriate antidiuretic hormone, cerebral salt wasting, and hypopituitarism/adrenal insufficiency) often are the result of direct or indirect pituitary and/or hypothalamus dysregulation, causing challenges with water and electrolyte regulation. The mainstays of treatment for these disorders are meticulous monitoring of fluid and electrolytes; fluid restriction or fluid replacement, diuresis, as well as electrolyte and hormone (e.g., desmopressin) replacement.[11]

TABLE 16.1 Physiologic Disturbance Correlated With Anatomic Level of Lesion						
Parameters	**Cerebral Cortex**	**Diencephalon**	**Thalamus**	**Midbrain**	**Pons**	**Medulla**
Mental status	Awake, alert, lethargic, obtunded	Light stupor	Deep stupor	Coma	Coma	Coma
Motor response	Appropriate	Focal response to pain	General response to pain	Decerebrate posturing, decorticate posturing	Flaccid	Flaccid
Pupil response	Normal size and reactivity	Small	Small	Midposition	Small	Small
Oculocephalic, oculovestibular reflex	Not testable	Normal response	Normal response	Abnormal	Abnormal	Abnormal[a]
Respiratory status	Variable	Variable	Cheyne–Stokes	Central neurogenic hyperventilation	Apneustic pattern	Apnea

[a]May be normal with isolated medullary injury.

Physical Assessment: Traumatic Brain Injury

A rapid yet comprehensive physical assessment is necessary when a TBI is suspected or confirmed. The clinician should be proactive in completing the neurologic examination prior to administering exam-altering medication; otherwise, valuable data will be lost. Examination of a patient who is experiencing an altered LOC requires noting the patient's: LOC, GCS score, cognitive status, pupillary function, cranial nerve examination, and their motor and sensory assessment. Patients with severe TBI require an airway and respiratory assessment (Table 16.1).

Level of Consciousness

The first indicator of neurologic dysfunction from TBI is LOC. The patient must have cerebral functioning in order to interact with their surrounding environment. The reticular activating system (RAS) within the brainstem regulates wakefulness. Therefore, for a patient to be alert and oriented, they must have an intact cerebral functioning and an intact RAS. Absence of both functions results in coma. Variation in function of either component results in a minimally responsive state, persistent vegetative state, or locked-in syndrome.[4,7] *Consciousness* is a state of arousal in which the person is aware of environmental stimuli. Consciousness is a spectrum in descending order from alert, to lethargic, obtunded, stuporous, and comatose (Box 16.1). However, do not assume a decreased LOC is caused solely by a head injury in absence of objective evidence. There is a plethora of pathological conditions outside the CNS that can decrease consciousness, such as hypoglycemia, hypotension, diabetic ketoacidosis, seizure, and intoxication.

For consciousness to be present, a stimulus must be presented to the CNS and must pass through the brainstem (except for visual stimulation) to the diencephalon. From there, the stimulus must reach the cerebral cortex, where it is recorded. The patient must have sufficient cortical function so that the stimulus can excite associations through memory, which lets the patient acknowledge the presence of the stimulus and make use of that stimulus to relate appropriately to the external environment.

Examination of the Pupils

The pupils are innervated by both the parasympathetic (third cranial nerve) and the sympathetic systems, with the former

Conscious State

Alert: Patient responds readily but may have some confusion, speech disturbance, or motor deficit.

Lethargic: Patient appears drowsy or sleepy but can be aroused to respond to questioning. If left alone, the patient will return to sleep or state of lack of attentiveness.

Obtunded: Patient is extremely drowsy, is difficult to arouse, and rarely answers in complete sentences; examiner may have to repeatedly stimulate to gain patient's attention.

Unconscious State

Stuporous: Patient does not verbalize appropriately or coherently; may moan and groan or utter monosyllables; responds to painful stimuli by moving extremities.

Comatose: Patient gives no evidence of awareness. May demonstrate decorticate or decerebrate posturing or flaccid motor response.

causing constriction and the latter causing dilation. The size of the pupil (measured in millimeters) depends on the degree to which each system influences the pupil at the time of examination. The normal pupil constricts promptly to light. Examination of the pupils consists of assessment of the size of the two pupils and their reactivity to light. It is also important to ascertain any preexisting conditions affecting the regularity of the patient's pupil size, e.g., anisocoria.

Injury to the parasympathetic system results in pupillary dilation caused by unopposed sympathetic response. Injury to the sympathetic system results in pupillary constriction because of the actions of the unopposed third nerve. If bilateral pupil abnormalities are seen, a lesion in the brain or brainstem has affected the nerve supply to the pupils. For example, bilaterally small pupils may very well be caused by a lesion within the brainstem that affects both descending sympathetic tracts. On the other hand, a unilaterally affected pupil can be expected to be caused by a lesion of the tracts outside the brain or brainstem (extraaxial). A unilaterally dilated pupil may be caused by compression of the third nerve by a herniating temporal lobe after it has exited the midbrain and as it crosses the floor of the skull. A unilateral small pupil that results from sympathetic denervation reacts more sluggishly to light. Bilaterally dilated and fixed pupils are generally caused by global hypoxia or by bilateral temporal lobe herniation from central cerebral edema with bilateral third-nerve compression. Bilaterally constricted pupils may be caused by central herniation of the posterior hypothalamus at the site of origin of the sympathetic fibers through the tentorial notch or by bilateral involvement within the brainstem, such as from pontine hemorrhage.

Brainstem Reflexes and Extraocular Cranial Nerves

The integrity of the brainstem can be evaluated with examination of certain cranial nerves, especially those related to conjugate gaze. In the patient who is awake, conjugate gaze is controlled by visual input through the complex system that coordinates the function of the extraocular muscles by way of cranial nerves III, IV, and VI. In the patient who is unconscious, however, visual input gives way to vestibular input to control conjugate gaze. This is best evaluated with examination of the oculocephalic or oculovestibular reflexes.[7,12]

The oculocephalic reflex is demonstrated by stimulating the vestibular system through movement of the head in reference to the neck. While the patient lies supine on the ground, stretcher, or bed, the person performing the assessment opens the patient's eyelids. In normal circumstances, the eyes should stare at the sky or ceiling. The clinician then rotates the head briskly but gently to one side or the other. In normal circumstances, the eyes may momentarily remain in their position in the orbits but immediately track conjugately to the side opposite the direction of the movement so that the eyes are directed once again toward the sky or ceiling. If conjugate activity cannot be observed (e.g., if one eye tracks and the other one does not or if neither eye tracks, also known as "doll's eyes"), this signals an abnormality and suggests a disturbance of the brainstem. This maneuver should never be performed in a patient with a TBI or multiple trauma until the cervical spine has been determined to be without injury.

The oculovestibular reflex is demonstrated by cold caloric stimulation, in which cold saline solution is irrigated into the external auditory canal. In a few seconds, the eyes conjugately deviate to the side of the irrigation and/or horizontal nystagmus occurs. If this response is not seen, an abnormality is present in the brainstem involving the medial longitudinal fasciculus, the vestibular system, or both (Fig. 16.5).

The midportion of the pons may be evaluated by the presence or absence of the corneal reflex. The corneal reflex can quickly be assessed by lightly touching the cornea with the corner of a soft gauze dressing and observing whether a blink reflex occurs.

Motor Examination

The motor system is best examined in conjunction with an examination of the patient's mental status or LOC. The awake patient can be asked to perform certain motor tasks, such as moving the legs or gripping. If the patient is unconscious, motor activity in response to pain is a good way to determine the level of unconsciousness, as previously described.

In the prehospital and transport environment, examination of gross motor function provides crucial data for prognostication, trending of condition, as well as areas of potential pathology. The acutely injured patient likely requires resuscitation and urgent transportation, neither of which should be delayed for an exhaustive neurologic examination. More detailed neurologic examinations are reserved for conscious patients, those able to follow commands, and those with focal deficits. In the gross motor examination, the

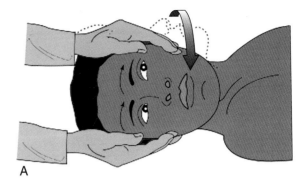

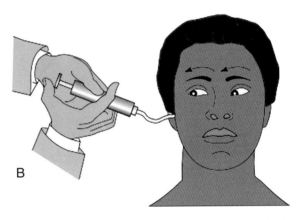

• **Figure 16.5 A.** "Doll's eye" maneuver (oculocephalic reflex). With an intact brain stem (cranial nerves 3–8), the eyes move opposite to the direction of head turning. **B.** Cold caloric test (oculovestibular reflex). With an intact brain stem, injecting cold water in the auditory canal results in tonic conjugate eye deviation toward the cold ear. (Reprinted from Marshall RS, Mayer SA. Ch. 5 – On call neurology. In: *Stupor and Coma.* 4th ed. Elsevier; 2021:68–87.)

clinician tests the strength of the patient's extremities against a 5-point scale. Box 16.3 can be used as a guide for evaluation of muscle strength and motor function. Strength and function are generally tested at the most distal aspect of the extremity; the clinician then moves proximally to determine if any deficits found distally are not present proximally. This elimination of deficits by a certain level in the extremity can help locate probably areas of pathology. See the section on Spinal Cord Injury examination for more detail on spinal and dermatomal distributions.

While examining the motor function of the patient, the clinician will also gather date for the GCS (see GCS section below). The clinician will first attempt to elicit motor function by verbal request. If the patient's LOC does not allow for following verbal commands, the clinician can first observe for any spontaneous movement in all four extremities. When verbal request fails, and no spontaneous movement is observed, the clinician may utilize noxious or painful stimuli to elicit a response. Pain stimuli can be applied centrally, such as with squeezing the trapezius muscle, or peripherally, by squeezing a pen or other small object against the proximal aspect of a finger or toe nail. The type of response observed can provide useful information on the severity of injury as well as outcome prognostication. In response to the stimuli, the patient may reach for the stimuli (localize), pull away from the stimuli (withdraw, or normal flexion), adduction or decorticate posturing (abnormal flexion), decerebrate posturing (abnormal extension), or no response (flaccidity). Although decorticate posture

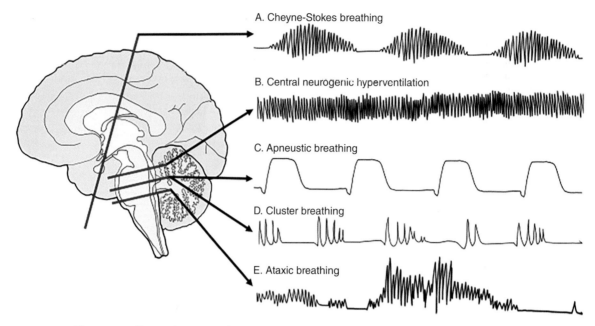

A. Cheyne-Stokes breathing

B. Central neurogenic hyperventilation

C. Apneustic breathing

D. Cluster breathing

E. Ataxic breathing

• **Figure 16.6** Abnormal patterns of respiration. (Reprinted from Prasad S, Pal PK, Chen R. Ch. 1 – Aminoff's neurology and general medicine. In: *Breathing and the Nervous System*. 6th ed. 2021:3–19, with permission from Elsevier.)

is serious, it is usually not as serious as a type of abnormal posture compared to decerebrate posture.

During examination of the pattern of motor response, the examiner must be aware of the possibility of primary motor system injury. For example, a left cortical lesion or a lesion in the left internal capsule may cause a contralateral hemiparesis that, even in the awake patient, may distort the motor response.

Respiratory Pattern

Many patients with significant head injuries have hypoventilation early after the injury. Later, the respiratory pattern may vary, depending on the level of the lesion. Patients with decorticate posturing often have an accompanying Cheyne–Stokes pattern of respiration with a regular crescendo–decrescendo change in the volume of inspiration, with the rate remaining rather regular. The patient with decerebrate posturing may have central neurogenic hyperventilation. Patients with brainstem lesions may have varying rates and depths of respiration, and an ataxic element is often noted. With lower brainstem lesions, the rate becomes more irregular, shallower, and less frequent, until medullary lesions result in respiratory paralysis. Often the transport team will need to intubate the patient for respiratory control (Fig. 16.6).

Glasgow Coma Scale

The GCS is the most widely used measure of coma severity in patients and can serve as an indicator of prognosis. Perhaps most important in the acute phase of care, the GCS is a useful tool in trending of patient condition. The trending of GCS in the acute phase can help the clinician determine the trajectory of the patient's likely clinical course and institute resuscitative measures accordingly. For trending of GCS to be a reliable indicator, there must be consistency amongst the raters. Therefore, it is beneficial to perform a GCS at the handoff of care with the receiving clinicians to assure mutual understanding of how previous GCS scores related to the patient's current state. Additional confounders, such as physiologic response or invasive interventions, can impact the scoring of the GCS. For example, eye-opening response may not be accurately assessed in patient with severe maxillofacial injuries or who is intubated and sedated. Similarly, verbal responses cannot be scored in the intubated patient.

The GCS score is out of 15, with the lowest score possible being 3. Table 16.2 outlines the GCS. Management of the TBI is often based on the severity of the injury, which is usually measured by

TABLE 16.2	Glasgow Coma Scale	
Circle the Appropriate Number and Compute the Total		
Best eye-opening response:	No response	1
	To pain	2
	To verbal stimuli	3
	Spontaneously	4
Best verbal response:	No response	1
	Incomprehensible sounds	2
	Inappropriate words	3
	Confused	4
	Oriented	5
Best motor response:	No response	1
	Abnormal extension (decerebrate rigidity)	2
	Abnormal flexion (decorticate rigidity)	3
	Flexion withdrawal from pain	4
	Localizes pain	5
	Obeys commands	6
		Total: _____ (3–15)

GCS, Glasgow Coma Scale.

the patient's GCS. A score between 13 and 15 represents a mild TBI, 9 and 12 is seen in moderate TBIs, and a score of 3–8 demonstrates a severe TBI.[4,8,13] GCS scores should be documented in the patient's medical record for the initiation of care, during transport, and at handoff.

After 40 years of use, the GCS was revised, creating the GCS-40. Small revisions were made to the Eye and Verbal sections. The terms used under eyer opening were changed from pain and sounds to pressure and speech, respectively. The terms under verbal response were changed from incomprehensible and inappropriate to sounds and words, respectively. More recently, an additional change was made to include pupillary response. Nonreactive pupils = 0, a single reactive pupil = 1, and both pupils reactive = 2. This pupillary score is allotted within the traditional 15-point scale and therefore makes the GCS-40 possible scale from 1 to 15.

Many additional scoring systems can be utilized, such as the Full Outline of Unresponsiveness (FOUR) score, and are often driven by local and regional practice.

Reexamination

Successful acute management of the TBI patient depends on frequent examination of the patient to determine the level of neurologic function and rate of deterioration. The information provided in Table 16.2 can be helpful in this analysis. When the transport team sees the injured patient for the first time, a baseline neurologic evaluation should be performed. Findings during subsequent examinations provide the transport team with an understanding of the intracranial injury. When a focal mass lesion such as a hematoma or focal contusion develops in a patient, the patient shows steady progression in depth of coma through the various levels depicted in Table 16.2.

Intracranial Pressure and Cerebral Perfusion Pressure

When considering ICP and cerebral perfusion pressure (CPP), clinicians may reference the Monroe-Kellie doctrine (hypothesis). This concept states that the sum of brain tissue, CSF, and circulating blood is maintained as a constant total volume. If one volume increases (e.g., brain tissue volume increase due to swelling from trauma), then one volume must consequently decrease (e.g., CSF pushed out, or circulating blood volume decreased) in order to maintain the desired consistent volume and pressure. If a given volume within the skull rises without commensurate decrease from another volume, ICP will increase. As the ICP increases, this pressure is exerted on structures and vasculature within the brain. If the ICP raises high enough, it will overcome the pressure of blood flow to the brain (CPP), and perfusion to those areas will be degraded. When the compensatory mechanisms of CSF and blood shunting are exhausted or inadequate, such as in the case of uncontrolled intracranial hemorrhage, brain tissue will be displaced and/or herniated through the foramen magnum. Normal ICP is near 5 to 10 mm Hg.

CPP is the pressure gradient representing the flow of blood to the brain (cerebral blood flow). CPP is defined as the difference of the mean arterial pressure (MAP) minus the ICP.[13] (CPP = MAP – ICP). The average CPP is between 60 and 80 mm Hg; however, this is dependent on average MAP relative to the patient's age and condition. Additionally, as MAP is a large contributor to CPP, decreases in MAP, from conditions such as hemorrhagic shock or vasoplegia, can degrade CPP and worsen cerebral ischemic injury.

TBI Interventions and Treatment

The management of TBI is based on both national and international guidelines (Box 16.2).[13] Each transport team should have protocols to guide the management of TBI. The primary focus of the transport team should be prevention and treatment of hypoxia, hypotension, and increased ICP, while optimizing CPP.[7,8,13] These core concepts guide several considerations in acute TBI management in the transport setting, including endotracheal intubation, reversal of anticoagulation, seizure prevention, use of osmotic therapies, and others.

Because the transport team may not always know the patient's primary diagnosis (i.e., subdural hematoma, epidural hematoma), management of patients based on GCS and the related physical examination results assists the team in providing the appropriate care to these patients. In addition to GCS, other clinical signs can be used to provide clues to rising ICP and worsening intracranial pathology. *Cushing's Triad*, consisting of bradycardia, irregular

---

• BOX 16.2 Summary of the Guidelines for the Management of Severe Traumatic Brain Injury That Affect Patient Transport

Initial Resuscitation
Complete and rapid physiologic resuscitation is the first priority, and no treatment should be directed toward intracranial hypertension in the absence of indications of deterioration in neurologic status or signs of impending herniation. However, when signs of neurologic deterioration are present, aggressive management must be initiated and should include:
- Controlled hyperventilation
- Administration of intravenous mannitol or HTS
- Sedation, analgesia, and neuromuscular blockade, used in a discretionary manner

Resuscitation of Blood Pressure and Oxygenation
Hypotension defined as a systolic blood pressure of less than 90 mm Hg or mean arterial pressure of 65 mm Hg must be avoided or aggressively managed.

At Pao_2 <60 mm Hg, apnea should be managed by securing the patient's airway and maintaining adequate ventilation.

Intracranial Pressure Treatment Threshold
Interpretation and treatment of ICP based on any threshold should be corroborated by frequent clinical examination and monitoring.

Controlled Hyperventilation
Avoid hyperventilation during the first 24 hours because reduced blood flow compromises cerebral perfusion. Ventilation management should be aimed at an end-tidal CO_2 goal of 35 to 40 mm Hg. If signs of impending herniation are present, controlled hyperventilation can be performed, yielding end-tidal CO_2 of 30 to 35 mm Hg, as a temporizing measure while en route to surgical intervention.

Use of Mannitol or Hypertonic Saline
Administration of mannitol or hypertonic saline may occur before initiation of ICP monitoring with signs of transtentorial herniations or deterioration of neurologic status.

ICP, Intracranial pressure.

respirations, and widening pulse pressures, is a critical finding. The patient's development of Cushing's Triad signifies increasing ICP and impending herniation. This sign is a late, deteriorating finding of severe TBI. Ideally, appropriate interventions for TBI management should be instituted prior to this development in order to prevent it; however, if the patient presents with these findings, then the clinician should institute aggressive measures immediately. Additional signs of impending herniation include[4,7,12]:

- Unilateral or bilateral pupillary dilation
- Asymmetric pupillary reactivity
- Motor examination results that show either extensor posturing or no response
- Other evidence of deterioration of the neurologic examination, such as a known midline shift or impending herniation on the CT scan results

General Management Considerations. There are several measures that should be considered in most patients with TBI. The patient who suffers trauma significant enough to injury cranial structures is also at risk for cervical spine injury. Therefore, application of a cervical collar should be strongly considered. When applying the collar, be sure not to apply it too tightly; a tight collar can impede venous outflow and the airway and increase ICP. Transport the patient with the head of bed at 30 degrees to promote venous outflow. When concern is present for thoracolumbar injury, the clinician may place the patient on a long spine board and transport in reverse Trendelenburg position. If the patient is being transported by fixed-wing aircraft, the patient should be positioned head forward to prevent gravitational forces from impacting venous outflow and ICP, particularly with ascent. Clinicians should try to reduce stimuli and provide comfort measures in order to decrease the ICP spikes that can accompany patients' discomfort and restlessness. Metabolic and electrolyte parameters, such as pH, sodium, potassium, and glucose, should be normalized.

Airway Management. The transport team's highest priority is establishing an adequate airway, providing oxygenation, and preventing or managing hypotension.[13] The awake patient may require supplemental oxygen in order to get oxygen saturation greater than 95%. If the patient is unable to maintain their airway, or the transport team anticipates the potential for deterioration during transport, the patient should be intubated. Care must be taken to maintain cervical spine protection while gaining access to the airway. A gastric tube should be inserted with care to prevent aspiration. Pulse oximetry and end-tidal CO_2 ($EtCO_2$) devices should be used throughout the transport process to monitor the patient's oxygenation and perfusion. $EtCO_2$ is discussed further in respiratory management.

Choice of medications used for rapid sequence intubation (RSI) of the patient with TBI requires a great deal of clinical experience, gestalt, and review of current literature.

Lidocaine as a pretreatment agent for patients undergoing RSI was in theory thought to be ideal for those who are at risk for increased ICP (i.e., intracranial hemorrhage). However, there is no high-quality evidence that directly addresses whether pretreatment with lidocaine effectively reduces the rise in ICP caused by laryngoscopy and endotracheal intubation. What little evidence exists consists of small trials that have reached contradictory conclusions.[14,15]

Fentanyl, another potential RSI pretreatment agent, is thought to prevent sudden elevations in blood pressure related to induction, thus preventing elevation of ICP. This effect requires higher drug dosing and should be avoided if the patient is hemodynamically unstable. Little current data exists regarding the beneficial effects of fentanyl on the ICP of patients with acute head injuries undergoing RSI.[15]

There has been off-label use of "push dose" vasopressor therapy in air medical transport practice, but there are no major studies supportive of this practice improving outcomes. This practice involves intravenous push administration of a small dose of a vasoactive medication in order to prevent hypotension during induction of hemodynamically unstable patients or those where procedurally induced hypotension is anticipated. More data is needed to identify the safety and efficacy of this treatment when performed as a preventative therapy for hypotension during RSI of the TBI patient.[16]

Blood Pressure Management. Patients with head injuries may lose cerebral autoregulation (Fig. 16.7). If this is the case, cerebral perfusion is directly related to mean systemic arterial pressure. Thus, hypotension may lead to under-perfusion, and hypertension may lead to vascular congestion and mass effect. Both extremes should be avoided.

Hypotension has been found to contribute to significant mortality and morbidity of patients with head injuries through its sequela of hypoperfusion of injured tissues, conversion of ischemic penumbra to nonsalvageable tissue, and worsening of secondary anoxic injury.[12,13,17] Fluids and blood products should be administered to maintain systolic blood pressure greater than 100 to 110 mm Hg.[13] Previous literature suggested a goal of greater than 90 mm Hg; however, given the severe impact of a blood pressure below 90 mm Hg has on morbidity and mortality, minimum blood pressure goals have been increased. Hypotension is rarely seen in isolated head injuries. When hypotension is seen in the multisystem trauma patient, hemorrhage should always be initially assumed and treated. Hypotension in patients with TBI is most often secondary to acute hemorrhage, impaired autonomic nervous system control, medication, spinal cord injury (SCI), or subacute diabetes insipidus. If euvolemia via fluid and blood product administration does not correct hypotension, infusions of norepinephrine or phenylephrine should be considered to maintain an adequate MAP and CPP.[13,17] Current consensus of the literature suggests maintaining a CPP of 60 to 70 mm Hg after TBI in adult patients.[13]

Anticoagulation Reversal. Patients receiving anticoagulation therapy are at a dramatically increased risk for uncontrolled hemorrhage within the cranial vault, even with minor TBI. This is seen more commonly in the elderly population where a low-impact injury such as a ground-level fall can be catastrophic. Careful consideration must be given to reversing anticoagulation

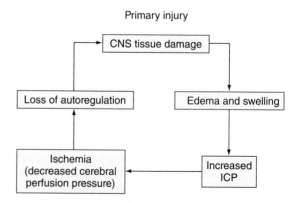

• **Figure 16.7** Sequence of pathophysiologic events initiated by primary injury.

TABLE 16.3	Anticoagulant Reversal Agents		
Class	**Agent**	**Preferred Tx**	**Secondary Tx**
Direct thrombin inhibitor	Dabigatran	Idarucizumab	PCC/dialysis
Direct Xa inhibitor	Rivaroxaban/apixaban	Andexanet alfa	PCC
Direct Xa inhibitor	Edoxaban	Andexanet alfa	PCC
Direct Xa inhibitor	Betrixaban	Andexanet alfa	PCC
AT-mediated inhibition of Xa	Fondaparinux	4 Factor PCC	PCC
Inhibition of thrombin; indirectly inhibits Xa	Unfractionated heparin	Protamine	-
Inhibition of thrombin; indirectly inhibits Xa	Enoxaparin/daltaparin	Protamine	-
Vitamin K antagonist	Warfarin	Vitamin K **and** 4 factor PCC	PCC/FFP

Current reversal strategies for common anticoagulants. (Baugh CW, Levine M, Cornutt D, et al. Anticoagulant reversal strategies in the emergency department setting: Recommendations of a multidisciplinary expert panel. *Ann Emerg Med*. 2020;76(4):470–485. doi:10.1016/j.annemergmed.2019.09.001)

therapy. Presence of active intracranial hemorrhage identified on radiologic imaging, clinical condition, and reason for chronic anticoagulation therapy are all factors used in this decision-making. The reversal agent used depends on what anticoagulant the patient is prescribed, what reversal agents are available, and the anticipated clinical course of the patient (Table 16.3). For example, for a patient receiving warfarin for anticoagulation, who is suffering from an intracranial hemorrhage, multiple reversal agents exist. Prothrombin complex concentrates (PCCs), fresh frozen plasma (FFP), and intravenous vitamin K can all reverse the effects of warfarin. However, PCCs will begin to reverse anticoagulation effects within minutes, FFP within a couple of hours, and vitamin K can take up to 12 to 24 hours for reversal of anticoagulation. Additionally, FFP requires a large volume of fluid to be administered to achieve effect, which can be troublesome in some populations such as congestive heart failure. Furthermore, the intrinsic INR of FFP is between 1.4 and 1.7, so reduction of INR to baseline is not possible with FFP. The agent(s) used will depend on agent availability and the severity of bleeding, as determined by the neurosurgeon. Given available evidence at this time (e.g., CRASH-3, CRASH-3 Trial Collaborators, 2019), tranexamic acid (TXA) is not currently accepted as common practice for control of intracranial hemorrhage. Beneficial effect of TXA in intracranial hemorrhage is controversial but treatment appears to be safe.

Seizure Management. Posttraumatic seizures that develop during transport should be promptly treated because they produce hypoxia, increase cerebral metabolic demand, risk rebleeding of vessels, and cause increased ICP. Intravenous administration of benzodiazepines is indicated for initial seizure management followed by an antiepileptic. If seizures are refractory to aggressive dosing of benzodiazepines and antiepileptic medications, developing status epilepticus, general anesthesia (i.e., propofol, etomidate, ketamine), and intubation will likely be necessary. Prophylactic use of antiepileptic medications may be considered, particularly in severe TBI and if the patient is receiving neuromuscular blocking agents[12,13]; however, data concerning the use of prophylactic antiepileptics in the post-TBI patient is controversial. Phenytoin and levetiracetam have been suggested to be equally beneficial in reducing early seizure rates. Also, these antiepileptic medications, especially phenytoin, are known to have adverse drug effects, including a potentially adverse effect on neurocognitive outcomes.[12,13]

Antibiotic Therapy. In the presence of isolated TBI, routine use of empiric antibiotics is not necessary. However, if the patient presents with penetrating injuries to the skull, open skull fracture, or is being transferred for neurosurgical intervention, antibiotics are then warranted. Infection is often seen in injuries caused by shell fragments because these fragments are likely to carry dirt, hair, and bone fragments into the brain. Infections develop most often from retained bone fragments, improper closure of the scalp and dura, and delay of definitive surgery beyond 48 hours. All patients with penetrating injuries should receive tetanus prophylaxis and intravenous antibiotics.[18] Transport teams should have protocols for this empiric antibiotic administration, such as with cefazolin or clindamycin.

Temperature Management. Hyperthermia in TBI is associated with worsened outcomes. It increases ICP, oxygen demand, glucose requirements, and much more. Thus, normal body temperature should be maintained. Central neurogenic fever occurs when there is hypothalamic dysfunction associated with TBI. This fever is noninfectious and will not respond to acetaminophen or antibiotics. Active cooling with cooling blankets and evaporative methods while controlling shivering is indicated. Meperidine has been used in the past to decrease the shivering response threshold, though dexmedetomidine is increasing in its popularity of use for this purpose. Close monitoring of the patient's temperature is also important if neuromuscular blocking agents are used because they inhibit the patient from shivering and alerting the clinician to hypothermia.

Respiratory Management. Routine hyperventilation is not recommended. Hyperventilation causes a drop in CO_2 which leads to vasoconstriction, ultimately depriving the brain of oxygen and essential nutrients. Maintain the CO_2 between 35 and 40 mm Hg to prevent secondary brain injury. However, controlled hyperventilation (CO_2 level of 30–35 mm Hg) may be useful as a temporizing method to reduce ICP when evidence of herniation is present while en route to a neurosurgical center.

The patient's CO_2 level should be maintained between 35 and 45 mm Hg throughout the transport. During the first 24 hours of TBI, cerebral blood flow is reduced by 50%. A CO_2 less than 30 mm Hg will impede cerebral perfusion and is associated with worsened neurologic outcomes.[13] With hyperventilation, the patient's $PaCO_2$ decreases, triggering cerebral vasoconstriction. This cerebral vasoconstriction leads to decreased cerebral blood volume, decreasing ICP; however, this decrease in cerebral blood volume can lead to cerebral ischemia, especially in the patient with a poor perfusion state postinjury.

$EtCO_2$ waveform capnography monitoring is the most appropriate method to monitor $EtCO_2$ in TBI patients. These patients should be placed on mechanical ventilation as soon as possible. Prolonged manual ventilation should be avoided due to the risk of CO_2 fluctuations.[19]

Osmotic Therapies. Hyperosmolar therapy, such as mannitol or hypertonic saline (HTS), may be used to treat increasing ICP, manifested as deterioration in the patient's neurologic status. Mannitol is an osmotic diuretic that decreases the patient's ICP by increasing the patient's serum osmolarity, thus creating an osmotic gradient in which water is drawn into the serum from the brain tissue. This act of cerebral dehydration reduces brain volume (reducing ICP), transiently increases plasma volume (until diuresed), and decreases blood viscosity (increasing cerebral blood flow). This mechanism requires an intact blood-brain barrier (BBB) to draw fluid across. Theoretically, if the BBB is severely disrupted, or after multiple doses of mannitol (which can contribute to breaking down the BBB), mannitol can leak into the parenchyma and cause a reverse gradient, worsening cerebral edema. The risk of this is minimal though. Mannitol should be administered through an intravenous filter.[4,7,13] It has been the "go-to" medication for this indication for decades; however, HTS has been increasingly utilized as an alternative to this long-standing drug.[20,21]

HTS, available in a wide array of tonicities (3, 7.5, 23.4%, etc.), has been studied for a couple of decades. Initially, research suggested there was no difference in effect when compared with mannitol. The latest research, however, suggests that HTS is just as effective, and potentially more effective, at lowering ICP than mannitol.[20,21] Although there is literature to support one treatment being superior to the other in reducing ICP, there is no literature to support a difference in outcomes based on choosing one agent over the other. HTS uses a similar mechanism as mannitol; it increases serum osmolarity and creates an osmotic gradient to decrease water content in the brain, reducing brain volume, and subsequently ICP. HTS has also been shown to dehydrate endothelial cells, in turn increasing internal vessel diameter; this, coupled with an increase in plasma volume, yields an improved blood flow. The key difference between HTS and mannitol is the diuretic effect. Because mannitol is an osmotic diuretic, one should consider avoiding this agent in the hypovolemic, multisystem trauma patient, and/or the hypotensive patient. HTS would likely be a better agent in this role, because its effects are less transient, and it does not cause an eventual loss of needed fluid volume.[20,21] Additionally, mannitol presents logistic challenges in the transport environment due to its sensitivity to temperatures and propensity to crystalize. Both solutions are vesicants and require close monitoring.

Analgesia and Sedation. Analgesia and sedation provide comfort for the TBI patient but also prevent ICP spikes related to pain and restlessness (e.g., pulling against interventions or restraints). The intubated patient who is restless or resists ventilatory support (ventilatory dyssynchrony) is increasing their ICP. These ICP spikes may be extremely deleterious. Intubated patients should be managed first with pharmacologically appropriate doses of sedation and analgesia, then, if needed, neuromuscular blocking agents.[12,22] Because of the effects of analgesic and sedation agents on the patient's hemodynamic status, the effects of these medications must be closely monitored by the transport team. However, pain can be a powerful stimulus to increasing physiologic metabolism and oxygen consumption, and its effects on the patient's ICP must be considered. Analgesia and sedation should be adequately provided before considering prolonged neuromuscular blockade, which should be avoided in patients at risk for posttraumatic seizures to maintain clinical assessment for seizure activity.

ICP Monitoring. There are a variety of noninvasive and invasive devices on the market for the management of patients with TBI and increased ICP. Devices are available to measure ICP, cerebral blood flow, and cerebral oxygenation. These devices are not common in transport because the facilities that have the resources available to insert and monitor these devices are likely the facilities to which the patients are being transported to, not from. However, it is imperative the clinician understands how to safely care for a patient with one of these devices when one is encountered. A few common devices include the following:

External ventricular drainage (EVD) catheter: A burr hole is drilled through the skull and a catheter is placed directly into the anterior horn of the lateral ventricle. The EVD is the gold standard in ICP management because it has the ability to directly measure ICP and can drain CSF to reduce ICP as needed.[20,23]

Subdural bolt: A hollow, fluid-filled screw is drilled through the skull to just below the inner table of the skull (the dura). Similar to other invasive pressure-monitoring devices, the fluid-filled screw is zeroed and transduced to measure the pressure within the cranial vault. Bolts are easier to place than EVDs and are less likely to become infected. However, a bolt can only measure ICP; it has no ability to reduce ICP.[23]

Lumbar drainage catheter: A catheter is placed in the subarachnoid space via needle puncture between lumbar vertebrae, similar to a lumbar puncture ("spinal tap"). This catheter can measure pressures within the space and drain CSF. These drains can be particularly helpful if there is a contraindication or hindrance to EVD placement, or as temporizing measure.[24] As with all CSF drains, caution should be maintained not to allow for inadvertent over-drainage of CSF. Historical teachings warn of the possibility of transtentorial herniation if pressures are dropped in the spinal canal, creating a pressure gradient, and allowing the brain to be squeezed from the high ICP cranium down toward the lower-pressure spinal canal.

Intraparenchymal fiberoptic catheter: Fiberoptic catheters can be used to measure ICP in nearly any space but are most commonly seen in the ventricular or intraparenchymal spaces. The tip of the catheter is pressure-sensitive and transmits a pressure-sensitive light up the catheter toward a mirror reflector and analyzer.[25] Though this catheter is unable to drain fluid to correct an elevated ICP, it can be useful in monitoring accurate ICPs in patients with severe brain swelling and compressed ventricles.

Transporting a CSF Drain. Similar to other invasive monitors, EVDs are transduced to a particular level in order to yield the desired, accurate measurement. The transducer is generally affixed on or near the collecting chamber and is leveled to the point of the tragus (or Foramen of Monro). The collection chamber will have a vertical measurement of cm H_2O and/or mm Hg (these two measurements are not interchangeable). After the transducer is leveled at the point of the tragus, a pressure is selected manually on the collection chamber by altering the height of its gauge. The pressure selected (i.e., 15 mm Hg) if the threshold for CSF to start draining. If the patient's ICP rises greater than this level, CSF will then begin to drain until the ICP is at or lower than the set pressure. It is important to remember when transporting a patient with a CSF drain that these drains are transduced to a particular level, are affected by gravity, and changes in position can dramatically alter the amount of CSF being drained. For example, raising or lowering the head of the bed will alter the transducer's relational position with the catheter tip and will consequently alter the rate at which CSF is drained. This could result in overdrainage when not needed or under-drainage when ICP spikes. Simply moving the patient from a head-elevated position to flat-lying can cause intervention-requiring rises in ICP.[26] For this reason, CSF drains should be clamped (stopcock to the "off" position) during movement and repositioning and reopened after motion is completed (Fig. 16.8).

Optic Nerve Sheath Diameter. Beneath the inner table of the skull, and surrounding the arachnoid space, is the thick membrane of the dura mater. As the optic nerves exit the skull toward the posterior eye, contiguous sections of dura mater surround and follow the optic nerves, making up the optic nerve sheath. As ICP increases, this pressure is similarly observed within the communicating optic nerve sheath. This communicating pressure is observed as dilation of the sheath's dura mater. The average optic nerve sheath diameter is about <5 mm. To measure the diameter, an ultrasound probe can be gently placed on a patient's closed eye (Fig. 16.9). The posterior aspect of the globe

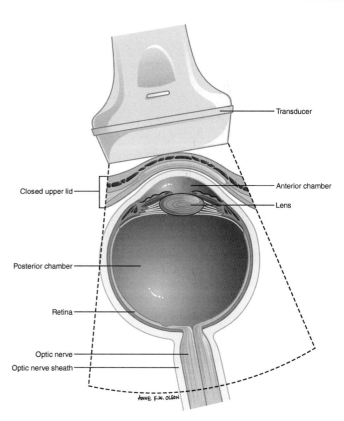

• **Figure 16.9** Diagram of sonographic evaluation through closed eyelid of eye and optic nerve sheath diameter. (Reprinted from Tayal VS, Neulander M, Norton HJ, Foster T, Saunders T, Blaivas M. Emergency department sonographic measurement of optic nerve sheath diameter to detect findings of increased intracranial pressure in adult head injury patients. *Ann Emerg Med.* 2007;49(4):508–514, with permission from Elsevier.)

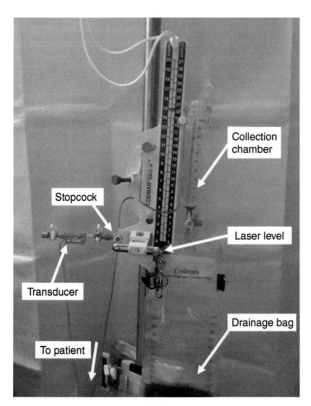

• **Figure 16.8** External ventricular drain (EVD) collection system. (Reprinted from Stout DE, Cortes MX, Aiyagari V, Olson DM. Management of external ventricular drains during intrahospital transport for radiographic imaging. *J Radiol Nurs.* 2019;38(e2):92–97, with permission from Elsevier.)

is identified, and using the ultrasound caliper measurement tool, measure the diameter of the vertical sheath identified deep of the globe. The measurement of the sheath should be taken about 3 mm deep of the posterior aspect of the globe (Fig. 16.10). There is some controversy and individual variance is what is determined as abnormal. However, many studies cite a measurement of >5.8 or 5.9 mm as likely abnormal, thus indicating increased ICP.[27]

Surgical Management. Finally, when ICP is refractory to medical management, surgical intervention may be necessary. Generally, this involves either a decompressive craniectomy or craniotomy. A craniotomy, such as a Burr hole, is a hole that is drilled into the skull to provide temporizing relief of elevated ICP. This is most commonly indicated for large epidural or subdural hemorrhages. A Burr hole may be performed in an emergency department by a trained, nonsurgeon provider. This is indicated if the patient is acutely deteriorating, or if neurosurgical intervention is several hours away.[13] Formal craniotomies include surgical evacuation of material (e.g., hematoma). For the TBI patient, the most common indication for a craniotomy is evacuation of an epidural or subdural hematoma. Surgical evacuation is improbable for subarachnoid and intracerebral hemorrhages. A craniectomy involves surgically removing a segment of the skull, commonly called a bone flap. This action permits the brain to swell outward rather than be compressed into the rigid skull which effectively reduces the risk of cerebral herniation. The bone flap is usually stored for reimplantation after the patient recovers. A patient with

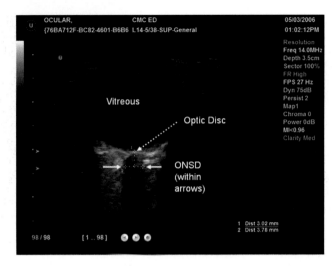

• **Figure 16.10** Ultrasonographic image of normal optic nerve sheath diameter measurement. Distance 1 is the distance (3 mm) behind the optic disc where the optic nerve sheath diameter (ONSD) is measured in its width. Distance 2 (between the *white arrows*) is the ONSD (3.78 mm). (Reprinted from Tayal VS, Neulander M, Norton HJ, Foster T, Saunders T, Blaivas M. Emergency department sonographic measurement of optic nerve sheath diameter to detect findings of increased intracranial pressure in adult head injury patients. *Ann Emerg Med.* 2007;49(4):508–514, with permission from Elsevier.)

a bone flap removal should be fitted with a rigid helmet to wear when out of bed to protect the brain that is now only covered by the scalp and meninges.

Spinal Cord Injury

All trauma patients, especially those with head or neck injury or neurologic deficits, are suspect for SCI and should be treated accordingly until ruled out.[28,29] The transport team should perform a baseline evaluation of the patient with potential spine injury before transfer and should monitor the patient closely for changes in neurologic status during the transfer process. The primary goal of the transport clinician in the care of SCI is to prevent further cord injury while providing supportive care.

Etiology and Incidence Rate

The incidence rate of SCIs that result in paralysis or debilitating weakness as a consequence of trauma to the spinal cord has been analyzed statistically in many different ways, in many different countries. An estimated 12,000 cases of SCIs occur per year in the United States.[1,2,30]

The age distribution of acute SCIs peaks in the 15- to 24-year-old age group. Frequency decreases in the middle-age group, with a second peak occurring at about the age of 55 years.[1–3,30] The incidence rate in women is lower for all age groups. Traffic accidents continue to be the most frequent cause of SCIs in all age groups. Motorcycles and bicycles cause 10% to 12% of SCIs. Excessive consumption of alcohol is a factor in one-third of cases involving accident victims with SCIs.[1–3,30]

More than half of work-related SCIs are caused by falls, and falls are the primary cause of SCIs in the home, particularly among the elderly, who fall down steps, fall from chairs, or fall off ladders. Approximately 7% of SCIs are caused by accidents that

occur during sporting and recreational activities and most commonly occur as a result of diving into shallow water.[1–3,30]

Most SCIs are incomplete injuries. Complete transection of the spinal cord is relatively rare. Incomplete SCIs commonly present with unique findings specific to the anatomic area of cord injury. These signs and symptoms are grouped into syndromes:

Anterior cord syndrome: Paraplegia below the level of injury, with loss of pain and temperature sensation.

Central cord syndrome: Motor impairment with some sensory impairment, usually to a worse degree in the upper extremities than the lower.

Brown-Séquard syndrome: Loss of motor function on ipsilateral side of injury, with sensory impairment to contralateral side of injury.

Complete cord transection: Complete loss of motor and sensory function below the level of injury; high-level injuries can be associated with spinal shock (Fig. 16.11).

The degree of functional loss with sudden spinal cord transection depends on the level of the injury. The higher the injury, the more function is lost. Complete sudden cord transection results in complete flaccid paralysis below the level of injury; areflexia (spinal shock) below the level of injury; urinary retention; and occasionally, in the male patient, priapism. A priapism is caused by a pooling of blood from a decrease in systemic vascular resistance. Incomplete sudden cord transections result in varying degrees of paralysis and sensory loss below the level of injury, areflexia (below the level of injury), and varying degrees of bladder or bowel paralysis.

Initial Assessment

Management of spinal cord trauma begins with the realization that the patient may have an unstable spine. Whether at the incident scene or at a local referring hospital, the transport team should conduct a thorough primary and secondary assessment of the patient with an SCI before transfer. This assessment provides a baseline for serial assessments and aims to identify development of commonly associated SCI complications, such as aspiration, neurogenic shock (bradycardia and hypotension), and poikilothermy.[4,8,12] Lifesaving treatment is priority before managing spinal injury, though it should be carried out with cautious movement if spinal injury is suspected.

Secondary Assessment

The secondary examination of a patient with SCI is similar to that of any trauma patient, gathering HPI, SAMPLE history, head-to-toe assessment, etc. Examination of the patient with an SCI should be performed with the patient maintained in a neutral position and the entire spine protected. A sensory and motor assessment helps the transport team determine the level and extent of injury.

Unless the cervical spine area has been already immobilized before arrival, the transport team should visually inspect and carefully palpate it to determine the presence of deformity, crepitus, pain, and muscle spasm, which are frequently associated with cervical spine injury. A second team member should maintain cervical spine in-line stabilization while this is performed and until an immobilization collar is applied.

Lower Spine Injuries

The patient should be asked to wiggle their toes. If the patient can move the toes of both feet, he or she should be asked to raise each

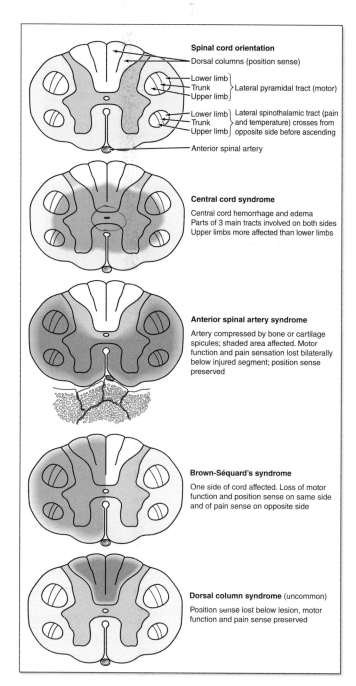

Spinal cord orientation
Dorsal columns (position sense)

Lower limb
Trunk   } Lateral pyramidal tract (motor)
Upper limb

Lower limb
Trunk   } Lateral spinothalamic tract (pain and temperature) crosses from
Upper limb   opposite side before ascending

Anterior spinal artery

Central cord syndrome

Central cord hemorrhage and edema
Parts of 3 main tracts involved on both sides
Upper limbs more affected than lower limbs

Anterior spinal artery syndrome

Artery compressed by bone or cartilage spicules; shaded area affected. Motor function and pain sensation lost bilaterally below injured segment; position sense preserved

Brown-Séquard's syndrome

One side of cord affected. Loss of motor function and position sense on same side and of pain sense on opposite side

Dorsal column syndrome (uncommon)

Position sense lost below lesion, motor function and pain sense preserved

• **Figure 16.11** Spinal cord syndromes. (Reprinted from Driel P. Textbook of adult emergency medicine. In: *3.3 – Spinal Trauma*. 5th ed. 2020: 76–87, with permission from Elsevier.)

leg slightly, one at a time. The patient's legs should not be raised if the prior examination revealed no movement or association. If the patient shows any obvious weakness, injury to the spinal cord must be assumed.

Cervical Spine Injuries

The patient should be asked to wiggle their fingers. If the patient can do so, the patient should be asked to raise each arm, one at a time. Again, substantial active movement of the upper extremity should be avoided if evidence exists of obvious fractures of the spine or extremity. The transport team should ask the patient to squeeze two fingers with both hands. In addition, the transport team should

ascertain the patient's dominant hand and cross over, matching the team member's dominant hand to the patient's dominant hand. The strength of the patient's grasp should be similar. If the patient cannot move his or her fingers and arms or has obvious weakness, SCI in the cervical region should be assumed.[4]

Patients with cervical spine injuries are at high risk for neurogenic or spinal shock and respiratory compromise. As mentioned earlier, these patients may require vasopressor and/or inotropic support; however, hypovolemia and hemorrhagic shock are significantly more common in the trauma patient and should be assumed until ruled out. These patients should be transported with cervical immobilization, cardiac and blood pressure monitoring, and respiratory function monitoring; nasal cannula $EtCO_2$ monitoring lends itself to significantly more rapid means of detecting respiratory decline than does SpO_2 monitoring.[19]

Classification of Cervical Spine Injuries by Mechanism of Injury

Flexion Injuries. *Anterior subluxation* (Box 16.3) is a flexion lesion characterized by disruption of the posterior ligament complex (Fig. 16.12). Because the anterior longitudinal ligament remains intact and the disk is not completely disrupted, this lesion is stable at the time of injury and is difficult to see radiographically.[31]

The stability of a *simple wedge fracture* depends on associated posterior ligament disruption. This flexion injury usually results from a compressive force on the anterior portion of the vertebral body with stretching of the posterior ligament complex. These fractures are generally in the mid or lower cervical segments and are considered stable fractures because of maintenance of posterior and anterior ligaments and the integrity of the interfacet points.[31,32]

Teardrop hyperflexion fracture dislocations are seen as a result of diving or traffic accidents and falls. This type of fracture is extremely unstable because the vertebra is displaced posteriorly as the person strikes an object, and displacement disrupts the apophyseal joint capsule disk below. The anterior margin of the

• BOX 16.3	Muscles to Be Tested for Evaluation of Motor Strength	
Actions to Be Tested	**Muscles**	**Cord Segment**
Abduction of the arm	Deltoid	C5
Flexion of the forearm	Biceps	C5, C6
Extension of the forearm	Triceps	C7
Flexion of digits 2–5	Flexor digitorum and profundus	C8
Opposition of metacarpal of thumb	Opponens pollicis	C8, T1
Hip flexion	Iliopsoas	L12
Knee extension	Quadriceps femoris	L3–L4
Dorsiflexion of foot	Deep peroneal	L5
Dorsiflexion of big toe	Extensor hallucis longus	L5
Plantar flexion of foot and big toe	Gastrocnemius flexor	S1

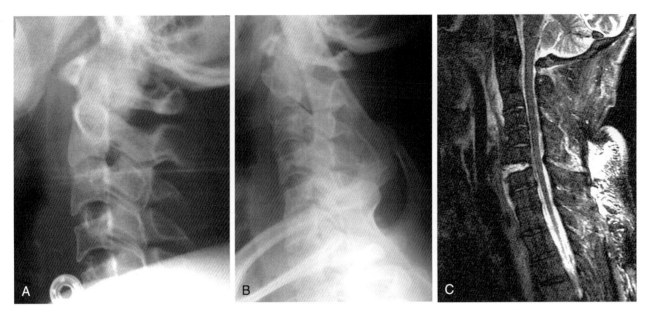

• **Figure 16.12 A.** Normal alignment of the cervical vertebrae in the lateral view. **B.** Subluxated position with narrowing of the intervertebral disk, anterior angulation, and widening of the space between the spinous processes. **C.** C5–C6 subluxation. Note the widened space between the spinous processes. (From Eiff PM, Hatch R. *Fracture Management for Primary Care.* 3rd ed. Elsevier Saunders; 1998.)

vertebra fractures in a teardrop-shaped fragment, and the fractured vertebra remains displaced posteriorly. Although often severe, the degree of neurologic deficit depends on the severity of hyperflexion compression. Patients who sustain teardrop flexion fractures frequently suffer acute anterior cervical cord syndrome.

Flexion-Rotation Injuries. Fractures that result from *flexion-rotation* are characterized by the displacement or fracture of one or more vertebrae. Fractured vertebrae may produce a unilateral facet dislocation with corresponding nerve-root compression. Severe distraction forces, those forces that cause separation of bone fragments, may cause an anterior displacement of the upper cervical body greater than 50%, which can result in bilateral locked facets and major cord injury, such as quadriplegia.[4,31,32]

Extension-Rotation Injuries. *Pillar fractures*, usually caused by motor vehicle accidents and falls, are the most common combined injury of the cervical spine. The mechanism of injury results in a force concentrated on the apophyseal joints of the mid and lower cervical segments and resultant vertical fractures of a lateral mass. A distraction of the fracture elements is probably caused by rebound flexion of the head and neck.[4,31]

Vertical Compression. *Compression cervical spine* injuries include the Jefferson fracture of the atlas and the bursting fracture of the lower cervical vertebrae. Compression fractures of the cervical spine are uncommon because the injury must occur from force transmitted vertically through the skull and occipital condyles of the spine at the precise moment the spine is straight.[31,32]

Extension Injuries. Most *hyperextension* injuries result from contact with a windshield or other structure in the interior of an automobile. Extension injuries can be of three types. The *extension teardrop fracture* is a rare extension injury that involves the anterior corner of the axis, the second cervical vertebra. This type of fracture is usually associated with preexisting degenerative arthritis of the cervical spine. The *hangman's fracture* is an unstable bilateral fracture of the pedicles of the axis. This fracture is often associated

with dislocation of the C2 or C3 cord segment and prevertebral soft tissue swelling.[31,32] *Hyperextension fracture-dislocation* injuries are associated with direct force backward or a backward and upward force without an axial loading force. The typical hyperextension-dislocation injury is accompanied by the following triad of signs: (1) midface skeletal or soft tissue injury, (2) varying degrees of central cord syndrome, and (3) a lateral cervical spine radiograph that appears normal with the exception of diffuse prevertebral soft tissue swelling (Fig. 16.13).[7,31,32] This type of extension injury is believed to be responsible for the quadriplegia in the rare patient whose cervical spine films appear normal. The probable mechanism of injury is cord compression between the posterior vertebral body, lamina, and ligamentum flavum during extension.

Atlas, Axis, and Dens Fractures

The first cervical vertebrae is also known as atlas and the second cervical vertebrae is called axis. Atlas is circular, and devoid of a vertebral body. The skull sits directly on this small vertebrae. Atlas sits atop axis, encircling the odontoid process (also known as the dens), the vertical bony prominence of axis. This arrangement allows for significant range of motion where the skull meets the neck. These vertebrae are commonly fractured independently, but they may also be fractured simultaneously. Simultaneous fracture and dislocation of these vertebrae can contribute significantly to SCI. This atlantoaxial dislocation, separation of ligaments connecting atlas and axis, should not be confused with atlanto-occipital dislocation, which represents ligamentous separation of the skull from the spine, effectively creating an internal decapitation. Fracture of the dens (odontoid processes of axis) is also commonly seen; typically, in one of three patterns. Type I involves an avulsion fracture of the tip of the dens, where the apical ligament connects it to the foramen magnum. Type II is a fracture at the base of the dens. Type III is a fracture of the dens as well as a fracture

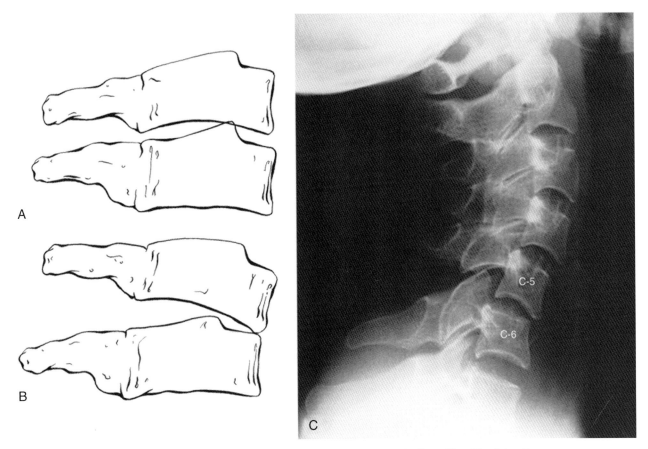

• **Figure 16.13** Hyperextension dislocation (hyperextension sprain). (From Hart BL. *Spine Surgery*. Elsevier; 2005.)

through the axis vertebral body. The energy necessary to fracture these vertebrae and processes decreases significantly with age.

Vertebral Artery Dissection

A potential complication in the presence of cervical spine injury is traumatic vertebral artery dissection. This vascular injury may also be present without cervical injury. The force of trauma, bending and manipulation of the neck, can lead to tears occurring in the walls of the vertebral arteries. These tears can lead to clot formation and subsequent impedance of blood flow to the brain. Further complications such as decreased perfusion to injured brain tissue or major stroke may occur.

Thoracic and Lumbar Spine Injuries

Injuries to the thoracic and lumbar spine vary in severity from muscle strains and ligamentous strain to fractures of the vertebral body, fractures of the dorsal elements, dislocation of the facets, and complex combination fracture dislocations. The spinal cord and the nerve roots may be injured by an encroachment into the spinal canal. Patients with stable compression fractures may sustain concomitant injury to the spinal cord, and patients with grossly unstable comminuted fractures may escape neurologic injury. Generally, the more comminuted, displaced, and unstable the spine fracture, the greater the likelihood of severe cord damage.[4,31]

Direct injuries to the spine and the spinal cord may occur as a result of a direct blow, such as from a falling tree limb or other heavy object, a stab wound, or a gunshot wound. Most injuries are caused by indirect trauma to the vertebral column resulting from energy generated by forces applied to the head, shoulders, trunk, or pelvis. These forces may contain an axial load as the main force with varying degrees of lateral bending, flexion, extension, or torsion. The thoracic and lumbar spine are most commonly injured by the kinetic energy produced by the person's body traveling through space and a sudden deceleration of the shoulders, upper trunk, or buttocks against an immovable object. The most common area is that of the thoracolumbar junction.

Rotational forces are commonly associated with fracture dislocations of the T12 to L1 levels. If the injury has more of an axial load than a rotational force, the body of L1 suffers a burst injury. In this type of injury, the posterior elements of the lamina, spinous process, and facet joints may be intact or may also be fractured. An example would be the lover's fracture, or jumper's fracture, where concomitant fracture of the calcaneus and burst fracture of a thoracolumbar vertebrae are seen, after the patient has fallen from a significant height, feet first.

The most common site of lumbar fractures is L2 or L3. Chance fractures, a specific type of flexion-distraction injury, occur when a person is restrained by a seat belt and experiences sudden deceleration, which causes sudden flexion and distraction centered at the mid-lumbar spine.[12] Patients with these fractures often escape spinal cord cauda equina damage, and the fracture may be overlooked in the presence of TBI or associated small intestinal injuries. Hence, presence of these fractures may increase the chance of intraabdominal injury.

Spinal Cord Injury Without Radiographic Abnormality (SCIWORA)

In around 1 in 10 patients with SCI, there are no findings suggestive of injury on radiographic imaging, usually CT scan. Though this is more common in the pediatric population (mostly under 8 years old), particularly due to the laxity of ligaments, SCIWORA does occur in adults. SCIWORA is chiefly seen in hyperflexion cervical spine trauma, due to its increased potential range of motion, though it has been observed in thoracolumbar trauma as well. Because of the relatively high incidence of SCIWORA, the transport clinician should consider instituting spinal motion restriction for transport of patients at risk of SCI to the receiving facility despite CT image clearance. The majority of SCIWORA cases are confirmed with MRI.

Sensory Examination

The presence of a sensory deficit confirms the suspicion of a cord or nerve-root injury. The transport team should test the patient's ankles and wrists and ask the patient if he or she can feel the touch. In the event that the patient cannot feel the touch in one or more places or reports numbness or tingling, SCI can be assumed. When injury occurs that affects one or more nerve roots, neurologic deficits will present in focal or radicular patterns: paresthesia, weakness, or paralysis to a given anatomic area of nerve distribution. Based on the presenting anatomic pattern of neurologic deficits, the clinician can often refer back to dermatome distribution to determine the likely area of injury (Fig. 16.14). Particular sets of clinical presentations on sensory examination can lead the transport clinician to a higher suspicion of a given type of spinal cord syndrome.

Neurologic Examination of the Unconscious Patient

Physical examination of the unconscious patient cannot reliably determine the presence or absence of SCI. Some data though may be obtained from the response to pricking the skin lightly on the soles of the feet or ankles with a sharp object. An involuntary muscle reflex and movement of the extremities should be observed, unless the patient is in a profound coma. If the cord is damaged, no such response will be seen. The lack of response to pinpricks in the upper extremities may indicate damage to the spinal cord in the cervical region. Failure of only the lower extremities to respond may indicate SCI in the thoracic or lumbar regions. Again, these findings cannot rule an SCI in or out, but they may be helpful to document for trending purposes. If an unconscious patient has any risk of SCI associated by mechanism of injury, SCO should be suspected and treated accordingly.

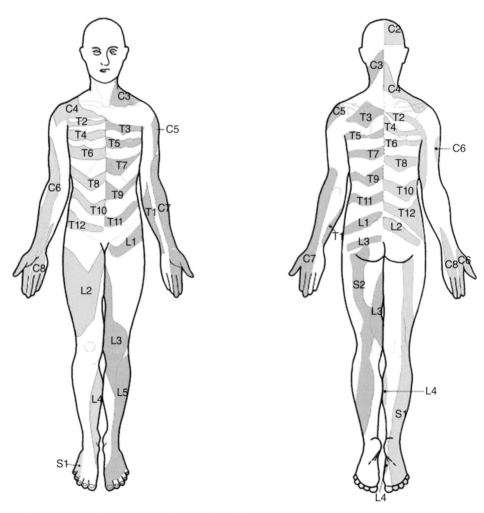

• **Figure 16.14** Dermatome map. (Reprinted from Swetal Patel. Chapter 34 – Human dermatomes. In: *Nerves and Nerve Injuries.* Vol. 1. 2015:477–483, with permission from Elsevier.)

Interventions and Treatment

Immobilization

These patients should be transferred supine, on a firm surface, and with the spine in good alignment. Log rolling of patients has been standard of practice when moving trauma patients, attempting to minimize spinal motion. However, some studies suggest that log rolling of patients with spine injuries is destabilizing at the fracture site and should be avoided if possible. Other methods of patient transfer, such as a six-person sheet lift, have been recommended. A scoop stretcher may also be used to transfer the patient onto the rigid transport stretcher to avoid the torsion effects produced by the logrolling maneuver.[33] Often, preferred methods of patient transfer with SCI require additional personnel or equipment not available to the transport clinician. All attempts should be made to restrict spinal motion during transfer of the patient, given the personnel and equipment available.

Current literature and recommendations are challenging the ingrained practices of emergency medical services (EMS) regarding use of the long backboard (spine board) for spinal immobilization. It is reported that of the over 1 million patients experiencing blunt trauma in the United States each year, only 0.5% suffer any form of SCI.[28] Additionally, use of a long backboard is not without harm. Adverse effects of backboard use include pain, induced discomfort leading to unnecessary radiologic imaging, respiratory compromise, and pressure sores.[28,33] Because of the low incidence, adverse effects, and lack of proof of benefit, the empiric use of backboards is under scrutiny. Many EMS systems are beginning to institute protocols to avoid use of backboards, except for during extrication, or for those patients at high risk for neurologic injury on assessment.[33] Decline in use is especially seen in the patients with penetrating trauma and those that were ambulatory on scene without significant pain.[28,33] The National Association of EMS Physicians and American College of Surgeons Committee on Trauma have released a position statement stating that spinal immobilization with use of a long backboard should be reserved for patients with the following:

- Blunt trauma and altered LOC
- Spinal pain or tenderness
- Neurologic complaint (numbness or motor weakness)
- Anatomic deformity of the spin
- High energy mechanism of injury *and:*
- Drug or alcohol intoxication;
- Inability to communicate; and/or
- Distracting injury.[33]

If the patient's potential spine injury has not been appropriately ruled out, the transport team must ensure that the patient remains immobilized or in motion restriction until arrival at the receiving facility. The backboard and cervical collar are the most common tools for spinal immobilization. When the backboard is used, the patient should be moved carefully onto the backboard, taking care to minimize spinal motion; techniques such as log roll and sheet lift can be utilized. For patients such as the elderly, where anatomic gaps are present from the backboard (e.g., severe kyphosis), padding should be applied to the voids in order to minimize motion. Additionally, padding should be applied between the backboard and bony prominences to prevent pressure ulcers, which can form in just 1 to 2 hours in the elderly population. In some circumstances, the backboard may be impractical given a patient's clinical condition. Alternative methods of immobilization and motion restriction, such as vacuum mattresses, are beginning to be available and utilized, which will hopefully decrease the risk of skin breakdown when a patient must remain immobilized for long transports.

With regard to cervical spine immobilization, a rigid cervical collar should be applied in any patient with concern or mechanism supporting possible cervical SCI. Exceptions may be made, usually in the circumstance of penetrating trauma, when it impedes care of other life threats (e.g., control of neck hemorrhage or airway obstruction). Decision-making with cervical sign immobilization and clearance can be aided by clinical decision algorithms, such as the National Emergency X-Radiography Utilization Study (NEXUS) or the Canadian C-Spine Rule. Though these rules are created to assist in determining the need for radiographic evaluation of the cervical spine to clear for injury, they are also useful in risk stratifying cervical spine injury likelihood. Even with low-risk scenarios, the clinician should err on the side of caution and utilize the cervical collar.

Airway

The patient's airway should be checked for patency and cleared of foreign matter or secretions. With the spine protected, the upper airway in a patient with an altered mental status should be opened with use of the modified jaw-thrust maneuver to allow spontaneous or assisted ventilation.[4] If a cervical collar is present, it may be opened, while maintaining manual stabilization, to better facilitate intubation.

Breathing

Breathing may be absent or inadequate in patients with high cervical cord injury (C5 or above), which results in loss of both diaphragmatic and intercostal phrenic nerve innervation and paralysis of respiratory muscles. Assisted ventilation with a bag-valve mask and tracheal intubation is indicated. If time and condition allow, a rapid motor and sensor exam should be conducted prior to induction and paralysis from RSI. Regardless of the method chosen to manage the patient's airway, the transport team must ensure proper, consistent protection of the entire spine.

Circulation

As with all critically injured patients, intravenous access is mandatory for patients with SCIs. Intravenous lines may be inserted on the scene or en route, depending on the patient's condition, distance of transfer, and institutional protocols. Isotonic solutions and blood products should be administered as indicated by patient condition. The rate and volume of infusion are based on the patient's cardiovascular response. Neurogenic shock may be present in patients with cervical or high thoracic spine injury. Neurogenic shock represents the interruption of sympathetic outflow below the level of injury, results in loss of autoregulation, a decrease in vascular tone (hypotension secondary to vasoplegia), and the inability of the heart to increase its intrinsic rate. The patient will present with bradycardia and hypotension, secondary to vasodilation.[4] A common mistake, *neurogenic shock* is notably different than *spinal shock*, which is observed when loss of muscle tone and reflexes occurs below the level of SCI and is not directly associated with circulatory compromise.

In the acute phase of multisystem trauma, the transport team should first assume hemorrhage as the source of any hypotension and transfuse blood products accordingly. If an isolated mechanism of injury does not support likely internal hemorrhage, or if radiologically cleared, the clinician should consider the presence of neurogenic shock and administer vasopressors accordingly. Vasopressors will likely be necessary to overcome the hypotension and vasoplegia associated with neurogenic shock. Additionally, excessive fluid administration can lead to pulmonary edema.

MAP should be maintained at greater than 85 to 90 mm Hg, although clinical research validating this goal is lacking, as there is not currently a method to measure blood flow to the spinal cord.[17]

This loss of sympathetic tone or injury-induced sympathectomy produces poikilothermy. In this state, the patient loses the ability to vasodilate and sweat in hot environments and the ability to vasoconstrict and shiver in cold environments. Thus, the patient's core body temperature often reflects the environment and must be considered if warming or cooling techniques are withheld.[12]

Vasovagal reflex with tracheal suctioning must also be considered for these patients. Preoxygenation is important to prevent vagal stimulation and severe bradycardia. This response is seen due to increased parasympathetic response to stimuli, triggered by activation of carotid baroreceptors. Subsequently, this response can be seen in other sources of stimuli, not limited to suctioning. In severe responses, decreases in CPP can be seen, even cardiac arrest.[12] Additional forms of sympathetic/parasympathetic dysregulation can be seen with complications of paroxysmal sympathetic hyperactivity (PSH) and autonomic dysreflexia (AD). PSH is an overactivation of the sympathetic response to stimuli, inducing tachycardia, hypertension, tachypnea, and hyperthermia. This sympathetic storm can occur in TBI or SCI. Treatment/prevention is aimed at decreasing stimuli and impeding sympathetic response with medication (e.g., fentanyl, propranolol, and/or gabapentin).[34] AD is similar to PSH in its unregulated sympathetic response to stimuli. AD usually occurs with cervical or high-thoracic spine injuries, and is noted by life-threatening hypertensive responses to noxious stimuli from below the level of injury. Most commonly, this is seen when the SCI patient has an occlusion of their urinary catheter and experiences the noxious stimuli of a distended bladder. Treatment is aimed at removal of the stimuli (e.g., draining the bladder) and prevention of future episodes.

Summary

The management of all neurologic traumatic emergencies includes rapid assessment, airway management with spinal protection, and serial examinations throughout the assessment and transfer phases. On completion of the transfer, the receiving caregivers must be provided with a thorough report of events, including the time of the incident, the mechanism of injury or preceding events, care rendered by the referring facility and the transport team, response of the patient to care initiated, medical history of the patient, and observed changes in the patient's condition. This thorough report provides the receiving caregivers with information to guide their management and ensure continuity of care for the patient with the best possible chance for a positive outcome.

References

1. Centers for Disease Control and Prevention. National Center for Health Statistics: Mortality Data on CDC WONDER. Accessed January 26, 2022. https://wonder.cdc.gov
2. Centers for Disease Control and Prevention, National Center for Injury Prevention and Control, Division of Unintentional Injury Prevention. Rates of TBI-related Emergency Department visits by age group – United States, 2001–2010. Accessed January 22, 2016. http://www.cdc.gov/traumaticbraininjury/data/rates_ed_byage.html
3. Huang KT, Bi WL, Abd-El-Barr M, et al. The neurocritical and neurosurgical care of subdural hematomas. *Neurocrit Care.* 2016;24:294–307.
4. Moore EE, Moore EE, Feliciano DV, Mattox KL. *Trauma.* 8th ed. McGraw-Hill Education; 2017.
5. Simon LV, Newton EJ. Basilar skull fractures (Updated February 4, 2022). In: *StatPearls [Internet].* StatPearls Publishing; Jan 2022. https://www.ncbi.nlm.nih.gov/books/NBK470175/
6. Salottolo K, Panchal R, Madayag RM, et al. Incorporating age improves the Glasgow Coma Scale score for predicting mortality from traumatic brain injury. *Trauma Surg Acute Care Open.* 2021;6(1). doi:10.1136/tsaco-2020-000641
7. Jallo J, Loftus C. *Neurotrauma and Critical Care of the Brain.* 2nd ed. Thieme; 2018.
8. Haydel M. Evaluation of traumatic brain injury, acute. Evaluation of traumatic brain injury, acute – differential diagnosis of symptoms. 2021. Accessed July 31, 2022. https://bestpractice.bmj.com/topics/en-us/515
9. Griswold DP, Fernandez L, Rubiano AM. Traumatic subarachnoid hemorrhage: a scoping review. *J Neurotrauma.* 2022 Jan;39(1–2):35–48. doi:10.1089/neu.2021.0007. Epub Apr 22, 2021.
10. Paul AR, Adamo MA. Non-accidental trauma in pediatric patients: a review of epidemiology, pathophysiology, diagnosis and treatment. *Transl Pediatr.* Jul 2014;3(3):195–207. doi:10.3978/j.issn.2224-4336.2014.06.01
11. Klein M. Post head injury endocrine complications. *Medscape.* July 14, 2022. Accessed July 31, 2022. https://emedicine.medscape.com/article/326123
12. McQuillan KA, Flynn MMB. *Trauma Nursing: From Resuscitation Through Rehabilitation.* 5th ed. Elsevier; 2019.
13. Carney N, Totten A, O'Reilly C, et al. *Guidelines for the Management of Severe Traumatic Brain Injury.* 4th ed. Brain Trauma Foundation; 2016. Accessed October 14, 2023. https://static1.squarespace.com/static/63e696a90a26c23e4c021cee/t/640b5e97fa1baa040e5c59af/1678466712870/Management_of_Severe_TBI_4th_Edition.pdf
14. Zeiler FA, Sader N, Kazina CJ. The impact of intravenous lidocaine on ICP in neurological illness: A systematic review. *Crit Care Res Pract.* 2015:12. https://doi.org/10.1155/2015/485802.
15. Kramer N, Lebowitz D, Walsh M, Ganti L. Rapid sequence intubation in traumatic brain-injured adults. *Cureus.* April 25, 2018;10(4):e2530. doi:10.7759/cureus.2530
16. Bakhsh A, Alotaibi L. Push-dose pressors during peri-intubation hypotension in the emergency department: A case series. *Clin Pract Cases Emerg Med.* November 2021;5(4):390–393. doi:10.5811/cpcem.2021.4.51161
17. Hawryluk G, Whetstone W, Saigal R, et al. Mean arterial blood pressure correlates with neurological recovery after human spinal cord injury: Analysis of high frequency physiologic data. *J Neurotrauma.* 2015;32(24):1958–1967. doi:10.1089/neu.2014.3778
18. Van Wyck DW, Grant GA. Penetrating traumatic brain injury: A review of current evaluation and management concepts. *J Neurol Neurophysiol.* 2015;06(06). doi:10.4172/2155-9562.1000336
19. Richardson M, Moulton K, Rabb D, et al. *Capnography for Monitoring End-Tidal CO_2 in Hospital and Pre-Hospital Settings: A Health Technology Assessment.* Ottawa (ON): Canadian Agency for Drugs and Technologies in Health; March 2016.
20. Bhardwaj A, Ulatowski JA. Hypertonic saline solutions in brain injury. *Curr Opin Crit Care.* 2004;10(2):126.
21. Kamel H, Navi BB, Nakagawa K, Hemphill JC 3rd, Ko NU. Hypertonic saline versus mannitol for the treatment of elevated intracranial pressure: A meta-analysis of randomized clinical trials. *Crit Care Med.* 2011;39(3):554–559.
22. Robba C, Poole D, McNett M, et al. Mechanical ventilation in patients with acute brain injury: Recommendations of the European Society of Intensive Care Medicine consensus. *Intensive Care Med.* 2020;46(12):2397–2410. doi:10.1007/s00134-020-06283-0
23. Nag DS, Sahu S, Swain A, Kant S. Intracranial pressure monitoring: Gold standard and recent innovations. *World J Clin Cases.* July 6, 2019;7(13):1535–1553. doi:10.12998/wjcc.v7.i13.1535

24. Evensen KB, Eide PK. Measuring intracranial pressure by invasive, less invasive or non-invasive means: Limitations and avenues for improvement. *Fluids Barriers CNS.* 2020;17:34. doi:10.1186/s12987-020-00195-3

25. Kawoos U, McCarron RM, Auker CR, Chavko M. Advances in intracranial pressure monitoring and its significance in managing traumatic brain injury. *Int J Mol Sci.* December 4, 2015;16(12):28979–28997. doi:10.3390/ijms161226146

26. Kleffmann J, Pahl R, Deinsberger W, et al. Intracranial pressure changes during intrahospital transports of neurocritically Ill patients. *Neurocrit Care.* 2016;(25):440–445. doi:10.1007/s12028-016-0274-6

27. Munawar K, Khan MT, Hussain SW, et al. Optic nerve sheath diameter correlation with elevated intracranial pressure determined via ultrasound. *Cureus.* February 27, 2019;11(2):e4145. doi:10.7759/cureus.4145

28. Nilhas A, Helmer SD, Drake RM, Reyes J, Morriss M, Haan JM. Pre-hospital spinal immobilization: Neurological outcomes for spinal motion restriction versus spinal immobilization. *Kans J Med.* April 29, 2022;15:119–122. doi:10.17161/kjm.vol15.16213

29. Wang TY, Park C, Zhang H, et al. Management of acute traumatic spinal cord injury: A review of the literature. *Front Surg.* December 13, 2021;8:698736. doi:10.3389/fsurg.2021.698736

30. Centers for Disease Control and Prevention, National Center for Injury Prevention and Control, Division of Unintentional Injury Prevention. Rates of TBI-related Deaths by Age Group – United States, 2001–2010. January 22, 2016. Accessed October 17, 2016. http://www.cdc.gov/traumaticbraininjury/data/rates_deaths_byage.html

31. Walters B, Hadley M, Hurlbert R, et al. Guidelines for the management of acute cervical spine and spinal cord injuries: 2013 update. *Neurosurgery.* 2013;60(CN_suppl_1):82–91.

32. Davenport M. Cervical spine fracture evaluation. June 21, 2021. Accessed August 8, 2022. https://emedicine.medscape.com/article/824380

33. White CC, Domeier RM, Millin MG, et al. Standards and Clinical Practice Committee, National Association of EMS Physicians. EMS spinal precautions and the use of the long backboard – resource document to the position statement of the National Association of EMS Physicians and the American College of Surgeons Committee on Trauma. *Prehosp Emerg Care.* 2014;18(2):306–314. doi:10.3109/10903127.2014.884197

34. Neurocritical Care Society. ENLS Protocols. Emergency Neurological Life Support. 2019. Accessed August 6, 2022. https://enls.neurocriticalcare.org/protocols

17

Thoracoabdominal Trauma

KYLE WILLIAMS

COMPETENCIES

1. Identify clinical indications of thoracoabdominal injuries.
2. Recognize signs and symptoms of life-threatening thoracoabdominal injuries.
3. State appropriate critical interventions to manage thoracoabdominal injuries.

Trauma remains the number one cause of death for Americans between 1 and 46 years old, and it is the number one cause of death overall. Its economic impact exceeds $671 billion annually. Each year more than 192,000 people lose their lives to trauma.[1]

Injuries to the chest and abdomen are common in trauma patients. Blunt trauma may be isolated to a specific location in the abdomen or involve a single organ, such as the liver. Frequently, injuries involve both compartments, and it is difficult in the field to differentiate exactly where the patient is injured or where is the source of bleeding. The diaphragm separates the thoracic and abdominal compartments and can be compromised itself, as in the case of a ruptured diaphragm.

The most common causes of penetrating trauma in the United States are gunshots and stabbings. One recent study found approximately 40% of homicides and 16% of suicides by firearm involved injuries to the torso.[2-4] In 2019, over 250,000 deaths were the result of firearms worldwide. Of these deaths, 65.9% occurred in six countries, listed in order: Brazil, United States, Venezuela, Mexico, India, and Colombia.[3-5] Penetrating injuries can easily involve both the chest and abdomen. The challenge remains: early assessment, recognition, and intervention by first responders. Rapid transport with advanced critical care teams providing diagnostic tools and life-saving interventions reduces time to the operating room and definitive care.

Thoracic trauma continues to be a leading cause of death in those younger than 40 years.[6] Thoracic injury is seen in nearly 50% of multiple trauma patients. With approximately 150,000 deaths per year in the United States alone, thoracic trauma is a common and potentially deadly injury in many cases can be corrected with tube thoracostomy and volume resuscitation.[7,8] Rapid recognition and early intervention are key. For the critical care transport team, special consideration is given to these patients regarding altitude changes as gas expands. Many transport teams may not be the first at the scene of an incident. It is imperative that emergency medical services (EMS) are familiar with these injuries so that rapid recognition and early interventions are

started and augmented on arrival of the critical care transport team. Outreach education by critical care transport teams will assist EMS and provide expert seamless transfer of care to the nearest trauma center equipped to care for these patients.

Thoracic injuries are broadly classified by mechanism as either blunt or penetrating. There are four mechanisms of blunt thoracic trauma: direct impact on thorax, thoracic compression, acceleration/deceleration injuries, and blast injuries.[9] An example of a common mechanism is an automobile traveling at 70 mph that strikes a telephone pole. There are three types of impacts: car versus pole, interior of the vehicle versus occupant, and internal organs versus stable structures of the chest. In this scenario, there may be multiple injuries to the lung, heart, great vessels, and mediastinum. Blunt injuries are also seen in falls, assaults, and sports. Penetrating trauma occurs because of gunshot wounds (GSWs), stab wounds, impalements, and bomb fragments. GSWs and blast injuries are ever-increasing in frequency leading to an injury pattern which are challenging to treat in the field and during transport.

Thoracic injury can be categorized into those who have life-threatening injury and a delay in recognition will lead to immediate deterioration or possible death versus those who are not detectable until assessed at hospital or specialty team. They are:

1. Airway obstruction
2. Open pneumothorax
3. Tension pneumothorax
4. Hemothorax
5. Flail chest
6. Cardiac tamponade
7. Blunt cardiac injury
8. Blunt thoracic aortic injury (aortic disruption)
9. Tracheal or bronchial injury
10. Diaphragmatic tears
11. Esophageal injury
12. Pulmonary contusion

The ABCDEs of resuscitation continue to serve as a framework for the management of complex trauma injuries. The primary survey can quickly help detect life-threatening injuries and initiate rapid interventions.

Airway Obstruction

An airway obstruction-threatening condition may be a result of blunt and penetrating injuries to the neck or chest which may injure the airway. There is no more important and critical intervention than recognition and proper treatment of airway obstruction or respiratory failure. In many cases, simple airway maneuvers such as a jaw thrust or elevation of the head of bed with avoidance of the head-tilt, chin lift maneuver in the presence or suspected cervical spine injury, will alleviate an airway obstruction.

Assessment

Maintenance of the airway is a priority in the trauma patient. Inadequate ventilation can lead to hypoxia and delivery of oxygen to tissue. Position of the tongue is important because of the potential for it to migrate backward and block the larynx in the unconscious person. Swelling of the oral cavity, laryngeal spasm or foreign bodies, fluids, and broken teeth are potential hazards to airway maintenance. While providing cervical spine mobilization to patients with facial injuries, be very careful of producing an airway obstruction with the procedure.

Intervention

The correct and appropriate bag-valve-mask technique in combination with basic airway adjuncts (such as oropharyngeal airway) and advanced adjuncts (such as endotracheal intubation, supraglottic airway devices) are crucial to successful ventilation and oxygenation. Patients requiring endotracheal intubation should be managed in a sequentially organized approach for optimal success. All providers performing rapid sequence intubation should be under strict medical control, and skills should be monitored and tracked. Intubation in the field has been associated with poor success rates in providers who are not properly and regularly trained.[10] Utilization of advanced airway equipment (videoscopic devices), end-tidal CO_2 ($EtCO_2$) detection, and pulse oximetry are the industry standards rather than the exception.

Open Pneumothorax

An open pneumothorax or "sucking" chest wound occurs when air accumulates in the pleural cavity between the chest wall and the lung due to a hole, open chest injury or physical defect caused by penetrating trauma. The larger opening of the chest wall can lead to a greater degree of lung collapse and difficulty of breathing. As the individual with the chest wound inhales, air enters both the lungs and the pleural cavity, and this places pressure on the lung. If the wound is large enough, it may draw enough air into the pleural cavity to make the lung collapse.

Assessment

The signs and symptoms of an open pneumothorax include decreased breath or absent breath sounds, shortness of breath, sudden chest pain, tachypnea or bradypnea, tachycardia, restlessness, agitation, and hypoxia. An open chest wound may be visible or audible hence the name "sucking" chest wound when air enters the wound. If air enters the pleural space without being able to escape, a tension pneumothorax may develop, which can lead to cardiovascular collapse, and death. If POCUS is available, lung sliding will be absent.

Intervention

In the prehospital setting, the open pneumothorax is covered with an occlusive dressing taped to the edges on three sides. This type of dressing will allow air to enter through the opening in the chest wall and exit or exhale with a flutter valve effect. There are some commercial products available to create the same concept. Avoid taping all four sides of the dressing over the "sucking" wound. A tension pneumothorax may be created because air is being prevented from leaving the pleural space. If a tension pneumothorax develops after the dressing has been applied, the dressing should be removed immediately, and the patient reassessed with a needle thoracostomy, possibly as a next step if a tension pneumothorax is not resolved (Figs. 17.1 and 17.2).

Continuous Assessment and Evaluation

Constant monitoring of the patient's vital signs, pulse oximetry, and end-tidal capnography is essential. Assessing for increasing

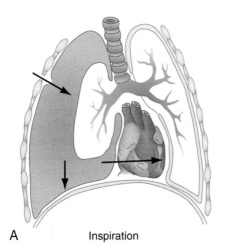
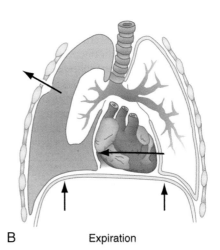

A Inspiration   B Expiration

• **Figure 17.1** Sucking chest wound. **A.** Inspiration. **B.** Expiration. (From Marx JA, Hockberger R, Walls R. *Emergency Medicine: Concepts and Clinical Practice.* 7th ed. Mosby; 2010.)

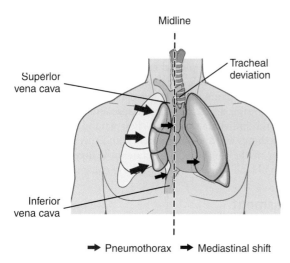

• **Figure 17.2** Tension pneumothorax. (From Sole ML, Klein D, Moseley M. *Introduction to Critical Care Nursing.* 4th ed. Saunders; 2004.)

dyspnea, subcutaneous emphysema, tracheal deviation, and changes in neurologic status alerts the transport team to critical changes and interventions required for treatment.

Tension Pneumothorax

Tension pneumothorax may be caused by blunt, penetrating, or iatrogenic trauma often defined as hemodynamic compromise which is a life-threatening condition that requires immediate intervention. There is a one-way "flap valve" mechanism created that allows a sizable amount of pressure of air into the pleural space with inspiration but then closes with expiration and traps the air. This progressive accumulation of air applies pressure to the heart, pushing great vessels and opposite lung tissue and displaces the trachea and mediastinum. The pressure increases to a point if untreated, it precipitates circulatory collapse and subsequent cardiac arrest.

Assessment

The patients may experience the following clinical signs and symptoms such as: severe shortness of breath and respiratory distress, shallow breathing, acute chest pain, hypoxia, tachycardia, hypotension, agitation and restlessness (if conscious), decreased or absent breath sounds upon lung auscultation, asymmetrical chest expansion, and with late signs of tracheal deviation, cyanosis, and subcutaneous air. If the patient is intubated, the peak inspiratory pressure (PIP) and plateau pressure (pPlat) would be elevated with distended jugular veins, however, the jugular veins could be flat if the patient is in severe hypovolemic shock. POCUS can also be used as an adjunct to confirm diagnosis, but this should be in combination with signs and symptoms of a tension pneumothorax. A POCUS should not delay a needle decompression if the signs and symptoms are present.

Interventions

A tension pneumothorax is a critical condition which requires the life-saving intervention of a rapid decompression of the pleural space. Needle decompression of the chest is also known as needle thoracostomy. Chest wall thickness in the adult patient must be considered for the decompression to be successful. Body mass

index (BMI) affects the chest wall thickness for both the mid-clavicular line (median thickness of 22 mm in lean, 27 mm in overweight, and 35 mm in obese) and anterior axillary line (median thickness of 22 mm in lean, 29 mm in overweight, and 39 mm in obese).[11] A large-bore needle 10 to 14 gauge longer than 3 inches should be placed in the second intercostal space, midclavicular line on the affected side, or lateral midaxillary line at the fourth or fifth intercostal space. The needle should be placed superior to the rib margin to avoid the intercostal artery. A "rush" of air may be present on insertion. If done in air transport, the rush of air may not be heard; instead, improvement in the patient's symptoms and a return to hemodynamic stability should be seen. The lateral midaxillary approach for a needle decompression has the lowest predicted failure rate of needle decompression effectiveness in multiple populations.[11] If the tension pneumothorax reoccurs, a simple thoracostomy (finger thoracostomy) or chest tube may be warranted if allowed per program's policy. As soon as available, a tube thoracostomy should be performed as a definitive measure. A large-bore intravenous (IV)/intraosseous access should be initiated as soon as possible to provide fluids and/or blood products for resuscitation. Administer supplemental oxygen to maintain oxygen saturations greater than 92%.

Continuous Assessment and Evaluation

Constant reevaluation of the patient's cardiopulmonary status is warranted. If the chest tube is placed and a persistent air leak occurs, the presence of tracheobronchial disruption must be considered.

Massive Hemothorax

Blunt or penetrating injury causes bleeding into the pleural space and a massive hemothorax is considered greater than 1500 mL of blood in the adult population.[12] This is mostly caused by rib fractures or parenchymal injuries, or venous injuries. Bleeding from arterial injuries is less common. The rapid and massive accumulation of blood and fluid in the pleural space can result in severe hemodynamic compromise. Large amount of blood causes the compliant lung to collapse and hypovolemic shock results (Fig. 17.3).

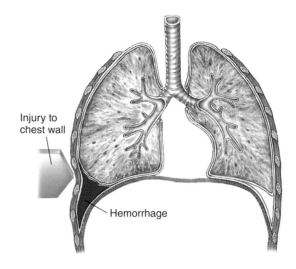

• **Figure 17.3** Hemothorax. (From Seidel HM. *Mosby's Guide to Physical Examination.* 7th ed. Mosby; 2011.)

Assessment

Dyspnea, tachypnea, chest pain, signs of shock, tracheal deviation, decreased breath sounds to the injured side (blood does not conduct sound), and dullness to percussion are signs and symptoms of a massive hemothorax. Neck veins are typically flat because of hypovolemia. In transport, ultrasound can readily detect hemothorax.

Interventions

Most hemothoraces simply need drainage with a chest tube. There are situations where aggressive resuscitation will be needed. These may include the following:

- High-flow oxygen should be administered to patients exhibiting respiratory distress , assessing the need for assisting ventilations and even need for endotracheal intubation with use of rapid sequence intubation.
- Large-bore IV lines should be initiated if there is a need for crystalloid or blood product resuscitation with warm fluids. Fluids should be carefully monitored, as aggressive fluids in the presence of thoracic trauma can lead to hypoxemia, especially in the presence of concurrent pulmonary contusions.
- Placement of chest tube drainage with greater than 200 mL/hr for 4 to 5 hours may require the chest tube to be clamped per protocols or medical direction in transport as a temporary measure to cause tamponade of the bleeding. This should be done after consultation with a physician or in the program protocols due to the increased risk of a tension pneumothorax developing. Surgery is likely for unresolved chest tube bleeding.

Small thoracostomy tubes (28 FR or smaller) are meant to treat pneumothorax over hemothorax secondary to the risk of clogging. Larger chest tubes, usually 28 French or larger, are needed for drainage of blood in adults. To promote drainage, keep the chest drainage system below the level of the patient's chest. The chest drainage system should be able to monitor water levels in the waterseal and suction-control chambers. Tidaling is fluctuation in the water-seal chamber with respiratory effort is normal. The water level increases during spontaneous inspiration and decreases with expiration. During positive pressure mechanical ventilation, tidaling fluctuations are the opposite: the water level decreases during inspiration and increases during expiration.[13] If tidaling doesn't occur, suspect the tubing is kinked or clamped, or a dependent tubing section has become filled with fluid. Tidaling does not complete lung expansion or with mediastinal tubes, because respirations don't affect tubes outside the pleural space.[13] Intermittent bubbling, corresponding to respirations in the water-seal chamber, indicates an air leak from the pleural space; it should resolve as the lung re-expands. If bubbling in the water-seal chamber is continuous, suspect a leak in the system. Assess for the leak's source, such as a loose connection or from around the site.

Continued output will require surgical intervention, such as a thoracotomy, which is based on initial chest tube drainage, hemodynamic status, and rate of ongoing blood loss. As a rule, avoid clamping a chest tube. Clamping prevents the escape of air or fluid, increasing the risk of tension pneumothorax.

Flail Chest

Flail chest occurs when three or more contiguous ribs are fractured in at least two locations and is usually caused by blunt trauma. Multiple rib fractures and flail segments can cause instability in the chest wall. Flail chest usually involves the anterolateral chest because of heavy posterior muscles and because the scapula protects the posterior chest wall. Paradoxical chest movement interferes with the normal function of the thoracic cage, causing inadequate ventilation. The instability of the chest wall and pain from rib fractures lead to hypoventilation and subsequent hypoxemia. The possibility of an underlying pulmonary contusion further contributes to hypoxia.

Assessment

Observation of the chest wall excursion is important. The patient will have respiratory distress, cyanosis, grunting, tachypnea, and use of accessory muscles. The patient will be in pain, so judicious use of pain medications is highly suggested.

Interventions

Management of a flail chest should address the major areas of concern. Maintaining adequate ventilation, fluid management, pain management, and management of the unstable chest wall. Stabilization of the affected side is accomplished with a gauze pad securing above and below the fracture sites.

Evaluation

Constant monitoring of the cardiopulmonary status is required. Pulse oximetry and EtCO$_2$ will assist in ventilator management. Pain control should be considered for patient comfort (Fig. 17.4).

Cardiac Tamponade

Cardiac tamponade is the result of an accumulation of blood in the pericardial sac from a medical condition or a blunt or penetrating trauma. Acute blood collection of less than 100 mL can cause a tamponade due to the intrapericardial pressure exceeding the intracardiac pressures, causing cardiac chamber collapse, and therefore reducing diastolic filling and cardiac output.[12] The collection of blood within the thick, fibrous pericardial sac causes pressure against the heart, decreasing function and cardiac output.

Assessment

The patient with acute cardiac tamponade shows signs of decreased cardiac output, such as altered mental status, cool clammy skin, tachycardia, and falling blood pressure. Beck's triad consisting of narrowed pulse pressure, jugular venous distention (JVD), and muffled heart sounds and/or pulsus paradoxus may be present. However, if the patient is severely hypovolemic, JVD may not be present. Decreased voltage of electrocardiogram (ECG) complexes may be present. Fluid will be identified in pericardial sac with POCUS (Fig. 17.5).

Interventions

Aggressive IV fluid management is used to keep systolic blood pressure elevated. If the ventricles do not overcome the fluid located intrapericardial, then the chambers will be compressed. The pressure inside the ventricles should be greater than the pressure beyond. There is a limit to how high the diastolic pressure can rise. In the case of severe hypovolemia leading to tamponade,

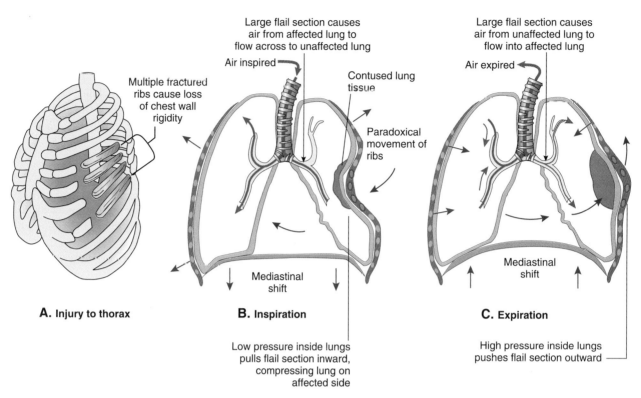

• **Figure 17.4** Flail chest. **A.** Normal lungs. **B.** Flail chest on inspiration. **C.** Flail chest on expiration. (Modified from Aehlert B. *Mosby's Comprehensive Pediatric Emergency Care.* 2nd ed. Mosby; 2007.)

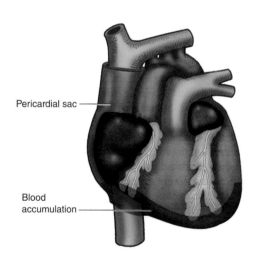

• **Figure 17.5** Cardiac tamponade. (From Sheehy SB. *Emergency Nursing: Principles and Practice.* 4th ed. Mosby; 1992.)

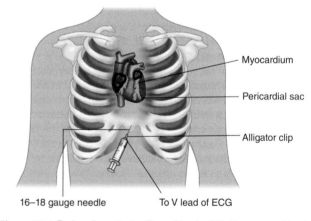

• **Figure 17.6** Pericardiocentesis. (From Sheehy SB. *Emergency Nursing: Principles and Practice.* 4th ed. Mosby; 1992.)

surgical intervention may be time critical and beyond the provider's capability. An emergent pericardiocentesis may be required. The catheter, preferably an 18G, 7 to 9 cm or bariatric 12 cm, is introduced through the left xiphocostal angle. The needle is at a 15- to 30-degree angle with the abdominal wall. The needle should be aimed toward the left shoulder and be advanced slowly while continuously aspirating. If no fluid is aspirated, the needle should be withdrawn promptly and redirected. A needle is placed into the pericardial sac to aspirate blood. Improvement in the patient's condition usually follows with improved function of heart and cardiac output. Ultrasound guidance has made pericardiocentesis more successful (Fig. 17.6). Refer to Chapter 20 for more information.

Evaluation

Aggressive management and continued monitoring of hemodynamics guide therapy. It is possible pericardiocentesis may have to be repeated during long transports.

Blunt Cardiac Injury

Blunt cardiac injury (BCI) are injuries associated with direct or indirect blunt trauma to the myocardium. These lesions may vary in size from small areas to large contusions and free-wall rupture.

Myocardial contusions have a prevalence of up to 86% in patients with chest wall trauma and many patients may not show any cardiac symptoms. Cardiac manifestations may include arrhythmias, myocardial wall rupture, and valve damage, with the most prevalent being myocardial contusion. The most common causes of a BCI include motor vehicle collisions with speeds above 30 miles per hour, direct injuries to the chest such as sports injuries (baseball to the chest), fall from great heights, crush injuries, and blast injuries.[14] Commotio cordis is a type of cardiac contusion in which there is structural damage to the heart with resultant arrhythmias that develop within 24 hours after chest impact. This type of contusion is considered a significant cause of morbidity and mortality on the sports field.

BCI can be the cause of coronary artery injuries that leads to myocardial ischemia due to coronary artery dissection. The most commonly involved artery is the left anterior descending (71.4%), followed by the right coronary artery (19%), left main (6.4%), and circumflex (3.2%).[14]

Indirect cardiac injury is significant cardiac damage that occurs because of a traumatic event that was directed toward the heart. This may be explained as an external force with secondary rise of the intrathoracic pressure creating stress on the cardiac tissue. This stress causes a surge of catecholamines release that will cause myocyte injuries, coronary spasms, or thrombosis.[14]

Assessment

If the patient has had a direct blow to the chest, he or she may have chest pain, hypotension, tachycardia, dysrhythmias, changes in heart tones, rales from pulmonary edema, heart failure, and cardiogenic shock. Cardiac enzymes may be elevated due to the traumatic injury; use in conjunction with EKG is suggested to identify patients at risk of complications secondary to myocardial contusion.[15] There may be ST segment changes on ECG, the only concern is the inability to distinguish the changes from a myocardial contusion or coronary lesion in this setting. There is always a need for repeating the EKG in chest trauma and having a look at prior tracings if available.[14] POCUS may demonstrate wall motion abnormalities (Fig. 17.7). Refer to Chapter 20 for more information.

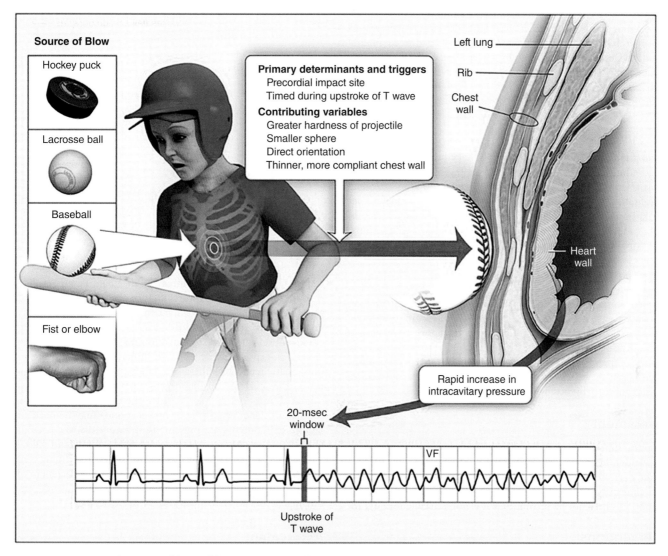

• **Figure 17.7** Myocardial contusion. (From Contaragyris C, Peytel E. Sudden death caused by a less lethal weapon chest-wall injury [Commotio cordis]. *Anaesthesia Critical Care & Pain Medicine.* 2012;31:5.)

Interventions

Patients presenting with multiple traumatic injuries, hypotension, and tachycardia require excluding internal hemorrhage as a main cause rather than BCI. Management is either stabilization efforts, aggressive resuscitation, or surgical interventions.

Blunt Thoracic Aortic Injuries

Blunt thoracic aortic injuries (BTAI) account for 1.5% of thoracic injuries, with high morbidity and mortality, with up to 80% of these patients die before hospitalization.[16] Causes of BTAI include: head-on or lateral collision impact, fall of more than four meters, twisting of the aorta at the ligamentum arteriosum, seat belt or steering wheel injuries, or ejection from a vehicle. Classification of BTAI includes Grade I: Intimal tear, Grade II: Intramural hematoma, Grade III: Pseudoaneurysm, and Grade IV: Rupture.[16]

Assessment

The patient may not exhibit any signs of external trauma. Signs and symptoms may include: hypotension, decreased level of consciousness, hypertension of the upper extremities, discrepancy between blood pressures in the upper extremities, decreased quality of femoral pulses compared with upper extremities, parascapular/upper back pain, chest pain, left apical cap due to pleural blood above apex of the left lung, and large hemothorax with widened mediastinum. Fracture of the first rib, sternum, flail chest and deviation of the trachea to the right indicate a high suspicion for aortic disruption.

Interventions

Secure the airway and insert two large-bore IV lines for fluid and/or blood administration. Do not over fluid resuscitate. Keep blood pressure around 90 and the heart rate below 100 after adequate resuscitation.[16] Consider a short-acting antihypertensive, per agency's policy or physician's order.[16] Insert a chest tube for hemothorax and consider TXA. Facilitate rapid transport to appropriate trauma center.

Tracheobronchial Injuries

Tracheobronchial disruptions are infrequent, but a life-threatening percentage of blunt thoracic chest trauma injuries are most likely in the cervical trachea area.[17] Injury to the trachea or large airways causes rupture or perforation. Blunt ruptures or tears of the lower trachea or mainstem bronchus are generally caused by a dashboard, steering wheel, or clothesline injury. Penetrating injuries are rare and usually occur in the proximal trachea.

Assessment

Dyspnea, subcutaneous and mediastinal emphysema fluctuating in size, stridor, hoarseness, recurrent pneumothorax, pneumomediastinum, decreased or absent breath sounds, and a continuous air leak with chest tube drainage are all signs of tracheobronchial injuries. Hemoptysis may not be present, but it is not a reliable finding.[7,18]

Interventions

If the patient has spontaneous breathing and adequate gas exchange, delay the intubation until fiberoptic bronchoscopy is available. Positive pressure ventilation may worsen the injury. Blind intubation may worsen the injury to include placement of the endotracheal tube outside of the tracheobronchial lumen.[18] It is desirable to go lower than the injury. At times, one-lung ventilation may be necessary. The patient will need surgical repair for large tears or if clinically unstable.

Esophageal Injuries

Blunt trauma injury to the esophagus is rare, with less than 1% of injuries. The primary mechanism of esophageal injury is GSWs accounting for 70% to 80%, followed by stab injuries in about 15% to 20%. Mortality is estimated at 20% to 30% due to the presence of other injuries.[19] Gastric contents and bacteria leaking into the mediastinum can lead to mediastinitis and to sepsis. Perforation also results in massive fluid loss and possibly hypovolemic shock.

Assessment

Hematemesis, hemoptysis, hoarseness, dysphagia, upper abdominal pain, subcutaneous emphysema, mediastinal air, bloody nasogastric (NG) drainage, and particulate matter in a chest tube may be seen. Saliva exiting through penetrating esophageal injuries assists in the diagnosis.

Interventions

Advanced airway management, nothing by mouth (NPO), NG tube, antiemetics, IV fluids, antibiotics, and possible chest tube placement may be used if gastric contents are in the pleura. These patients usually require surgical repair of the defect.

Diaphragmatic Injury

Diaphragmatic rupture occurs around 0.5% of all trauma patients. The diaphragm separates the thoracic cavity from the abdominal cavity and is responsible for changes in intrathoracic pressure that causes respiration. It is one of the strongest muscles in the human body. Penetrating injury is the most common cause compared to blunt injury, 63% versus 37%, respectively.[20] Typically, blunt trauma exerts tremendous force on the diaphragm, resulting in rupture. These tears or ruptures are usually on the left side because the spleen is smaller than the liver and is less protected. Herniation of bowel contents into the thoracic cavity can cause respiratory compromise. Intestinal strangulation may also develop.[7,21]

The transport team may have difficulty in diagnosing a diaphragmatic tear. On a chest x-ray, there may only be an irregularity in the level of the diaphragm. If abdominal contents have migrated into the thoracic cavity, there may be absent breath sounds on the effected side or bowel sounds may be heard if the abdominal contents are present. Respiratory distress is common with herniation because of decreased tidal volume and pain.

Herniation of abdominal contents into the thoracic cavity causes compression of the ipsilateral lung and displacement of the mediastinal structures. Cardiopulmonary insufficiency results, causing significantly reduced respiratory efficiency.

Assessment

The patient may show signs of dysphagia, dyspnea, and abdominal pain. Sharp epigastric pain radiating to the left shoulder (Kehr's sign) also occurs, which is the result of splenetic bleeding affecting the phrenetic nerve, which is felt in the shoulder. Bowel sounds may be present in the chest, decreased breath sounds on the affected side, and possibly a scaphoid abdomen caused by loss of abdominal contents into the chest.

Interventions

Interventions include advanced airway management, making the patient NPO, establishing an IV and NG/OG tube for decompression, and eventually surgical repair.

Pulmonary Contusion

The incidence of pulmonary contusions can be up to as many as 75% of patients with blunt thoracic trauma. This is a direct injury to the parenchyma resulting in edema and hemorrhage without laceration. Three quarters of patients with pulmonary contusions have accompanying rib fractures, however, not always present.[9] Hypoxia is caused by loss of the ability to exchange gases at the cellular level. This is one of the most problematic issues, especially for the long-term patient. These patients can spend weeks on ventilatory support and are complex to manage. Using advanced ventilators is desired in the transport of these patients.

Assessment

These patients usually exhibit dyspnea, tachycardia, hemoptysis, hypoxia, and respiratory insufficiency. They may also have chest pain from chest wall contusions or abrasions.

Interventions

Provide advanced airway management and pulmonary toilet as needed. If intubation is needed, expect higher pressures and increased positive end-expiratory pressure. The use of bilevel positive airway pressure and continuous positive airway pressure has shown to be beneficial, especially if the patient is awake and cooperative. Judicial use of IV fluids is recommended. If faced with fluid overload, consider diuretics.

Resuscitative Endovascular Balloon Occlusion

Internal hemorrhage requires rapid recognition and surgical intervention. Aortic occlusion is part of thoracic management and allows for an opportunity for definitive hemorrhage control. Resuscitative endovascular balloon occlusion involves placement of an endovascular balloon in the aorta to control hemorrhage and to augment afterload in traumatic arrest and hemorrhagic shock states (Fig. 17.8). The London Air Ambulance service was the first in the world to perform the procedure in 2014. It is similar to open cross-clamping of the aorta during emergency thoracotomy in the emergency department or operating room.

Abdominal Trauma

The mechanism of abdominal injury is the same as that of thoracic trauma. Abdominal injury is the most frequent cause of potentially preventable death. The abdominal cavity can hold large amounts of blood and may or may not be distended. Blunt trauma results from compression after being crushed between solid objects such as a steering wheel and vertebrae or a shearing force causing a tear or rupture at points of attachment of involved organs. Penetrating trauma can be caused from stab wounds, GSWs, or foreign objects. A far more common mechanism of injury (MOI) is blast injuries from explosions.

Assessment

Abdominal trauma is subtle, and signs and symptoms are difficult to detect. Classic signs of injury include decreased bowel sounds (blood and fluid are poor conductors of sound) and pain or

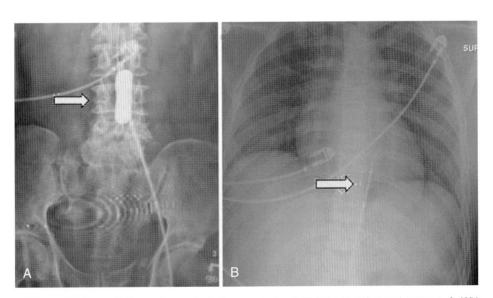

• **Figure 17.8** Resuscitative endovascular balloon occlusion (REBOA) with saline and contrast. **A.** With saline only. **B.** In Pelvic Trauma. (From Brenner ML, Moore LJ, DuBose JJ, et al. A clinical series of resuscitative endovascular balloon occlusion of the aorta for hemorrhage control and resuscitation. *J Trauma Acute Care Surg.* 2013;75(3):506–511.)

guarding on assessment over the specific injured area. Organ injuries are associated with location and MOI. In recent years the use of POCUS has enhanced detection of abdominal injuries. Refer to Chapter 20 for more information.

Intervention

Patients with abdominal injuries can have symptoms that vary from altered mental status and tachycardia to shock and a distended abdomen. Any patient that has sustained blunt abdominal trauma with profound shock and without obvious signs or symptoms should be suspected of having a significant intraabdominal injury, and aggressive management should be instituted with crystalloid followed by blood products. Securing the airway with spinal precautions and providing ventilator support, wound management, IV access, fluids, and rapid transport to definitive care remains critical to optimal outcome.[22] Patients who are interfacility transfer and have radiologic studies with an indication of pneumoperitoneal should be flown at the safest lowest altitude as defined by the pilot in command.

Specific Abdominal Injuries

Spleen

The spleen is the most injured organ from blunt (25%) and penetrating (7%) trauma.[23] Forty percent of all spleen injuries have no symptoms. They may exhibit Kehr's sign or referred shoulder pain from left hemidiaphragm irritation.[24–26] Patients may exhibit signs of hemorrhagic shock such as altered mental status, tachycardia, delayed capillary refill, and hypotension. The abdomen may be tender to palpation over the left upper quadrant or may be distended and painful.

Liver

The liver is the largest organ in the abdominal cavity and the second most injured intraabdominal organ in blunt trauma.[23] It is extremely vascular and at any time holds 30% of the cardiac output. Liver injuries are usually from direct trauma to the liver itself causing fractures to the liver tissue. Deceleration forces may avulse vasculature-supplying blood flow to the liver, resulting in significant bleeding. Penetrating trauma to the liver accounts for 37% of injuries and carries a 10% mortality rate.[25] Any penetrating injury below the fourth intercostal space may have directly injured the liver and or spleen.

Assessment

Patients with blunt and penetrating injuries can have symptoms that vary from altered mental status and tachycardia with slight abdominal distention to profound shock and a markedly distended and taut abdomen. A distended abdomen may indicate severe bleeding from either liver and/or spleen. When these patients are assessed, inspection and palpation of the abdomen should be done to locate contusions, abrasions, and pain. Other injuries, such as rib and scapular fractures, are associated with liver trauma. The amount of force in blunt abdominal injuries and the MOI and location of wounds in penetrating trauma are important indicators of liver injuries. Ultrasound findings include fluid in Morison's pouch. Refer to Chapter 20 for more information.

Pancreas and Duodenum

Lying in the retroperitoneal space, the pancreas and duodenum are in close proximity to each other and are typically injured together. The rate of injury is low with less than 3% of all abdominal injuries.[27,28] Complications of infection, fistula formations, gastrointestinal disorders, and pancreatitis contribute to the majority of deaths in these injuries.

Assessment

Symptoms of isolated blunt pancreatic and duodenal injuries may be difficult to observe in the prehospital environment. If duodenal digestive juices and blood are contained within the peritoneal space, the patient may not have any abdominal symptoms. Assessment usually shows tenderness over the area of the pancreas and absence of bowel sounds. The patient may be hemodynamically stable, with symptoms associated only with peritonitis or no symptoms at all. These injuries are difficult to diagnose, but careful history taking can assist in identification. Neither serum amylase nor lipase is useful in the evaluation of acute abdominal trauma. Normal levels do not exclude a major pancreatic injury, and elevated values may have other causes such as chronic liver disease or excessive alcohol use.[23]

Treatment

The transport treatment for these patients includes a high index of suspicion for injury when the patient has vague abdominal symptoms after trauma. Treatment includes any procedures necessary for patient stabilization and supportive care for the patient's respiratory and cardiovascular status if the patient remains stable. If duodenal injury is suspected, gastric tube insertion reduces the gastric and duodenal juice infiltration of the peritoneal space. Outlying hospitals may transfer these patients several days after injury when isolated pancreatic and duodenal symptoms occur.

Colon and Small Intestine

Colon and small intestine damage usually occur more frequently in penetrating than in blunt trauma. In many cases, the liver, spleen, and other organs are injured. Ninety percent of colon injuries are caused by penetrating trauma.[7,29,30] The small intestine is the most injured organ in penetrating injuries because of the volume it occupies in the abdomen. Blunt injury to the small intestine occurs with crushing of the bowel against the spinal column. Improper use of seat belts, steering wheel impact, or blunt object applied to the abdomen can produce the crushing effect. If the victim has a transverse bruise across the lower abdomen from a lap belt, rupture of the small intestine should be considered. Bowel evisceration may occur with penetrating trauma or blast injuries. Bowel contents should be covered with sterile saline solution during transfer.

Assessment

A thorough assessment for abdominal trauma should be done for any suspected intestinal injury. It is important to inspect, locate, and identify all wounds from penetrating trauma. Remember that documentation should focus on the location of wounds and not to classify them as entrance and exit wounds. This should be done by other experts to prevent conflicts in legal findings. For interfacility transports, transport crews may find paper clips covered with tape to identify the location of holes to determine projection. Examination of the back, buttocks, and perineum (small-caliber bullets can bounce and travel anywhere) is essential. Evisceration of bowel may be found with penetrating and blast injuries. The color and size of the protruding bowel should be noted on initial examination.

Symptoms of isolated colon injury are associated with peritoneal irritation from blood and fecal matter. Blood is extremely irritable to the peritoneum. Pain on palpation and guarding may be present on examination. Symptoms of small bowel injury include tenderness, patient's reluctance to change position, rebound tenderness, and guarding. Radiographic films may reveal free air in the peritoneum or a small bowel ileus. The transport crews should notify the pilot to fly at a lower safe altitude to prevent expansion of air in the peritoneum.

Treatment

Most injuries of the intestine are associated with more life-threatening injuries, and transport management should be prioritized accordingly. While airway and cardiovascular systems are being stabilized, saline solution dressings should be applied to any eviscerated bowel or dry dressings to open wounds. The amount of blood loss should be noted at the scene. Most complications of bowel injuries occur later in the patient's course of recovery. The major factors related to morbidity and mortality are sepsis, abscess formation, wound infection, and intraabdominal peritonitis.[31]

Abdominal Evisceration

Evisceration of abdominal contents occurs after a penetrating wound to the abdominal area. The intestines, liver, spleen, and stomach are commonly involved in eviscerations which are outside of the body.[32] These injuries are dangerous as they expose the organs to the outside environment, unprotected and risking injury due to dehydration and infection.[32] In the case of eviscerations, do not attempt to replace organs back inside the body. Instead, cover all exposed abdominal contents with moist, sterile towels and occlusive dressing, and control bleeding if necessary.[32]

Gastroesophageal Trauma

Injuries to either the stomach or esophagus are uncommon. Both are well protected within the upper abdominal cavity. The pliability of the stomach does reduce the chances of injury. However, if the stomach is full during blunt trauma, it is more likely to rupture. Most injuries to these structures arise from penetrating trauma. Peritoneal signs will be present on assessment. Gastric tube drainage may be blood tinged or frank blood may be present. Radiologic studies may show free air in the abdomen.

Abdominal Vascular Injuries

Penetrating abdominal wounds account for 90% to 95% of all abdominal vascular injuries.[25] In blunt vascular injuries, the MOI is usually compressive or deceleration forces that result in avulsion of small vessels from larger vessels and intimal tears in the larger vessels. Intimal tears can result in thrombus formation, and avulsions can result in exsanguination. Penetrating injuries result in lacerations of tissues and free bleeding. The major vessels include the aorta and vena cava and the renal, mesenteric, and iliac arteries and veins. Vascular system injuries are a primary cause of death in patients with GSWs and stab wounds to the abdomen. Mortality rates are high even if the patient presents with no signs of shock.

Assessment

Assessment of patients who have a vascular injury to the abdomen may have no active external bleeding but show signs of severe shock. Bleeding can be profuse and not respond to fluid bolus or replacement. With arterial injuries, the femoral pulse may not be present on the affected side. Major venous injuries may produce profound shock, but signs may be delayed up to 30 minutes after injury. Bleeding from these injuries may be controlled with direct pressure to the area or compression.

Treatment

Rapid transport to surgical intervention is key in the survival of abdominal vascular injuries. Direct pressure is the initial treatment if visible. The use of TXA and blood and blood products in transport has gained momentum from the experience of the military while treating patients with multiple injuries.

Genitourinary Trauma

Genitourinary trauma includes injuries to the kidneys, bladder, ureters, urethra, and genitalia. Although not usually immediately life-threatening like the injuries previously discussed, these have specific causes for concern for the transport team. Because of the position of the urinary and reproductive organs within the abdominal cavity, a high index of suspicion for trauma to the genitourinary organs should be maintained when regions of the abdomen and/or back are injured.

Renal and Ureter Trauma

Renal trauma is frequently associated with abdominal injury; the kidney is the third most commonly injured abdominal organ. Renal injuries sustained from blunt mechanisms such as motor vehicle collisions (63%), falls (43%), contact sports (11%), and pedestrian injuries (4%).[33] Blunt injuries sustained from sudden deceleration or acceleration can result in the stretching of the ureters and renal arteries and veins with the weight of the kidneys. Contusions are generally from a direct blow to the flank. Of all renal and ureter blunt traumas, 85% are minor contusions; the remaining 15% consist of vascular injury, deep cortical lacerations, or shattered kidneys.[33]

Penetrating injuries are usually caused by GSWs (83%–86%) or stabbings (14%–17%) to the back and/or abdomen, with high incidence rate of associated injury to other abdominal organs.[33] Low-velocity bullet injuries are more common than high-velocity injuries (79% vs. 8%); the damage is typically parenchymal laceration.[33] Often, high-velocity GSW injury results in nephrectomy because the kidney explodes on impact or passage of the bullet. Most renal injuries (80%–85%) are minor and consist of contusions and minor lacerations, and 10% are major and extend into the medulla, collecting system, or both with possible result of extravasation of urine. Vascular injuries occur in 1% to 3% of renal injuries, and retroperitoneal hematoma formation is likely.[33]

Urethral injury, although rare, is generally a result of penetrating trauma such as GSWs or stab wounds. Rapid deceleration injuries may result in avulsion of the ureter from the renal pelvis.

Assessment

During the secondary assessment, any contusions, abrasions, or stab penetrations to the back or flank area should alert the transport team to the possibility of renal trauma. The patient may have flank pain. Kidney damage should always be suspected with GSWs to the abdomen. Hematuria is a marker for both renal and extrarenal abdominal injuries after blunt trauma. All patients with gross hematuria should be evaluated after transfer for both renal and associated abdominal injuries. In addition, patients in shock or with a history of shock and microscopic hematuria after blunt trauma should be suspected of abdominal injuries. Studies show that patients with microscopic hematuria, but no shock do not have any major renal injury and are treated conservatively without surgical intervention. Patients should be adequately hydrated to assure clear urine to prevent acute kidney injury (AKI).

Treatment

Renal injuries are not usually immediately life-threatening, the transport team should give supportive care and identify the patient's risk for kidney injury when other life-threatening injuries are absent. If a urinary catheter is present, the transport team should transport with gravity drainage and monitor urinary output. Ureter injury will probably not be diagnosed until full evaluation is completed in the trauma center; therefore, no specific intervention exists in transport. At the receiving center, surgery may be indicated for major kidney injuries, urethral tears, or renal vascular damage. Many of these injuries are managed without surgical intervention.

Bladder and Urethral Trauma

Blunt trauma to the bladder is commonly associated with pelvic fracture (90% of cases). The bladder lies within the pelvic girdle, and bone fragments from the pelvis can penetrate the bladder. This can result from the compressive and/or shearing forces seen in blunt trauma. Rupture occurs with a direct blow to the lower abdomen. A distended or full bladder increases the risk of bladder rupture during blunt trauma. Rupture of the bladder can cause extravasation of urine into the peritoneal cavity. Although urine is sterile, no symptoms may be noticed for several days. Ultrasound may be able to detect bladder rupture, and injury may be identified sooner. Urethral injuries are associated with bladder rupture and pelvic fractures. These injuries occur much more frequently in men than women because of the length of the urethra. The urethra may be torn at the level of the prostate gland by pelvic fractures. Straddle injuries such as horseback riding, bicycle riding, and gymnastics as well as direct penetrating trauma may cause injuries to the lower or more external urethra.

Assessment

Identification of patients at risk is the best way for the transport team to determine bladder and urethral injuries in the field. Subjective symptoms that are common in both bladder and urethral injuries are lower abdominal pain, groin tenderness, and the inability to void. Hematuria is likely in bladder trauma. Shock is usually associated with other visceral or vascular injuries. Blood at the meatus is the single most important sign of urethral injury.

Treatment

Transport treatment of patients with bladder and urethral injuries should emphasize a high index of suspicion for their injuries, and life-threatening injuries should take priority. Urinary catheters should not be inserted when blood is found at the meatus until after a urethrogram has confirmed an intact tract. Further damage can be done with the insertion of a urinary catheter. If transport times are prolonged and a full bladder is suspected, controlled insertion may be accomplished. Discussion with a physician is suggested prior to this. Autonomic hyperreflexia is a potentially life-threatening medical condition that occurs with T spinal cord injury (SCI) when there is pain or discomfort below the level of injury, even if the pain or discomfort cannot be felt. It can cause hypertension, diaphoresis, bradycardia, and increased intracranial pressure. The transport team should keep these symptoms in mind when transporting patients diagnosed with urethral tears and inability to void. Transport to trauma centers should be done without delay. Further diagnosis and treatment will be accomplished with retrograde cystography for bladder trauma and retrograde urethrography for urethral injuries (Fig. 17.9).

Genital Trauma

Genital trauma is more common in men than in women. The female reproductive tract is well protected within the pelvis. Injuries to female genitalia are infrequent with either blunt or penetrating trauma. Bone fragments from a pelvic fracture may pierce female reproductive organs. Injuries to the external female perineum from straddle accidents can result in hematoma formation. In men, penetrating trauma to the penis and scrotum is caused most often from GSWs. Urethral disruption may accompany these injuries. Other causes of blunt injury are MVA, industrial accidents, and assault. Of scrotal injuries, 50% are caused by blunt trauma, and patients usually have contusions, hematomas, avulsions, laceration, or testicular rupture on examination.

Assessment

Assessment of the patient with genital injury includes a thorough history and visual inspection. Reports of the event can be a source of embarrassment to the patient, so the transport nurse must listen without judgment. Discrepancies between the history and MOI should be noted and reported. On physical examination, visually inspect the perineal area hematoma formation anywhere on the perineum, scrotum, or penis. If the scrotum is swollen and painful, ruptured testis should be suspected. Rectal injury can be identified when the perineum is examined. The transport nurse should look for any signs of injury and document any lacerations or avulsions, including the presence and amount of any vaginal bleeding. Menstrual history is important for female patients.

Treatment

Unless bleeding is profuse, injuries to the genitals are not immediately life-threatening. Treatment should consist of saline-soaked gauze to the avulsion and lacerations, particularly those to the scrotum. Ice packs to the scrotum and penile hematomas help reduce swelling and pain; direct pressure should be applied to areas of penile injury. In the case of penile or scrotum amputation, the recovered parts should be transported in saline-soaked gauze on ice without direct contact between the ice and tissue.

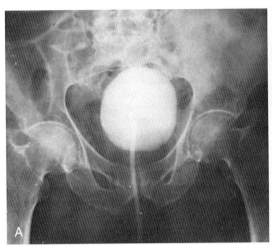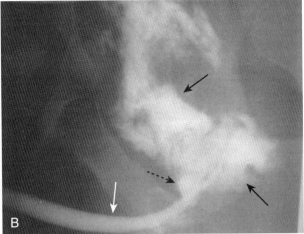

• **Figure 17.9 A.** Cystogram. **B.** Urethral trauma. Contrast instilled retrograde through the penile urethra *(solid white arrow)* is seen to leak from the posterior urethra secondary to a perforation *(dotted black arrow)* and collects outside of the urinary system in the perineum and extraperitoneal bladder spaces *(solid black arrows)*. (**A.** From Herring, W. *Learning Radiology: Recognizing the Basics.* Saunders Elsevier; 2012. **B.** From Ehrlich RA, McCloskey ED, Daley JA. *Patient Care in Radiography: With an Introduction to Medical Imaging.* Mosby; 2004.)

Vaginal bleeding is difficult to control, and a pressure dressing should be applied if possible. Exsanguination can occur with major vaginal tears because of the rich blood supply. When severe bleeding and shock are present, transport to the nearest center capable of treating gynecologic emergencies should be the first priority. Impaled objects should be left in place and immobilized. The success rate of repair of genital injuries is high, even penile reimplantation has been successful with microvascular surgery. Immediate treatment after advanced airway management should include resuscitation with crystalloid then blood products and TXA.

Bariatric Considerations

Classified at a body mass index greater than 35, the bariatric trauma patient presents some unique characteristics in patient management when the thoracic or abdomen is injured. The chest wall compliance is decreased because of increased abdominal cavity contents, which makes location for insertion of a chest tube challenging. The transport provider may have to insert the chest tube higher than normal to avoid hitting abdominal structures. Because of the declining functional capacity due to size, lung volume is lost in patients who lie flat. Therefore "ramping" or reverse Trendelenburg position is encouraged during preoxygenation and intubation if sitting up is contraindicated. The effects of preoxygenation markedly decrease with obesity. Significant soft tissue injuries may occur because of excessive tissue, and injuries may hide in folds. In the bariatric patient, the ultrasound waves have farther to travel and are attenuated along the way. In resuscitation of the hypotensive episodes, bariatric patients are under resuscitated.[34]

Summary

The transport of the thoracoabdominal trauma patient presents many challenges to the critical care transport team. These injuries can be potentially lethal. The transport team must maintain a high index of suspicion for occult injuries as well as injuries that are obvious on examination. Sources of bleeding in both the thoracic and abdominal cavities may make it difficult to assess just how much blood a patient has lost. The use of blood and TXA and rapid transport to an appropriate trauma center is vital. Early recognition, aggressive management, and integration of technology, such as ultrasound and rapid transport to qualified trauma centers, have proven to enhance patient survival and the return as a productive member of society.

References

1. American College of Surgeons Committee on Trauma. *Thoracic Trauma: Advanced Trauma Life Support for Doctors.* 9th ed. American College of Surgeons; 2012.
2. Nishimura T, Sakata H, Yamada T, et al. Different patterns in abdominal stab wound in the self-inflicted and assaulted patients: An observational analysis of single center experience. *Kobe J Med Sci.* Jul 20, 2017;63(1):E17–E21.
3. https://www.boneandjointburden.org/fourth-edition/vb23/penetrating-injuries. Accessed November 14, 2022.
4. https://publichealth.jhu.edu/sites/default/files/2022-05/2020-gun-deaths-in-the-us-4-28-2022-b.pdf. Accessed November 14, 2022.
5. Richardson EG, Hemenway D. Homicide, suicide, and unintentional firearm fatality: Comparing the United States with other high-income countries, 2003. *J Trauma.* 2011;70:238–243.
6. Meredith JW, Hoth JJ. Thoracic trauma: When and how to intervene. *Surg Clin North Am.* 2007;87(1):95–118, vii. doi:10.1016/j.suc.2006.09.014
7. Pollack AN. *Critical Care Transport.* 2nd ed. Jones and Bartlett; 2017.
8. Marx JA, Hockberger RS, Walls RM, et al. *Rosen's Emergency Medicine: Concepts and Clinical Practice.* Mosby/Elsevier; 2010.
9. Dogrul BN, Kiliccalan I, Asci ES, Peker SC. Blunt trauma related chest wall and pulmonary injuries: An overview. *Chin J Traumatol.* 2020;23(3):125–138. doi:10.1016/j.cjtee.2020.04.003
10. Gnugnoli DM, Singh A, Shafer K. EMS field intubation. In: *StatPearls.* StatPearls Publishing; July 26, 2022.
11. Azizi N, Ter Avest E, Hoek AE, et al. Optimal anatomical location for needle chest decompression for tension pneumothorax: A multicenter

prospective cohort study. *Injury.* Feb 2021;52(2):213–218. doi:10.1016/j.injury.2020.10.068

12. Edgecombe L, Sigmon DF, Galuska MA, et al. Thoracic trauma [Updated May 29, 2022]. In: *StatPearls.* StatPearls Publishing; Jan 2022. https://www.ncbi.nlm.nih.gov/books/NBK534843/

13. https://www2.getinge.com/us/education/chest-drain-education/. Accessed November 20, 2022.

14. Fadel R, El-Menyar A, ElKafrawy S, Gad MG. Traumatic blunt cardiac injuries: An updated narrative review. *Int J Crit Illn Inj Sci.* 2019;9(3):113–119. doi:10.4103/IJCIIS.IJCIIS_29_19

15. Farahani AA, Shahali H. Myocardial contusion: A case of fatal cardiac dysrhythmias during air medical transportation. *Air Med J.* 2021;40(6):446–449.

16. Hazrati E, Shahali H. Blunt thoracic aortic injury: A life-threatening emergency on air medical transportation. *Air Med J.* 2021;40(6):450–454.

17. Mattox KL, Moore EE, Feliciano DV. *Trauma.* McGraw-Hill Medical; 2013.

18. Carretta A, Ciriaco P, Bandiera A, Negri G. Diagnostic and therapeutic approach to post-traumatic tracheobronchial injuries. *Signa Vitae.* 2021;17(2):10–19.

19. Sudarshan M, Cassivi SD. Management of traumatic esophageal injuries. *J Thorac Dis.* Feb 2019;11(Suppl 2):S172–S176. doi:10.21037/jtd.2018.10.86

20. Furák J, Athanassiadi K. Diaphragm and transdiaphragmatic injuries. *J Thorac Dis.* Feb 2019;11(Suppl 2):S152–S157. doi:10.21037/jtd.2018.10.76

21. Gould J, Vedantham S. The role of interventional radiology in trauma. *Semin Intervent Radiol.* 2006;23(3):270–278.

22. Raza M, Abbas Y, Devi V, et al. Non operative management of abdominal trauma – a 10 years review. *World J Emerg Surg.* 2013;8:14.

23. Walls R, Hockberger R, Gausche-hill M, Erickson TB, Wilcox SR. Rosen's Emergency Medicine – Concepts and Clinical Practice E-Book [Pageburstls]. Elsevier; 2022. https://pageburstls.elsevier.com/#/books/9780323757911/

24. McQuillan KA, Makic MB, Whalen E. *Trauma Nursing: From Resuscitation Through Rehabilitation.* Saunders/Elsevier; 2009.

25. American College of Surgeons. *Advanced Trauma Life Support: Student Course Manual.* American College of Surgeons; 2012.

26. Gurney D. *Trauma Nursing Core Course (TNCC): Provider Manual.* Emergency Nurses Association; 2014.

27. Hardy M, Snaith B. *Musculoskeletal Trauma: A Guide to Assessment and Diagnosis.* Churchill Livingston; 2011.

28. Smith WR. *Management of Musculoskeletal Injuries in the Trauma Patient.* Springer-Verlag; 2016.

29. Zalstein S, Pearce A, Scott D, Rosenfeld J. Damage control resuscitation: A paradigm shift in the management of haemorrhagic shock. *Emerg Med Australas.* 2008;20(4):291–293.

30. Lamb CM, MacGoey P, Navarro AP, Brooks AJ. Damage control surgery in the era of damage control resuscitation. *Br J Anaesth.* 2014;113(2):242–249.

31. Como J, Bokhari F, Chiu WC, et al. Practice management guidelines for selective nonoperative management of penetrating abdominal trauma. *J Trauma.* 2010;68(3):721–733.

32. https://accessemergencymedicine.mhmedical.com/content.aspx?bookid=2969&sectionid=250456703. Accessed November 28, 2022.

33. Erlich T, Kitrey ND. Renal trauma: The current best practice. *Therapeutic Advances in Urology.* October 2018:295–303. doi:10.1177/1756287218785828

34. Uppot RN. Impact of obesity on radiology. *Radiol Clin North Am.* 2007;45(2):231–246.

18

Musculoskeletal and Soft Tissue Trauma

DANA FLIEGER

COMPETENCIES

1. Compare and contrast assessment findings consistent with arterial and venous bleeding.
2. Distinguish between compressible and noncompressible bleeding.
3. List hemorrhage control measures to stop compressible bleeding.
4. Demonstrate appropriate assessment steps for the injured extremity.
5. Identify and treat potential complications related to musculoskeletal emergencies.

Introduction

Soft tissue and orthopedic injuries can be life-threatening, resulting in rapid exsanguination and death; fortunately, most of these types of injuries are not life-threatening. However, a simple soft tissue injury, fracture, or dislocation can become a devastating injury resulting in severe, permanent disability. Even a moderate sprain, if inadequately treated, can result in an unnecessarily extended disability and can lead to recurrent injuries.

Although soft tissue and musculoskeletal injuries are rarely fatal, they often result in long-term disabilities that account for millions of dollars lost to the economy each year.[1] The first care provided to a patient with a fracture, dislocation, or severe sprain often determines the ultimate results that occur as a consequence of the injury.[1] The transport team can often prevent permanent disability with prompt temporary measures, such as hemorrhage control, basic wound care, immobilization, or splinting, especially in patients with multiple traumas, when more definitive management must be postponed until life-threatening injuries have been treated.

Musculoskeletal System and Soft Tissue

A basic understanding of the composition and function of musculoskeletal and soft tissues is essential to the proper management of traumatic emergencies and ultimately to the welfare of the patient as a whole. *Soft tissue* structures include tissues that connect, surround, or support the bones and organs of the body, including skin, fascia, blood vessels, nerves, and fat. The term *soft tissue* also encompasses the nonbone tissues of the musculoskeletal system including tendons, ligaments, and muscles. The *musculoskeletal system* is composed of bones, ligaments, muscles, joints, tendons, blood vessels, and nerves. The function of the musculoskeletal system is to allow movement, provide support, and protect internal organs.[1-3]

Various soft tissues have differing functions, but all share a number of commonalities. Soft tissues rely on nerves for sensation and direction, as well as vasculature for continuous blood supply. As a result, soft tissue disruption results in pain and hemorrhage.

Bone is a living structure with its own neurovascular innervation and capacity to heal. It is a specialized connective tissue with a calcified collagenous intercellular substance and is either cancellous or compact. The calcium content of bone depends on many factors such as parathyroid hormone and estrogen levels, dietary intake, and stress. An acid–base imbalance resulting in a decreased pH can cause bone demineralization.[1-3]

Definitions

Minor *orthopedic injuries,* or injuries to the axial skeleton, are not typically emergencies but do require urgent care. However, some fractures in isolation can cause life-threatening hemorrhage. Pelvic and femur fractures can result in massive blood loss. Isolated open fractures with significant collateral vessel damage and external hemorrhage can also be life-threatening, as are multiple fractures when the cumulative blood loss is significant. The amount of blood loss associated with individual fractures can vary based on the location. According to the American College of Surgeons in 2018, tibia or fibula fractures can cause up to 750 mL of blood loss, femur fractures around 1500 mL, and pelvic fractures can cause several liters of blood accumulation in the retroperitoneal space.[4]

Soft tissue and orthopedic injuries associated with underlying organs increase injury burden. For example, rib fractures with underlying pulmonary contusion or liver injury result in a more complex course and higher injury burden than the same rib fractures without underlying injury. Even among extremity injuries, a fracture or dislocation of the knee or elbow can cause permanent damage to nerves and vessels distal to the injury

TABLE 18.1	Urgent Complications of Orthopedic Injuries
Injury	**Possible Complications**
Clavicle fractures	Brachial plexus compression or damage; pneumothorax or hemothorax
Humerus fractures	Injury to brachial artery or radial nerve
Pelvic fractures	Injury to bladder, urethra, rectum
Distal femoral shaft fractures	Femoral or popliteal vessel injury
Proximal tibia fractures	Compression of the anterior tibial compartment; tibial nerve injury
Clavicular head dislocation	Compression of trachea, subclavian, and carotid arteries
Posterior elbow dislocation	Compression of brachial artery
Posterior hip dislocation	Aseptic necrosis of the femoral head and sciatic nerve damage
Knee dislocation	Compression of the popliteal vessel
Ankle dislocation	Compression of the pedal artery

From Perdue P. Abdominal injuries and dangerous fractures. *RN*. 1981;44(7):35,84.

treated immediately. Table 18.1 lists various orthopedic injuries and possible complications.

A soft tissue *injury* is any injury that results in the disruption of soft tissue. Soft tissue injuries can be categorized as open and closed. Examples of closed injuries include contusions, sprains, and strains; open injuries include lacerations, punctures, abrasions, avulsions, amputations, and burns.

Mechanisms of Injury

Various mechanisms may cause injury to the musculoskeletal system or soft tissue, including blasts, penetrating injuries, blunt force, motor vehicle collisions, falls, sports, and even routine activities. Either accelerating or decelerating forces may cause injury to bones or soft tissue. When a force is applied to the musculoskeletal system and causes an injury, the surrounding tissue and organs may be injured along with the bones and muscles.[3,5,6] The mechanism of injury must be kept in mind when assessing the patient and considering potential secondary injuries.

Hemorrhage Management

Soft tissue injury management must start with immediate identification of the presence or absence of active bleeding. If active bleeding is present, it must be categorized as life-threatening or non-life-threatening bleeding. Life-threatening bleeding may be of arterial or venous origin. Early exposure of the patient's entire skin surface is critical to ensure that a source of major bleeding is not missed.

Historically, trauma resuscitation has been taught in a stepwise paradigm with the first focus on the airway, then breathing, followed finally by circulation assessment and management (which includes assessment for life-threatening hemorrhage). Experts now advocate for a reprioritization to Circulation, Airway, and then Breathing (CAB), to quickly address any active, life-threatening

bleeding that may be present before completing the rest of the assessment. Reducing the risk of hypothermia is also an important part of resuscitation care.

Nearly half the patients that die of major trauma die in the first hour of injury. Of these patients, nearly half die of major hemorrhage. As a critical care transport clinician, it is essential to understand that all major bleeding must be stopped as fast as possible. It also is critical to understand that all major hemorrhages should be categorized as either compressible or noncompressible. This understanding should fundamentally impact resuscitation and transportation priorities. Noncompressible bleeding includes bleeding in the cranium, thorax, abdomen, retroperitoneum, pelvis, great vessels, and liver that requires surgical intervention for hemorrhage control. Patients with noncompressible bleeding require prioritization and urgent transportation to a facility that can perform emergent surgical or endovascular hemorrhage control. Resuscitative efforts should be aggressive, with a goal mean arterial pressure (MAP) of 65 or greater, especially with traumatic brain injury involvement. In severely hypotensive multisystem trauma patients with multiple injuries and lack of complete advanced diagnostic imaging, critical care transport clinicians should consider that at least some element of total blood loss may be the result of noncompressible injury.

In contrast, compressible life-threatening bleeding includes any major hemorrhage that occurs in a part of the body in which hemorrhage control can be achieved by direct compression, or by compression of the major vessels proximal to the injury site. Examples of compressible hemorrhage include major vascular injuries to the extremities and scalp. Patients with compressible injuries primarily need immediate hemorrhage control. Although patients with compressible hemorrhage also need rapid transport to a major trauma center, the rush to transport should not inhibit what these patients need most: aggressive, immediate hemorrhage control. If the focus on rapid movement to a trauma center results in substandard hemorrhage control and additional blood loss during transport, care is substandard.

Most compressible bleeding can be stopped with a dry sterile dressing and dedicated attention to direct pressure on the bleeding surfaces of the wound. Commercial hemostatic dressings with impregnated chemicals that promote hemostasis may be preferable to simple dry sterile dressings. Current Tactical Combat Casualty Care (TCCC) guidelines call for early use of hemostatic dressings and authorized tourniquets, where appropriate. This is the standard of care for forward-deployed personnel; however, some civilian protocols call for the provider to attempt hemorrhage control with direct pressure first and to apply a tourniquet if direct pressure does not stop bleeding promptly.[7]

In the prehospital environment, the critical care transport team may need to accomplish multiple priorities simultaneously with limited resources. Compressible major bleeding should be managed first with direct pressure if adequate resources are available to ensure undivided continuous direct pressure *in* the wound. Pressure on the surface of the skin while wound edges remain open will do little to stop major bleeding. Similarly, the application of bulky dressings to the skin surface, or undedicated direct pressure, which becomes lost because of provider distraction, will have similar, ineffective results. If a patient has major extremity hemorrhage, and inadequate personnel are available to maintain direct pressure, a tourniquet should be applied early. Once other priorities are managed (i.e., airway protection, ventilation, movement to transport vehicle), providers may be able to dedicate additional resources to provide direct pressure.

When a tourniquet is used, it should be placed 2 to 3 inches proximal to the sight of major bleeding, but be mindful of reassessment to ensure there are no injuries under the tourniquet.[7] The tourniquet should be tightened until bleeding stops. If a single tourniquet is tightened to maximum capability, but distal pulses are still present or bleeding remains uncontrolled, a second tourniquet may be placed proximal to the first tourniquet. Tourniquets applied ineffectively may have a counterproductive effect on those patients who have also suffered a venous injury alongside an arterial injury. Initial application of a tourniquet to a conscious or semiconscious person causes extreme pain from the compression of the tourniquet. It is not uncommon for the patient to resist adequate tightening of the tourniquet. Tourniquet application should not be delayed until the patient is hypotensive or in shock; rather, it should be applied immediately on recognition of severe hemorrhage. After application, it is critical to reassess tissue distal to the tourniquet frequently for return of pulses or bleeding. Ongoing resuscitation interventions may raise blood pressure to a point where the tourniquet no longer occludes distal blood flow. In this case the tourniquet may need to be tightened further. Tourniquets should not be loosened by the transport provider. It is important to note the time of application by writing it in permanent ink on the tourniquet.

Soft Tissue Wound Management

Local wound care is initiated by assessing the wound for evidence of hemorrhage, debris, or the presence of bone ends protruding through the skin. These findings should be noted on the chart, and a dry sterile dressing should be applied. No attempt should be made to pull bones back beneath the skin. Open wounds without active hemorrhage but with significant contamination might require irrigation before dressing. Saline or tap water work equally well. Extensive irrigation, debridement, and exploration should be deferred until arrival at the receiving hospital. Patients with large wounds, especially those that may be tied to an open fracture, should receive early intravenous antibiotics, including a first-generation cephalosporin (such as cefazolin) and an aminoglycoside (such as gentamicin). Proper wound care is as essential to a positive outcome as good splinting. This technique should not be overlooked. Tetanus status should be assessed and updated, if necessary, at some point during patient care.

Traumatic Amputations

Complete *traumatic amputations* of extremities may occur from various kinds of trauma, such as motor vehicle collisions, explosions, entanglements in farm or industrial machinery, or crushes caused by heavy objects. For traumatic amputations with massive hemorrhage, hemorrhage control should be followed by blood resuscitation. Low titer type O whole blood is preferred.[7] For transport clinicians who do not carry blood, 1 L of warmed crystalloid solution should be administered to the patient.[8] The American College of Surgeons states that administering more than 1.5 L of crystalloid solution results in increased mortality.[8]

Depending on unit protocol, the transport clinician should consider the use of tranexamic acid (TXA). To be most effective, TXA must be administered early and within 3 hours of the injury. TXA is a medication that blocks the breakdown of clots and can be administered IV or IO. According to the National Library of Medicine, "TXA is a synthetic reversible competitive inhibitor to the lysine receptor found on plasminogen. The binding of this receptor prevents plasmin (activated form of plasminogen) from binding to and ultimately stabilizing the fibrin matrix."[9]

TXA should be strongly considered for any patient who will need a blood transfusion, as well as patients with signs and symptoms of a traumatic brain injury (TBI) with an associated blast or blunt injury.[7]

If there is not massive hemorrhaging associated with an amputation, as with a digit injury, the transport clinician should irrigate the wound, apply a dry sterile dressing secured by a mild pressure gauze wrap, and immobilize and elevate the extremity. As the patient is warmed and fluid resuscitated, there is significant potential that retracted or spasmed vessels will reopen and hemorrhage will ensue. Traumatic amputations, specifically those proximal to a joint, should be monitored closely by the crew and/or have preemptive tourniquets applied prior to departing the scene. Special care should be taken to remain vigilant in those transport vehicles that have limited access to areas of the lower body if the lower extremities are involved. Amputation sites must be reassessed upon any movement, and frequently during transport. It may be advantageous to place a light-colored pad under the amputated extremity during transport to more easily identify rebleeding.

To care for the amputated body part, the transport team should irrigate it with crystalloid solution, wrap it in saline-moistened gauze (if unavailable, use a clean sheet), and place it in a plastic bag or container. Then, the severed part should be put in another container and cooled with another plastic bag that contains ice. Dry ice should not be used because it increases necrosis. As with any acute vascular injury, the expediency with which the patient and amputated part reach definitive care directly correlates with the success of reimplantation. The decision to proceed with reimplantation should only be made by a surgeon capable of performing the procedure.

Classification of Orthopedic Injuries

When force is applied to a limb, the energy of the impact dissipates and affects supporting structures. An excessive amount of force may damage more than one structure in the line of force.[5] This type of stress to the axial skeleton and its supporting structures can cause various types of injuries, including fractures, dislocations, sprains, tendon injuries, and strains.

Fractures

A *fracture* is defined as any break in the continuity of the bone or cartilage, and it may be either complete or incomplete, depending on the line of fracture through the bone.[5,10] Fractures generally are classified as closed or open. If the skin is unbroken, then the fracture is *closed,* regardless of the number of fractures. If the skin is broken, then the fracture is *open,* although it may be simple and minor in nature. Any broken skin in the area of a fracture must be included in the report. An open fracture is more serious because of the risk of infection. Fig. 18.1 illustrates nine different types of fractures as defined by radiographic appearance.

Fractures of the long bone may produce steady, slow bleeding and can result in 750 mL of blood loss from the humerus or tibia and 1500 mL of blood from each femur.[11,12] Ongoing blood loss from open bone ends poses a significant risk to the patient. Open long bone fractures that have been dressed before flight crew arrival or shortly after arrival should be closely monitored during transport. The risks for the development of significant hemorrhage

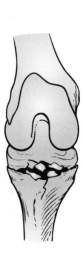
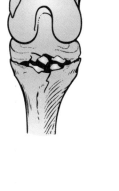
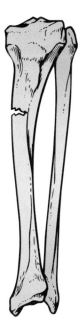
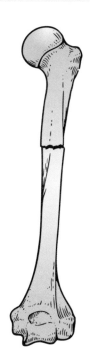
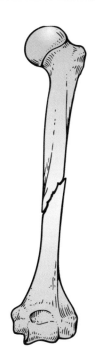
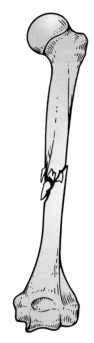
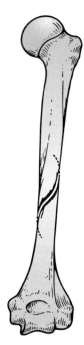

Impacted Fracture

The broken ends of the bones are forcefully jammed together.

Greenstick Fracture

The bone remains intact on one side, but broken on the other, in much the same way that a "green stick" bends; common in children, whose bones are more flexible than those of adults.

Transverse Fracture

The break occurs perpendicular to the long axis of the bone.

Oblique Fracture

The break occurs diagonally across the bone; generally the result of a twisting force.

Comminuted Fracture

The bone is splintered or shattered into three or more fragments; usually caused by an extremely traumatic direct force.

Spiral Fracture

The bone is broken into a spiral or S-shape; caused by a twisting force.

• **Figure 18.1** Fractures According to Radiographic Appearance. (From Shiland BJ. *Medical Assistant: Digestive System, Nutrition, Financial Management and First Aid—Module C.* 2nd ed. Elsevier.)

from exposed long bone ends mirror those risks associated with nonbleeding traumatic amputation. As rewarming and fluid resuscitative efforts are undertaken, the patient is at high risk of significant hemorrhage. Wrapping bone ends in hemostatic dressings before bulky dressing application may be considered.

These patients must be monitored closely for shock, and the long bone fracture should be immobilized for comfort. Care should be taken to ensure the fractured extremity is not touching the side of the transport platform, as vibrations can increase pain and discomfort. Another risk associated with fractures, even uncomplicated ones, is that of fat embolism, which can cause varying degrees of respiratory distress, including respiratory failure. Signs and symptoms of fat embolism are petechial rash, diffuse pulmonary infiltrates, hypoxemia, confusion, fever, tachycardia, and tachypnea. Patients at highest risk for fat embolism are those with long bone fractures of the lower extremity.[4,5,13] Fat embolism is discussed in more detail later in this chapter.

Dislocations

A *dislocation* is the displacement of the normal articulating ends of two or more bones. A *complete dislocation* causes a tearing of the ligaments. A dislocation may also be described as *compound* when the joint is exposed to the outside air. A dislocation is referred to as *subluxated* when the displacement is incomplete. Joints that are frequently dislocated are shoulders, elbows, fingers, hips, and ankles.

Less frequently seen are dislocated wrists or knees. Patellar dislocations are also common and should not be mistaken for a knee dislocation. Knee dislocation can be considered an emergency due to the potential for vascular injury and compartment syndrome.[14] Reduction of knee dislocation can be difficult, and orthopedic surgery should be consulted at the receiving treatment facility.

Assessment of an Orthopedic Injury

For adequate assessment data, a thorough history is important. This information can be obtained by talking to first responders on the scene or by reading the medical record. As previously discussed, an injury can often be anticipated by knowing the mechanism of injury and the circumstances under which it was sustained. To document a musculoskeletal assessment, certain orthopedic terms may be used. Box 18.1 lists common orthopedic terms.

Open fractures produce greater blood loss and risk of infection than closed fractures; thus they demand more immediate attention. However, closed fractures also must be carefully monitored.[4] The examination for fractures should be organized by body areas, with observation first for obvious deformities. If conscious, the patient should be asked to try to move each extremity. If a fracture or dislocation exists, movement or attempted movement is almost always painful, or extremely limited in dislocations. Range of motion, or lack of it, needs to be recorded. The extremities should be palpated proximally to distally, with evaluation for pain, displacement, crepitus, sensation,

Abduction: movement of a body part away from the body's midline.

Adduction: movement of a body part toward the midline.

Ankylosis: decreased range of motion caused by stiffening of the joint.

Dorsiflexion: movement of the hand or foot upward.

Eversion: movement of the ankle outward.

Extension: movement of the joint to open it or to maximally increase its angle.

External rotation: outward rotation.

Flexion: bending of the joint.

Hyperextension: extension past neutral.

Internal rotation: inward rotation.

Inversion: movement of the ankle inward.

Kyphosis: round back; increased flexion of the spine.

Lordosis: sway back; increased hyperextension of the spine.

Plantar flexion: movement of the foot downward.

Pronation: movement of the forearm to place the palm downward.

Rotation: movement of one bone turning on another.

Scoliosis: lateral curvature of the spine.

Supination: movement of the forearm to place the palm upward.

Torsion: twisting of the bone on its axis.

Valgus: deformity that causes an outward turning of the foot or toe (e.g., genu valgus or knock-kneed).

Varus: deformity that causes an inward turning of the foot or toe (e.g., genu varus or bowlegged).

---

and decreased or absent pulses. The sternum and rib cage are palpated to determine stability of the ribs. Lastly, the transport team should gently press laterally inward on the iliac crests and downward on the symphysis pubis to assess for increased pain and to determine pelvic stability.[15]

The classic signs of musculoskeletal trauma include deformity, localized swelling, pain, pallor, diminished or absent pulses, paresthesia, and paresis or paralysis.[11] If the patient is conscious, the transport team can ask about the patient's pain and its location. Peripheral pulses (especially those distal to the fracture site) should be checked bilaterally for presence and quality. Paresthesia should be checked in the conscious patient by touching or pinching the affected extremity and assessing for altered sensation. Always compare patient responses on each side.

Capillary refill should be monitored, and skin temperature noted.[6,11,12] Paralysis at the time of the injury, or ensuing paralysis on repeated examination, increases the severity and may determine the transport destination.

Joints above and below the fracture site or point of injury need to be evaluated. Neurovascular status assessments of the affected extremity should be done frequently, but especially before and after splinting.

Children deserve special consideration when evaluated for musculoskeletal injuries. Because their bones are more flexible than those of adults, greater force is often necessary to cause a fracture. Therefore, a child who has sustained even minor rib fractures must be assumed to have sustained serious internal injuries, until proven otherwise. The transport team should suspect splenic or diaphragmatic injury in a child with low rib fractures. Injury to the flexible skeleton of a young child may cause different outcomes than in an adult patient.[6,11,12]

Management of Orthopedic Injuries

Improper handling of a patient with an injury to the musculoskeletal system may convert a simple problem into a much more serious one. A closed wound may become an open one, a clean wound may become grossly contaminated, or blood vessels and nerves may be seriously injured. The five basic principles for management of fractures and dislocations are to (1) avoid unnecessary handling; (2) immobilize; (3) apply clean dressings to wounds; (4) control hemorrhage with direct pressure; and (5) check for the "5 Ps" distal to the injury – pain, pulselessness, paresthesia, pallor, and paralysis.[1,6,11,12]

Splinting

Proper emergency care rendered to a patient with any type of orthopedic injury may shorten hospital stay, accelerate recovery, and decrease the chance of serious complications. Because the extent of an injury is difficult to assess initially, the best approach is to assume a fracture is present and immobilize it until further evaluation can be made with radiography.

The primary objective of splinting is to prevent the motion of fractured bone fragments or dislocated joints, preventing the following complications[1,6,11,12]:

1. Laceration of the skin by broken bones, which can increase the risk of contamination and infection.
2. Damage to local blood vessels, which can cause excessive bleeding into surrounding tissue, ischemia, and even tissue death.
3. Restriction of blood flow to an area due to pressure of bone ends on blood vessels.
4. Damage to nerves by inadvertent excessive traction, contusion, or laceration, which can result in permanent loss of sensation and paralysis.
5. Damage to muscles, with possible subsequent necrosis, scarring, and permanent disability.
6. Increased pain associated with movement of bone ends.
7. Hypovolemic shock.
8. Delayed union or nonunion of fractured bones and dislocated joints.

Basic principles of management for any type of orthopedic injury must be considered in splint application. These include the following[1,6,11,12]:

1. Visualize the injured area by cutting off all clothing in the surrounding area, which is especially important when the size of the transport vehicle may challenge one's ability to easily see the entire patient during transport. If the fracture is caused by a bullet, be mindful not to cut through the hole.
2. Check and document neurovascular assessment before applying the splint; marking the location of a palpated pulse makes consistent evaluation of the injured extremity easier.
3. If an extremity is extremely angulated and a distal pulse cannot be palpated, gentle traction may be applied to attempt to reduce the fracture. A fracture should never be forced.
4. All open wounds should be covered with a dry dressing.
5. A splint should be applied to immobilize the joint above and below the fracture.
6. Padding should be placed in the splint to prevent pressure against bony areas and to reduce the risk of additional injury to the skin.
7. Bone ends should never be pushed back into a wound. Bone ends should be padded and covered. Keeping an open fracture clean may assist in decreasing infection.
8. Rapid transport of a patient with an unstable condition may override any attempts to splint fractures.
9. If an orthopedic injury is suspected, then apply a splint.
10. Reassess neurovascular status after the splint has been applied.

When splinting a patient's injuries and preparing the patient for transport, the clinical team should consider the size of the transport vehicle, the transport vehicle's configuration, and changes in altitude as they relate to the use of air splints.

Soft Splint

A *soft splint* is one that has no inherent rigidity, such as a pillow or a rolled blanket. Both can provide considerable support when wrapped around an injured part and bandaged.

Rigid Splint

A *rigid splint* is solid and inflexible. It is placed along the side, front, or back of the injured extremity, and when used correctly, it immobilizes the fracture. Rigid splints are effective only when they are long enough to immobilize the entire fractured bone, are padded sufficiently, and are secured firmly to an uninjured part.[10,15]

Many items, such as rolled newspapers or pieces of wood, can be used to make a rigid splint. Whatever is used, however, must be long enough to immobilize the injured area and one joint above and below the injured area (Box 18.2).

Traction Splint

Traction splints are rigid splints that apply gentle force to align and immobilize the bone to prevent further damage during movement and transportation.[9] Traction splints are indicated only for midshaft femur fractures.[16] Traction splints are contraindicated in possible fractures of the pelvis, fractured knee, fracture or serious wound to the tibia/fibula, and severe injuries in which a wound and loss of bone continuity exist. Examples of traction splints are the Thomas half-ring, the Hare traction splint, the Kendrick traction device, and the Sager splint.[13] Traction splints immobilize by pulling on the distal portion of the entire extremity below the fracture. The time necessary to apply a traction splint should be weighed against the need for rapid transport.

• BOX 18.2 General Principles of Splinting

- Expose and examine the injured extremity. Look for a wound, tenting of the skin, or obvious discoloration that may indicate the presence of or potential for an open fracture.
- Support the body part.
- Remove jewelry and constrictive items of clothing.
- Assess and document sensory and circulatory status before immobilization. If no palpable distal pulse is found, medical control may recommend application of gentle traction along the long axis of the extremity (distal to the injury) until the distal pulse is palpable.
- Immobilize the extremity so that the splint includes the joints above and below the fracture or the bones above and below the dislocation. Avoid excessive movement of the body part. (Movement may increase bleeding into the tissue space, increase the risk of fat embolism, or convert a closed fracture to an open fracture.)
- Note: immobilization requires a minimum of two rescuers.
- When applying splints to the hand or foot, leave the fingers or toes exposed to provide for inspection and evaluation of neurovascular status.
- Reevaluate and document sensory and circulatory status after immobilization. If a nerve or pulse deficit develops after splinting, remove the splint and place the extremity in its original position.

From Sanders MJ. *Mosby's Paramedic Textbook*. Mosby; 1994.

Splinting Fractures of the Upper Extremities

Fractures of the clavicle usually occur at the middle and distal thirds of the bone from a blow to the shoulder. Pain, swelling, and deformity are generally evident. Supporting the arm in a sling and binding it against the chest with a swathe sufficiently immobilizes the fracture. However, injuries that occur in motor vehicle collisions may fracture the bone more medially, pushing it into the thoracic outlet and possibly injuring the long subclavian artery or vein or the brachial plexus.[1]

Fractures of the upper end of the humerus may or may not involve the shoulder joint. Pain and tenderness are seen, but severe angulation is less commonly observed. The goal in the treatment of the humeral fracture is to maintain shoulder function. This goal can best be achieved by treating the problem as a soft tissue injury that happens to involve bone.[13] If gross deformity is found at the fracture site, the arm should be splinted in the position in which it is found with padded boards and pillow splints. In most cases, however, little gross angulation occurs, and the arm may be splinted with a sling and swathe.[1,11,12]

Fractures of the midshaft of the humerus endanger the radial nerve. The transport team can check for damage to the radial nerve by observing the patient's ability to spread the fingers. If damage has occurred, pain on movement and tenderness at the fracture site are seen. If angulation is present, a transport clinician should use gentle constant traction, apply a sling, and, with traction still held, place a padded board along the outer border of the humerus. A swathe is applied around the sling, the padded board, and the injured arm, binding the arm to the chest. A fracture without angulation may be splinted in the same manner.

Fractures of the elbow endanger the radial, ulnar, and median nerves and the brachial artery. The transport clinician should check for a pulse, movement, and sensation distal to the injury (Fig. 18.2). The fracture should be splinted in the exact position found, with a rigid splint above and below the fracture. If possible, the arm should be bound to the side to offer additional support.

After gentle traction has been applied to any severe angulation of a fracture of the radius or the ulna, a rigid splint should be applied, immobilizing both the elbow and the wrist.

Fractures of the wrist without angulation should be splinted in the same manner as the radius and the ulna. Those fractures with severe angulation, however, should be splinted in the position found.

Severe hand injuries often involve both soft tissue and bone injury. In most cases, the hand should be splinted in the position of function, with the fingers slightly bent and a bulky fluff dressing in the palm of the hand. A rigid splint should also be used to immobilize the wrist.[11,12]

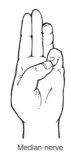 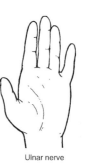 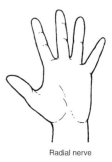

Median nerve   Ulnar nerve   Radial nerve

• **Figure 18.2** Testing for Neurologic Function in the Upper Extremities.

Splinting Dislocations of the Upper Extremities

When a shoulder is dislocated, the normal rounded appearance of the shoulder is flattened. There are three types of shoulder dislocations: anterior, posterior, and inferior.

Most dislocations are anterior. In the anterior dislocation, the patient holds the arm away from the body, and a bony prominence is seen in the front of the shoulder.[11,12,17] A pillow splint and frequently the help of a second person to hold the arm are used for maximal stability without changing the deformity. With a posterior dislocation, little deformity is evidenced, and the arm is held against the chest or abdomen. A sling and swathe are all that are necessary to maintain position. A rare inferior dislocation (the humerus is dislocated downward from the shoulder) may cause the patient to hold the arm above the head. The transport critical care transport clinician splints it in the position found. These patients should be transported in a sitting position when possible.

A dislocated elbow may appear as a posterior or anterior dislocation. With a posterior dislocation, which is more common, the arm is flexed. A long splint with the flexion maintained should be applied. A sling helps to maintain stability. This patient should also be transported in a sitting position if possible. With an anterior dislocation, the arm is extended, and the joint is immovable because of pain. Again, the transport team splints the injury in the position found.

A dislocated wrist has an obvious deformity, and a well-padded splint should be used. The index finger is the most commonly dislocated finger, with the deformity being obvious and the fingertip slightly cyanotic and cold. A splint helps to control pain. Immobilization is all that is needed for both injuries.

Splinting Fractures of the Lower Extremities

Fractures of the hip and proximal femur are anatomically divided into two types: fractures of the neck of the femur (transcervical) and fractures through the trochanters (intertrochanteric). Both present identically, with pain and swelling around the hip, pain on hip motion, and various degrees of shortening and external rotation.[13,17] The fractured hip is best splinted with pillows in the position found. In assessment of a hip injury, associated injuries to the knee and sciatic nerve as well as ipsilateral femoral shaft fractures may be seen.

With fractures of the shaft of the femur, a strong contraction of the gluteus medius muscle occurs, with a tendency to pull the proximal fragment of the femur outward as adduction causes bowing at the fracture point.[17,18] These fractures should be splinted immediately with a traction splint and kept in the splint until definitive orthopedic care is rendered. Femoral shaft fractures can cause extensive blood loss that can lead to hypovolemic shock, so these patients should be carefully monitored for early signs of shock.

Fractures of the knee should be splinted as they are found, with no attempt made to correct any angulation. Checking for and reporting changes in pulse, movement, and sensation is especially important with any type of knee injury. Fractures of the patella are recognizable as swelling of the anterior knee with little or no resistance to extension of the joint. A transport clinician should splint this kind of fracture with a rigid splint and the patient's knee in extension.

Fractures of the tibia or fibula are managed with a rigid splint. The splint should immobilize both the ankle and knee joints and is best when carried as high as the groin. Great care must be taken with these fractures to prevent penetration of bone ends through the skin because the skin is thinner in this area of the leg.[12,13,18]

Severely angulated fractures of the ankle should be straightened while applying traction to the heel and forefoot. A rigid splint should then be applied to immobilize the foot and ankle. If any question of a sprain or fracture exists, the injury should be splinted until a diagnostic radiograph can be made. Pain management should be considered prior to manipulation or traction, if possible.

Splinting Dislocations of the Lower Extremities

Differentiating between a dislocated hip and a fractured hip is often impossible, although, with a dislocated hip, the patient's thigh is sometimes flexed to some extent and turned slightly inward. Treatment for either one is the same. The transport team should splint, with pillows or sheets and blankets, in the position found. Because of the close proximity of the sciatic and femoral nerves, an immediate neurologic assessment of the affected limb is of utmost importance (Fig. 18.3). A rapid reduction within 8 hours should be performed by a physician to minimize avascular necrosis of the femoral head causing destruction of the hip joint.

Dislocations and fractures of the knee are treated the same. Any resistance to attempts to straighten an angulation indicates that it should be splinted in the position found, again paying heed to pulse, movement, and sensation. A rigid splint, preferably a padded board, should be used. All patients with a knee injury should be considered at high risk for popliteal artery injury. Distal pulses, skin color, and capillary refill should be checked frequently. The ankle brachial index (ABI) can be measured by obtaining an upper extremity blood pressure, followed by a second blood pressure on the calf of the injured extremity just above the ankle. To determine the ABI, divide the lower extremity systolic blood pressure by the upper extremity systolic blood pressure. An ABI greater than 0.9 has been associated with a low risk of popliteal artery injury.

Ankle dislocations rarely occur without associated fractures and should be aligned and splinted the same as ankle fractures. Dislocations of the foot are rare but generally involve more than one joint. They also should be treated the same as a fracture of the foot. Toe dislocations are innately stable and need no splinting.[12]

Whenever possible, after splinting a dislocation or a fracture, the transport team should elevate the affected extremity and apply ice to the location of the injury. This improves patient comfort and can make the splinting of the extremity easier.

Pelvic Fractures

A pelvic fracture can be one of the most serious injuries that a patient can sustain. Arterial injuries occur in 20% of patients with pelvic fractures; however, disruption of large venous structures in the pelvis frequently results in fatal hemorrhage as well. Posterior fractures are more likely than anterior fractures to cause hemorrhage. The major cause of death is hemorrhage from arteries and veins torn by the fracture or dislocation.[1,6,11,12]

The most common form of pelvic fracture results from a severe external force applied directly on the pelvis or from an indirect force transmitted upward along the shaft of the femur. Minor fractures of the pelvis include breaks of individual bones

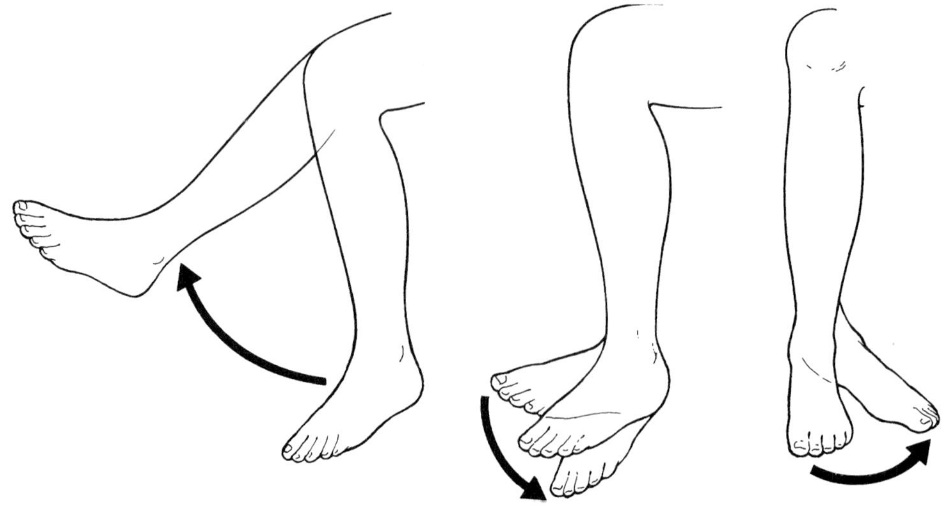

Femoral nerve   Sciatic nerve   Peroneal nerve

• **Figure 18.3** Testing for Neurologic Function in the Lower Extremities.

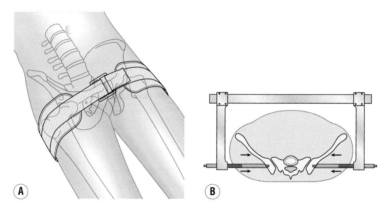

(A)   (B)

• **Figure 18.4** Proper Placement for Pelvic Binders. **A.** Pelvic binders. **B.** G-clamp. (Mackenzie SP, Gray AJ, White TO. *McRae's Orthopaedic Trauma and Emergency Fracture Management.* 3rd ed. Elsevier; 2016.)

without a break in the continuity of the pelvic ring. These fractures are relatively stable and rarely necessitate hospitalization. Major pelvic fractures are generally fractured in at least two separate places, and a separation of one or both sacroiliac joints may be found. These fractures are commonly seen in patients with multiple traumas.

Approximately 60% of pelvic fractures should be considered major because of the complications of injury to the structures lying within the pelvis.[1,6,11,12] Along with the danger of damage to the major blood vessels within the pelvic girdle, fractures of the pubic ramus may lacerate the urethra, fractures of the brim of the pelvis may disrupt the ureters, and the bladder itself may rupture.[1,6,11,12] Open fractures of the pelvis occur with direct communication between fracture fragments and a laceration of the skin, vagina, or rectum. This uncommon fracture is caused by a high-velocity injury, and subsequent massive hemorrhage occurs with a 50% mortality rate. Even small amounts of blood on vaginal or rectal examination may indicate the possibility of an open fracture.[1,6,11,12]

Control of bleeding is a top priority.[13,15] All patients with an unstable pelvis, and those with a significant mechanism of injury and pelvic pain on palpation, should be immobilized with a commercial pelvic binder. If a commercial binder is not available, critical care transport clinicians can use a sheet to bind the pelvis. The goal of pelvic binding is not so much to "splint" the fracture but to decrease the pelvic ring space, thus creating a smaller space for blood loss. The landmark for the placement of pelvic binders is the greater trochanter.[19] Of note, there is clinical evidence that pelvic binders adequately stabilize the pelvis and reduce hemorrhaging, though it is unknown whether survival rate is improved by their use.[20] It is still, however, the standard of care for both military and civilian treatment of unstable pelvic fractures. Fig. 18.4 illustrates the landmark and proper placement for a pelvic binder. A diagnosis of a pelvic fracture with hemodynamic instability should ideally be treated with blood transfusions, although resources and policies of the transportation agency will dictate resuscitation efforts. In a large multicenter study, Lustenberger and colleagues found inaccuracies in the detection of clinically unstable pelvic injuries in a prehospital environment.[21] Therefore, if a patient is hypotensive, resistant to resuscitation, and severely injured from blunt trauma, you must assume there is bleeding in the pelvis and apply a binder. Taping or tying knees and ankles together will also decrease the pelvic ring space by internal rotation. Care should be taken to ensure the pelvic binder is not too tight, as this may cause overreduction.

Fat Embolism

Fat embolism is a complication that may occur with large bone, pelvic, and rib fractures. It is generally not seen until 12 to 72 hours after injury. The transport team may encounter a patient with fat emboli, especially in delayed transports.[11,12]

Clinical signs of fat emboli include respiratory failure, shock, and elevation in serum lipase levels. Thrombocytopenia (count <150,000) can also occur, and patients may have petechiae present.

Long bone fractures should be appropriately immobilized. Patients should be closely monitored for respiratory distress, especially lack of improved oxygenation despite increasing the FiO_2. If the patient is intubated, positive end-expiratory pressure may be used to maintain an adequate PO_2 during transport.[11,12] Although there is no specific treatment for fat embolism syndrome, supplemental oxygen may be indicated to support respiratory symptoms.[22]

Compartment Syndrome

Compartment syndrome develops when there is increased pressure within the compartment space of an extremity or other area of the body from bleeding, soft tissue swelling, fluid accumulation (such as in a burn injury), or because of external sources such as splinting.[11,12] Fractures, crush injuries, burns, and pit viper snake bites may put a patient at risk for compartment syndrome, as may prolonged compression of an extremity in a splint.

The diagnosis of compartment syndrome does not require advanced imaging or laboratory testing. A clinical diagnosis can be made using the six Ps of compartment syndrome: pain, pallor, pulselessness, paresthesia, paralysis, and poikilothermia (cool skin).[23] Suspicion of compartment syndrome is warranted in any patient with extremity trauma and pain out of proportion to the injury. Patients often describe compartment syndrome pain as deep, burning, or unrelenting. Pain out of proportion with passive movement of the affected extremity is a hallmark symptom of compartment syndrome. Patients may also complain of neurologic symptoms such as paresthesia in the effected extremity. Clinical signs of compartment syndrome include pallor, cool skin, decreased capillary refill, and weak or absent distal pulses.[23] These changes are suggestive of decreased blood flow and are very late signs of compartment syndrome.

If an external dressing or immobilization device contributes to compartment syndrome, then it should be loosened or removed. Ideally compartment pressure should be measured by an intracompartmental pressure monitor system. If the compartment pressure is greater than 30 mm Hg or is within 30 mm Hg of the patient's MAP, a fasciotomy may be indicated. Emergency fasciotomy must be done within 4 hours to prevent irreversible damage to muscles and nerves. However, fasciotomy is a sterile surgical procedure requiring in-depth knowledge of surgical anatomy and should not be done without consulting medical control.[13,18]

Maxillofacial Trauma

Trauma to the face can occur by many mechanisms. Most frequently it is seen in sports injuries, recreational activities, and more seriously in motor vehicle collisions and assaults. Treatment of these injuries is best performed at a trauma center because these injuries typically require the involvement of numerous specialty services. Injuries to the face can impact the patient's mortality, as well as their psychosocial well-being and activities of daily living. Changes in the way we eat, speak, laugh, kiss, see, smell, and experience the world can be detrimental to the patient's psychological health. However, in the acute phase of injury, and during transport, attention should be focused on immediate life threats.

Injuries to the face and jaw can produce significant airway compromise. Complications such as blood, bone, dirt, and debris in the upper airway can cause immediate or delayed obstruction and subsequent hypoxia, followed by death or disability. When caring for a patient with maxillofacial trauma, the care provider should be hypervigilant in assessing for airway compromise. These injuries often need prompt airway management and may require atypical approaches.

The patient that presents after a shotgun injury to the lower face, or after a fall from 40 feet, face down, onto cement may not be easily intubated by direct laryngoscopy. Adjuncts and alternatives such as the gum elastic bougie, fiber-optic or video-assisted laryngoscopy, inverse intubation procedure, retrograde intubation, and so forth may be required. Nasotracheal intubation may be considered, but only after basilar skull fracture has been ruled out radiographically. Also, the procedure is rarely done in critical care transport as an advanced airway procedure. When caring for patients with maxillofacial trauma, surgical cricothyrotomy is an essential skill. A surgical airway is needed in approximately 5% of patients suffering gunshot wounds or blast injuries to the face, especially when affecting the jaw or lower third of the face.[5]

Facial fractures can also lead to other issues. In addition to airway obstruction, facial fractures can cause significant pain, damage to facial or cranial nerves, or laceration of many facial vessels. This can lead to significant hematoma formation, or even exsanguination in extreme cases. The formation of hematomas in key areas can be devastating. One such example is a retrobulbar hematoma (blood accumulating posterior to the eye), which causes the optic nerve to become stretched and impedes optic vasculature. A retrobulbar hematoma is an ophthalmic emergency and can lead to blindness if pressure is not relieved by rapid surgical intervention. Immediate transport to a provider who can perform an emergent lateral canthotomy is essential to salvaging the patient's sight. Facial fractures caused by significant force should also lead the provider to consider the patient at high risk for intracranial injuries, and appropriate precautions should be applied. These patients, including those with complicated facial fractures, such as Le Fort fractures, should be transported to a trauma center for evaluation.

There are three types of Le Fort fractures, numbered I, II, and III. Type I results after significant downward force on the upper teeth.[24] Type II results from midface force, and Type III results from force to the nasal bridge and upper maxilla.[24] Fig. 18.5 illustrates the different types of Le Fort fractures. Use of a bag valve mask may be complicated by the unstable or absent facial bones allowing for difficulty with ventilation. Nasopharyngeal airways should be avoided in patients with suspected facial fractures, as they may cause further damage to the surrounding tissues and vasculature. With the absence of stable facial bones in Le Fort injuries, the soft tissue may cause airway obstruction if

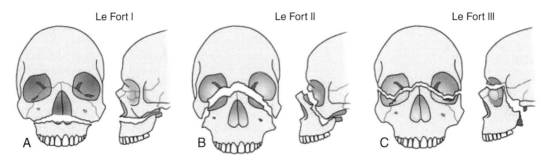

Le Fort I Le Fort II Le Fort III

A B C

• **Figure 18.5** Different Types of Le Fort Fractures. (From Avery LL, Susarla SM, Novelline RA. Multidetector and three-dimensional CT evaluation of the patient with maxillofacial injury. *Radiol Clin North Am.* 2011;49(1):183–203, Fig. 13.)

the patient is placed in a supine position. A reverse Trendelenburg or elevated head of bed position is a more appropriate position if the cervical spine is addressed. Use of gastric tubes (NG/OGT) should be used with caution and may require radiography at the accepting facility.

Crush Injuries

Crush injuries occur when parts of the body, typically extremities, are entrapped by a heavy object. Crush syndrome is a potential life- and limb-threatening condition that can occur with crush injuries.[25] It is characterized by reperfusion injury, which occurs when the entrapped limb is freed, causing myoglobin and potassium to be released into the bloodstream. This results in traumatic rhabdomyolysis, damaging the kidneys and increasing the risk of hyperkalemia.[25] Patients suffering from crush syndrome also experience hypocalcemia due to calcium being absorbed by injured muscle cells. Hyperkalemia and hypocalcemia cause cardiac instability, leading to arrhythmias. In addition to renal injuries and electrolyte disturbances, other complications can include hypovolemia and acidemia.[25] The severity of crush syndrome depends on how much of the extremity or extremities are entrapped and the length of time under entrapment.

As with all patients, the ABC algorithm should be used when assessing a patient with a crush injury. Close cardiac monitoring should be conducted throughout the transport, with EKG tracings obtained before, during, and after transport. Peaked T waves, prolonged PR interval, prolonged QRS, frequent Premature Ventricular Contractions (PVCs), and bradycardia should all be noted, as they are indicative of hyperkalemia. Fig. 18.6 depicts T wave progression as potassium levels increase. Insulin and 50% dextrose (D50) should be administered to patients experiencing EKG changes indicative of hyperkalemia.[25] Typically, regular insulin is administered by Intravenous Push (IVP) and followed by 50 mL D50.[25] Insulin carries potassium with it into the cells and is followed by D50 to ensure stable blood glucose levels. Albuterol can

also be used to lower potassium levels, as it too drives potassium back into the cells. Calcium can be administered to aid with cardiac stability. Calcium gluconate or calcium chloride can be used; however, the transport clinician should be cautious when administering calcium chloride via peripheral IV as it can be highly irritating. Each of these medications may have to be redosed depending on the length of transport. The administration of IV sodium bicarbonate, before or after pressure release, may be considered, according to local protocol.

Aggressive fluid administration is the main treatment for crush syndrome, as this dilutes the concentration of potassium. IV or IO access and fluid administration should be started prior to extrication if possible, and fluid rate should be titrated to a urine output goal of 100 to 200 mL per hour.[25] Also prior to extrication, the use of a tourniquet on the limb should be considered if it has been crushed for greater than 2 hours, especially if fluid administration is not able to be initiated prior to extrication.[25] Patients who experience a crush injury should be monitored closely for compartment syndrome following a crush injury. Antibiotics such as ertapenem or cefazolin should be administered for wounds caused by the crush injury.[25]

Summary

In most cases, orthopedic and soft tissue injuries are not life-threatening; however, the long-term outcome for patients who sustain these injuries is greatly influenced by the initial care that they receive. The transport team should approach soft tissue and orthopedic emergencies with these goals in mind: (1) identify life-threatening bleeding and aggressively manage major hemorrhage; (2) minimize the complications associated with dislocations and fractures, both open and closed; (3) decrease complications of immobility caused by these injuries; (4) facilitate the delivery of more definitive care; and (5) help to preserve and restore the complete function of the affected extremity.[7,8]

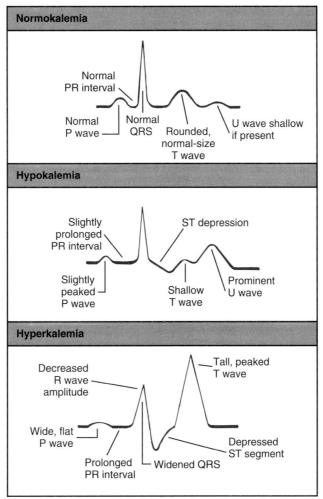

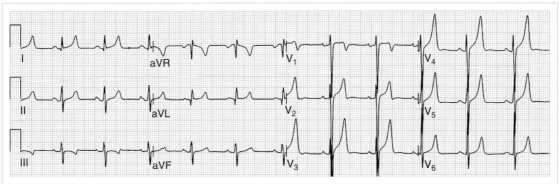

• **Figure 18.6** T Wave Progression as Potassium Levels Increase. (From Felver L. The cellular environment: Fluids and electrolytes, acids and bases. In: Rogers JL, ed. *McCance & Huether's Pathophysiology: The Biologic Basis for Disease in Adults and Children.* 9th ed. Elsevier; and From Olshansky B, et al. *Arrhythmia Essentials.* 2nd ed. Elsevier; 2017.)

References

1. Smith W, Stahel P. *Management of Musculoskeletal Injuries in the Trauma Patient.* Springer-Verlag; 2014.
2. Skinner HB, McMahon PJ. *Current Diagnosis & Treatment in Orthopedics.* McGraw-Hill Medical New; 2014.
3. Clarke S, Santy-Tomlinson J. *Orthopaedic and Trauma Nursing: An Evidence-Based Approach to Musculoskeletal Care.* Wiley Blackwell; 2014.
4. American College of Surgeons. *Advanced Trauma Life Support: Student Course Manual.* 10th ed. American College of Surgeons; 2018.
5. Hardy M, Snaith B. *Musculoskeletal Trauma: A Guide to Assessment and Diagnosis.* Churchill Livingstone; 2011.
6. McQuillan KA, Makic MB, Whalen E. *Trauma Nursing: From Resuscitation Through Rehabilitation.* 5th ed. Saunders/Elsevier; 2019.
7. Deployed Medicine. TCCC Guidelines. 2021. https://www.deployedmedicine.com/market/11/content/475#:~:text=The%20TCCC%20Guidelines%20are%20the,a%20substitute%20for%20clinical%20judgment. Accessed August 10, 2022.

8. Henry S. ATLS 10th Edition Offers New Insights into Managing Trauma Patients. 2021. https://bulletin.facs.org/2018/06/atls-10th-edition-offers-new-insights-into-managing-trauma-patients/. Accessed August 10, 2022.

9. Chauncey J, Wieters J. Trancxamic Acid. StatPearls Publishing LLC; 2022. https://www.ncbi.nlm.nih.gov/books/NBK532909/. Accessed August 10, 2022.

10. Sanders MJ, Lewis LM, Quick G, McKenna K. *Mosby's Paramedic Textbook*. Elsevier/Mosby Jems; 2012.

11. Mattox KL, Moore EE, Feliciano DV. *Trauma*. McGraw-Hill Medical; 2013.

12. Marx JA, Hockberger RS, Walls RM, et al. *Rosen's Emergency Medicine: Concepts and Clinical Practice*. Mosby/Elsevier; 2010.

13. Campbell J, ed. *International Trauma Life Support for Prehospital Care Providers*. 6th ed. Pearson Prentice Hall; 2008.

14. Mohseni M, Simon L. Knee Dislocation. StatPearls Publishing LLC; 2022. https://www.ncbi.nlm.nih.gov/books/NBK470595/. Accessed August 10, 2022.

15. Bracey A. *Guidelines for Massive Transfusion*. American Association of Blood Banks; 2005.

16. Davis D, Ginglen J, Kwon Y, Kahwaji C. EMS Traction Splint. StatPearls Publishing LLC; 2021. https://www.ncbi.nlm.nih.gov/books/NBK507842/. Accessed August 10, 2022.

17. Andrew N. *Critical Care Transport*. Jones and Bartlett; 2011.

18. Proehl J, ed. *Emergency Nursing Procedures*. 4th ed. Saunders/Elsevier; 2009.

19. Fisher A. Pelvic Binders in Trauma Resuscitation. 2019. https://nextgencombatmedic.com/2019/06/11/pelvic-binders-in-trauma-resuscitation/. Accessed August 06, 2022.

20. Shackleford S, Hammesfahr R, Morissette D, et al. The use of pelvic binders in tactical combat casualty care. *J Spec Oper Med*. 2017; 17:135-147.

21. Lustenberger T, Walcher F, Lefering R, et al. The reliability of the pre-hospital physical examination of the pelvis: A retrospective, multicenter study. *World J Surg*. 2016;40(12):3073–3079.

22. Adeyinka A, Pierre L. Fat embolism. [Updated September 5, 2022]. In: *StatPearls [Internet]*. StatPearls Publishing; January 2022. https://www.ncbi.nlm.nih.gov/books/NBK499885/

23. Pechar J, Lyons MM. Acute compartment syndrome of the lower leg: A review. *J Nurse Practice*. 2016;(4):265–270. doi: 10.1016/j.nurpra.2015.10.013

24. Patel B, Wright T, Waseem M. Le Fort Fractures. 2022. https://www.ncbi.nlm.nih.gov/books/NBK526060/. Accessed August 06, 2022.

25. Walter T, Powell D, Penny A, et al. Crush syndrome – prolonged field care. *Joint Trauma System Clinical Practice Guideline*. 2016. Accessed August 01, 2022. https://jts.health.mil/assets/docs/cpgs/Crush_Syndrome_PFC_28_Dec_2016_ID58.pdf

19

Burn Trauma

CHRISTOPHER P. STEVENSON AND MICHAEL J. FELDMAN

COMPETENCIES

1. Identify the pathophysiology of burn wounds.
2. Describe the initial assessment of the patient with burns.
3. Describe the management of the patient with burns during transport.

Etiology and Epidemiology

Burn injuries are a leading cause of traumatic injury in the United States. Over 450,000 people seek care in emergency departments annually.[1] Annually, 4000 people die from burn-related injuries, with most deaths being at the scene or in transport.[1] Injury patterns for burn patients vary with age. The most common burn injury for children under 5 is scald, while the most common in older children and adults is flame. Burn mortality has improved with advances in burn resuscitation and the trend to early excision. With these advances, the survival rate has improved to around 96%.[1] The World Health Organization estimates that 265,000 fire-related deaths occurred worldwide in 2014, with most of these in developing countries.[1–3]

A *burn wound* is an injury caused by the interaction of an energy form (thermal, chemical, electrical, or radiation) and biologic matter like skin, subcutaneous tissue, or muscle and other body parts. Burn injuries are differentiated by mechanism including thermal, chemical, electrical, and radiation.

Thermal: The most common mechanism includes flame and flash burns, scalds, or contacts with hot substances (Fig. 19.1). Flame and flash burns are the most prevalent, accounting for approximately 40% of hospital admissions. Scalds are the second most common overall and the most common in children under 5 years old.[1,2] *Chemical* injuries occur when a strong acid or alkali comes in contact with skin. An acid will cause an injury of coagulation necrosis, whereas an alkali will cause liquefication. Chemical burns account for a lower total proportion of burns but may account for up to 1/3 of burn deaths.[3] Burns from household chemicals are common in pediatric patients, related to inadequate storage and poor labeling.[3,4]

Electrical burns occur when contact is made with an electrical current. This current may be alternating, direct, or by lightning which contains both alternating and direct current properties. The current itself is not considered to have any thermal properties while traveling through material of low resistance; however, the potential energy of the current is transferred into thermal energy when it meets resistance with biologic tissue and is dispersed

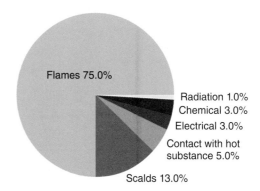

• **Figure 19.1** Causes of burn injuries.

throughout that tissue. As the electrical current flows through increasingly narrow areas, such as joints and distal extremities, resistance, heat, and subsequent damage increase.[3,5]

Radiation injuries can be caused by both ionizing and nonionizing radiation. This can be from medical device exposure, lab spill, or up to the scale of weapon detonation. Damage is caused by both direct cell damage and alteration of DNA. Radiation injuries make up a small percentage of burn injuries.[3]

Pathophysiology of Burn Wounds

The causes of burns may vary, but the local and systemic responses are generally similar. The extent of the injury is influenced by three factors: (1) the intensity of the energy source, (2) the duration of exposure to the energy source, and (3) the amount of tissue exposed.[1,3,6] The relationship between the duration of exposure to and intensity of the energy source is significant in determining the magnitude of the injury. Increased intensity with increased exposure causes increased amounts of tissue damage. The larger the surface area involved, the greater the systemic impact. Systemic changes are most noted in patients with a total body surface area (TBSA) of greater than 20%. Significant factors that determine severity of electrical injury are (1) voltage and amperage, (2) resistance of internal body structure and tissue, (3) type and pathway of current, and (4) duration and intensity of contact.[3,5]

For a better understanding of the pathophysiology of burn wounds, one must know the anatomy and functions of the skin, the largest organ of the body. Skin is composed of two layers: the epidermis and the dermis. The *epidermis,* the outer layer, consists of the basement layer of cells that migrate upward to become surface keratin. It contains melanocytes, Langerhans cells, Merkel cells, and inflammatory cells.[3] The inner layer, the *dermis,* consists of collagen and elastic fibers and contains hair follicles, sweat and sebaceous glands, nerve endings, and blood vessels. Beneath the cutaneous layers is a layer of subcutaneous tissue that consists primarily of connective tissue and fat deposits; this layer overlies fascia, muscle, and bone.

The primary functions of skin include (1) the regulation of body temperature through dilation and constriction of the dermal and subcuticular vessels in response to environmental temperature, (2) protection against injury and bacterial invasion, (3) prevention of body fluid loss, and (4) sensory contact with the environment including temperature and pain perception. Skin is also an important factor in appearance and identity and may have a great impact on confidence in interpersonal relationships. A burn injury interrupts and compromises these functions, and these changes can be permanent and life-altering.[3]

Thermal Burn Injury

The physiologic response of the body to thermal injury consists of varying degrees of tissue damage, cellular impairment, and fluid shifts from loss of plasma membrane integrity. Locally, a brief initial decrease in blood flow to the area occurs, followed by a marked increase in arteriolar vasodilation. Release of toxic mediators of inflammation is activated with the burn, creating a complex circulatory dysfunction. These mediators include histamine, serotonin, kinins, oxygen-free radicals, prostaglandins, thromboxanes, and interleukins.[3] Although inflammatory activity is a necessary part of the healing process, excess production of mediators, especially oxidants and proteases, causes more capillary endothelial and skin cell damage.[3,6] This increases capillary permeability, particularly once the burned area reaches a size that is approximately 20% TBSA, which causes intravascular fluid loss and wound edema.[1,2]

Hypoproteinemia that results from the increase in capillary permeability, aggravates edema in the unburned tissue. Myocardial contractility is thought to be decreased because of the cell-mediated inflammatory response. Insensible fluid loss from the burn wound and increases in basal metabolic rate along with fluid shift leads to hypovolemia, hypotension, and inadequate end-organ perfusion without appropriate resuscitation.[1,3]

The decrease in circulating plasma causes hemoconcentration, which in turn can cause hemoglobinuria when the hemoglobin is filtered through the kidneys and can contribute to renal failure. Increased peripheral vascular resistance leads to a decrease in venous return to the heart, decreased cardiac output, impaired tissue perfusion, and a decrease in renal perfusion, which can also contribute to renal failure.[1,3]

A decrease in splanchnic blood flow occurs, which increases the occurrence of mucosal hemorrhages in the stomach and duodenum. An increased risk of sepsis from bacterial translocation may also be seen because of diminished mucosal barrier function in the intestine. Patients with burns on more than 20% of the BSA can also develop an ileus, which can be of special concern for the patient transported by air at high altitudes and require decompression.[1-3]

Decreased immune response in both cell-mediated and humoral pathways increases the patient's susceptibility to infection.[3] Thus the transport team must take precautions to prevent further injury to the burn victim through exposure to contaminated environments.

Thermal burns and pregnancy should be considered in any female of reproductive age. The outcome of the pregnancy is determined by the extent of the mother's burn injury. Spontaneous abortions can be anticipated with burns greater than or equal to 60% of BSA. The incidence rate of preterm labor or spontaneous abortion is reduced with adequate oxygenation, fluid resuscitation, and electrolyte imbalance correction. Appropriate care of the mother is the priority and provides the greatest viability for the fetus.[1-3]

Electrical Injury

Electrons flowing through the body produce injury by depolarizing muscles and nerves. They can also disrupt electrical rhythms in the brain and heart. Electrical energy is also converted to thermal energy when it meets resistance from tissues. Resistance is described as the degree of hindrance to electron flow. Those tissues that contain the most electrolyte media, nerves, blood vessels, and muscles transmit current most easily because they have the least resistance. Tendons and fat are most resistant and do not allow conduction, which causes burning and surrounding deep muscle damage. The intensity of the electrical current that passes through victims shows a direct correlation to the tissue damage produced.[1,3,5]

Voltage is defined as the force with which electrical movement occurs. High-voltage injuries (>1000 V) and low-voltage injuries (<1000 V) are both common, and either type can cause death. High voltage exposure causes more significant injury to the patient and results in tissue charring and extensive blistering. The type of current, alternating or direct, can also determine the significance of injury.[7,8] Alternating current (AC) produces a tetanic contraction of muscles. Generally, flexor contraction is stronger than extensor and may cause a victim to "hold on" – to the source. This reaction is not seen with DC; therefore, low-voltage AC exposure, such as to a household current of 110 V, can be more dangerous than a DC exposure (Table 19.1).[1,3,5]

The current pathway is critical because it may determine the severity of injury. Current passing through the head and thorax involves the respiratory center or heart and is likely to produce

TABLE 19.1	Effects of Amperage by Household Currents (60-Hz Alternating Current)
mA	**Effect**
>1	Current is perceptible through skin
3–5	The "let go" current, or maximum a child can overcome tetany
<15	Adult "let go" current
50–120	Ventricular fibrillation

Compiled from Zemaitis MR, Foris LA, Lopez RA, et al. Electrical injuries. [Updated 2022 May 1]. In: *StatPearls [Internet].* StatPearls Publishing; Jan 2022. https://www.ncbi.nlm.nih.gov/books/NBK448087/

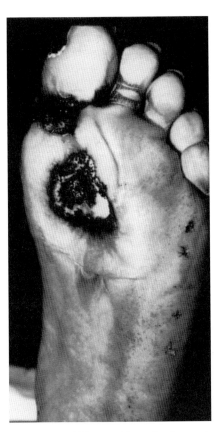

• **Figure 19.2** Exit wound from direct current.

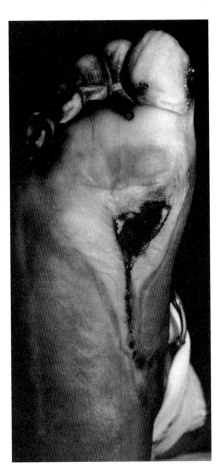

• **Figure 19.3** Exit wound from alternating current.

instant death. Current passing from hand to foot may not affect the respiratory center but may damage the heart. From the entry point, the electrical current follows the path of least resistance, causing one or more tracks of damage. The energy collects at the grounding point, causing significant tissue necrosis, subsequently causing an explosive exit through the skin.[1,3] The mortality rate of hand-to-hand current passage is reported to be 60%, hand-to-foot current passage is 20%, and foot-to-foot current passage is 5%. DC has been noted to leave a discrete exit wound (Fig. 19.2), whereas AC tends to be more explosive (Fig. 19.3).

With electrical injury, flame burns can occur as the result of the secondary ignition of clothing or other items by the current known as an arc injury. The ignition of clothing usually occurs with high-voltage injuries that are greater than 350 to 1000 V. Frequently, high-voltage injuries cause combinations of all types of electrical burns.[1,3,5]

As electrical current passes through the body, severe dysrhythmia may occur. Ventricular fibrillation is frequently induced as a 60-cycle AC passes through the ventricles.[3,5] DC injuries predominantly result in asystole by depolarizing the entire myocardium. In addition to those fatal rhythms, other dysrhythmias may occur, such as atrial fibrillation, sinus bradycardia, ventricular and atrial ectopy, supraventricular tachycardia, bundle branch block, and first- and second-degree block. These arrythmias can occur in both high- and low-voltage injuries. Coronary artery spasm, coronary endarteritis, and direct myocardial injury are thought to be the cause of these dysrhythmias. Damage to the myocardium, including myocardial rupture, is also a result of an electrical injury. These injuries are believed to be caused by the heat generated by the current. Myocardial damage manifests similarly to ischemia.[1,3,5]

Entry through the skull can affect the brainstem, leading to respiratory arrest and cerebral hemorrhage or edema. Nervous system tissue is an excellent conductor of electrical current, so central nervous system damage is common. Effects of electrical injury to the central nervous system are manifested by unconsciousness, seizures, disorientation, or amnesia. Other neurologic complications that have been identified are spinal cord injuries, particularly those associated with electrical current traversing a hand-to-hand or head-to-foot course, and local nerve damage with peripheral neuropathies.[1,3,5] These injuries have the potential for numerous long-term complications. Patients may suffer from headaches, memory and behavior changes, and gait and balance disturbances, as well as paresthesias and neuropathies.[5]

Extensive necrosis over vessels resulting from electrical injury may precipitate delayed hemorrhage from large blood vessels. Arterial thrombosis, deep vein thrombosis, and abdominal aortic aneurysms may also result. A major vessel that has been only partially damaged may cause difficulty with homeostasis in open or newly closed wounds. Injuries to the abdominal cavity commonly identified after electrocution are submucosal hemorrhages in the bowel, liver failure, pancreatitis, nausea and vomiting, paralytic ileus, and various forms and degrees of ulcerative disease.[3,5]

High voltage injury and subsequent tetanic contraction may lead to tendon and muscle avulsion, protein coagulation, hemolysis and thrombosis, and tissue edema.[3,5] When severe, this may lead to compartment syndrome, myoglobinuria, hyperkalemia, and rhabdomyolysis. This puts the patient at high risk for acute kidney failure.[1,3]

Immediate burns to the eyes, optic atrophy, and the development of cataracts are not uncommon, particularly if the entrance or exit wounds appear on or around the head. Cataracts may develop unilaterally or bilaterally and occur as soon as 4 months or as late as 3 years after the injury.[3,5]

For the pregnant patient, the hand-to-foot pathway of current invariably passes through the fetus. The amniotic fluid and abundant uteroplacental vascularity have a low resistance to current flow, and the fetus becomes an easy victim of electrical injuries. Regardless of how slight the injury may appear, the mother must be transported to a hospital in which appropriate fetal monitoring can be done.

Acute renal failure is a complication that results from direct damage to the kidney by the electrical current or blunt trauma to the kidney or from myoglobinuria. Myoglobin is released because of extensive muscle necrosis, and myoglobinuria is proportionate to the amount of muscle damage incurred.[1,3,5]

Chemical Injury

Chemical burns, like thermal burns, involve denaturing of proteins. Strong acids, with a pH less than 2, or bases with a pH greater than 11 impact cells by altering physiologic pH, which in turn weakens the hydrogen bonds holding proteins together. They may also dissolve surrounding lipids, disrupting protein function. The severity of chemical injury is based on numerous factors including concentration of the agent, extent of penetration, duration of contact, and amount of body exposed.[3] Chemical agents may be further broken down by their mechanism of action: reduction, oxidation, corrosive, protoplasmic, vesicant, or desiccant.[1,3,4]

Acids cause coagulation necrosis, precipitating protein and resulting in a layer of leathery eschar. Alkali agents penetrate deeper into tissue by creating a Liquefaction necrosis. Alkali injuries to the eye are of notable concern. They can easily penetrate the cornea, resulting in opacification; immediate and copious irrigation must be initiated.[1,3,4]

While the identification and mechanism for each agent is beyond the scope of this text, there are some notable and common agents worth discussing including hydrofluoric acid, cement, gasoline, and tar.[1]

Hydrofluoric acid is a corrosive agent used for a variety of industrial and household applications. It is found in numerous industrial cleaning agents, the manufacture of computer processors, glass etching compounds, and industrial dyes. It is particularly dangerous due to its action as an acid in combination with its properties as a metabolic poison. Hydrofluoric acid has a unique ability to chelate positively charged ions, particularly in calcium and magnesium. This causes intracellular ions to leave cells resulting in cell death and may be so overwhelming that they cause systemic impacts including cardiac dysrhythmias and death.[1,3,9]

Cement injury is due to its action as both an alkali and desiccant. It contains calcium oxide, which becomes calcium hydroxide when exposed to water. Cement injury can be insidious as it may be initially painless. The cement dust may adhere to skin and be activated by perspiration, with injury not becoming evident until hours later.[1,3,10]

Gasoline and other hydrocarbons are corrosive agents. Prolonged exposure may cause cell membrane damage to lipid cell membranes causing dissolution and resulting in cell death. Rapid evaporation can additionally cause cellular dehydration and cold injury from heat loss.[3]

Tar and asphalt are long-chain hydrocarbons. Because they are heated in application, they may cause both thermal and chemical injury. The immediate concern is for thermal injury as they retain heat for a prolonged period and may require extensive cooling. After cooling, tar can be removed with mineral oil, medical solvent, antibiotic ointments, or baby oil.[7,8]

Assessment

The assessment of the patient with burn injuries begins with the ABCDEs of the primary assessment. Burn wounds are often dramatic in appearance, becoming a significant distraction, and can take the transport team's attention away from more immediate life-threatening problems.

The subjective assessment includes as thorough a history as circumstances permit. Obtain as much information as possible from the patient or bystanders and family. The history should include the mechanism and time of the injury and a description of the surrounding environment, such as injuries incurred in an enclosed space, the presence of noxious chemicals, the possibility of smoke inhalation, and any related trauma. The time of the injury is especially important in the calculation of fluid resuscitation. Information regarding tetanus immunization status, allergies, past medical history, and medications should also be obtained with the history.[1,2]

Thermal Burns

Assessment of a thermal burn includes estimating the burn size and depth, associated inhalation injuries, and calculation of fluid resuscitation needs. The size of a burn wound is most frequently estimated with the rule of nines[1-3] method, which divides the body into multiples of 9% (Fig. 19.4). A more accurate assessment can be made of the burn injury, especially for pediatric patients, with a Lund and Browder chart[1-3] which considers growth changes (Fig. 19.5). For estimating scattered burns, an approximation can be made with the patient's entire palmar surface including the fingers, extended and joined with thumb along the hand, to represent 1% of the total TBSA and visualization of that palm over the burned area. Use of electronic assessment tools is becoming popular because these tools not only increase the accuracy of assessment but also enhance continuity of care because they are easily transmitted to each level of caregiver.[1-3]

Primarily, the temperature of the burning agent, the duration of exposure, and the conductance of the tissue involved determine the depth of a thermal burn wound. Initially, the estimation of injury depth is difficult. An accurate determination of depth is often not possible until the wound is cleaned and debridement has occurred. Products of combustion may impair evaluation and overlying blisters may hide an underlying full-thickness injury. This presents a significant challenge in the out-of-hospital environment and may explain the common disparity between initial estimates and those obtained in tertiary care.

Burn wounds typically present in a bull's-eye pattern, with each ring representing a different zone of intensity, first described in 1953 and referred to as Jackson's zones of injury, where zones of necrosis, stasis, and hyperemia were described.[3] The zone of necrosis is the area of nonviable tissue and is the area of greatest damage. The zone of stasis is an area of tissue that is at risk of becoming nonviable but may recover. The zone of hyperemia is at the periphery of the wound and consists of viable, perfused tissue.[3]

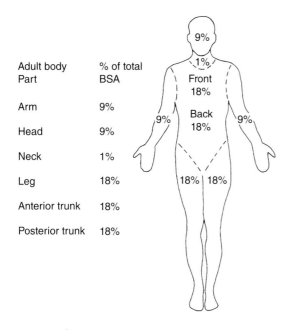

Adult body Part	% of total BSA
Arm	9%
Head	9%
Neck	1%
Leg	18%
Anterior trunk	18%
Posterior trunk	18%

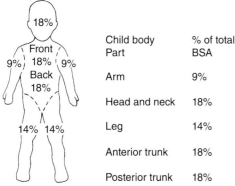

Child body Part	% of total BSA
Arm	9%
Head and neck	18%
Leg	14%
Anterior trunk	18%
Posterior trunk	18%

• **Figure 19.4** Rule of nines.

Burn depth describes the extent of tissue damage and is related to the zones of stasis. A *superficial* injury, or first-degree burn, involves the epidermis and is represented by the outermost ring, the zone of hyperemia. This type of injury is usually red in appearance, is painful, and heals in a matter of days. As discussion progresses to burn resuscitation, it is critical to note these areas are not included in calculation of TBSA for resuscitation.[1,3]

A *partial-thickness* injury, or second-degree burn, involves both the epidermis and dermis. This burn is representative of the zone of stasis, which is potentially viable tissue, despite the heat injury. This wound is characterized by reddened skin that is wet or blistered, is painful, and may heal in 14 to 21 days.[3] However, overlying blisters may be misleading because a full-thickness burn can be evident beneath. As this tissue is at risk, it may also convert to a full-thickness burn, especially in the presence of infection or hypoperfusion.[1,3]

Full-thickness or third-degree burn injuries are the center ring, called the zone of coagulation. These injuries encompass wounds that consist of both dermal layers and extend into the subcutaneous tissue. Subdermal burns destroy both layers of tissue and extend into fat, muscle, and bone. These are sometimes referred to as fourth-, fifth-, and sixth-degree burns, respectively.[3] Full-thickness injuries may appear leathery in appearance or white and waxy, with thrombosed vessels that are easily visible under the surface.[1,3] They are painless because of destruction of sensory nerves, with no epithelial

growth for healing. These wounds necessitate surgical excision and grafting to reduce scarring and contractures.

Inhalation Injuries With Thermal Burns

The three types of identifiable inhalation injuries are (1) carbon monoxide and or cyanide poisoning; (2) supraglottic injury, which is primarily thermal in nature; and (3) subglottic injury, which is primarily chemical in nature. Inhalation injuries are the primary cause of death at the scene of a burn injury, and they contribute significantly to the overall morbidity and mortality rates of burn patients.[1–3]

Carbon monoxide poisoning occurs because the affinity for carbon monoxide to hemoglobin is markedly greater than that of oxygen (approximately 200 times greater); therefore, the carbon monoxide displaces the oxygen and binds with the available hemoglobin to form carboxyhemoglobin, with resultant hypoxia.[1] The signs and symptoms of carbon monoxide poisoning include tachycardia, tachypnea, headache, dizziness, and nausea. Carboxyhemoglobin levels are necessary in determining the management approach for these patients. Levels of 0% to 15% rarely cause symptoms and may be normal, especially for a heavy smoker. Levels of 15% to 40% cause varying amounts of central nervous system disturbances, such as confusion and headache. Levels greater than 40% can cause mental status changes and coma. Any patient with suspected carbon monoxide injury should be given 100% oxygen; this would include any patient involved in an enclosed space fire such as a structure or vehicle.[1–3,11] If carbon monoxide poisoning is present, pulse oximetry becomes inaccurate as it does not differentiate oxygen from carbon monoxide bound to hemoglobin.[1] The half-life of carbon monoxide is approximately 4 hours. This is decreased to around 40 minutes by breathing 100% oxygen, either by mask or endotracheal intubation.[1,3,11] As carbon monoxide is not differentiated by pulse oximetry, patients may be hypoxic with a normal SpO$_2$. When carbon monoxide poisoning is present or suspected, delivered oxygen cannot be down-titrated without using a carboxyhemoglobin level.

Hyperbaric oxygen therapy (HBOT) remains a topic that requires additional study. High-flow oxygen at 100% is agreed to be the most important initial treatment. Several studies have shown benefits in the reduction of long-term neurological sequala with the use of HBOT, but high-quality prospective studies are needed before definitive guidelines can be established.[11] Careful consideration should be given in cases of cardiac ischemia, pregnancy, unconsciousness, neurologic deficits, and very high carboxyhemoglobin levels.[11] As many hyperbaric centers are not burn centers and many burn centers lack hyperbaric capability, flight crews should be familiar with local resources and transport destinations guided by program guidelines.

Hydrogen cyanide is given off when man-made materials are burned. Inhaled cyanide interferes with mitochondrial function, altering ATP production by aerobic metabolism and may produce profound metabolic acidosis. Patients may present with agitation, altered mental status or loss of consciousness, profound acidosis that is unresponsive to resuscitation, or be found dead at the scene. While a confirmatory readily available test does not exist, a number of indicators including lactate level greater than 10 mmol/L, TBSA <15% with smoke inhalation, and/or decreased level of consciousness (GCS <14) should be considered a presumptive positive. Given the lack of confirmatory test and the catastrophic damage that may ensue, treatment with hydroxycobalamin should be initiated early based on index of suspicion.[1,3,12]

Age	0–1	1–4	5–9	1–14	15
A – ½ of head	9 ½ %	8 ½ %	6 ½ %	5 ½ %	4 ½ %
B – ½ of one thigh	2 ¾ %	3 ¼ %	4%	4 ¼ %	4 ½ %
C – ½ of one thigh	2 ½ %	2 ½ %	2 ¾ %	3%	3 ¼ %

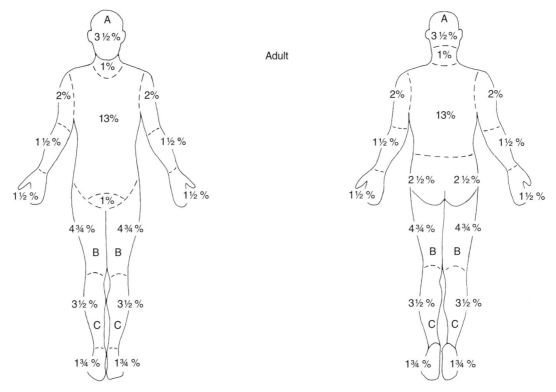

• **Figure 19.5** Lund and Browder method for calculating percentage of burned body surface area.

Supraglottic injury should be suspected when deep facial burns, singed facial hair, or carbonaceous sputum are present. Other signs and symptoms of upper airway injury include the presence of redness or sloughing of mucosal tissue in the oropharynx, stridor, wheezing, or any other sign of respiratory difficulty. Absence of these signs and symptoms initially does not exclude the possibility of inhalation injury because upper airway edema may not be present until after the onset of fluid resuscitation.[1,2]

Subglottic injury is often more difficult to diagnose because the injury is progressive in nature and not visible to the prehospital provider. Apart from steam, it is caused by the inhalation of the particulate by-products of combustion. The resultant chemical injury leads to impaired ciliary function, inflammation, mucous hypersecretion, inactivation of surfactant, bronchospasm, and microemboli, which combine to lead to a ventilation/perfusion mismatch. The primary symptom is hypoxemia that is resistant to oxygen therapy. Severity of injury is difficult to assess initially as the process may worsen over time. Any patient with suspected inhalation injuries should be closely observed for 24 hours for onset of respiratory complications.[1,2]

Electrical Injuries

If the patient becomes part of the circuit, they may incur direct-contact burns. These wounds may appear devastating, and they frequently resemble a crush injury rather than a burn (Fig. 19.6). The most common point of entry is the hand or skull, and the most common exit site is the feet. The sizes of these entrance and exit wounds are no real indicator of the amount of damage done to internal tissue. When the current leaves the body on its course to the ground, arc burns occur. The arcing current produces extremely high energies, ranging from 3000°C to 20,000°C.[3] Wounds are deeper because the heat intensity is closer to the body. Deep partial-thickness and full-thickness thermal burns may be indistinguishable when the heat source is more distant from the body.

Cutaneous injuries from electrical contact are frequently apparent because the skin is the first point of contact with the electrical current. Dry skin has a greater resistance than wet skin, producing greater generation of heat and subsequently a larger burn. AC produces overriding tetanic contractions of the flexor muscle of the upper extremities, causing prolonged exposure. As a result, the patient may present with contractures and the inability to be positioned in positions of extension, especially after high voltage injury. Destruction of muscle tissue from deep injury may lead to compartment syndrome and rhabdomyolysis. Tissue necrosis can lead to dangerous hyperkalemia, hypocalcemia, and the resulting electrolyte imbalance can precipitate cardiac dysrhythmia. High levels of myoglobin can cause renal tubular obstruction and lead to renal failure.[1–3,5]

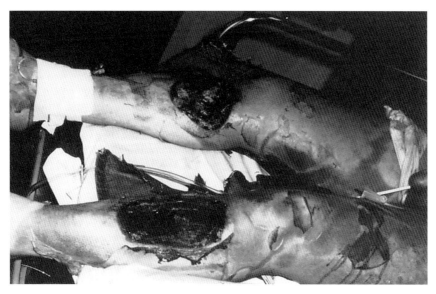

• **Figure 19.6** Direct-contact burns resembling crush injuries.

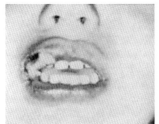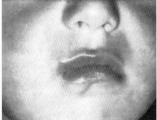

• **Figure 19.7** Oral commissure burns in a child less than 2 years of age.

Oral commissure burns are commonly seen in children under the age of 2 years. These burns are typically caused by a child chewing or sucking on a household (110-V) electrical cord. This type of burn is frequently localized but can cause associated injuries to the tongue, palate, and face (Fig. 19.7).

Lightning Injuries

Lightning injuries are dissimilar to those caused by high-voltage contact; therefore, the effects and injuries differ. A lightning bolt may have a voltage of up to 1 billion volts and induce currents greater than 200,000 A. Although the intensity of lightning is much greater than high-voltage electricity, the duration of exposure is much shorter, ranging from 1/10 to 1/100 of a second. Because of this shorter duration, skin burns are less severe than those burns seen with high-voltage injuries.[1,13,14] Linear and punctate burns are frequently seen with lightning injuries, and feathering burns are pathognomonic to lightning injuries.[15] With a lightning strike, the electrical current turns moisture on the skin to steam and frequently blows off or shreds clothing or shoes (Fig. 19.8). Blunt trauma is frequently associated with lightning injuries and is caused when the victims are hurled to the ground by the current.[1,13,14] A victim may suffer a direct strike from a lightning bolt or may experience a splash injury. The splash injury occurs when lightning strikes an object and the stroke jumps to another object that acts as a better conductor. This mechanism causes multiple lightning strikes in people standing in close proximity to an object or to another individual who has been struck.

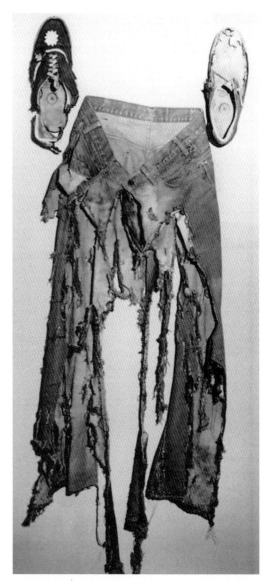

• **Figure 19.8** Clothing of a patient struck by lightning.

Patients with minor injuries usually are conscious; however, they may have lost consciousness transiently and are frequently confused and amnesic. Patients with moderate lightning injuries show more obvious altered mentation and may be combative or comatose. They may fall or be thrown down forcibly from the current, which may cause fractures and dislocations. Therefore, associated trauma such as thoracic or abdominal injury should be considered. Superficial and deep partial-thickness burns may be apparent with a moderate lightning strike injury as well as tympanic membrane rupture caused by the explosive force of the lightning strike. Difficulty in palpating peripheral pulses and a mottled appearance of the patient's lower extremities is caused by arteriospasm and is frequently characteristic of a moderate injury. The condition usually clears in a few hours. Severe lightning injuries can be more dramatic. If the lightning current passes through the brain, the DC or blast effect caused by the strike may damage the brain. The patient is comatose and may possibly be undergoing a seizure. A closed head injury caused by a fall must also be considered in these cases.[1,2,13,14]

Lightning may cause paralysis to the medullary respiratory center, first causing respiratory arrest and then cardiac arrest. If immediate ventilation does not occur, a subsequent cardiac arrest follows, and brain death occurs from anoxia. Multiple dysrhythmias are associated with lightning strikes, including ventricular tachycardia, premature ventricular contractions, and atrial fibrillation. ST changes associated with ischemia are also common. Many ocular injuries have been reported, including detached retina, hyphema, direct thermal burn, corneal lesion, and cataract. As with electrical injuries, cataracts may appear as late as 2 years after the strike, but they are most commonly present in the first few days after the injury. Patients must be assessed for other signs of trauma caused by the impact of the strike and for life-threatening injuries.[1,13,14] For the pregnant victim of a lightning strike, the prognosis of the unborn child is difficult to determine. As with all burn injuries, resuscitation of the mother is the primary concern.[1,2]

Chemical Burn Injuries

Chemical burns differ from thermal burns in that the burning process continues until the agent is inactivated by reaction with the tissues, is neutralized, or is diluted with water. The degree of damage by a chemical agent depends on the concentration and quantity of the agent, its mechanism of action, the amount of body surface area involved, and the duration of contact. Alkalis cause deeper and more significant wounds than acids.[1,3,4]

Radiation Burn Injuries

Exposure to radiation can damage cellular DNA, cause erythema and thermal appearing injury as well as contamination by ingestion, inhalation, or absorption. The degree of injury depends on the type of radiation, duration of exposure, distance, and shielding, as well as the sensitivity of the exposed tissue. While alpha particles may be stopped by the skin and only pathologic if consumed, beta particles may cause burns up to full thickness. The eye is especially susceptible to radiation injury. Gamma particles may penetrate the skin and cause diffuse cellular damage (total burn). Early effects of radiation injury may start with nausea and vomiting in combination with cutaneous injury. With larger doses, there may be early cardiovascular collapse.[3]

Management of Burn Injury

Transport of a burn patient requires an orderly prioritized approach. Equipment and supplies should be organized in advance, when possible, to expedite assessment and stabilization of the burn patient. Although supplies and equipment vary among transport programs, depending on protocols and primary service populations, little is needed beyond the standard emergency medical supplies to provide quality burn care. Sheets and blankets should be carried even in the summertime to prevent hypothermia during transport.

Scene Safety

If transport of the burn patient involves scene response, the safety of all responders must be ensured. Safety precautions may include vigilance for toxic substances with the victim of a chemical burn, extinguishing sources of flame for the thermal burn, or use of special personnel and equipment for removal of electrical lines. In the case of chemical injury, thorough decontamination and donning of appropriate personal protective equipment should take place before patient contact by transport team. This is especially important for drivers and pilots of the vehicles. Communication with ground personnel regarding the type of scene and landing zone is mandatory before approaching.

Removing the victim from any source of electrical current may place rescuers at risk. Wooden poles, rubber gloves, and ropes are not without risk and should be used only by those trained to work with electricity. The transport team must not assume that a downed wire is not dangerous because it is not producing sparks and because the surrounding areas are dark. Extrication is safe only when the power is turned off and confirmed by utility specialist. If victims must be removed immediately because of injury, only trained individuals should attempt to do so.

Primary Survey

Management of the burn patient begins with the ABCDEs of the primary survey, including airway, breathing, and circulation, with a brief baseline neurologic examination. During assessments and interventions for life-threatening problems in the primary survey, the transport team should take precautions to maintain cervical spine immobilization if trauma is suspected. The transport team must be sure that the burning process has been stopped, which may require copious irrigation of the burn wound, as in the case of chemical burns, or simple removal of clothing and jewelry from the patient. The patient must be protected from further injury, and the safety of the transport team members must be ensured. The primary survey should then be performed.[1,2]

Airway/Breathing/Inhalation Injury Management

Intubation may need to be accomplished early because it could become impossible later with the onset of edema after the initiation of fluid replacement to manage the burned patient's airway. Assessment for dyspnea is more difficult during transport because of the noise and vibration, so the transport team should learn to rely on other parameters for assessment of respiratory status.[1,2] Securing an endotracheal tube (ETT) may be difficult because tape, which is most often used, does not adhere to burned skin. Commercial ETT holders should be the standard in the out-of-hospital environment.

Inhalation injury is considered one of the most frequent causes of death in burn patients.[1,3] Management includes careful assessment of the airway and rapid early intervention for signs of obstruction. Early intubation, before massive edema formation, may be required in patients with supraglottic injury. Administration of humidified oxygen helps minimize inspissation of secretions, and frequent suctioning helps remove accumulated secretions. Use of bronchodilators may be helpful for minimizing bronchospasm and encouraging mucociliary clearance. Other medications that may be used include N-acetylcysteine alone as a mucolytic agent or in combination with heparin as scavengers for oxygen-free radicals that are produced by activation of alveolar macrophages or nitric oxide to decrease pulmonary vasoconstriction. Heparin may also reduce the incidence of microemboli, use of inhaled heparin has little systemic uptake,[3] and the use of these is driven by regional protocols, and it may be more appropriate to start them in an in-patient setting. Mechanical ventilation during transport should begin with low tidal volumes and low airway pressures to minimize ventilator-associated lung trauma.[3]

Circulation/Fluid Resuscitation

Two intravenous (IV) lines should be initiated peripherally with large-bore catheters. The fluid of choice for initial resuscitation is LR, but normal saline may be used initially if LR is not available.[1–3] LR most closely mimics intravascular fluid. The use of LR also avoids causing metabolic acidosis associated with large volume administration of normal saline.[1,3] Ideally, lines should be placed in nonburned areas, but they may be placed through the burn if they are the only veins available for cannulation. IO lines are also acceptable, preferentially through nonburned skin. IV lines should be well secured because venous access may not be available peripherally after the onset of generalized edema. The goal of initial fluid resuscitation is to restore and maintain adequate tissue perfusion and vital organ function, in addition to preserving heat-injured but viable tissue in the zone of stasis while preventing complications of over or underresuscitation.[1–3] Fluid needs are based on the size of the patient and the extent of the burn. As there is a predominance of overresuscitation prior to arrival at tertiary burn care, the American Burn Association (ABA) now recommends a simplified resuscitation during EMS care and transport and during the primary survey on hospital arrival. If the burn is estimated to be greater than 20% TBSA, the following rates should serve as a starting point.[1]

- 14 years and older: 500 mL/hr of LR
- 6 to 13 years old: 250 mL/hr of LR
- 5 years and younger: 125 mL/hr of LR

These rates are a simple starting point to resuscitation. Once weight in kilograms is established and an accurate TBSA can be calculated, these rates are adjusted, and fluid rate is titrated based on urine output.[1,2] Fluid resuscitation approach may vary regionally. The formulae most used for estimating fluid needs are the Parkland formula, which is 4 mL × kg × % total BSA (TBSA) burned, and the modified Brooke, which is 2 mL × kg × % TBSA burned. In both, one-half of the total amount of fluids should be given over the first 8 hours from the time of the injury, with the second half to be given over the following 16 hours.[3] The reduction in fluid rate, however, is not automatic after the eighth hour. The formulas only represent estimates of fluid needs; fluid rates are titrated based on urine output throughout the resuscitation.[1,3] The commonality in resuscitation formulas is that resuscitation is focused on fluid replacement over time, based on weight and TBSA, and guided by urine output. The replacement of fluid matches the

loss of fluid from the burn, as this is a gradual loss over time that is proportionate to weight and TBSA. Additionally, focus is on greater fluid loss over the first 8 hours post burn. This is due to the increase in capillary permeability being greatest in this timeframe. Until the 8-hour mark post burn, colloids should be avoided. The difference in the formulae centers on the amount of fluid per kg of body weight. Currently, the ABA recommends varying rates based on age and mechanism. All resuscitation formulae are a starting point only; regardless of the formula used, urine output guides fluid titration.

Adult (14 years and older) Thermal and Chemical Burns should receive 2 mL × weight in kg × TBSA % of second- and third-degree burns in the first 24 hours. Half of the volume is given over the first 8 hours and the remainder over the next 16 hours.[1]

Example:

An adult with 30% TBSA burns (excluding first degree) with a weight of 85 kg:

2 mL × 30 × 85 = 5100 mL in the first 24 hours

Half in the first 8 hours = 2550

The hourly rate if the burn just occurred would be 319 mL/hr. If the resuscitation start was delayed by 2 hours, the hourly rate would be divided by the remaining 6 hours = 425 mL/hr.

Pediatric Patients (13 years and younger) should receive 3 mL × weight in kg × TBSA % of second- and third-degree burns in the first 24 hours. Half of the volume is given over the first 8 hours and the remainder over the next 16 hours.[1]

Example:

A 10-year-old with 50% TBSA burns (excluding first degree) with a weight of 35 kg:

3 mL × 50 × 35 = 5250 mL in first 24 hours

Half in the first 8 hours = 2625

Hourly rate = 328 mL/hr

Children weighing less than 30 kg are recommended to have an additional infusion of D5 LR at a maintenance rate. This is due to their increased metabolic demands and decreased ability to store glycogen.

Adult patients with high voltage electrical injury and evidence of myoglobinuria Should receive 4 mL × weight in kg × TBSA % in the first 24 hours. Half of the volume is given over the first 8 hours and the remainder over the next 16 hours.[1]

Example:

An adult with 35% TBSA second- and three-degree burns from a high voltage electrical injury and myoglobinuria with a weight of 100 kg.

4 mL × 35 × 100 = 14,000 mL in the first 24 hours

Half in the first 8 hours = 7000 mL

Hourly rate = 875 mL/hr

These adjusted rates are a starting point. The rate must be adjusted based on hourly urine output, measured with an indwelling catheter. Target urine output for adults is 0.5 mL/kg/hr or 30 to 50 mL/hr. Target urine output for pediatric patients is 1 mL/kg/hr. Patients with high voltage injury and myoglobinuria should have a target rate of 75 to 100 mL/hr until the pigmentation has cleared. If the urine output is below the goal, the resuscitation infusion should be increased by up to one-third every hour until the target output is achieved. If urine output is above goal, the resuscitation fluid should be decreased by up to one-third hourly until urine output is at the target volume.[1]

It is important to continue this titration even past the eighth hour. Resuscitation fluids should not be automatically cut in half but should continue to be titrated based on the urine output. Titration based on urine output assumes normal baseline renal function. Preexisting renal disease complicates resuscitation and may be driven by a variety of other data points. This should be done in collaboration with the receiving burn center.

Both over- and underresuscitation have negative outcomes for the patient. The current theory of "fluid creep" (fluid administered in excess of predicted amounts) would suggest that patients are frequently being overresuscitated by more than 1.5 times the highest recommended amount of fluid. Often fluids are overprescribed and overdelivered prior to arrival at tertiary burn care.[16] Overresuscitation can lead to excessive edema formation, damaging viable tissue, contributing to cerebral and pulmonary edema/ARDS, and compartment syndromes of the extremities and abdomen. Underresuscitation may lead to increased capillary permeability, acute kidney injury related to hypovolemia, shock, and organ failure.[1,3]

Burn Wound Management

Care of the burn wound includes covering the burned area with a dry, clean dressing and, in the case of a large burn wound, placing the patient on one dry, clean sheet and covering with blankets added over the sheets as needed. Wet dressings should not be used because they provide an open pathway for bacteria, cause additional tissue injury, and leave the patient at risk of hypothermia because of loss of skin integrity from the burn injury. Hand burns should not be submerged in water beyond the initial cooling. This can lead to wound conversion from partial to full thickness and wound maceration.[1,3]

The burn patient should be covered with blankets to avoid hypothermia, and IV fluids should ideally be warmed. There are some commercial wound care products are available. These should not be used without consulting a burn center.

Circumferential burns to the chest or extremities represent the more easily recognizable complications in burn care. Circumferential burns to the chest wall decrease chest wall compliance, creating respiratory insufficiency and hypoxia, especially in the pediatric population in which chest walls are more pliable. This problem can be further aggravated by generalized edema, especially in overresuscitation. In patients receiving mechanical ventilation, the decreased compliance to the chest wall may result in high peak airway pressures. Prior to the availability of advanced mechanical ventilation modes in transport, there may have been a greater need for chest wall escharotomies prior to arrival in tertiary burn care. With the common availability of advanced modes of ventilation outside the hospital, this need has been lessened. Utilization of ventilation and oxygenation strategies such as higher peep, lower tidal volumes with higher respiratory rates, inverse I:E ratio, and advanced pressure modes of ventilation should be attempted first. If unable to oxygenate and ventilate despite attempts to optimize ventilation mechanically, chest wall escharotomy may be necessary with consultation from receiving burn center.[1]

Circumferential burns to the extremities or digits can be equally threatening to the circulatory stability of the affected limb, producing the "5 Ps" that represent the signs and symptoms of compartment syndrome: pain, pallor, pulselessness, paresthesia, and paralysis. A Doppler scan device may be helpful in locating pulses in a particularly edematous area, but loss of pulses is a late sign of compartment syndrome. Circumferential burns should be elevated above the level of the heart to prevent compartment syndrome. IV access should be avoided, if possible, in extremities with circumferential burns. If no other access is available, monitor the limb carefully and keep elevated. Blood pressure cuffs should be avoided on limbs with circumferential burn wounds.[1,3]

Escharotomies are the definitive way to deal with compression from circumferential burns (Figs. 19.9 and 19.10). However, because

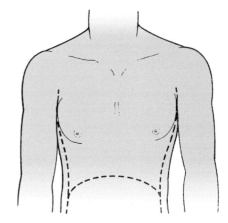

• **Figure 19.9** Chest escharotomy sites.

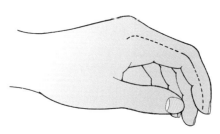

• **Figure 19.10** Escharotomy site on the finger.

this skill is difficult to teach and maintain, some recommendations are that a decompression technique should not be used until a skilled provider is available. This method should be used in patients with concern for compartment syndrome secondary to circumferential burn injury. Consider performing escharotomies as soon as possible; however, it should be performed by a trained provider who can manage the potential complications as well as assess the adequacy of the procedure. (See Box 19.1 for possible escharotomy sites.) Major vessels, nerves, tendons, ligaments, and joints should be avoided because future range of motion can be adversely affected. Results of the escharotomy should be carefully monitored. In most cases, relief of the constriction should be immediate.[1,3]

Patients with circumferential extremity burns can sometimes have their edema managed through elevation of the limb, avoiding compressive dressings, and avoiding IV access in the limb. This is a temporary response to the problem and requires constant clinical reassessment. When in doubt, coordinate care with the closest verified burn center.

For those burn patients who may not be transported until later in the disease process or those who may need long-distance transport to receive care, some debriding and dressings may be necessary. Mild soap and water may be used to clean simple burns. Blisters should be managed according to the burn center's wound care protocols, or in direct collaboration with medical control from the receiving burn center.

When cleaning burns that are the result of contact with tar or asphalt, after the burning process has been stopped, there is little urgency to remove tar in the prehospital environment. The removal of these substances helps decrease the patient's pain.[7] Removal of tar may be considered if transport is delayed and does not interfere with other priorities. Several methods are described in literature. Mineral oil and antibiotic ointment are two readily available products to help facilitate tar removal.[4,9]

•BOX 19.1   Possible Escharotomy Sites

Chest

Anterior axillary incisions bilaterally joined with a transverse incision along the costal margin (Fig. 19.9).

Extremities

Axially on medial or lateral aspect; if a single incision is insufficient to relieve the constriction, then an incision on both sides should be performed.

Elbow

Medial aspect anterior to the medial epicondyle.

Hand

Axially on the dorsum, between the tendons rather than across them.

Fingers

Midlateral axial (Fig. 19.10).

Ankle

Medial aspect anterior to medial malleolus.

Foot

Axially on the dorsum between the tendons rather than across them.

Pain Management

Burn pain varies depending on the burn injury type, body parts involved, depth, and size. Partial-thickness burns are more painful than full-thickness burns, as the full-thickness burn has damaged the pain receptors, while a partial-thickness burn has not. Factors that can affect burn pain include actual stimulation of nociceptors, fear of procedures, and anxiety regarding change in body image. Regardless of what types of medications are administered, they should all be given IV in the initial management.[1] The generalized edema during this time allows for only sporadic absorption of the medication if given intramuscularly. As fluid shifts reverse, a "dumping" and potential overdose of any medications that were given intramuscularly can occur.[14] The exception to this is a tetanus booster, which can be given intramuscularly.

For acute burn injury pain, opioids are the analgesic of choice, with or without anxiolytic sedatives, such as benzodiazepines.[1,3] Nonopioid analgesics that have proven effective include medications such as ketamine and dexmedetomidine for short periods for procedures. Additional pain management techniques, such as diversion, reassurance, and repositioning, may also be beneficial.

Antibiotics

Antibiotics should be given only at the direction of the receiving burn center. Systemic antibiotics are not indicated in the initial care of burns. In cases of delayed presentation with signs of cellulitis, they may be considered with medical direction. Infection prevention is centered around wound care, keeping open wounds clean and dry.[3,17]

Other Transport Considerations

Electrocardiographic monitoring should be instituted on any patient with a large burn, an electrical injury, or preexisting heart disease.[7,14] Electrode patches may be a problem to place because the adhesive does not stick to burned skin. A urinary catheter with a urometer should be placed to accurately monitor urinary output. As with intubation, the catheter should be inserted early, especially for the patient with perineal burns, because edema may make later insertion impossible.

To combat the problem of adynamic ileus, the transport team should consider insertion of a gastric tube in all burn patients with significant burns to decompress the stomach. This process is especially important for the patient being transported at high altitudes or for extended transport times. Initial diagnostic studies should include hematocrit and electrolyte levels, urinalysis, chest radiograph, arterial blood gases with carboxyhemoglobin levels as indicated, and electrocardiography.[1,3]

Accurate documentation of all treatment provided before and during transport of the burn patient is essential. This information provides the necessary history of the incident and its initial treatment to allow for consistent and quality planning of patient care at the receiving facility. Documentation of time of injury and accounting for all fluids received prior to arrival at the burn center are required for continuation of fluid resuscitation.

Electrical Injury Management

As soon as the scene is secured, and the patient is away from the current, primary and secondary assessment can proceed. Dysrhythmias should be treated with advanced cardiac life support algorithms or the transport program's individual protocols. Evaluation for cardiac injury is important because of the high incidence of dysrhythmias and autonomic dysfunction with electrical exposure.[1,5]

Cervical spine injury is of special concern for victims of electrical injury because of possible blunt trauma and because of severe tetanic contractions caused by the electrical current; therefore, the cervical and thoracic spine must be immobilized.[1]

Assessment of the area of surface burns is difficult because deep injury may be produced. Adequate volume replacement, treatment of acidosis, and management of myoglobinuria must also be initiated. Fluid replacement should start with the prehospital recommendations based on age. Once a more accurate evaluation is made, resuscitation is adjusted with the electrical injury formula.

Higher rates of urinary output are essential to maintain because hemoglobinuria and myoglobinuria are common with electrical injuries.[1,3,5] The fluid resuscitation must be based on actual urine flow. A minimum urine output of 100 mL/hr should be maintained for adults and 1.5 to 2.0 mL/kg/hr for children until myoglobinuria has cleared.[1,3,5]

Lactic acidosis is common because of significant muscle damage caused by electrical injury. Sodium bicarbonate may be used to alkalinize the urine. Mannitol may be considered in the resuscitative phase to increase urinary output and to minimize acute tubular necrosis, but this may complicate urine output–driven fluid resuscitation by artificially increasing urine output.[3]

Lightning Injury Management

Primary survey does not differ with the victim of a lightning strike. The patient's cardiopulmonary status must be assessed immediately, and cardiopulmonary resuscitation should be initiated on finding the patient in cardiac arrest. As with any unknown injury, the cervical spine must be immobilized before intubation and transport. The patient's cardiac status must be monitored continuously to evaluate for potential dysrhythmias.

Cutaneous burns seen with lightning injuries are often not as extensive as those seen with high-voltage injuries, unless there is secondary ignition of clothing or surrounding environment. If significant cutaneous burns are present resuscitation should take place based on electrical injury guidelines.

In cases where multiple victims are present, reverse disaster triage may be performed with patients in arrest receiving immediate treatment. Cardiac arrest after lightning strike may be reversible with immediate treatment and favorable postarrest outcomes have been noted. Patients may suffer a respiratory arrest that leads to cardiac arrest and assisted ventilation and airway management may prevent this.[1,3,13,14]

Chemical Injury Management

Treatment of chemical injuries necessitates removal of all saturated clothing and a copious irrigation of the burn wound, with providers undertaking appropriate personal protection. In the patient with an otherwise stable condition, wound irrigation, and decontamination takes priority over transportation to prevent the spread of contamination to transport vehicles and providers.[1,4] Duration of irrigation has not been established as a standard but recommended times span 30 minutes to 1 hour. Evaluation of wound pH has been used as a tool to verify adequacy but may not be available in the prehospital environment.[1,4] Thermoregulation should be guarded during decontamination to prevent complications of hypothermia.

Dry chemicals such as lime should be brushed off before irrigation. Water with low pressure can be used for wound irrigation.[1,4] Neutralizing agents may be more harmful than simply irrigating with water. The exogenous heat production by neutralization reaction can cause further tissue destruction. In the treatment of chemical burns, the transport team must be aware of the possibility of exposure to the noxious agents and don appropriate protective gear before coming into contact with the patient or the patient's clothing.[1,3,4]

Burns involving hydrofluoric acid present a special consideration due to the agent's ability to bind calcium and systemic potential for hypocalcemia that may produce dysrhythmias. After irrigating the wound, dressings containing calcium may be applied. Combining calcium chloride, gluconate, or carbonate with a water-soluble gel, applying to the wound, and covering with a dressing should be considered if available and time permits. In severe cases, replacement of IV calcium may be necessary as indicated by ECG changes or if serum monitoring is available.[1,4,9]

Radiation Injury Management

Radiation burns are treated like other kinds of burns as the initial injuries occur from the heat of the explosion. Victims of radiation injury should initially be treated by those trained in managing hazardous materials and transport by specially trained teams may be required. The focus beyond the lifesaving measures is to avoid contaminating the transport team and the transport vehicle and limiting further damage. Contaminated clothing must be removed and prolonged gentle irrigation with water or saline with gentle cleansing of intact skin. Resuscitation should be undertaken in the same manner as thermal injury and guided by urine output.[3]

Evaluation

Evaluation of the burn patient consists primarily of assessment of the effectiveness of problem intervention and the recognition of future potential complications. Not all complications are, however, predictable, or correctable.

Vital signs are not the most accurate method of monitoring a patient with a large burn because of the pathophysiologic changes that accompany such an injury. Blood pressure may be difficult to ascertain because of increasing generalized edema. An invasive monitoring device may not be accurate because of the peripheral vasoconstriction caused by release of vasoactive mediators such as catecholamines. Tachycardia of 100 to 120 is common in patients with major burn injuries.[1-3] This may be a product of catecholamine response, inflammatory mediators, hypovolemia, concurrent trauma, pain, or systemic poisons. Unexpected relative bradycardia warrants further investigation, as there may be confounding preexisting medications such as beta-blockers or preexisting cardiac disease. Tachycardia beyond 120 beats per minute also warrants investigation of the adequacy of resuscitation, concurrent trauma, or systemic poisoning. A decrease in level of consciousness not associated with trauma may also be indicative of hypoxia or hypovolemia. This problem should be alleviated with appropriate adjustments in ventilatory and circulatory support. If the level of consciousness does not improve with increased hydration and oxygenation, other problem sources such as carbon monoxide/cyanide poisoning or electrolyte imbalance should be suspected and investigated.[1,3,12]

The urinary output should be maintained at 30 to 50 mL an hour in adults and 1 to 1.5 mL/kg/hr for children less than 30 kg. Electrical injury with myoglobinuria should have a target urine output of 75 to 100 mL an hour.[1] Oliguria is an indication of inadequate fluid volume and should be easily corrected by increasing the rate of fluid administration. When this method is ineffective and fluid volume needs have been accurately assessed and administered, other causes should be investigated. If urine output does not respond to volume resuscitation, consult the receiving burn center for direction. Myoglobinuria that occurs from the release of myoglobin after deep muscle damage can precipitate in the renal tubules and cause acute renal failure. This problem is especially common after electrical burns, and urine should be monitored in such cases for color changes (dark tea color) that indicate the presence of myoglobin. Alkalinization of the urine through the addition of bicarbonate to the IV fluids is done to prevent the myoglobin from progressing to its nephrotoxic metabolites. Osmotic diuretics such as mannitol may help dilute the urine and flush the renal tubules, but they may confound burn resuscitation by artificially inflating urine output. In transport, this should only be done at the request of the receiving burn center.

Pulmonary edema can occur from either overzealous fluid resuscitation or smoke inhalation injury, and the transport team should be careful to monitor respiratory function as fluid administration progresses. This problem is especially apparent when the transport of the burn patient has been delayed.[3]

Hyperkalemia from potassium released from the damaged tissues can be reversed in several ways, including administration of sodium bicarbonate, glucose and insulin, or ion exchange resins. Hypoglycemia is a complication that frequently occurs in infants and young children because of their inability to maintain adequate glycogen stores. Blood glucose should be assessed frequently for pediatric patients. Maintenance rate lactated Ringer's solution with 5% dextrose should be administered in patients <30 kg to prevent hypoglycemia.[1]

Impact of Transport

The prehospital care of patients with major burns can have a significant impact on their outcomes. The initial management, if done properly, can prevent the complication of over- and underresuscitation, improving the survivability of salvageable tissue.

As these injuries can be dramatic and severe, the expertise of a well-trained transport team can be an asset to the prehospital providers and community hospital emergency departments.

Incorrect resuscitation, burn estimation, and management of inhalation injuries are common prior to admission to tertiary burn care. Fluids are often overprescribed and over delivered and this phenomenon is not benign. Appropriate resuscitation is necessary to prevent the complications of over- and underresuscitation; transport team members familiar with burn resuscitation principles and guidelines can lessen the deleterious impact and optimize the patient's long-term outcomes.

The decision to transport to a burn center is made based on the condition of the patient; the size of the burn; and, in the case of scene response, the distance to the burn center. Patients with concurrent traumatic injuries should first be evaluated at a trauma center if the traumatic injuries present the greatest immediate risk. If the burn injury is the greater risk to the patient and initial burn care can be facilitated en route, the initial transport to a burn center may be appropriate. The ABA has identified criteria for the transfer of burn patients to a burn center (Box 19.2).

Summary

Burn and electrical injuries can present a major challenge to transport team members, but an orderly, prioritized approach can improve patient outcomes. Patients may exhibit a wide spectrum of injuries from minor cutaneous burns to multiple traumatic injuries with deep cutaneous burns. The quality of treatment that the patient initially receives may impact overall outcome. A clear understanding of the pathophysiology of burn injuries is essential in providing quality burn care. Transportation of these patients to an appropriate hospital and early involvement of a burn care specialist are invaluable.

References

1. American Burn Association. *Advanced Burn Life Support Course Provider Manual.* Author; 2018.
2. American College of Surgeons. *Advanced Trauma Life Support for Doctors. Student Course Manual.* 10th ed. Author; 2018.
3. Herdon, David N. *Total Burn Care.* 5th ed. Elsevier; 2018.
4. Chai H, Chaudhari N, Kornhaber R, et al. Chemical burn to the skin: A systematic review of first aid impacts on clinical outcomes. *Burns.* May 14, 2022:S0305-4179(22)00113-9. doi:10.1016/j.burns.2022.05.006. Epub ahead of print.
5. Zemaitis MR, Foris LA, Lopez RA, et al. Electrical injuries. [Updated May 1, 2022]. In: *StatPearls [Internet].* StatPearls Publishing; Jan 2022. https://www.ncbi.nlm.nih.gov/books/NBK448087/
6. Schaefer TJ, Tannan SC. Thermal burns. [Updated Sep 18, 2021]. In: *StatPearls [Internet].* StatPearls Publishing; Jan 2022. https://www.ncbi.nlm.nih.gov/books/NBK430773/
7. Carta T, Gawaziuk J, Liu S, Logsetty S. Use of mineral oil fleet enema for the removal of a large tar burn: A case report. *Burns.* Mar 2015;41(2):e11–e14. doi:10.1016/j.burns.2014.07.007. Epub Oct 11, 2014.
8. Hohl DH, Coltro PS, Gonçalves HOC, et al. Comparison between two strategies of topical treatment in tar burn: A case report. *J Burn Care Res.* May 7, 2021;42(3):590–593. doi:10.1093/jbcr/iraa197
9. Wang S, Dai G. Hydrofluoric acid burn. *CMAJ.* Mar 18, 2019;191(11):E314. doi:10.1503/cmaj.181078
10. Lacy AJ, Freeman CL, Sexton MK. CEMENT BURNS. *J Emerg Med.* Nov 2021;61(5):533–535. doi:10.1016/j.jemermed.2021.03.019. Epub Jun 2, 2021.
11. Eichhorn L, Thudium M, Jüttner B. The diagnosis and treatment of carbon monoxide poisoning. *Dtsch Arztebl Int.* Dec 24, 2018;115(51–52):863–870. doi:10.3238/arztebl.2018.0863
12. Maclennan, L, Moiemen, N. Management of cyanide toxicity in patients with burns. *Burns.* Feb 2015;41(1):18–24. doi:10.1016/j.burns.2014.06.001
13. Blumenthal R. Injuries and deaths from lightning. *J Clin Pathol.* May 2021;74(5):279–284. doi:10.1136/jclinpath-2020-206492. Epub Aug 12, 2020.
14. Rotariu EL, Manole MD. Cardiac arrest secondary to lightning strike: Case report and review of the literature. *Pediatr Emerg Care.* Jan 2020;36(1):e18–e20. doi:10.1097/PEC.0000000000001255
15. Mutter E, Langley A. Cutaneous Lichtenberg figures from lightning strike. *CMAJ.* 2019;191(9):E260. doi:10.1503/cmaj.181221
16. Harshman J, Roy M, Cartotto R. Emergency care of the burn patient before the burn center: A systematic review and meta-analysis. *J Burn Care Res.* Feb 20, 2019;40(2):166–188. doi:10.1093/jbcr/iry060
17. Ramos G, Cornistein W, Cerino GT, Nacif G. Systemic antimicrobial prophylaxis in burn patients: Systematic review. *J Hosp Infect.* Oct 2017;97(2):105–114. doi: 10.1016/j.jhin.2017.06.015. Epub 2017 Jun 16.

• BOX 19.2   Burn Unit Referral Criteria

1. Partial thickness burns greater than 10% of the total body surface area.
2. Burns that involve the face, hands, feet, genitalia, perineum, or major joints.
3. Third-degree burns in any age group.
4. Electrical burns, including lightning injury.
5. Chemical burns.
6. Inhalation injury.
7. Burn injury in patients with preexisting medical disorders that could complicate management, prolong recovery, or affect mortality.
8. Any patients with burns and concomitant trauma (such as fractures) in which the burn injury poses the greatest risk of morbidity or mortality. In such cases, if trauma poses the greater immediate risk, the patient may be stabilized initially in a trauma center before being transferred to a burn unit. Physician judgment is necessary in such situations and should be in concert with the regional medical control plan and triage protocols.
9. Burned children in hospitals without qualified personnel or equipment for the care of children.
10. Burn injury in patients who need special social, emotional, or long-term rehabilitative intervention.

From *American Burn Association: Advanced Burn Life Support Referral Criteria.*

20

Point-of-Care Ultrasound

ARTHUR BROADSTOCK, KELLY TILLOTSON, SARDIS HARWARD, TYLER CHRISTIFULLI, AND RYAN WYATT

Introduction

Point-of-care ultrasound (POCUS) has revolutionized clinicians' ability to assess patients at the bedside, as it provides a timely and dynamic view of the patient's anatomy, physiology, and pathology. Since its introduction, diagnostic ultrasound has been used in a vast scope of clinical applications. A subset of these is POCUS, where the clinician performs an ultrasound examination, interprets the results, and integrates the findings to answer a focused clinical question or perform a bedside procedure. Large machines that were once tethered by power cables have been transformed into lightweight, battery-powered, handheld devices.[1] Ultrasound has several advantages for prehospital patient care in that it is portable and safe and can be performed quickly.

Since the first described use of prehospital ultrasound in the early 2000s, prehospital ultrasound has been implemented in many countries, including France, Germany, Italy, Denmark, and the United States.[2] The literature surrounding the use of these devices is heterogeneous, largely in part due to the differing practice patterns of individual emergency medical systems, varying transport times, and differing levels of training and providers involved.[2-4] However, studies demonstrate that the use of prehospital ultrasound has led to more accurate triage of trauma patients, changes in hospital management including decreased time to operative intervention, decreased use of computed tomography, decreased hospital cost, and overall decreased length of stay.[5,6] Furthermore, multiple studies show that prehospital providers can acquire quality thoracic and abdominal POCUS images with good interrater reliability and are also capable of interpreting the results with appropriate accuracy.[5-9] Adequate proficiency in these skills can be achieved with a brief training session, making it a highly useful and accessible addition to the prehospital provider's clinical skill set.[10]

Fundamentals of Point-of-Care Ultrasound

Possessing a basic understanding of the physical principles of ultrasound is integral to the interpretation of ultrasound images. Ultrasound is a type of mechanical energy that produces sound waves at a frequency above the spectrum of human hearing, typically between 1 and 20 megahertz (MHz). Ultrasound waves are created by applying an electric current to a piezoelectric crystal or other material within the transducer. These ultrasound waves are transmitted through the body and are reflected from body tissues back toward the transducer. The ultrasound probe absorbs the reflected sound waves to generate an electrical signal which is interpreted by the ultrasound's computer processor to create a visual ultrasound image. In newer ultrasound machines, the piezoelectric crystal has been replaced by silicon chips, which are cheaper to manufacture and have allowed ultrasounds to become more portable.

The brightness of the structures within the image is determined by how reflective that tissue is to sound energy and how much of that reflected energy is sensed by the transducer. Bright or white structures viewed on ultrasound reflect a high proportion of the sound waves, and these structures are called "hyperechoic," which represent highly reflective materials (e.g., bone, calcium, air). Black structures are tissues that allow all ultrasound beams to pass through and are called "anechoic," which typically represent fluid-filled structures. The varying degrees of grey in between are called "hypoechoic" and represent tissues with differing densities that reflect varying degrees of sound waves. As the sound waves travel through tissues, some sound energy is lost and is not reflected back to the transducer. This can occur due to absorption in the tissues, refraction, reflection, and scatter.

An important component of sound is its frequency, which is a measure of how many sound waves or cycles occur in 1 second. High-frequency ultrasound will produce more cycles per second with shorter wavelengths, which can produce a higher-resolution image. However, it is also more susceptible to energy loss as it travels through tissue and cannot image structures deep within the body. Conversely, low-frequency ultrasound consists of longer wavelengths and travels a longer distance but does not provide the same degree of image clarity as high-frequency ultrasound. In an ultrasound machine, frequency can be selected in two ways. Different probes will have different frequency ranges (Fig. 20.1). The curvilinear probe utilizes a lower frequency range and a wide footprint, suiting it best for abdominal and some lung applications. The phased array probe also utilizes a lower frequency range but possesses a smaller footprint to allow for easier positioning between ribs for cardiac views. The linear probe has a smaller footprint and a higher frequency range, suiting it best for soft tissue, musculoskeletal, vascular studies, and procedural guidance. Some portable ultrasound systems possess a variable frequency probe,

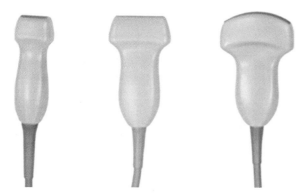

• **Figure 20.1** Phased Array Probe, Linear Probe, Curvilinear Probe (Left to Right). (From Ultrasound 101-Part 1 Transducers. Accessed November 1, 2022. https://123sonography.com/blog/ultrasound-101-part-1-transducers)

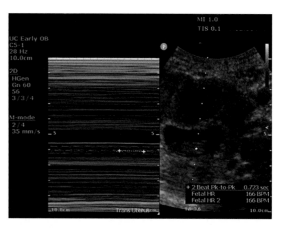

• **Figure 20.3** M-Mode Demonstrating a Calculation of a Fetal Heart Rate. (Courtesy UC Emergency Medicine.)

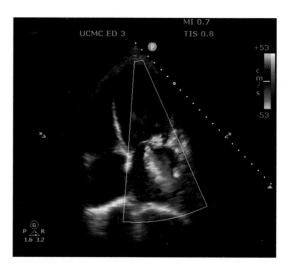

• **Figure 20.4** Color Doppler Demonstrating Mitral Regurgitation. (Courtesy UC Emergency Medicine.)

where the frequency range can be changed depending on the study indication while maintaining the same probe footprint. Secondly, after selecting a probe with a given frequency range, the exact frequency can be further adjusted using the manual settings to optimize image quality. When performing a particular study, most ultrasound machines will have a set list of "presets" for a given indication (e.g., cardiac, lung, biliary, renal) for each probe, which adjust settings like the frequency, artifact filtering, and other image processing to optimize image quality for that type of study.

Additionally, ultrasound has multiple modes that provide varying types of information to the clinician. B-mode ("brightness mode") is the standard grayscale 2D image (Fig. 20.2). M-mode ("motion mode") displays the motion of one vertical line of the image over time and provides a means to compare the motion of structures within the image (Fig. 20.3). M-mode is useful for multiple applications in echocardiography and lung ultrasound. Doppler ultrasound is a mode that uses the Doppler effect to characterize the movement of fluids, usually blood, through the body. There are multiple types of Doppler imaging, including color Doppler, spectral Doppler (e.g., continuous and pulse wave), and power Doppler, all of which provide different information on the velocity and/or direction of fluids within the body (Fig. 20.4).

Lastly, the ultrasound machine has various adjustable parameters to optimize image quality. The focal zone designates the area

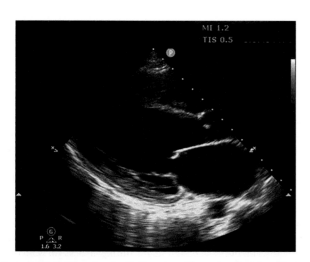

• **Figure 20.2** B-Mode Image of a Parasternal Long Cardiac View. (Courtesy UC Emergency Medicine.)

of narrowest intersection of ultrasound waves, which confers higher resolution. This can be adjusted vertically on the screen. The gain provides an overall level of "brightness" to the image. The depth parameter allows for deeper structures to be visualized but sacrifices image resolution.

Applications of POCUS in Prehospital and Transport Medicine

POCUS can be used to diagnose and monitor an array of pathology in the transport environment. The remainder of this chapter will discuss the potential applications of POCUS and how it may be used to aid in clinical decision-making.

Trauma: The FAST Exam

Trauma patients have a high likelihood of rapid decompensation from their underlying injuries during transport. Standardized use of POCUS has helped providers identify life threats in an efficient and timely fashion.

The use of ultrasound in the evaluation of abdominal trauma was initially described in 1971 and the term Focused Assessment with Sonography in Trauma (FAST) was coined in 1996.[11,12] The exam can be completed with a singular curvilinear probe for most patients and usually takes less than 2 minutes to complete after basic training. The FAST exam is also recommended by advanced trauma life support (ATLS) after the initial primary assessment. The FAST exam is used to evaluate life threats from traumatic causes, namely internal hemorrhage, pericardial effusion/tamponade, and pneumothorax. The protocol has been validated in blunt trauma and has become the standard of care for evaluation of hypotensive traumatic patients. The traditional FAST exam interrogates four anatomic regions: the right upper quadrant (RUQ), left upper quadrant (LUQ), pelvis, and cardiac view.

Right Upper Quadrant

The anatomic landmarks in the RUQ consist of the liver, right kidney, and diaphragm. To evaluate the RUQ, place the curvilinear probe with indicator pointed toward the head in the anterior axillary line at the bottom of the rib cage and scan until the border of the liver and right kidney is identified (Fig. 20.5). For complete evaluation of the RUQ, scan from the superior portion of the liver through hepatorenal interface (Morison's pouch) and visualize the most inferior aspect of the liver.

When the patient is supine, the RUQ is the most dependent position in the abdomen, and is often the location where free fluid will accumulate first. This fluid can be seen on ultrasound in the Morison's pouch, which is the potential space between the liver and the kidney (Fig. 20.6). Studies show that the Morison's pouch is the most common and the most sensitive location for identification of free fluid using ultrasound.[13]

While fluid most often collects in Morison's pouch, it can also collect between the diaphragm and the liver and around the liver tip, thus necessitating a full evaluation of the RUQ by fanning and scanning through the quadrant. Other fluid-filled structures in the RUQ have the potential to be misidentified as abdominal free fluid. Renal cysts, liver cysts, gallbladder, inferior vena cava (IVC), and intraperitoneal fat can be mistaken for free fluid. However, free fluid typically fills a whole potential space, including "nooks and crannies" that often fill triangular spaces, whereas fluid-filled organs/vessels are often circular in shape. If there is question, however, it is prudent to assume that an anechoic/hypoechoic structure is free fluid due to the consequences of ignoring intraabdominal free fluid.

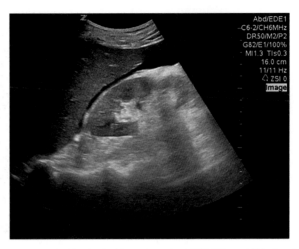

• **Figure 20.6** Positive Right Upper Quadrant FAST Exam With Anechoic Fluid Between the Liver and Kidney. (From Clinical Ultrasonography 101: Where Right Upper Quadrant Scans Go Wrong. Accessed November 1, 2022. https://canadiem.org/right-upper-quadrant-scans-go-wrong/)

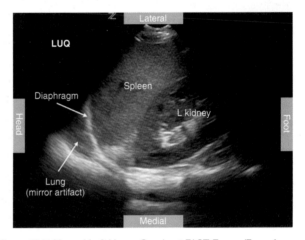

• **Figure 20.7** Normal Left Upper Quadrant FAST Exam. (From Accessed November 1, 2022. https://www.pocus101.com/efast-ultrasound-exam-made-easy-step-by-step-guide/)

Left Upper Quadrant

The LUQ is the second region interrogated in the FAST exam. This view includes the left kidney, spleen, and diaphragm (Fig. 20.7). To obtain the view, move the probe to the left side of the patient at the base of the ribs, indicator pointed toward the head. As the left kidney and spleen are more posterior (owing to the stomach's anterior location), the practitioner will need to move the probe posteriorly to identify these landmarks. The saying "knuckles to the bed" is a good reminder of how to position the hand posteriorly to scan the LUQ.

The spleen is a smaller organ than the liver and may be more challenging to identify, with the left kidney often coming into view first. The sonographer may also need to move the probe up or down one rib space to appreciate the entire view. Once the kidney is identified, locate the interface of the kidney and the spleen, the splenorenal recess. Fluid most often collects between the spleen and the diaphragm but can also collect in the splenorenal recess (Fig. 20.8).

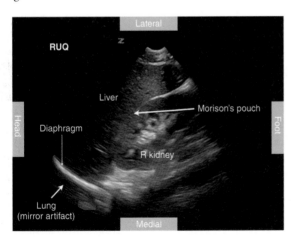

• **Figure 20.5** Normal Right Upper Quadrant FAST Exam. (From Dinh V. eFAST Ultrasound Exam Made Easy: Step-By-Step Guide. Accessed November 1, 2022. https://www.pocus101.com/efast-ultrasound-exam-made-easy-step-by-step-guide/)

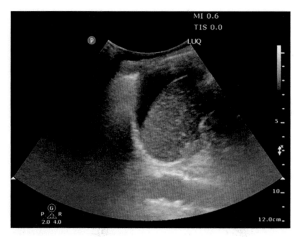

• **Figure 20.8** Positive Left Upper Quadrant FAST Exam With Anechoic Fluid Between the Spleen and Diaphragm. (From The Pocus Atlas. Trauma. Accessed November 1, 2022. https://www.thepocusatlas.com/trauma-atlas)

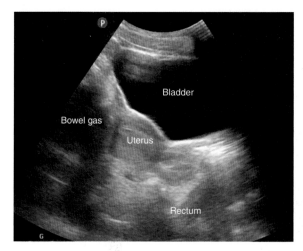

• **Figure 20.9** Normal Longitudinal Pelvis FAST View in a Female Patient. (From eFast Ultrasound Exam Made Easy: Step-by-Step Guide. Accessed November 1, 2022. https://www.pocus101.com/efast-ultrasound-exam-made-easy-step-by-step-guide/)

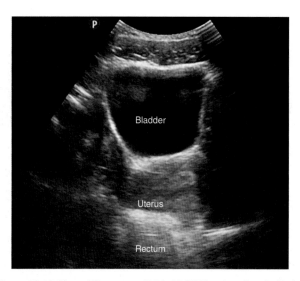

• **Figure 20.10** Normal Transverse Pelvis FAST View in a Female Patient. (From eFast Ultrasound Exam Made Easy: Step-by-Step Guide. Accessed November 1, 2022. https://www.pocus101.com/efast-ultrasound-exam-made-easy-step-by-step-guide/)

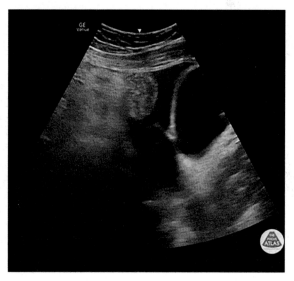

• **Figure 20.11** Positive Pelvic FAST Exam With Anechoic Fluid Superior to the Bladder. (From The Pocus Atlas. Trauma. Accessed November 1, 2022. https://www.thepocusatlas.com/trauma-atlas)

Pelvic View

In patients who have been upright or those with pelvic trauma, the pelvic view often demonstrates free fluid in patients with hemoperitoneum. The pelvic view will include the bladder, bowel, the uterus in female patients and seminal vesicles and the prostate in male patients.

The pelvic view is evaluated in the transverse and longitudinal view (Figs. 20.9 and 20.10). Two views are used to fully evaluate the anatomic structures as well as the potential spaces they create. In males, free fluid collects behind the bladder, the rectovesical pouch. In females, free fluid collects between the bladder and the uterus, the rectouterine pouch or pouch of Douglas (Fig. 20.10).

To obtain the longitudinal view, place the probe with the indicator pointing toward the head on the top of the pelvis, resting the inferior edge of the probe on the pubic symphysis. The bladder will be a fluid-filled organ directly above the pubic symphysis. In females, the uterus can be observed behind the bladder. In males, the prostate and seminal vesicles can be seen deep into the bladder. To obtain the transverse view, rotate the probe until the indicator is pointed to the patient's right. Then, the practitioner fans through the entire bladder and pelvic organs (Fig. 20.11).

The bladder, being a fluid-filled organ, allows excellent transmission of sound waves, thus creating a clear image of pelvic anatomy. The seminal vesicles, ovarian cysts, and blood vessels may look like free fluid in the pelvis. Additionally, many females have trace free fluid in the pelvis that is nonpathological. However, as stated previously, it is advisable to assume a positive finding rather than miss a potentially life-threatening finding.

Cardiac View

A subxiphoid view is obtained to evaluate for the presence of a pericardial effusion, usually in the setting of penetrating chest injury. A pericardial effusion should appear as an anechoic or hypoechoic

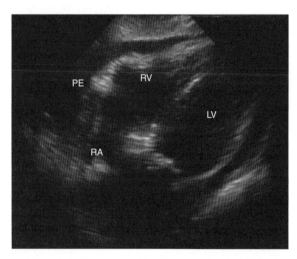

• **Figure 20.12** Subxiphoid view of the heart with pericardial effusion (PE). (From Singh G, Sabath B. Over-diuresis or cardiac tamponade? An unusual case of acute kidney injury and early closure. *J Community Hosp Intern Med Perspect.* 2016;6(2):31357. doi:10.3402/jchimp.v6.31357)

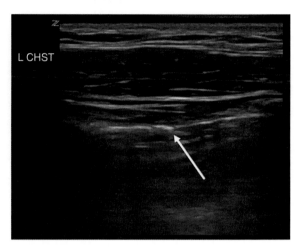

• **Figure 20.13** Lung Point (*arrow*) Demonstrating Aerated Lung on the Left and a Pneumothorax on the Right. (From UC Emergency Medicine. Accessed November 1, 2022. https://www.tamingthesru.com/us/scanning-school/lung-main)

circumferential structure around the heart (Fig. 20.12). While it is often anechoic, coagulated blood can appear hypoechoic and is often difficult to distinguish from surrounding tissues. The main objective is to evaluate for hemopericardium or tamponade, which carries a high degree of mortality if untreated.

EFAST – Lung Ultrasound

The extended FAST exam, or the EFAST, in addition to the abdominal and cardiac views, interrogates the lungs in search of a pneumothorax. The "E" stands for extended view, which includes the addition of bilateral lung ultrasound to evaluate for pneumothorax.

A pneumothorax of sufficient size to displace mediastinal structures and compress the superior and inferior cava will diminish right heart preload and, consequently, left heart preload and stroke volume. Ultrasound findings in pneumothorax are largely based on the presence or absence of artifacts that result from visceral-parietal pleural contact.[14] Lung sliding, or the shimmering appearance of the visceral pleura moving with the underlying lung parenchyma against the static parietal pleura of the chest wall, is lost with the accumulation of air within the pleural space.[15–17] It is important to note that while the presence of lung sliding definitively excludes the presence of pneumothorax at the level examined, the absence of lung sliding does not definitively confirm the presence of pneumothorax. Any condition that limits movement at the pleural interface may result in loss of lung sliding, including apnea, single lung or esophageal intubation, or lung adhesions to the chest wall.[17] The simultaneous presence and absence of lung sliding identifies a lung point, or the point of loss of contact between the visceral and parietal pleura, and is highly specific to pneumothorax.[17,18] This is a dynamic examination requiring the assessment of moving pleura with inspiration and therefore is not able to be assessed by a still image. However, Fig. 20.13 demonstrates the relative depth of the exam and the pleural line visible under subcutaneous tissue and muscle layers of the chest wall.

Investigations of the use of ultrasound to diagnose pneumothorax during prehospital and critical care transport are limited and suggest that accuracy may be slightly lower than when performed in the emergency department or intensive care unit.[19–22] With that in mind, ultrasound for pneumothorax provides an additional

method of patient assessment during transport, when typical exam maneuvers (such as lung auscultation) may be hindered.

Limitations of the Fast Exam

The fast exam is a highly validated protocol with sensitivities of 85% to 96% and specificities of 98% to 100% (ref 6–10). As stated previously, the FAST exam has been validated in blunt hypotensive trauma patients. However, it has not been validated in penetrating trauma. Furthermore, a negative FAST exam does not exclude internal bleeding. The retroperitoneal space cannot be evaluated by the fast exam, and thus patient may have hemorrhage from an extraperitoneal source. Additionally, normal anatomic structures are commonly mistaken as free fluid by the novice sonographer. Importantly, a negative FAST exam does not exclude intraperitoneal hemorrhage. Multiple studies have suggested that the average volume of free fluid needed to be detected by the FAST exam ranged from 250 to 620 mL.[23] Naturally, with more experience, less free fluid is needed for the user to feel confident in calling a positive FAST. Studies have shown that it may take over 100 examinations until a clinician is competent to diagnose smaller volumes of fluid.[23,24] While FAST is a specific test and can rule in pathology, it is not a very sensitive test used for ruling out pathology. It is not intended to replace the use of computed tomography (CT) but rather expedite an unstable patient to the operating room or potentially modify your transport dispositions.

Cardiac Ultrasound

The Views

Point-of-care echocardiography is a powerful tool that can lend crucial insight into a patient's cardiovascular system and elucidate potential causes of shock.

Parasternal Long Axis

The parasternal long axis (PSLA) view provides a lengthwise image of the heart from the base to the apex (Fig. 20.14). This view is helpful to obtain a sense of the patient's systolic function and can also assess for pericardial effusions.

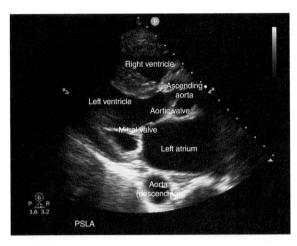

• **Figure 20.14** Parasternal Long Axis View of the Heart. (Courtesy UC Emergency Medicine.)

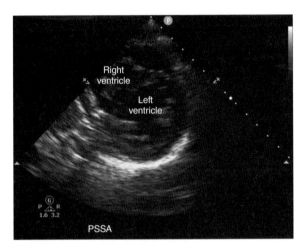

• **Figure 20.15** Parasternal Short Axis View of the Heart. (Courtesy UC Emergency Medicine.)

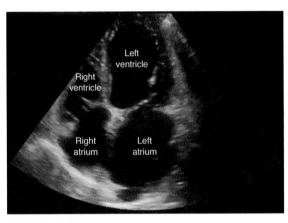

• **Figure 20.16** Apical Four Chamber View of the Heart. (Courtesy UC Emergency Medicine.)

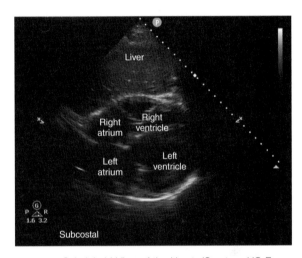

• **Figure 20.17** Subxiphoid View of the Heart. (Courtesy UC Emergency Medicine.)

Parasternal Short Axis

The parasternal short axis (PSSA) view provides a widthwise or axial cross-section through the midportion of the heart. This view is best obtained at the level of the papillary muscles and yields a cross-section of the right and left ventricle (Fig. 20.15). The PSSA view provides a clear comparison of the relative sizes of the left and right ventricles. The right ventricle is typically no larger than two thirds the size of the left ventricle. However, conditions like pulmonary embolism, pulmonary hypertension and right heart failure can increase the size of the right ventricle and may cause deviation of the interventricular septum towards the left ventricle during systole, which is best appreciated in this view. The overall function of the left ventricular is also assessed easily from this view.

Apical Four Chamber

The apical four chamber (A4C) view provides a coronal cross-section through the heart from the base to the apex, yielding a view of the right and left atria, the tricuspid and mitral valves, and the right and left ventricles (Fig. 20.16). This view is useful for evaluating right and left ventricular systolic function, assessing valvular function, identifying the presence of a pericardial effusion, comparing the relative sizes of the left and right ventricles, and may provide insight into wall motion or structural abnormalities.

Subxiphoid/Subcostal

The subxiphoid view is commonly used in cardiac arrest due to the probe placement not interfering with hand placement during cardiac compressions. This view is acquired by placing the probe inferior to the xiphoid and transmitting ultrasound beams superiorly, often using the liver as an acoustic window. The ideal view is a four-chamber view that includes both atria and ventricles as well as the mitral and tricuspid valves (Fig. 20.17). The subcostal view is also useful in identifying pericardial effusions (Fig. 20.12).

Inferior Vena Cava

The IVC provides clinicians with a sense of the patient's fluid status. A collapsible IVC with greater than 50% collapsibility with inspiration signifies volume depletion that will likely improve with administration of fluids. In contrast, a plethoric IVC that does not change with respiration can signify volume overload or potentially clue the clinician into a downstream obstructive

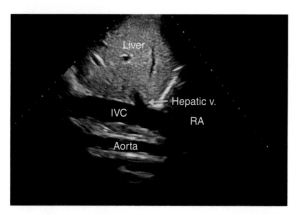

• **Figure 20.18** Coronal View of the IVC Entering the Right Atrium. (From Renal Fellow Network. Inferior Vena Cava POCUS: The Basics of Image Acquisition. Accessed November 1, 2022. https://www.renalfellow.org/2020/03/20/inferior-vena-cava-pocus-the-basics-of-image-acquisition/)

process like pulmonary embolism (PE), cardiac tamponade, or tension pneumothorax in the correct clinical setting (Fig. 20.18).

Pathology

Left Ventricular Systolic Function

Poor left ventricular systolic function can lead to decreased cardiac output and ultimately cardiogenic shock. Systolic function is measured by the ejection fraction or the amount of blood ejected in each cardiac cycle. This can be visually estimated by comparing the size of the LV in systole and diastole and estimating the percent change between the two. A normal ejection fraction is a 50% to 70% decrease in the LV chamber size. This can be assessed from a PSLA, PSSA, or A4C view. Point-of-care echocardiography is instrumental in identifying reductions in a patient's ejection fraction to guide the clinician's therapeutic interventions.

Right Ventricular Size and Function/ Pulmonary Embolism

PE, the most lethal manifestation of venous thromboembolism, typically occurs whena thrombus embolizes from a deep vein to a pulmonary artery. Submassive PE is defined as any PE that results in right heart dysfunction or ischemia, and a massive PE impedes right ventricular function to the point of hypotension.[25] Although the embolism itself is unlikely to be visualized unless it extends to the level of the right ventricular outflow tract, standard echocardiographic views may be used to evaluate right ventricular function in massive and submassive PE.[26,27] Similarly, the presence or secondary signs of a deep venous thrombosis (DVT) on ultrasound of the deep venous system significantly increases the probability of PE in a dyspneic patient.[26,27] The ability to deduce the presence of a PE from secondary findings has been utilized in both the prehospital and critical care transport settings to inform resuscitation and maximize prenotification of receiving providers.[27,28]

Findings suggestive of PE on standard echocardiographic views include RV dilation, flattening of the interventricular septum, decreased systolic function of the RV, and hypokinesia of the right ventricular free wall that spares the apex.[25,29,30] Normally, the right ventricle should be about two-thirds the size of the left ventricle. Enlargement of the right ventricle such that it is an equal size to the left ventricle is highly suggestive of right heart strain and can be adequately assessed on bedside echocardiogram.[31]

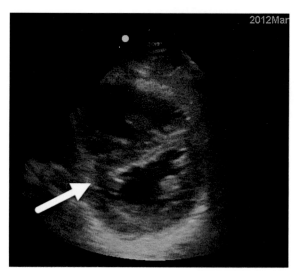

• **Figure 20.19** Parasternal Short Axis View Demonstrating Flattening of the Interventricular Septum Concerning for Right Heart Strain. (From Pocus Atlas. Accessed November 1, 2022. https://www.thepocusatlas.com/echocardiography-2)

Flattening of the interventricular septum visualized in the PSSA – colloquially known as D sign – reflects elevation of right ventricular pressure to equal or exceed left ventricular pressure due to vascular resistance within pulmonary circulation (Fig. 20.19). Hypokinesia of the RV free wall with normal wall motion at the apex seen in the AP4 view is known as McConnell's sign. The mechanism behind McConnell's sign is not completely understood but may be due to focal ischemia of the ventricular free wall or apical tethering to a hyperdynamic left ventricle.[32]

Three-point compression POCUS for the diagnosis of lower extremity DVT is performed by exerting external compression of the lower extremity veins with the ultrasound probe to visualize the collapse of the walls of the venous structure. Complete wall collapse indicates the absence of a thrombus. Occasionally, a hyperechoic structure may be seen within the vessel lumen, suggesting the presence of a thrombus. Images are obtained at the common femoral vein, the junction of the great saphenous and common femoral veins, intersection of the femoral and deep femoral veins, and the popliteal vein at the level of the popliteal fossa.[33,34] While these methods have been found to be over 90% sensitive and specific for the presence of DVT, sensitivity drops to 43% when the presence of DVT alone is used to extrapolate a diagnosis of PE.[29,30,35]

Cardiac Tamponade

Cardiac tamponade is a physiologic phenomenon defined by elevated pressure within the pericardium due to the accumulation of percardial fluid, which impairs ventricular preload and results in hemodynamic instability.[36] Diagnosis is classically made by a combination of physical exam findings, chest imaging, and characteristic EKG changes. Over the past decade, bedside ultrasound has become the preferred method for diagnosing tamponade due to the relative efficiency of obtaining diagnostic images at bedside and the opportunity for procedural guidance during pericardiocentesis.[37–40]

The typical findings of pericardial tamponade include a pericardial effusion plus RV diastolic collapse, RA systolic collapse, and a large IVC. Although many measurements may be obtained to determine the extent of hemodynamic compromise in cardiac tamponade, right ventricular diastolic collapse is often considered a pathognomonic finding on bedside echocardiogram due to its direct translation to decreased ventricular preload.[37,38,41] Ventricular collapse may be apparent in any cardiac window but is best appreciated in the PSLA in both B mode and M mode.[38,39,41] Impaired cardiac filling secondary to increased intrapericardial pressure is additionally reflected in elevated central venous pressure, and IVC plethora may be present despite profound hypotension.[39,41] This is the most sensitive sonographic finding for pericardial tamponade. The parasternal long axis, apical four-chamber, and subxiphoid views may be used to examine the intrapericardial space and identify the etiology of the pericardial effusion: hypoechoic fluid is more likely to reflect a simple pericardial effusion, clotted hemopericardium may have an isoechoic or heterogenous echotexture, and loculated fluid collections form from purulent or fibrinous material in the setting of infection or inflammation.[41,42] While most cardiac tamponade management during transport is focused on aggressive resuscitation and hemodynamic support, there is at least one published case study of in-flight ultrasound-guided pericardiocentesis to relieve tamponade physiology during transport.[43]

Lung Ultrasound

Lung ultrasound can rapidly identify causes of dyspnea. In addition to pneumothorax, which was previously discussed, ultrasound can quickly reveal pulmonary edema, pneumonia, and pleural effusions, which may account for a patient's shortness of breath. Pulmonary edema is easy to identify on ultrasound and appears as "B-lines," which are hyperechoic lines that originate from the pleura and travel into the far field of the screen (Fig. 20.20). Greater than three B-lines per one sonographic field is abnormal and is suggestive of interstitial fluid. Pleural effusions appear sonographically as anechoic fluid pockets at the base of the lungs, often with atelectatic lung visible within the fluid space (Fig. 20.21).

Aortic Ultrasound

Ruptured abdominal aortic aneurysm (rAAA) is a time-sensitive diagnosis, and mortality with this condition increases steeply with prolonged interval between symptom onset and definitive management.[44] Such management, however, is best performed by multidisciplinary interventional teams that rarely exist outside of

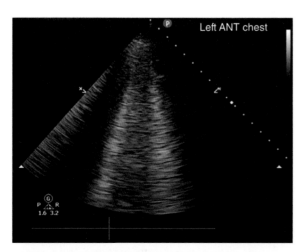

• **Figure 20.20** B-lines Consistent With Interstitial Fluid Within the Lung. (From https://www.tamingthesru.com/us/scanning-school/lung-main, CC BY-NC-SA 4.0. Accessed November 1, 2022.)

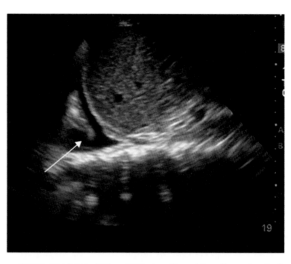

• **Figure 20.21** Right-Sided Pleural Effusion. (From https://www.tamingthesru.com/us/scanning-school/lung-main, CC BY-NC-SA 4.0. Accessed November 1, 2022.)

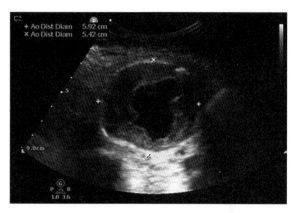

• **Figure 20.22** Enlargement of the Abdominal Aorta Consistent With Aortic Aneurysm. (Courtesy UC Emergency Medicine.)

regional referral centers. Consequently, early identification of rAAA aids in triage to facilities capable of providing collaborative medical and surgical care and guides the resuscitation of affected patients during transport by air or ground.[45]

Although visualization of the abdominal aorta may be limited by bowel gas, ultrasound has been demonstrated to have high sensitivity and specificity for identifying aneurysmal segments even when performed by operators with limited training.[46] Identifying an enlarged aortic diameter in the setting of hypotension or abdominal pain lends a high clinical suspicion for this diagnosis (Fig. 20.22). Once rAAA is suspected, prehospital providers must initiate rapid transport to facilities with capable vascular or cardiothoracic surgery services.[44,47]

Obstetric Ultrasound

Obstetric ultrasound in the prehospital setting may determine the timing of transport, necessity of specific interventions prior to or during transport, and the appropriateness of the receiving facility. With the exception of the pregnant trauma patient (who is best served by the nearest level 1 trauma center), pregnant patients should only be transported to facilities with maternal and neonatal services. Outcomes among high-risk patients are significantly improved when they are managed at regional referral centers capable of providing high levels of obstetric care.[48–51] Outcomes are best when transport occurs during the antenatal period rather than immediately postpartum.[52–56]

Determining Pregnancy Status

Palpation of the uterine fundal height may determine presence and age of pregnancy, but this method is not accurate in patients with large body habitus and gestational growth abnormalities.[57,58] POCUS can be used to rapidly assess for the presence of pregnancy and approximate gestational age. The physiologic changes associated with pregnancy make resuscitation of the pregnant patient uniquely challenging. This is particularly true during the second and third trimesters of pregnancy when the gravid uterus reaches a sufficient size to compress the IVC and compromise venous return from the lower extremities.[59] Manual displacement of the gravid uterus to the patient's left and/or left lateral decubitus positioning during transport can improve venous return in hypotensive patients. In these cases, POCUS may be used to rapidly assess for intrauterine pregnancy of sufficient fetal size to compromise maternal caval venous return and/or to detect fetal heart tones for assessment of fetal viability.[60,61] In the event of cardiac arrest, patients at a gestational age of at least 20 weeks may benefit from resuscitative hysterotomy to definitively relieve pressure on the IVC, and a fetus of at least 24 to 25 weeks' gestation may benefit from emergent perimortem cesarean delivery to allow aggressive postdelivery resuscitation.[62–64]

Risk of Imminent Delivery

Delivery during transportation has significant potential to compromise outcomes for both mother and neonate, as both are at risk of requiring some degree of resuscitation following delivery.[65,66] Methods to evaluate the anticipated progression of labor are therefore necessary to optimize patient care regardless of the setting in which it is provided. POCUS assessment of amniotic fluid volume and fetal presentation provides important clinical information that may not be readily apparent on initial physical examination. The Fetal Evaluation for Transport by Ultrasound (FETUS) exam – an assessment of fetal heart rate (FHR), position and movement, and general placental condition – has been proposed as a screening examination prior to and during maternal transport.[56] If amniotic fluid is markedly reduced or absent (indicating rupture of membranes) and a patient is experiencing regular uterine contractions, POCUS may be further used to determine the fetal presenting part and anticipate potential complications of delivery.[67]

Fetal Heart Rate

Assessment of FHR prior to or during transport is of limited utility unless subspecialty providers with the requisite qualifications to provide fetal interventions have accompanied the transport team. With that said, POCUS evaluation of FHR is easily performed by placing an M-mode cross-sectional beam over the fetal heart and noting the frequency of echogenic deflections over time at the corresponding depth (Fig. 20.3).

Cardiac Arrest

Current estimates for out-of-cardiac arrest survival indicate an 11% survival rate to hospital discharge, with rates of survival more abysmal for patients with nonshockable rhythms.[68] As such there is extensive research performed in this area with the goal of increasing survival. Sadly, in cardiac arrest, often the only piece of objective data available to the provider is the cardiac rhythm. However, using ultrasound, the provider can gain incredible information that assists in the management of a cardiac arrest.

While ultrasound provides a robust set of information during cardiac arrest, it is paramount that the use of ultrasound does not detract from high-quality chest compressions and does not cause pulse check time to exceed a maximum of 10 seconds.[69] Typically, the subcostal view is used as it is away from the chest compression device or the hands of those providing chest compressions. While compressions are ongoing, the ultrasound operator obtains a subcostal view of the heart using either the phased array or the curvilinear probe. On the pulse check, the image is obtained, and compressions are resumed at the end of the pulse check. The image should be reviewed after compressions are resumed. The image should be interrogated for pericardial tamponade/pericardial effusion, signs of right heart strain, and cardiac activity.

In cardiac arrest, pulseless electrical activity (PEA) and asystole are nonshockable rhythms per ACLS protocol. As part of managing these arrests, one must evaluate for and treat reversible causes. These are traditionally described as the "H's and T's" (Table 20.1). With ultrasound, some of these reversible causes may be identified and treated, namely hypovolemia, cardiac tamponade, tension pneumothorax, PE, and acute coronary syndrome.

The definition of PEA is organized cardiac electrical activity without the ability to generate a palpable pulse. However, with the advent of POCUS, we have noted the presence of what is now termed pseudo-PEA. In pseudo-PEA, there is visualization of organized electrical activity and organized cardiac activity, but these in conjunction fail to generate a palpable pulse. Visualizing the cardiac activity on ultrasound distinguishes these two entities. Pseudo-PEA, as it involves myocardial activity, is managed differently than true PEA. Pseudo-PEA is considered a state of profound shock with some underlying pathology. Treatment of pseudo-PEA is directed at improving cardiac output and addressing other potential types of shock, including obstructive, hypovolemic and distributive causes that may be further evaluated with additional POCUS investigation. Thus, prompt recognition of pseudo-PEA with ultrasound has potential to change patient outcomes substantially.

In cardiac arrest, it is critical to identify cardiac activity. Absence of cardiac activity, also known as true asystole, denotes absent movement of the atria, ventricles, or heart valves noted on ultrasound. During cardiac arrest, some cardiac activity may be noted during a pulse check. This activity may be irregular and/or disorganized. The presence of visible organized cardiac activity noted during the initial pulse check during cardiac arrest has been found to correlate with increased likelihood of obtaining ROSC.[70,71] Similarly, absence of cardiac activity, particularly in the later minutes of a cardiac arrest, is a poor prognostic indicator. Thus, cardiac activity is a critical piece of data to guide further interventions or to

TABLE 20.1 Reversible Causes of Cardiac Arrest

H's	T's
Hypovolemia	Tamponade
Hypoxia	Tension Pneumothorax
Hydrogen Ions (acidosis)	Thrombosis (MI)
Hypo/hyperkalemia	Thrombosis (PE)
Hypothermia	Toxins

Bolded items are identifiable using POCUS

terminate resuscitative efforts. The practitioner should be cautious when determining absence of cardiac activity. While the concept of cardiac activity sounds simple, interpreting the activity observed is more nuanced. The definition of cardiac activity is organized myocardial contractions. The mitral or tricuspid valve may be seen slightly fluttering on ultrasound during asystole or PEA from blood swirling in the heart chambers immediately after ceasing chest compressions. This is not synonymous with cardiac activity and requires resumption of chest compressions.

The RUSH Protocol

With any critically ill patient, rapid diagnosis is paramount to patient stabilization. Using the skills discussed in this chapter, ultrasound can provide an expedited bedside assessment of multiple causes of hypotension and shock to guide resuscitative interventions. The Rapid Ultrasound for Shock and Hypotension (RUSH) exam is a protocol developed in 2006 by Dr. Scott Weingart that combines an assessment of reversible causes of shock including hypovolemic, obstructive, and cardiogenic etiologies. The components of a RUSH exam are listed in Table 20.2.

Ultrasound-Guided Procedures

With the advances in POCUS, the use of this imaging modality has become standard of care for performing many procedures. Arterial lines and central venous line placement are safer and more successful when ultrasound is used to visualize access to the desired blood vessel. Ultrasound is also used for many other procedures such as foreign body removal, thoracentesis, and paracentesis. In the prehospital setting, ultrasound can be used in two critical procedures: intravenous (IV) access and pericardiocentesis.

Intravenous Access

For many patients, IV access presents a challenge due to their underlying medical conditions, hypovolemia, age (pediatrics), sclerotic veins, or obesity. There can be an initial steep learning curve to starting a patent IV using ultrasound; however, with practice it can be quickly and safely accomplished.[72] In these cases, ultrasound may be used to identify and access patients' veins. Placing the linear probe on the limb of interest, you may scan along the limb and identify blood vessels. With downward pressure on the vessels, the veins will collapse while the artery will remain open and pulsate. Once you have identified a vein, you can gain access to the vein via two techniques; in-plane or out-of-plane. For in-plane technique, place your probe parallel with the vessel in long axis, which should allow the vessel to have a rectangular appearance on the screen. You

may need to fan the probe left and right to find the point at which the vessel has the largest caliber, indicating that the transducer is directly over the center of the vessel. Then, the probe is held still while a needle is inserted at the skin next to the indicator mark on the probe. The needle is then visualized as it traverses the soft tissue and enters the vessel. The needle tip will appear as a hyperechoic linear structure traveling toward the vessel (Fig. 20.23). Once the needle tip punctures the vessel and is visualized within the center of the vessel, the catheter may be advanced over the needle in standard fashion.

For out-of-plane (short axis) technique, the probe is positioned perpendicularly to the vessel so that it shows the vessel in a transverse view, producing a circle on the screen. This view may be helpful for vessels that are torturous or difficult to visualize in an long axis view. Once the vessel is identified, it should be centered in the middle of the screen. A needle is then inserted into the skin in front of the probe, aligned with the center of the probe. As the needle is slowly advanced, the hyperechoic needle tip will come into view. With the tip in view, advance the probe distally until the needle tip is out of view. Then advance the needle tip with a downward angle until the needle tip returns into view. Continue this until the needle tip "tents" the wall of the vessel. Advance the needle and enter the vein; at this point, the needle tip should be seen in the center of the vessel, creating a "bullseye" effect, as shown (Fig. 20.24). The catheter can then be threaded over the needle as is standard, gaining IV access.

Pericardiocentesis

Few procedures spark more anxiety than pericardiocentesis. In the prehospital setting, this procedure is typically attempted in cardiac arrest or in a patient with hemodynamic instability from cardiac tamponade. Traditionally, this procedure is taught in a landmark-based approach and is a blind procedure. However, this leads to potential complications including puncture of the myocardium, inadequate decompression of fluid, and inappropriate placement of the needle leading to potential pulmonary or cardiac complications. Ultrasound has changed the way this procedure is performed, allowing the proceduralist to visualize their needle throughout the procedure and reducing complications.

To perform the procedure, first one must obtain an optimal image demonstrating the pericardial effusion. Typically, the procedure may be performed using the PSLA view or subcostal view, though it is also possible to perform the procedure using the A4C view. These views are obtained using the phased array probe or the curvilinear probe.

After obtaining the appropriate view, the needle is inserted in an in-plane technique, following the needle as it enters the pericardium and into the pericardial effusion.

Conclusion

Point-of-care ultrasound offers prehospital clinicians an unparalleled array of diagnostic abilities. However, transport crews should continue to limit ground time with the use of this technology. Using the device in the vehicle in transit may limit ground time and expedite transport to the trauma center. As devices become less expensive and more portable, ultrasound will become more prevalent in the prehospital care of patients. Providers and medical directors alike should be aware of this technology and the advantages it can offer to the care of patients in their region.

TABLE 20.2	Components of RUSH Exam
Component	Relevant Findings
Echocardiogram	Heart failure, cardiac tamponade, right heart strain (PE)
FAST	Intraabdominal fluid
Aorta	Abdominal aortic aneurysm
IVC	Decreased intravascular volume
Lungs	Tension pneumothorax

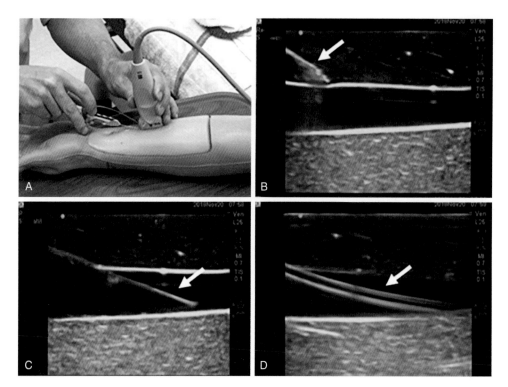

• **Figure 20.23** Long Axis Technique for IV Placement, *Arrow* Demonstrating Needle and Catheter. (From Millington SJ, Hendin A, Shiloh AL, Koenig S. Better with ultrasound: Peripheral intravenous catheter insertion. *Chest*. 2020;157(2):369–375. doi:10.1016/j.chest.2019.04.139)

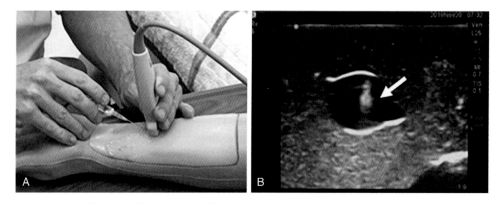

• **Figure 20.24** Short Axis Technique for IV Placement, *Arrow* Demonstrating Needle Tip. (From Millington SJ, Hendin A, Shiloh AL, Koenig S. Better with ultrasound: Peripheral intravenous catheter insertion. *Chest*. 2020;157(2):369–375. doi:10.1016/j.chest.2019.04.139)

References

1. Busch M. Portable ultrasound in pre-hospital emergencies: A feasibility study. *Acta Anaesthesiol Scand*. 2006;50(6):754–758. doi:10.1111/j.1399-6576.2006.01030.x
2. Nelson BP, Chason K. Use of ultrasound by emergency medical services: A review. *Int J Emerg Med*. 2008;1(4):253–259. doi:10.1007/s12245-008-0075-6
3. Jørgensen H, Jensen CH, Dirks J. Does prehospital ultrasound improve treatment of the trauma patient? A systematic review. *Eur J Emerg Med*. 2010;17(5):249–253. doi:10.1097/MEJ.0b013e328336adce
4. Bøtker MT, Jacobsen L, Rudolph SS, Knudsen L. The role of point of care ultrasound in prehospital critical care: A systematic review. *Scand J Trauma Resusc Emerg Med*. 2018;26(1):51. doi:10.1186/s13049-018-0518-x
5. Walcher F, Weinlich M, Conrad G, et al. Prehospital ultrasound imaging improves management of abdominal trauma. *Br J Surg*. 2006;93(2):238–242. doi:10.1002/bjs.5213
6. Melniker LA, Leibner E, McKenney MG, Lopez P, Briggs WM, Mancuso CA. Randomized controlled clinical trial of point-of-care, limited ultrasonography for trauma in the emergency department: The first sonography outcomes assessment program trial. *Ann Emerg Med*. 2006;48(3):227–235. doi:10.1016/j.annemergmed.2006.01.008
7. Heegaard W, Hildebrandt D, Spear D, Chason K, Nelson B, Ho J. Prehospital ultrasound by paramedics: Results of field trial. *Acad Emerg Med*. 2010;17(6):624–630. doi:10.1111/j.1553-2712.2010.00755.x
8. Pietersen PI, Mikkelsen S, Lassen AT, et al. Quality of focused thoracic ultrasound performed by emergency medical technicians and paramedics in a prehospital setting: A feasibility study. *Scand J Trauma Resusc Emerg Med*. 2021;29(1):40. Published Feb 25, 2021. doi:10.1186/s13049-021-00856-8

9. Brooke M, Walton J, Scutt D, Connolly J, Jarman B. Acquisition and interpretation of focused diagnostic ultrasound images by ultrasound-naive advanced paramedics: Trialling a PHUS education programme. *Emerg Med J.* 2012;29(4):322–326. doi:10.1136/emj.2010.106484

10. Walcher F, Kirschning T, Müller MP, et al. Accuracy of prehospital focused abdominal sonography for trauma after a 1-day hands-on training course. *Emerg Med J.* 2010;27(5):345–349. doi:10.1136/emj.2008.059626

11. Kristensen JK, Buemann B, Keuhl E. Ultrasonic scanning in the diagnosis of haematomas. *Acta Chir Scand.* 1971;137:653–657.

12. Rozycki GS, Ochsner MG, Schmidt JA, et al. Prospective study of surgeon-performed ultrasound as the primary adjuvant modality for injured patient assessment. *J Trauma.* 1995;39(3):492–498 [discussion: 498–500].

13. Lobo V, Hunter-Behrend M, Cullnan E, et al. Caudal edge of the liver in the right upper quadrant (RUQ) view is the most sensitive area for free fluid on the FAST exam. *West J Emerg Med.* 2017;18(2):270–280. doi:10.5811/westjem.2016.11.30435

14. Staub LJ, Biscaro RRM, Kaszubowski E, et al. Chest ultrasonography for the emergency diagnosis of traumatic pneumothorax and haemothorax: A systematic review and meta-analysis. *Injury.* 2018;49:457–466. doi:10.1016/j.injury.2018.01.033

15. Helland G, Gaspari R, Licciardo S, et al. Comparison of four views to single-view ultrasound protocols to identify clinically significant pneumothorax. *Acad Emerg Med.* 2016;23(10):1170–1175. doi:10.1111/acem.13054

16. Lee FCY. Lung ultrasound – a primary survey of the acutely dyspneic patient. *J Intensive Care.* 2016;4(1):57. doi:10.1186/s40560-016-0180-1

17. Bhoil R, Ahluwalia A, Chopra R, et al. Signs and lines in lung ultrasound. *J Ultrason.* 2021;21(86):e225–e233.

18. Mojoli F, Bouhemad B, Mongodi S, et al. Lung ultrasound for critically ill patients. *Am J Respir Crit Care Med.* 2019;199(6):701–714. doi:10.1164/rccm.201802-0236CI

19. Avila J, Smith B, Mead T, et al. Does the addition of M-mode to B-mode ultrasound increase the accuracy of identification of lung sliding in traumatic pneumothoraces? *J Ultrasound Med.* 2018;37(11):2681–2687. doi:10.1002/jum.14629

20. Quick JA, Uhlich RM, Ahmad S, et al. In-flight ultrasound identification of pneumothorax. *Emerg Radiol.* 2016;23(1):3–7. doi:10.1007/s10140-015-1348-z

21. Oliver P, Bannister P, Bootland D, et al. Diagnostic performance of prehospital ultrasound diagnosis for traumatic pneumothorax by a UK helicopter emergency medical service. *Eur J Emerg Med.* 2020;27(3):202–206. doi:10.1097/MEJ.0000000000000641

22. Griffiths E. Helicopter emergency medical services use of thoracic point of care ultrasound for pneumothorax: A systematic review and meta-analysis. *Scand J Trauma Resusc Emerg Med.* 2021;29(1):163. doi:10.1186/s13049-021-00977-0

23. Gracias VH, Frankel HL, Gupta R, et al. Defining the learning curve for the Focused Abdominal Sonogram for Trauma (FAST) examination: Implications for credentialing. *Am Surg.* 2001;67(4):364–368.

24. Berger S. Survival from out-of-hospital cardiac arrest: Are we beginning to see progress? *J Am Heart Assoc.* 2017;6(9):e007469. doi:10.1161/JAHA.117.007469

25. Sista A, Kup WT, Schiebler M, et al. Stratification, imaging, and management of acute massive and submassive pulmonary embolism. *Radiology.* 2017;284(2):5–24. doi:10.1148/radiol.2017151978

26. Fields JM, Davis J, Girson L, et al. Transthoracic echocardiography for diagnosing pulmonary embolism: A systematic review and meta-analysis. *J Am Soc Echocardiogr.* 2017;30(7):714–723.e4. doi:10.1016/j.echo.2017.03.004

27. Kuttab HI, Flanagan E, Damewood SC, et al. Prehospital echocardiogram use in identifying massive pulmonary embolism in unidentified respiratory failure. *Air Med J.* 2021;40(1):73–75. doi:10.1016/j.amj.2020.10.004

28. Robinson AE, Simpson NS, Hick JL, et al. Prehospital ultrasound diagnosis of massive pulmonary embolism by non-physicians: A case series. *Prehosp Emerg Care.* 2022; online ahead of print. doi:10.1080/10903127.2022.2113190

29. Falster C, Jacobsen N, Coman KE, et al. Diagnostic accuracy of focused deep venous, lung, cardiac and multiorgan ultrasound in suspected pulmonary embolism: A systematic review and meta-analysis. *Thorax.* 2022;77(7):679–689. doi:10.1136/thoraxjnl-2021-216838

30. Dwyer KH, Rempell JS, Stone MB. Diagnosing centrally located pulmonary embolisms in the emergency department using point-of-care ultrasound. *Am J Emerg Med.* 2018;36(7):1145–1150.

31. Taylor RA, Moore CL. Accuracy of emergency physician-performed limited echocardiography for right ventricular strain. *Am J Emerg Med.* 2014;32(4):371–374. doi:10.1016/j.ajem.2013.12.043

32. McConnell MV, Solomon SD, Rayan ME, et al. Regional right ventricular dysfunction detected by echocardiography in acute pulmonary embolism. *Am J Cardiol.* 1996;78(4):469–473. doi:10.1016/S0002-9149(96)00339-6

33. Needleman L, Cronan JJ, Lilly MP, et al. Ultrasound for lower extremity deep venous thrombosis: Multidisciplinary recommendations for the Society of Radiologists in Ultrasound Consensus Conference. *Circulation.* 2018;137:1505–1515. doi:10.1161/circulationaha.117.030687

34. Varrias D, Palaiodimos L, Balasubramanian P, et al. The use of point-of-care ultrasound (POCUS) in the diagnosis of deep vein thrombosis. *J Clin Med.* 2021;10(17):3903. doi:10.3390/jcm10173903

35. García JP, Alonso JV, García PC, et al. Comparison of the accuracy of emergency department-performed point-of-care-ultrasound (POCUS) in the diagnosis of lower-extremity deep vein thrombosis. *J Emerg Med.* 2018;54(5):656–664. doi:10.1016/j.jemermed.2017.12.020

36. Kearns MJ, Walley KR. Tamponade: Hemodynamic and echocardiographic diagnosis. *Chest.* 2018;153(5):1266–1275. doi:10/1016/j.chest.2017.11.003

37. Nagdev A, Stone MB. Point-of-care ultrasound evaluation of pericardial effusions: Does this patient have cardiac tamponade? *Resuscitation.* 2011;82(6):671–673.

38. Goodman A, Perera P, Mailhot T, et al. The role of bedside ultrasound in the diagnosis of pericardial effusion and cardiac tamponade. *J Emerg Trauma Shock.* 2012;5(1):72–75. doi:10/4103/0974-2700.93118

39. Ceriani E, Cogliati C. Update on bedside ultrasound diagnosis of pericardial effusion. *Intern Emerg Med.* 2016;11:477–480. doi:10.1007/s11739-015-1372-8

40. Osman A, Chuan TW, Rahman JA, et al. Ultrasound-guided pericardiocentesis: A novel parasternal approach. *Eur J Emerg Med.* 2018;25(5):322–327. doi:10.1097/MEJ.0000000000000471

41. Alerhand S, Carter JM. What echocardiographic findings suggest a pericardial effusion is causing tamponade? *Am J Emerg Med.* 2019;37(2):321–326. doi:10.1016/j.ajem.2018.11.004

42. Vakamudi S, Ho N, Cremer PC. Pericardial effusions: Causes, diagnosis, and management. *Prog Cardiovasc Dis.* 2017;59(4):380–388. doi:10.1016/j.pcad.2016.12.009

43. Darvishi M, Shahali H. Acute cardiac tamponade: A case of life-threatening coronavirus disease 2019 complication during air medical transportation. *Air Med J.* 2021;40(3):179–181. doi:10.1016/j.amj.2021.01.004

44. Chaikof EL, Dalman RL, Eskandari MK, et al. The Society for Vascular Surgery practice guidelines on the care of patients with an abdominal aortic aneurysm. *J Vasc Surg.* 2018;67(1):2–77.e2. doi:10.1016/j.jvs.2017.10.004

45. Mell MW, Starnes BW, Kraiss LW, et al. Western Vascular Society guidelines for transfer of patients with ruptured abdominal aortic aneurysm. *J Vasc Surg.* 2017;65(3):603–608.

46. Mai T, Woo MY, Boles K, Jetty P. Point-of-care ultrasound performed by a medical student compared to physical examination by vascular surgeons in the detection of abdominal aortic aneurysms. *Ann Vasc Surg.* 2018;52:15–21. doi:10.1016/j.avsg.2018.03.015

47. Mikati N, Phillips AR, Corbelli N, et al. The effect of blood transfusion during air medical transport on transport times in patients with

ruptured abdominal aortic aneurysm. *Prehosp Emerg Care.* 2022; 26(2):255–262. doi:10/1080/10903127.2020.1868636

48. Jensen EA, Lorch SA. Effects of a birth hospital's neonatal intensive care unit level and annual volume of very low-birth-weight infant deliveries on morbidity and mortality. *JAMA Pediatr.* 2015; 169(8):e151906. doi:10.1001/jamapediatrics.2015.1906

49. Snowden JM, Cheng YW, Emeis CL, et al. The impact of hospital obstetric volume on maternal outcomes in term, non-low-birthweight pregnancies. *Am J Obstet Gynecol.* 2015;212(3):380.e1–380.e9.

50. Clapp MA, James KE, Kaimal AJ. The effect of hospital acuity on severe maternal morbidity in high-risk patients. *Am J Obstet Gynecol.* 2018;219(1):111.e1–111.e7. doi:10.1016/j.ajog.2018.04.015

51. Shah KP, deRegnier RAO, Grobman WA, et al. Neonatal mortality after interhospital transfer of pregnant women for imminent very preterm birth in Illinois. *JAMA Pediatr.* 2020;174(4):358–365. doi:10.1001/jamapediatrics.2019.6055

52. Stewart MJ, Smith J, Boland RA. Optimizing outcomes in regionalized perinatal care: Integrating maternal and neonatal emergency referral, triage and transport. *Curr Treat Opt Pediatr.* 2017;3:313–326.

53. Horak TS, Sanborn A. The need for reliable robust maternal transport program to improve maternal outcomes in rural America. *Clin Obstet Gynecol.* 2022; online ahead of print. doi:10.1097/GRF.0000000000000722

54. DeSisto CL, Oza-Frank R, Goodman D, et al. Maternal transport: An opportunity to improve the system of risk-appropriate care. *J Perinatol.* 2021;41(9):2141–2146. doi:10.1038/s41372-021-00935-9

55. Ohara M, Shimizu Y, Satoh H, et al. Safety and usefulness of emergency maternal transport using helicopter. *J Obstet Gynaecol Res.* 2008;34(2):189–194. doi:10.1111/j.1447-0756.2008.00756.x

56. Polk JD, Merlino JI, Kovach BL, et al. Fetal evaluation for transport by ultrasound performed by air medical teams: A case series. *Air Med J.* 2004;23(4):32–34. doi:10.1016/j.amj.2004.04.005

57. Jelks A, Cifuentes R, Ross M. Clinician bias in fundal height measurement. *Obstet Gynecol.* 2007;110(4):892–899. doi:10.1097/01.AOG.0000282758.28533.d9

58. Peter JR, Ho JJ, Valliapan J, et al. Symphysial fundal height (SFH) measurement in pregnancy for detecting abnormal fetal growth. *Cochrane Database Syst Rev.* 2015;9:CD008136. doi:10.1002/14651858.CD008136.pub3

59. Jeejeebhoy FM, Zelop CM, Lipman S, et al. Cardiac arrest in pregnancy: A scientific statement from the American Heart Association. *Circulation.* 2015;132(18):1747–1773. doi:10.1161/CIR0000000000000300

60. Brun PM, Chenaitia H, Dejesus I, et al. Ultrasound to perimortem caesarean delivery in prehospital settings. *Injury.* 2013;44(1):151–152. doi:10.1016/j.injury.2012.08.029

61. Tommila M, Pystynen M, Soukka H, et al. Two cases of low birth weight infant survival by prehospital emergency hysterotomy. *Scand J Trauma Resusc Emerg Med.* 2017;25(1):62. doi:10.1186/s13049-017-0407-8

62. Capobianco G, Balata A, Mannazzu MC, et al. Perimortem cesarean delivery 30 minutes after a laboring patient jumped from a fourth-floor window: Baby survives and is normal at age 4 years. *Am J Obstet Gynecol.* 2008;198(1):e15–e16. doi:10.1016/j.ajog.2007.09.007

63. Lott C, Truhlar A, Alfonzo A, et al. European Resuscitation Council Guidelines 2021: Cardiac arrest in special circumstances. *Resuscitation.* 2021;161:152–219. doi:10.1016/j.resuscitation.2021.02.011

64. Moors XRJ, Biesheuvel TH, Cornette J, et al. Analysis of prehospital perimortem caesarian deliveries performed by helicopter emergency medical services in the Netherlands and recommendations for the future. *Resuscitation.* 2020;155:112–118. doi:10.1016/j.resuscitation.2020.07.023

65. Shipway T, Johnson E, Bell S, et al. A case review: In-flight births over a 4-year period in the Northern Territory, Australia. *Air Med J.* 2016;35(5):317–320. doi:10.1016/j.amj.2016.04.005

66. Jones AE, Summers RL, Deschamp C, et al. A national survey of the air medical transport of high-risk obstetric patients. *Air Med J.* 2001;20(2):17–20.

67. Ghi T, Eggebo T, Lees C, et al. ISUOG practice guidelines: Intrapartum ultrasound. *Ultrasound Obstet Gynecol.* 2018;52(1):128–139. doi:10.1002/uog.19072

68. Berger S. Survival from out-of-hospital cardiac arrest: Are we beginning to see progress? *J Am Heart Assoc.* 2017;6(9):e007469. doi:10.1161/JAHA.117.007469

69. Huis In 't Veld MA, Allison MG, Bostick DS, et al. Ultrasound use during cardiopulmonary resuscitation is associated with delays in chest compressions. *Resuscitation.* 2017;119:95–98. doi:10.1016/j.resuscitation.2017.07.021

70. Masoumi B, Azizkhani R, Heydari F, Zamani M, Nasr Isfahani M. The role of Cardiac Arrest Sonographic Exam (CASE) in predicting the outcome of cardiopulmonary resuscitation; a cross-sectional study. *Arch Acad Emerg Med.* 2021;9(1):e48. Published June 28, 2021. doi:10.22037/aaem.v9i1.1272

71. Gaspari R, Weekes A, Adhikari S, et al. Emergency department point-of-care ultrasound in out-of-hospital and in-ED cardiac arrest. *Resuscitation.* 2016;109:33–39. doi:10.1016/j.resuscitation.2016.09.018

72. Stolz LA, Cappa AR, Minckler MR, et al. Prospective evaluation of the learning curve for ultrasound-guided peripheral intravenous catheter placement. *J Vasc Access.* 2016;17(4):366–370. doi:10.5301/jva.5000574

21

Legal and Professional Issues in Critical Care Transport

CHRISTOPHER TAYLOR

COMPETENCIES

1. Integrate the concepts related to professional practice, including discussion on the laws, rules, and regulations affecting critical care transport.
2. Discuss medical direction during interfacility transports as well as differentiating between scope of practice and standard of care.
3. Discuss additional legal issues regarding transport to include transport decisions as well as the role of the family.
4. Briefly discuss civil litigation.

Introduction

Critical care transport team members can, at times, work in situations and environments that require the ability to work in an independent fashion, making clinical decisions with other medical providers who may not have specialized training to address the care that the patient may require. In addition, these same teams often practice critical care in environments where contact with online medical control is limited or inaccessible. Decision-making by critical care transport team members during these times requires proficiency in life-saving skills and understanding of required professional standards and basic legal principles. Their interactions with other healthcare providers, the patient, and family members require, at minimum, being familiar with complicated concepts and staying aware of the changes that both define and refine our understanding of patient care.

This chapter addresses some of the common professional issues faced by transport teams including legal topics that surround patient care and medical direction, as well as providing an understanding of scope of practice and standards of care. In addition, this chapter will provide a basic overview of the legal process that the medical professional may encounter when concerns about the care that was provided are raised.

Legal Issues

An understanding of the law, legal principles, and regulations that are specific to transport is essential to protecting both critical care transport team members as well as the patient during transport. Clinical scope of practice, regulations by the Federal Aviation Administration regarding air transport, online medical control, the Federal Communication Commission as well as state and local rules and regulations that govern and direct ground transport vehicles represent a portion of the education and training that transport team members must maintain to provide safe and competent patient care.

An Overview of the Law

Law comprises all the rules and regulations by which our society is governed. Statutes are laws made by the legislative branch of a governmental body at either the state or federal level. Statutes can vary from state to state and can be changed, modified, or repealed by the same governmental body that enacted them. Statutes declare policy that is used to prevent harm and frequently require written rules and regulations for enforcement. Administrative agencies write administrative law as well as the rules and regulations that enforce the statute. Statutory laws are used to define laws that have been enacted and can be in the form of regulatory and administrative laws that are used to regulate the care provided and provide the power to enforce them. The State Boards of Nursing are administrative agencies that oversee aspects of licenses, discipline, and education of nurses through interpretation of statutory laws. Another common example would be State EMS agencies or Public Health Departments. Case law, or judicial law, varies from state to state and is based on judicial decisions in previous court rulings. Questions of law that may come about such as in cases involving medical malpractice, are decided in court, where questions of facts are the responsibility of a jury.

A crime can be defined as committing or omitting an act in violation of the law forbidding or commanding it. An individual can be charged with a crime which can either be a felony or a misdemeanor depending on the type of violation that has occurred. It is legal action taken by the government for behavior that is considered offensive or harmful to society. *Civil injury law*, in contrast to criminal law, is when physical harm or damage occurs through negligence or breach of duty. It permits an action to be filed by an individual for monetary compensation. Civil tort law is a broad area of law that covers harm or injury other than a breach of contract. Most lawsuits involving transport teams fall into this category and are related to medical and nursing care.

Elements of Malpractice

The most common civil law that may involve critical care transport teams is malpractice. While the terms negligence and malpractice are sometimes used interchangeably, there are distinctions between the two. While anyone can be liable for negligence, only a professional can be liable for malpractice. Generally, negligence occurs when a person fails to act as an ordinary or reasonable person would under similar circumstances. Malpractice is more specific and looks at a standard of care as well as the professional status of the caregiver. The elements of malpractice that must be present are shown in order of priority in Box 21.1.

First, a *duty* must be present. This usually occurs when a transport team member accepts responsibility for the care and treatment of the patient. Because of this relationship, the team member is obligated to act in a prescribed manner to care for the patient.

Once a duty is established to exist, the second element is a *breach of duty*. A breach of duty may occur as a result of malfeasance (act of commission) or nonfeasance (act of omission).[1-12] Administration of the wrong medication is malfeasance, whereas failure to follow a standard operating procedure is nonfeasance.[1-12]

The third element is *foreseeability*. Foreseeability involves whether one could reasonably expect certain events to cause specific results.[1-12]

The fourth element is *causation*. A link must be proven between the breach of duty and the injury that is alleged to be suffered.[1-12]

The fifth element is *injury*. The patient must be harmed physically, financially, or emotionally in a discernible way.[1-12]

The sixth element in malpractice are *damages*. Damages are compensatory in nature and may be of different types. *General damages* are inherent to the injury itself. *Special damages* are losses and expenses incurred as a result of stress and emotional pain produced by the injury. *Punitive damages* are requested for an alleged malicious intent or willful or wanton misconduct.[1-12]

Damages can be in the form of any of the following, but not limited to, noneconomic damages including pain and suffering, mental anguish, disfigurement, emotional distress, or loss of chance of survival. An individual also may recover economic damages including past, present, and future medical expenses as well as past, present, and future loss of wages or earning capacity.

In malpractice cases, all six elements must be proven by a "preponderance of the evidence" to prevail. Some potential sources of malpractice exposure for transport teams include patient assessment and triage, patient rescue and handling, and failure to properly use or maintain equipment. Delays in transport, condition changes, admissions, discharges, and transfers are other common areas that have given rise to malpractice suits.

Statute of Limitations

Filing a lawsuit is under a *statute of time limitations*. Generally, if malpractice is alleged after a traumatic injury, the statute of limitations is 2 years; in cases of disease, it is at the time discovered. The exception is in pediatric cases. The statute of limitations is extended until the minor is emancipated or reaches the age of majority (established by state law).[1-12]

Discussion of Liability

Intentional Torts or Criminal Acts

Intentional torts involve conduct in which an individual is reasonably certain that harm will result from his or her actions. In other words, the conduct is not accidental but involves a level of intent. Several intentional torts may affect transport team members. The terms assault and battery are often used together in a criminal context. In civil law, these terms carry different definitions and connotations. Assault is an intentional tort that causes fear or apprehension that a person will be touched in a harmful or offensive manner. The basis of this tort is simply fear and the apparent present ability that harmful touching may result. Assault can stand alone as a tort but is often accompanied by a battery.

Battery is the actual physical contact with a person, without his or her consent, that results in an offensive contact or injury. Battery is not a beating but is as simple as unwanted touching. Medical battery occurs when a medical procedure was performed without obtaining the proper informed consent before the treatment or procedure was performed. For example, a surgeon who has a signed consent form from a patient to amputate the patient's right arm but incidentally amputates the left arm. The patient will likely file a claim for a tort based on medical negligence. However, in addition, a claim for medical battery (an unwanted touching) also could be claimed.

Other types of intentional tort are false imprisonment, which is the unjustifiable detention of a person without his or her consent. Invasion of privacy, which is a key concept in issues related to confidentiality, is another example of an intentional tort. The patient has the right to the privacy of medical information. Photographs may not be taken, and information may not be released without consent. Some situations are newsworthy, and the public's right to know can exceed the patient's right to privacy. Knowledge of statutes and knowledge of relevant laws related to consent is vital. Defenses often used against intentional torts are consent (discussed later in this chapter), self-defense, defense of others, and necessity.[1-20]

Quasi-Intentional Torts

A *quasi-intentional tort* protects an individual's interest in a person's reputation, privacy, and freedom from unfounded legal action. It is a legal action that arises from damage inflicted on a person's

---

• BOX 21.1   Elements of a Malpractice

Presence of duty
Breach of duty
Foreseeability
Causation
Injury
Damages

reputation or privacy. Quasi-intentional torts are not based on negligence. For example, libel and slander (defamation) are quasi-intentional torts, as these involve the false intentional communication of information to a third party that causes harm to that individual. The act or intent is the key component of this tort. Whether or not the action was designed to cause harm or was malicious is not an issue. Tort law does not actually protect a person; it just provides an avenue through the courts to seek compensation for damages done.[1-20]

Vicarious Liability

Vicarious liability is defined as one party being responsible for the actions of another. The doctrine of *respondeat superior,* "let the master respond," has been used frequently when nurses are accused of malpractice. As a result of this doctrine, the employer has an obligation to ensure that employees perform duties in a competent, safe manner. Two elements must be shown: (1) the injured party must prove that the employer had control over the employee and (2) the negligent act occurred in the scope and course of the employment. Vicarious liability can be found with either malfeasance or nonfeasance of the employee.[1-20]

Courts have attached judgments directly against institutions for corporate negligence. Hospitals have found themselves accountable as an entity when the duty is owed directly to the patient and not through employees. Types of corporate duties attached directly to the institution are outlined in Box 21.2.[1-20]

Legal Issues in Critical Care Transport

Abandonment

The principles related to abandonment are important to transport provider practice. *Abandonment* occurs with unilateral termination of the provider–patient relationship without the consent from the patient. Abandonment is sometimes defined as the unilateral termination of the provider–patient relationship at a time when continuing care is needed and is a form of negligence. Abandonment can also occur if the care of the patient is transferred to a provider of lesser training when the patient needs a higher level of training. Transport teams can also be liable for abandonment if they deliver a patient to a medical facility and fail to give a verbal report specific to the patient and the care that was provided during transport, which may involve interventions/changes in condition. Transport issues concerning the assumption of care and release of such should be defined within policies and protocols of the transport program and with the review and guidance of legal counsel. It has been suggested that the act of dispatching an ambulance was presumptive of voluntary assumption of a duty to a patient.[5] In essence, those who have requested, or have had requested on their

---

• BOX 21.2   Examples of Corporate Duties Owed Directly to the Patient

Duty of reasonable care in maintenance and use of equipment
Availability of equipment and services
Duty of reasonable care in selecting and retaining employees
Adoption and assurance of compliance with rules related to administrative responsibility for patient care
Selection and retention of medical staff

---

behalf, medical assistance can be considered patients. In addition, a patient can also be considered those that have complaints suggestive of injury or illness, evidence of such, or who have experienced a situation or event that may precipitate injury or illness in the broadest sense can constitute a patient. This assumption should be considered in the development of communication center protocols in discussion with local medical direction.[14,17]

Consent Issues

Many medical tort claims are related to *consent issues.* They draw on the decisional capacity of the patient which means that they understand their current medical condition, the risks and benefits, and the alternatives of a proposed treatment plan and have the legal ability to provide consent. *Informed consent* requires more than a patient's signature on a consent form. The suggested treatment must be presented to the patient with a discussion of all material risks, consequences, and available alternatives. If the patient refuses the first treatment option, other treatment options should be explained. Informed consent requires understanding on the part of the patient.[1-20]

Consent can be written or oral. Providers are frequently asked to obtain signatures on consent forms. Before the patient signs, the provider should determine that the patient understands the purpose of the consent. *Expressed consent* exists when a patient with decisional capacity agrees to or requests evaluation, treatment, and/or transport. *Implied consent* exists when a patient is compliant with a request (extending arm for phlebotomy, allowing placement of nasal prongs, etc.). Implied consent also exists when a patient's current medical condition prevents them from being able to provide expressed consent or when a third party is not present to provide Third Party Consent. When the patient does not have the decisional capacity, or it is in question, then the use of a prehospital cognitive evaluation, which is used to evaluate the neurological and mental status, can assist in determining capacity. If the patient passes the evaluation and there is still concern regarding their decisional capacity, or if a medical condition exists that may affect their judgment, such as a head injury, then the transport professional should engage their medical director and law enforcement for on-scene guidance. In some cases, the lack of decisional capacity and their current medication condition may require involuntary care and transport. Through established state statutes, treatment protocols, online medical direction, and the assistance of law enforcement, transport professionals may have legal options which would allow for involuntary care and transport if the patient does not have the decisional capacity to make their own healthcare decisions or their current medical condition calls into question their decisional capacity. Consent for the treatment of minors is reserved for a parent or legal guardian. Implied consent is used for minors with life-threatening emergency conditions. The parents or legal guardian should be contacted as soon as possible for notification and consent. Most states have laws related to emancipated minors who can consent before the age of majority. In addition, minors may be allowed to consent to treatment of certain conditions, such as sexually transmitted diseases, pregnancy, and substance abuse.[1-20]

Refusal of care, or the withdrawal of consent to care, are areas that pose increased liability to both medical providers as well as medical direction, who ultimately oversee the care of the patient. Patients have the right to refuse part or all of an evaluation, as well as treatment and/or transport, if they have the decisional capacity to do so. As previously discussed, some states have laws that can provide a legal avenue for involuntary transport, such as those patients who present with complicated neurological conditions, mental disorders, or drug/alcohol intoxication. In an effort to avoid what would likely be considered a high-risk refusal, given some of these conditions mentioned, explaining in detail the risks involved as well as considering involving family and friends may help. Knowing that each situation confronted by transport personnel is unique, inquiring help from both family and friends is not without its risks. Involving medical direction as well as law enforcement can also provide support and offer rationality that not refusing treatment and transport is important. Some patients can have decisional capacity and knowledge of the seriousness of their medical condition yet still refuse treatment. It is important for transport professionals to thoroughly document the interaction and ensure that the patient is with family or friends who can provide support, and let them know that the transport professionals will return if needed. The court tends to support the right of the patient to make a knowing choice in refusing consent. The exception is in the case of minors. If the court is convinced a child needs life-saving measures, the compelling state's interest in the child usually overrides the parent's interest.[1–20]

Documentation

The trend toward increasing specialization means patients are assessed, cared for, and treated by more healthcare professionals than ever before. Thus, complete, accurate, and timely documentation is not only crucial to the continuity of care, but the record of treatment may form the basis of a defense against a claim for professional negligence. As documentation has become increasingly scientific and complex, the quality and precision of documentation have greater legal significance. Medical records provide contemporary proof of the nature and quality of care provided. A factual, timely, consistent, and complete patient care record will assist in proving that transport team members' actions were within the standard of care. The patient care record also establishes a record of the patient care continuum for the purpose of continuing education and research, provides data for cost analysis and containment, and establishes a standard for future documentation necessary to legally protect the provider. Documentation of care has become synonymous with care itself. Failure to document often implies that the care was not provided. One supposition of the legal system is that if the action was not written down, it did not happen. More specifically, if it was not properly documented, then it was not done. Although this may be a supposition of the legal system, medical practice and practical experience reveal that it is impossible to document everything done for a given patient. Courts in recent years have been moving toward greater acceptance of usual and customary practices and procedures when determining if a conduct not documented indeed took place. Transport team members should carefully document all positive and negative findings in order to ensure treatment rendered is in compliance with program protocols and guidelines. Essential components of a patient care record include an ongoing account and trending of patient complaints, signs, and symptoms, as well as a clear statement of the patient's condition before treatment and the response to treatment. The record should show evidence of provider judgment and critical thinking, not just a list of completed tasks and interventions; rather, it should document both why patient data were interpreted in a specific way and the outcome of the interventions.

Documentation in the medical record should be based on objective data and be:

- Concise, accurate, and thorough
- Include all interventions performed and response to interventions
- Clearly written and legible
- Without judgmental terms
- Timely

Illegible, poorly written, incorrect spelling, and missing or inaccurate records can serve as a reflection of the care that was provided. It can be used in a manner to try to label the care as inadequate and reduce the credibility of the members involved. Errors in documentation and a lack of attention in documenting can have unforeseen consequences years later when the provider needs to review their report during a deposition or when on the stand in a court of law. Charts must be timely and concurrent with care and written as soon as possible after transport. Most state laws indicate that a medical record must be delivered to the receiving facility within 24 hours of patient delivery. To avoid documentation pitfalls, using clear and concise information on a consistent basis can help to reduce the chance of errors. The use of abbreviations is strongly discouraged unless they are approved by organizations such as the Joint Commission or local medical control. Frequently, documentation is full of general phrases that lack supportive information and may be interpreted as biased or opinionated. Communication among emergency providers and the use of common terminology is critical. Understanding common medical terminology is important for effective communication and for documentation purposes. The key points of documentation are that it documents care and treatments given, validates continuity of care between health professionals, establishes a record of patient care so that it can be reviewed for continuity, continuing education and research, provides data for reimbursement and cost analysis, and legally protects the caregiver.

Health Insurance Portability and Accountability Act

The Health Insurance Portability and Accountability Act (HIPAA) was enacted by Congress in 1996. It is a federal law intended to protect patient health information and simplify the means by which healthcare providers electronically file and transmit healthcare claims. These safeguards currently apply to all protected health information, including electronic, written, verbal, and photographic forms. The HIPAA law has three different rules with specific compliance guidelines. The *Transaction and Code Set Rule* is primarily related to billing and requires that the transport team ensure that the appropriate information is documented to enhance this process. The *Privacy Rule* designates that private health information (PHI) about the patient be safeguarded and restricted. Finally, the *Security Rule* outlines how PHI should be protected, including encryption of transmitted data and physical security of a facility in which PHI is stored. HIPAA has presented a challenge to transport teams who must be careful and consistent in how information about the patient is provided and used. Implications for transport teams include the following:

- Transport team members must undergo mandatory HIPAA training.
- Oral and written information about the patient must be protected. Information about the patient should be appropriately stored.
- Patients should receive a Notice of Privacy Practices. This notice is not given during the transport process but should be provided after the emergency has passed.

Transport teams may share PHI about the patient with providers at a scene and at a referring hospital without a patient's consent, contact a base station and provide radio reports, provide follow-up on the patient for quality improvement purposes, and provide selected information with involved law enforcement.[16,17,23,25,33]

Information may also be shared without the patient's consent when information is needed related to the monitoring and controlling of communicable disease, injury, or disability; disclosure for compiling statistics, such as for births and deaths; reporting of adverse events to the Food and Drug Administration and disclosure to government oversight committees; disclosure to evaluate workplace injuries; and organ donation programs and certain law enforcement personnel. Examples of information that may be shared with law enforcement personnel include child maltreatment, PHI sought through the court system, and disclosure of limited information in the process of identifying a suspect. Transport team members must become aware of the implications of HIPAA to the patients that they transport and their practice.[16,17,23,25,33]

Consolidated Omnibus Budget Reconciliation Act/Emergency Medical Treatment and Active Labor Act[16]

The Emergency Medical Treatment and Active Labor Act (EMTALA) was enacted by Congress in 1986 to provide a path to access to emergency medical services notwithstanding their ability to pay or insurance status and has often been referred to as an "antidumping" law. EMTALA states that a hospital must provide treatment to stabilize a patient's medical condition or appropriately transfer the patient to another hospital that is able to provide appropriate management that otherwise could not have been provided at the medical facility that they originally presented at. The essential components of the EMTALA include the following:

1. All patients who present to an emergency department (ED) should receive a nondiscriminatory medical screening to determine whether a medical emergency is present.
2. A patient with a medical emergency must be stabilized within the capabilities of the transferring hospital and within reasonable probability that no material deterioration in the patient's clinical condition will occur.
3. If the patient must be transferred for further care, a receiving hospital must have accepted the patient and have the appropriate equipment and staff available to care for the patient.
4. The referring hospital must send all copies of medical records, diagnostic studies, and informed consent documents, and the patient must be transported with the appropriate vehicle and personnel.

If the patient's condition is unstable, the transfer certification must address the following[16]:

• Patient's condition
• Benefits of transfer
• Risk of transfer
• Specific information about the receiving facility, including that patient report was called to the receiving facility
• Description of the mode of transportation
• Patient or designate must sign a consent and certify how the transfer was initiated (patient request, physician request, or other)
• The form should be witnessed, and the patient or designee must sign that he or she understands the risks and benefits of transfer

In 1990, the COBRA law underwent further revisions that broadened the scope of who is subject to the law. The law now includes all participating physicians and any other physician responsible for the examination, treatment, or transfer of the patient at the participating hospital.[16] Further clarifications of EMTALA were released by the Department of Health and Human Services, Centers for Medicare and Medicaid Services in September 2003. The document was titled "Clarifying Policies Related to the Responsibilities of Medicare-Participating Hospitals in Treating Individuals with Emergency Medical Condition (Final Regulation)."[1–3,13–15,21–32] Violations of COBRA/EMTALA legislation include financial penalties and potential loss of government funding.

Use of Hospital Helipads

In 2004, site review guidelines from EMTALA helped to clarify the use of hospital helipads by Emergency Medical Services (EMS) personnel.[1,17] It is not uncommon to have Fire/EMS agencies use a hospital helipad as a means to transport a critical patient to an appropriate medical facility such as a trauma or burn center. In circumstances such as these, the patient handoff is not considered an EMTALA violation by the hospital, as there was never any intention that the patient would receive an examination or treatment at the medical facility where the helipad is at.

If medical assistance is requested by the ambulance crew, then it is likely that the hospital could become responsible for EMTALA compliance. If the hospital is the principal owner of the ambulance that requests the assistance of the helicopter on the helipad, then the hospital has a potential EMTALA obligation if the patient is transported from the scene of an emergency, as the patient must be transported to the owner-hospital. This specific scenario is subject to the exceptions under the "ambulance rule," such as if the patient meets transport to a specialty center such as for trauma or for management of a STEMI.[1,16,17]

Diversion

Over the past 15 years, EDs and hospital patient *diversion* have become an issue of concern for healthcare providers in the United States. Initially, it was seen in larger cities, but it has now become an issue across the entire country and even the world.[15,22,25,27] Causes of diversion include use of EDs for nonurgent cases; inadequate staffing; decrease in the number of EDs that are available in given areas of the country; use of ancillary services, such as computed tomographic or magnetic resonance imaging scans; and hospital bed shortages. Recent healthcare crises such as COVID-19 and variants of such have added to an increase in frequent hospital diversions, staff shortages, and limited resources to deal with the complex medical issues that are associated. Originally the implementation of freestanding emergency rooms in rural areas helped to provide a need where emergency services were limited. In some locations, freestanding emergency rooms provide a service outside of a hospital campus and are generally not located near the hospital that they are owned by. Although most illnesses can be managed at these locations, they generally require transfer to the main affiliated hospital for further management and care. Locations such as these have helped with overcrowding and providing available resources for transport teams. No matter the cause, diversion does have an impact on transport programs.[1,2,4,12,16,17,30,34] According to EMTALA, hospitals with specialized services, such as trauma and burn centers, do not have a "right" to divert; however, they can use diversion to help manage patient flow. The intent here is that diversion assists with keeping patients safe and improving quality of care.[15]

Transport teams, as well as stakeholders in healthcare, must be aware of diversion policies in the communities in which they serve and be a part of how these policies are developed. This can include a structured system that allows transport teams to bypass hospitals in order to prevent overcrowding or where these locations have limited beds available during times of increased EMS call volume. This selective bypass process should involve medical control as well as transport teams so that there is a mechanism to alter or change locations based on the patient's acuity. This awareness also includes the role of the transport program in the event of a disaster.

Similar to the resource issues identified in emergency room overcrowding and diversion, there are many times when a transport program may have to direct limited resources to meet multiple responses. While *Mission diversion* is not specifically involved with EMTALA regulations,[9] transport programs should have written policies and procedures about how and when missions are diverted, what priorities are used to determine which missions are diverted, who makes the decision to divert or redirect the patient, how transport teams are notified, and what type of documentation is required when a diversion occurs.

Medical Direction During Interfacility Patient Transfers

In the United States, transport team members' actions in the field are governed by state regulations, local regulations, and the policies of their organization. A physician medical director, often with the advice of a medical advisory committee, guides the development of these policies. Patient care generally falls within the responsibility of transferring personnel before the transfer and to the receiving team after the transport team releases the patient. Three possible sources of authority apply once the transport team and the patient leave the premises of the transferring hospital; transferring physician orders, transport teams protocols from their supervising physicians, and the wishes of the receiving physician. Written protocols should be available for transport teams, in the form of medical operations manuals or standard orders, to reference and follow. Medical directors should write or oversee the development of these protocols, to help give guidance to team members when physician presence is not available. Medical directors can also give guidance on patient care through direct consultation or online medical control. Under this paradigm, transport professionals effectively assume the role of out-of-hospital field agents to regional physicians who use standing orders and protocols to help guide their clinical decision-making.

The practice of critical care transport differs from the practice of emergency medicine. Likewise, emergency medicine differs from EMS, and interfacility transport differs from providing prehospital care. Each is a distinct specialty with focused knowledge, skills, and abilities. This may require several physicians working together to provide the experience and expertise required for a comprehensive medical transport service.

Physicians in a medical specialty usually practice in the hospital and may not be familiar with the operational aspects of critical care transport. Specialists are more likely to require additional training to function efficiently in the prehospital environment and for them to function in a medical direction capacity. It may be easier for physicians/medical directors who are familiar with EMS and/or critical care transport to assume leadership of transport programs.

Physicians who have completed a fellowship in Emergency Medicine, or who have obtained board certification in EMS, are generally more familiar with what is involved in caring for patients outside hospital settings.

Treatments and procedures administered by transport team members generally fall under one of two categories: online medical orders or offline medical orders (standing orders). Online medical control provides the unique perspective and knowledge of medical personnel to assist with critical decision-making during patient care such as with treatment options and deviations from standard treatment outlines. In addition, certain situations may post specific medicolegal concerns and risks that are best addressed by the guidance of online medical staff. This type of communication is generally conducted through voice communication, which should be recorded to allow for review purposes and quality assurance.

Offline medical control is generally known as protocols or standing orders and provides the standards of treatment expected for patient care. These orders are considered an extension of care by the medical control physician. It is a delegated medical practice that also provides the guidelines for high-risk procedures such as rapid sequence intubation, cricothyrotomy, and chest tube insertions which, due to their seriousness and due to time constraints, may not allow for direct communication with medical control staff prior to them being performed. Although not every circumstance or situation encountered by critical transport providers can be covered, standing orders can be used as a guideline during times of limited communication, such as during natural or manmade disasters.

Scope of Practice and Standards of Care

Scope of practice and standards of care for transport team members may vary based on whether a transport program is hospital based, provided by a private vendor, or a governmental entity. Local medical communities and practices may affect how transport team members provide medical care. Scope of practice does not define a standard of care, nor does it define what should be done in a given situation. It defines what is legally permitted to be performed by the licensed individuals at that level, not what must be done. The scope of practice addresses the question of what providers are allowed to do legally, as established by state statutes, or rules and regulations. Standard of care addresses whether the right thing was performed and, if so, whether it was done properly. This is often determined by the scope of practice, literature, and expert witnesses to evaluate professional judgment.

Scope of practice defines the parameters of various duties or services that may be provided by an individual with a specific licensure. Whether regulated by rule, statute, or court decision, it represents the limits of services an individual may legally perform. Scope of practice identifies the activities and procedures that represent illegal activity if performed without licensure. In addition to drawing boundaries between the professionals and the lay public, scope of practice also defines the boundaries among professionals, creating either exclusive or overlapping domains of practice. Scope of practice, however, does not define every activity of a licensed individual. Rather it delineates specific activities regulated by law, including technical skills that, if performed improperly, represent significant harm to the patient and therefore must be kept out of the hands of untrained individuals. With respect to the scope of practice, a medical director cannot increase it for transport team members or discipline unless the state regulatory agency allows for such change. The medical director assumes the risk and responsibility that they have overseen training and that transport team members are able to safely perform the specific procedures.

Critical care transport medicine is a specialized practice environment that differs in many ways from other areas of critical care medicine. Transport team members must possess highly complex decision-making skills to assess, manipulate and support vital organ system function and/or prevent further life-threatening deterioration of a patient's condition during transport. These differences include an unstructured work environment, working in a multidisciplinary team, limited supplies, limited support, and altered assessment approaches.

Critical care transport team members often are held responsible for knowing the normal and expected course for a patient having a specific condition or undergoing a specific procedure, knowing what is not normal and not expected within their area of specialty practice. Actions taken must be consistent with what a reasonable and prudent specialty provider would do under the same or similar circumstances, based on scope and standards commonly recognized by members of the professional specialty. Critical care transport medicine requires professionals to assess and prioritize patient care in an environment that is often noisy and chaotic. They must be able to function under different degrees of stress before, during, and after patient transport, while applying expertise in clinical decision-making and acting professionally and autonomously. Team members are accountable for functioning within their scope of practice despite distractions in the environment.

To discuss the scope of practice and standards of care that is expected of critical care transport, it is also prudent to provide an overview of the practice requirements, which include the education, certification, licensure, and the credentialing aspects.

Education for transport team members is generally obtained through postsecondary schooling as part of the requirement to obtain the initial discipline-focused licensure. Specific education requirements vary by discipline.

Training for transport team members should include a comprehensive orientation program that includes both didactic and clinical instruction is essential to achieving a level of competence. Transport team members must possess skills in both critical care and emergency medicine in order to effectively assess, plan, implement, and evaluate actual and potential patient problems.

Licensure represents permission granted to an individual by the state to perform certain restricted activities that the individual could not legally do without such permission. Licensure provides a certain amount of autonomy in delivering care but must also satisfy ongoing requirements that ensure a certain minimum level of competency.

Certification is essentially an external verification of the competencies that an individual has achieved and typically involves an examination process. Certifications specific to critical care or advanced practice care providers ensure that a basic understanding of topics and treatment related to critical patients has been achieved. In some cases, transport team members who are new or recently assigned to critical care transport may lack this certification. On-the-job training as the new provider prepares for the certification exam is an effective way to gain firsthand practical experience which can help to make some topics related to critical care medicine understandable.

Credentialing is generally conducted by healthcare organizations on a local level and is used to verify qualifications, education,

and skills of licensed providers. It is a form of protection that assures organizations maintain the highest standards and safety for patient care.

Ethical Issues

Today, transport team members are faced with many ethical dilemmas, including whom to transport and by what method; when not to transport, especially if patient resuscitation is futile; and being asked or forced to transport patients in unsafe environments, for example, when the weather is less than optimal. Some transport teams are forced to make decisions about whether to transport a patient with equipment or problems that they have inadequate experience handling because of competition or fear of revenue loss.[4,26,27,29,35–42]

Ethical Decision-Making in the Transport Environment

Ethical decisions are generally made based on a set of specific values, which include the following[27,35]:
- *Patient autonomy:* Allowing patients to make decisions about their healthcare.
- *Beneficence* versus *malfeasance:* The benefit of the transport outweighs the potential harm the transport could cause.
- *Veracity:* Honesty, telling the truth, open patient care, and healthcare provider relationships; veracity should also extend to statement of purpose for the transport program.
- *Justice:* Fairness for the patient and, at times, the community that the transport program serves.

Unfortunately, multiple demands may influence the transport decision, including competition, lack of experience, and concern about employment.

The availability of equipment, advanced life support skills, and personnel has contributed to the development of a *technologic imperative.*[4,27,29,35–42] In other words, because it exists, it must be used. Patients, families, and communities have come to expect access to the newest and best technologies and everything should be available for everyone.

In 1995, Iserson and colleagues[37,38] developed a model that is still pertinent to making ethical decisions in the transport environment. This model includes the following:
- Problem perception: Is there a problem?
- List alternatives: Identify solutions and barriers.
- Choose an alternative.
- List the consequences of the actions chosen.
- Consider one's own personal beliefs when making the decision.
- Evaluate the decision.

Ethical decision-making is a dynamic process. The transport team cannot ignore previous experience or the personal beliefs of the team members and those with whom the team is working. These things are never easy, but they cannot be overlooked.

Additional Legal Issues Regarding Transportation

Transport Decisions

As healthcare costs continue to increase, the cost of patient transport and appropriate use of services have become important issues that many transport programs must address. Deciding when to transport a patient who has sustained cardiac arrest, whether as a result of trauma or a medical problem, continues to be one of the most difficult dilemmas faced by many transport programs. For a patient who is in the emergency room in cardiac arrest, transport teams generally would not consider transport until the patient is relatively stable to tolerate transport. For the patient who needs specialized care that is not available at the emergency room, such as with a ruptured spleen, chest tube placement, or other intervention, critical care transport staff would need to evaluate whether the patient is stable enough for transfer versus the desires of the referring facility staff to transfer the patient regardless of condition. Other factors contributing to the determination of transport include those surrounding the transport personnel themselves, such as the duration of their current shift or the number of highly complex transports they have completed previously.

Patient- and Family-Centered Care

Patient care during transport is generally focused on meeting the physiologic needs of an acutely ill or injured patient. However, the patient is generally a part of a family, although the definition of the term may vary. A family may be described in legal, cultural, religious, or personal terms. The families of today are as diverse as the people who live in them.[22,31,32,34,43–45]

Although transport team members are accustomed to the transport environment and process, they should not forget that this experience is new and often frightening for the family members of a seriously ill or injured person. The transport team must consider care of the family to be an extension of patient care and not an additional task that needs to be accomplished. The support that healthcare professionals provide to a patient's family during the initial stages of the patient's crisis can be invaluable. Contact with a transport team or ED staff may be the family's first interaction with healthcare personnel in this emergency. The family's perception of the response of these healthcare providers can be the impetus to either healthy or ineffective coping. Ideally, early interventions aimed at decreasing the family's stress should be performed to prevent the breakdown of the family structure.[10,24,31,32,43,44]

Unfortunately, death is an inherent part of the transport process. Some patients die before transport, and the role the family may play in this dying process can make patient care particularly arduous for the transport team.

Family Considerations in the Transport Environment

Family members of critically ill or injured patients are already under stress,[22,31,32,34,43–45] and the need to transport the patient on a fixed-wing aircraft, helicopter, or ground vehicle adds to that level of stress.[22,31,32,34,43–45] Decisions concerning care must be made quickly, and the patient's family members often feel uninformed and unsure, especially if they have limited medical knowledge. Because time is a factor, the family has no opportunity to elicit medical information and request second opinions.

Family members may feel uncomfortable relaying concerns about the transport to the healthcare providers and transport team. Some concerns are related to the medical treatment rendered or even the safety of transport. Other concerns may include the following[10,24,31,32,43,44]:

- Separation from their loved one for the duration or distance of the transport

- Uncertainty about the events that necessitated transfer and transport of the patient
- Lack of understanding of the medical diagnosis
- The referring physicians, nurses, and transport team members are unfamiliar to the family and patient

Because most patients who need critical care transport have injuries or illnesses that are sudden and unplanned, family members usually do not have time to prepare for the emergency. If they have never been exposed to this type of crisis, they may not have the coping skills needed to effectively manage the stress entailed.[10,24,31,32,43,44]

Transporting Family Members

Family members frequently ask whether they can travel to the receiving facility with the patient. Research continues to show that patients, families, and healthcare providers can benefit from family presence.[43]

The decision to transport a family member is based on multiple factors, some more important than others. The entire transport team should provide input, but safety should always be the overriding principle. In air transport, the pilot has the final word and has to consider how additional passengers will affect both the weight and balance of the aircraft. The extent of care that will be needed during transport also must be taken into consideration. With certain transports, there may not be sufficient room to accommodate a family member. Other factors include the emotional state of the family members. Safety for the entire team is the primary factor on which to base this decision when concern exists about the possibility of transporting a family member.

Other factors the team may take into consideration when deciding whether to transport members of the patient's family are the patient's age, the seriousness of the patient's condition, other transportation available to the family, and the length of the transport time. Box 21.3 provides examples of inclusion and exclusion criteria for transport of family members.

Some transport vehicles, particularly air medical, are not capable of carrying an additional passenger because of performance factors or space limitations. Although the aircraft may have the capability of carrying extra passengers, some limitations, including engine power, effects of weather on equipment performance, and the amount of weight the aircraft can safely carry, determine whether an additional passenger can be brought aboard.

When transporting family members, they must be transported in the passenger seat of the vehicle, properly fastened according to the laws of the state. Transport programs should have in place policies to support the decision-making process regarding sibling transport, with safety being a priority. Ultimately the final decision always rests with the vehicle operator and medical team, taking into consideration what is best for the patient and the safety of all concerned.

Orders and Giving Report

Documentation of orders regarding patient care that are received or discussed should include the time and full name of the physician providing such. The documentation of orders that are denied is just as important as those that are approved or authorized. This helps to establish the thought process of the clinician at the time that care was being provided. Verbal communications, especially those requiring medical orders, should be done in a way to allow for the conversation to be recorded for review, clarification, and

CHAPTER 21 Legal and Professional Issues in Critical Care Transport

• BOX 21.3 Examples of Inclusion/Exclusion Criteria for Determination of Whether Family Members Should Accompany a Patient During Air Medical Transport

Inclusion of family members during air medical transport may be desirable in the following cases:
- The referring facility is far from the receiving facility, and the family has no other means of transportation.
- The patient is near death, and the family wishes to be with the patient during his or her last moments.
- The patient is a child and would benefit from being accompanied by a parent.
- The family and the patient both strongly want the family to accompany the patient.

Exclusion of family members during air medical transport may be desirable in the following cases:
- Inclusion of the family member will interfere with patient care.
- The family member's weight exceeds permissible parameters.
- The family member is overly anxious and poses a danger to the safety of the transport.
- The landing zone is walled in on three sides, and the pilot must do a vertical takeoff.
- A crew member has a concern about a family member.
- Weather conditions are marginal.
- The family member has a fear of flying.
- The family member gets motion sickness.
- The distance between the two facilities is short.
- The patient's condition is unstable and requires extensive care.

quality assurance purposes. The patient care report and to whom it was provided should also be documented as well. If radio reports are performed, they should be brief, clear, and concise. When giving a report, it should include, at a minimum, a history of the present illness/mechanism of injury, assessment findings, and treatment initiated. If orders are given by online medical control, they need to be acknowledged and repeated for verification purposes. If other transport team members are present, discuss with them in a cross-check format, whether it pertains to medications or procedures, that it is agreed that the intervention is the right thing to do for the patient. This will help to reduce the chance of errors. A completed patient care report is the only verification that all relevant care performed, as well as the handoff of the patient to the receiving facility, has been accomplished.

Litigation

Professional clinicians, by the very nature of the work performed and at times life-threatening interventions that may have been performed, may be called upon to testify as a fact or expert witness in a claim involving allegations of professional negligence. Professional negligence, or malpractice, is a more complicated claim than simple negligence. The claimant has the burden of proving by a preponderance of evidence that the actions of the healthcare provider were not consistent with what is generally accepted as the standard of care. The professional standard of care for a given healthcare provider is that the level of care, skill, and treatment while considering all relevant surrounding circumstances, is recognized as acceptable and appropriate by reasonably similar healthcare providers. The elements of a lawsuit can be vast and complex to the layperson and can invoke fears of the amount of liability that the transport professional may be responsible for.

To understand the elements of a lawsuit and how much direct involvement the transport professional has is best answered by legal advice from a licensed attorney and would be too broad to discuss here.

Conclusion

The role of the transport professional as well as the expectations to be efficient in the job require that we undertake a continuous fact and evidence-based approach by furthering our education through researching and reviewing these important topics discussed here. Legal and professional issues that the transport professional may encounter are vast and although not every topic can be presented and discussed in this chapter, it should help to serve as the first blocks of a strong foundation furthered by staying current on both the legal and professional issues that are encountered daily. This can be achieved through legal journals specific to the medical community or discussing case studies that can help to establish a framework for a resolution if such situations are encountered through the course of our day-to-day job.

References

1. American College of Emergency Physicians (ACEP). Appropriate interfacility patient transfer. *Ann Emerg Med*. 2016;67(5):690.
2. Burt CW, McCaig LF, Valverde R. Analysis of ambulance transports and diversions among US emergency departments. *Ann Emerg Med*. 2006;47(4):317–326.
3. Commission on Accreditation of Air Medical Transport Systems (CAMTS). *Accreditation Standards*. 10th ed. CAMTS; 2015.
4. Geiderman J, Marco CA, Moskop J, et al. Ethics of ambulance diversion. *Am J Emerg Med*. 2015;33(6):822–827.
5. George JE. *Law and Emergency Care*. Mosby; 1980.
6. Hoot NR, Aronsky D. Systematic review of emergency department crowding: Causes, effects and solutions. *Ann Emerg Med*. 2008; 52(2):126–136.
7. Kelen G, Peterson S, Pronovost P. In the name of patient safety, let's burden the emergency department more. *Ann Emerg Med*. 2016; 67(5):737–740.
8. Magauran BG. Risk management for the emergency physician: Competency and decision-making capacity, informed consent, and refusal of care against medical advice. *Emerg Med Clin North Am*. 2009;27(4):605–614, viii.
9. Williams A. Legal issues in air and ground transport. In: Blumen I, ed. *Principles and Directions of Air Medical Transport*. Air Medical Physicians Association; 2015:170–194.
10. William J. Family presence during resuscitation: To see or not to see. *Nurs Clin North Am*. 2002;37(1):211–220.
11. York-Clark D, Stocking J, Johnson J, eds. *Flight and Ground Transport Nursing Core Curriculum*. Air & Surface Transport Nurses Association; 2006.
12. York-Clark D, Johnson J, Stocking J, Treadwell D, Corbett P, eds. *Critical Care Transport Core Curriculum*. Air & Surface Transport Nurses Association; 2017.
13. American Academy of Pediatrics. *Air and Ground Transport of Neonatal and Pediatric Patients*. 3rd ed. AAP; 2007.
14. Beahan S. Legal issues in medical records/health information management. In: Thomas Payne, ed. *Practical Guide to Clinical Computing Systems*. 2nd ed. 2015:167–178.
15. Cushing M. *Nursing Jurisprudence*. Appleton & Lange; 1988.
16. Emergency Medical Treatment and Active Labor Act, as established under the Consolidated Omnibus Budget Reconciliation Act (COBRA) of 1985 (42 USC 1395 dd) and 42 CFR 489.24; 42 CFR 489.20 (EMTALA regulations).

17. Fanaroff J. Legal issues in pediatric transport. *Clin Pediatr Emerg Med.* 2013;14(3):180–187.

18. Requarth JA. Informed consent challenges in frail delirious, demented, and do-not-resuscitate adult patients. *J Vasc Radiol.* 2015; 26(11):1647–1651.

19. Thibeault SM, ed. *Transport Professional Advanced Trauma Course.* 6th ed. Air & Surface Transport Nurses Association; 2015.

20. Treadwell D, James S, Arndt K, Werth R. *Standards for Critical Care and Specialty Transport.* Air & Surface Transport Nurses Association; 2015.

21. Agency for Healthcare Research Quality. 2016. Accessed June 19, 2016. http://www.ahrq.gov/

22. American Heart Association. *Family Support.* 2015. Accessed June 18, 2016. https://eccguidelines.heart.org/index.php/circulation/cpr-ecc-guidelines-2/part-3-ethical-issues/?strue=1&id=5-1

23. Baker EF, Moskop JC, Geiderman JM, et al. Law enforcement and emergency medicine: An ethical analysis. *Ann Emerg Med.* 2016; 68(5):599–607.

24. Beachley M. Evolution of the trauma cycle. In: McQuillan KA, Makic MB, Whalen E, eds. *Trauma Nursing: From Resuscitation to Rehabilitation.* 4th ed. Saunders; 2009:1–18.

25. Ben-Assuli O. Electronic health records adoption, quality of care, legal and privacy issues and their implementation in emergency departments. *Health Policy.* 2015;119(3):287–297.

26. Boehringer BK, Tilney P. An elderly man in cardiac arrest on a ski slope. *Air Med J.* 2015;34(2):62–63.

27. Campbell TW. Do death attitudes of nurses and physicians differ? *Omega.* 1983;14(1):43–49.

28. Carruba C. Role of medical director in air medical transport. In: Blumen I, ed. *Principles and Directions of Air Medical Transport.* Air Medical Physicians Association; 2015:89–96.

29. Chester A, Harris T, Hodgetts T, Keefe N. Survival to discharge after cardiac arrest attended by a doctor-paramedic helicopter emergency medical service: An Utstein-style multiservice review of 1085 activations. *J Emerg Med.* 2015;49(4):439–447.

30. Clark J. That transport was appropriate, wasn't it? *Air Med J.* 2015;35(1):16–18.

31. Doyle CJ. Family participation during resuscitation: An option. *Ann Emerg Med.* 1987;16(6):673–675.

32. Dwyer T. Predictors of public support for family presence during cardiopulmonary resuscitation: A population based study. *Int J Nurs Stud.* 2015;52(6):1064–1070.

33. Lazar RA. *EMS Law: A Guide for EMS Professionals.* Aspen; 1989.

34. Emergency Nurses Association. *Trauma Nursing Core Course.* 7th ed. Emergency Nurses Association; 2014.

35. Erler CJ, Thompson CB. Ethics, human rights and clinical research. *Air Med J.* 2008;27(3):110–113.

36. Guyette F, Reynolds J, Frisch A, Post Cardiac Arrest Service. Cardiac arrest resuscitation. *Emerg Med Clin North Am.* 2015;33(3):669–690.

37. Iserson K, Sanders A, Mathieu D. *Ethics in Emergency Medicine.* Galen Press; 1995.

38. Kraus C, Marco C. Shared decision-making in the ED: Ethical consideration. *Am J Emerg Med.* 2016;34(8):1668–1672.

39. Lu D, Guenther E, Wesley A, Gallagher T. Disclosure of harmful medical errors in out-of-hospital care. *Ann Emerg Med.* 2013; 61(2):215–221.

40. U.S. Department of Health and Human Services Food and Drug Administration Office of Good Clinical Practice Center for Drug Evaluation and Research Center for Biologics Evaluation and Research Center for Devices and Radiological Health. *Guidance for Institutional Review Boards, Clinical Investigators, and Sponsors. Exception From Informed Consent Requirements for Emergency Research.* March 2011, Updated April 2013. Accessed June 19, 2016. http://www.fda.gov/downloads/RegulatoryInformation/Guidances/UCM249673.pdf

41. Venkat A, Huckstein JV, Dhindson HS. Ethical issues in air medical transport. In: Blumen I, ed. *Principles and Directions of Air Medical Transport.* Air Medical Physicians Association; 2015:32–38.

42. Von Vopelius-Feldt J, Coulter A, Benger J. The impact of prehospital critical care team on survival from out-of-hospital cardiac arrest. *Resuscitation.* 2015;96:290–295.

43. Flanders SA, Strasen JH. Review of evidence about family presence during resuscitation. *Crit Care Clin North Am.* 2014;26(4):533–550.

44. Fultz JH. Air medical transport: What the family wants to know. *J Air Med Transp.* 1993;12(11–12):431–435.

45. Joyce C, Libertin R, Bigham M. Family centered care in pediatric critical care transport. *Air Med J.* 2015;34(1):32–36.

22

Quality

MICHAEL A. FRAKES AND BRIAN M. WILSON

The World Health Organization defines quality of care as the degree to which health services for individuals and populations increase the likelihood of desired health outcomes. Quality is subjective, a concept for which each consumer of a good or service has a unique expectation. Broadly, quality can be considered as freedom from defects and the ability of a good or service to satisfy stated or implied needs. Different stakeholders have different perceptions, such as economic efficiency for insurers, revenue for investors, clinical knowledge and technical performance for providers, and, for patients, interpersonal elements of the care experience and the avoidance of harm. Increasing the challenge is that perceptions of quality are dynamic – changing as products, services, people, processes, and environments vary.

History

The modern quality profession began when Walter Shewhart described statistical process control for measuring variance in production systems. His methods are still used today. Dr. W. Edwards Deming and Dr. Joseph Juran drew on Shewhart's work and recognized that system problems could be addressed through three fundamental managerial processes – planning, control, and improvement. Deming is also closely associated with the use of the Plan–Do–Check–Act (PDCA) cycle, a systematic approach to improving work processes.

Deming, Juran, and others championed the idea that quality means meeting customer requirements and that increased productivity is the result of quality improvement. They advocate for management commitment and employee involvement to improve systems and avoid problems, prioritizing identification of the most critical problems and the use of statistics and other problem-solving tools. Deming wrote about the need for transformational approach to business and quality, summarized in his 14 points of management, which are listed in Box 22.1.

Kaoru Ishikawa enlarged the scope of the quality team to include employees, not just managers. In 1987, the criteria for the first Malcolm Baldrige National Quality Award were published. At the same time, the ISO 9001, Quality Systems – Model for quality assurance in design, development, production, installation, and servicing was published. Both established standardized measurement systems to benchmark organizations against comprehensive quality rubrics.

• BOX 22.1   Deming's 14 Points

1. Create constancy of purpose.
2. Adopt the new philosophy.
3. Cease dependence on mass inspection.
4. Constantly and forever improve the system.
5. Remove barriers.
6. Drive out fear.
7. Break down barriers between departments.
8. Eliminate slogans, exhortations, and targets.
9. Eliminate work standards, quotas, and numerical goals.
10. Institute modern methods of supervision and leadership.
11. Institute training on the job.
12. Institute a program of self-improvement and retraining.
13. End the practice of awarding business on price alone.
14. Put everybody to work to accomplish the transformation.

Domains of Quality

Donabedian famously described broad categories of measures looking at structures, processes, and outcomes. Those domains are easily overlaid on the four environments in which we operate – direct patient care, the microsystem of our care delivery operation, the mesosystem which supports the care delivery operation, and the macrosystems of healthcare, business, and vehicle operations (see Fig. 22.1). An optimal quality structure incorporates the three Donabedian categories across the four environments.

Systems are sets of interrelated processes, and processes are interacting activities that transform inputs into outputs. Process management, then, relies on an organization's ability to identify processes and, for each process, understand their stakeholders and know the inputs and outputs. There is variation in all processes, but quality and efficiency are best when variation is minimized. Process monitoring and evaluation for special causes lends itself to the use of statistical process controls. Special cause variation results from unexpected or unusual occurrences that are not inherent in the process and identifies a need for improvement. Using statistical process controls in monitoring helps to distinguish normal or common cause variation from special cause variation (Box 22.4). This is important because making minor adjustments

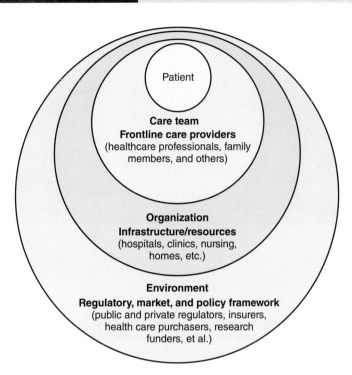

• **Figure 22.1** Healthcare Environments.

to a process when normal variation is misperceived as special variation, called tampering, can paradoxically worsen variation.

Process improvement extends monitoring to improving systems and products by using problem-solving approaches to understand the root causes of barriers to optimal performance, then to identify the best way to remove those barriers. This may be directed at improving a process that is performing as expected but for which a higher level of performance is desired, or it can be directed at reducing variation. Like tampering with a controlled process, trying to "fix" problems may paradoxically worsen them while seeking to understand root causes and using that learning to reduce variation and to diminish non-value-added activities will improve outputs.

In addition to evaluating internal performance, opportunities for improvement are also identified by comparing performance against external benchmarks. It is in the identification of performance measures that an organization has the biggest opportunity to be boundary-spanning and to show a true organizational approach.

Practically, one approach is to consider the core business of each department in the organization as viewed by internal and external customers. For example, external customers want the Communications Center to answer the phone quickly and politely, to send a vehicle in a timely fashion, and to offer an accurate ETA. Internal customers need accurate data capture, accurate location tracking, rapid detection of overdue vehicles, and technically correct responses to vehicle emergencies.

Specific indicators and goals can come from a wide array of sources, and casting a broad net is helpful to the organization. The Malcolm Baldrige Foundation describes how the best organizations compare themselves not with similar organizations or best-in-class organizations but against the best organizations in the area of interest. It makes sense to aspire to provide the same performance quality as national and world leaders. Don't be afraid to be great.

For our medical transport systems, we certainly want to consider health quality initiatives, industry performance databases, scientific literature, and best-practice patient management guidelines. Particularly for operational and administrative service lines, regulatory requirements, accreditation requirements, contractual obligations, professional society standards, and internal policies can be good sources of performance measures.

Integrated Quality Systems

Organizations work to create a climate of excellence, personal growth, and organizational growth. The organization is strongest when employees at all levels are empowered to utilize their talents fully, to take actions (within boundaries) without prior approval, and to be involved fully in organizational processes, including performance improvement teams. Employees in environments providing this training and support understand that they are valued for their minds, not just their work.

Quality is not a stand-alone element of an entity but must be integrated with all three levels of the organization: strategic planning, tactical planning, and operations. Consistent quality planning, monitoring, and reviewing are required in each of those three levels. Quality planning includes understanding changing customer needs and expectations, support of and alignment with strategic plans, linking goals with tactics and operations, and balancing short- and long-term requirements. The quality system helps assure that performance measures, process monitoring, and initiatives are deployed through all parts of the organizational structure and that there is boundary-spanning integration across functional areas in the organization. The quality system must include structures for evaluation and process improvement and ultimately should integrate quality activities into the regular front-line work.

Kaizen reflects the practice of implementing small, gradual changes across the whole organization, for the long time horizon of the organization. When fully deployed, everyone in the organization participates. It is driven by a basic belief that when quality becomes ingrained in the organization's people, the quality of products and services will follow. Key factors are the initiation of operating practices that lead to the uncovering of waste and non-value-added steps, the involvement of everyone in the organization, extensive training in the concepts and tools for improvement, and a management that views improvement as an integral part of the organization's strategy.

Quality system philosophies coalesce around eight traits of a total quality structure, given as follows.

1. Strategically based: organizations have a comprehensive strategic plan that contains at least the elements of vision, broad objectives, and activities to complete the broad objectives. The plan is to give substantial competitive advantage in the marketplace.
2. Focus on internal and external customers: the customer is the driver. External customers define the quality of the product or service delivered, whereas internal customers help define the quality of people, processes, and the environment associated with the product services.
3. Obsession with a quality product: an organization must be obsessed with exceeding the customer's definition of quality – perfect the product you deliver most often.
4. Scientific approach: use hard data for establishing benchmarks, monitoring performance, and making improvements.
5. Long-term commitment: creating an ongoing culture of total quality improvement is essential.

6. Teamwork: internal enthusiasm and energy helps to improve quality and the success of quality measures, thereby improving external competitiveness.
7. Continual process of improvement: this is necessary to improve the process. Products are delivered by processes, developed by people who can change and improve the product.
8. Employee empowerment: simultaneously brings more minds into the decision-making process and increases ownership.

Improvement Frameworks

Improvements in structure, process, and outcome are classically accomplished through iterative Plan–Do–Check–Act (or Plan–Do–Study–Act) improvement cycles (Fig. 22.2).

In planning, a process is selected and a clear improvement objective defined. The project team involves stakeholders representing elements of the process. It is important to understand the process and stakeholders well in order to avoid erroneous assumptions and oversimplification. It is often helpful to define processes with a flowchart, which will help both with understanding participants and the efficiency of steps in the process. From that deep understanding, the team develops a data collection and measurement plan. Baseline data is gathered to illuminate the problem and for future use to evaluate improvement. A 1-year "lookback" is a common timeframe for establishing an effective baseline; however, quality teams are encouraged to extend this interval as far as necessary to acquire meaningful and useful data.

Clear operational definitions are key to assuring that data collection is accurate and comparisons are consistent. This can be extraordinarily challenging. A classic medical example is, "What counts as an airway management attempt?" Operationally, how do you ensure that vehicle arrival and departure times are consistently and accurately recorded? If you are relying on provider radio reports, does each operator key the radio at the same part of the transport? Does the pilot report "overhead," which incorporates a variable time left for the descent, or "skids down?" Does

the ground vehicle operator report when the vehicle is on property, in the ambulance bay, or in park?

It is at this point where the team uses quality and data management tools, described later, to identify special cause variation and to identify the root causes of problems. A simple root cause tool is the "five whys," the technique of asking "why" after each successive response to peel away layers of "symptoms" and ultimately to understand the cause of those symptoms. From the determined causes, the improvement team can develop a plan for implementing possible changes.

As the improvement team progresses to "Do," the proposed change is tested in so-called rapid cycle improvements. Changes are made and tested over periods of 3 or months or less, often in a separable subset of the organization, like a location or shift.

Changes are implemented using the principles of effective change management. A full treatment of change management is beyond the scope of this chapter but briefly involves five elements, summarized in Box 22.2.

Results are analyzed as the cycle progresses and when it is complete, looking for improvements compared with the baseline and for unintended consequences both in the studied process and in affected processes. Successful changes are implemented on a larger scale, and the improvement cycle continues as other iterative changes, identified in the planning phase or illuminated by the pilot test, are put through a new PDCA cycle. There must also be an element of ongoing monitoring of implemented changes in the data gathering plan.

Particularly for process improvements, the rubrics of Lean and Six-Sigma are commonly considered. Lean is a system for developing process improvement that is continuous and focuses on reducing and eliminating waste, defined as anything that does not increase value to the customer. The classic domains of waste are summarized in the acronym DOWNTIME (Box 22.3). Six-Sigma makes use of statistics and data analysis to analyze and reduce errors or defects. The purpose is to reduce defects to no more than 3.4 per million units or events. Both Lean and Six-Sigma have significant overlap with the general quality management

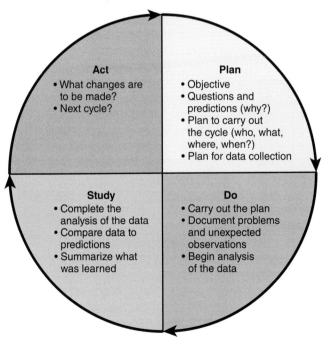

• **Figure 22.2** PDSA Cycles.

• BOX 22.2 Tenets of Change Management

- Provide supportive resources: Infrastructure, equipment, and software systems. Consider also the tools needed for reeducation, retraining, and rethinking priorities and practices.
- Communication. Groups have established skill sets, knowledge, customs, and experiences. Providing clear and open lines of communication throughout the process is a critical element in all change modalities. This involves transparency and two-way communication structures that provide avenues to vent frustrations, applaud what is working, and seamlessly change what doesn't work.
- Monitor and manage resistance. Resistance is a very normal part of change management, but it can threaten the success of a project. Most resistance occurs due to a fear of the unknown and because of the risk associated with change. Anticipating and preparing for resistance by arming leadership with tools to manage it will aid in a smooth change lifecycle.
- Celebrate success. When managing a change through its lifecycle, recognize the success of teams and individuals involved. This will help in the adoption of both your change management process as well as adoption of the change itself.
- Review and revise. As much as change is difficult, it is also an ongoing process. Like communication, ongoing monitoring and adaptation should be woven through all steps to identify and remove roadblocks.

- Defects: mistakes that require additional time, resources, and money to fix.
- Overproduction: production when those who receive their output either are not ready for it or do not need it.
- Waiting: work has to stop to wait for a bottleneck to be cleared.
- Not utilizing talent: not or underutilizing people's talents, skills, and knowledge.
- Transportation: waste caused by moving things around.
- Inventory excess: supply in excess of real customer demand.
- Motion waste: excess movement caused by employees or machines, which does not add value.
- Excess processing: processing more than is required or as a result of long-winded, poorly designed processes.

principles of customer focus, attention to added value, continuous improvement, and interest in employee engagement.

Quality Tools

Understanding performance against a measure requires some structure and, often, some math. There are seven classic quality tools, originally developed by Kaoru Ishikawa and implemented as Japan's postwar industrial complex turned to statistical quality control as a means of quality assurance. These tools help to clarify current understanding of performance and to uncover root causes.

Stratification. Stratification sorts data into distinct groups to help reveal patterns that might not otherwise be visible when it is viewed overall. Examples are days of the week, per-base, per-shift, or air vs. ground. As with operational definitions, considering stratification early is important to assure that segmentation information is included.

Histogram. A histogram aids in representing data frequency distributions across different stratified sample groups, allowing you to quickly and easily identify areas of improvement within your processes. With a structure similar to a bar graph, each bar within a histogram represents a group, while the height of the bar represents the frequency of data within that group (see Fig. 22.3).

Check sheet (tally sheet). Check sheets collect quantitative or qualitative data. A check sheet collects data in the form of check or tally marks that indicate how many times a particular value has occurred, allowing you to quickly zero in on defects or errors within your process or product, defect patterns, and even causes of specific defects. These are often preliminary data analysis tools.

Cause-and-effect diagram. Also known as Ishikawa or fishbone diagrams, these tools help identify factors leading to an outcome. A fishbone diagram's causes and subcauses are usually grouped into six main groups: measurements, materials, personnel, environment, methods, and machines. In many cases contributing factors can be identified in each group; however, it should be noted that there are instances where not all groups will be applicable. Planned and thoughtful analysis of these categories helps assure full evaluation for true causes and to avoid oversimplification (see Fig. 22.4).

Pareto chart. The Pareto chart operates according to the 80-20 rule: 80% of a process's or system's problems are caused by 20% of major factors, sometimes called the "vital few." The remaining 20% of problems are caused by 80% of minor factors. The goal of the Pareto chart is to highlight the relative importance of a variety of parameters, allowing you to identify and focus your efforts on the factors with the biggest impact on a specific part of a process or system. Targeted high-impact interventions or countermeasures are time, effort, and resource efficient and produce the highest yield. A combination of a bar and line graph, the Pareto chart depicts individual values in descending order using bars, while the cumulative total is represented by the line (see Fig. 22.5).

Scatter diagram. The scatter diagram is most useful in depicting the relationship between two variables, which is ideal for identifying cause-and-effect relationships. Dependent values are on one axis and independent values on another, and then each dot

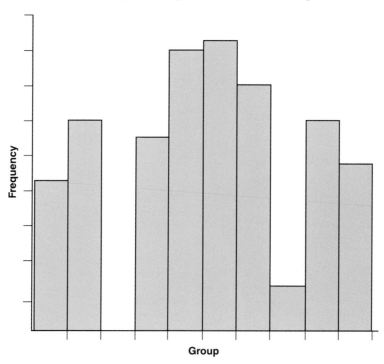

• **Figure 22.3** Histogram.

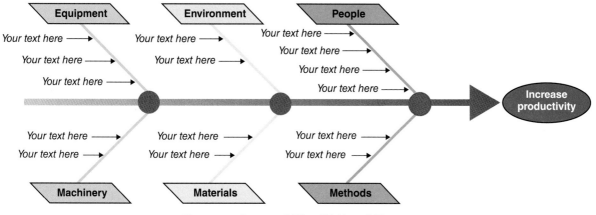

• **Figure 22.4** Cause-and-Effect ("Fishbone") Diagram.

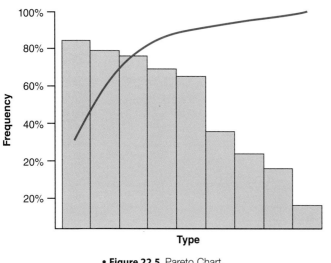

• **Figure 22.5** Pareto Chart.

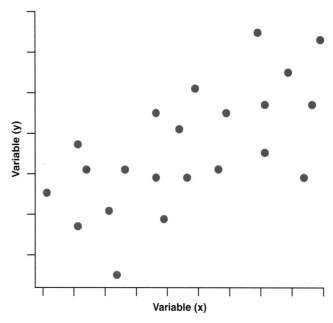

• **Figure 22.6** Scatter Diagram.

represents a common intersection point. When connected by a best-fit line, the relationship between the variables is described. The stronger the correlation in the diagram, the stronger the relationship between variables (see Fig. 22.6).

Control chart. This tool helps determine whether or not a process is stable and predictable or if the variation in a process is the result of "special causes" instead of normal or "common cause" variability. Control charts use a central line to depict a mean, with an upper and lower control limit around that mean. The control limits, based on historical data, and movements around the mean, describe the stability of the process. Box 22.4 shows particular rules for identifying special cause variation in a control chart. Control charts are designed to prevent two common mistakes: (1) adjusting the process when it should be left alone (tampering) and (2) ignoring the process when it may need to be adjusted (see Fig. 22.7).

Run chart. A run chart is the simplest of charts. It is very helpful but not included in the traditional list of seven tools. A run chart is a single line plotting some value over time, allowing you to evaluate trends and to have a general picture of a process. Run charts lack the benefit of statistical control limits, so they do carry risk of adding variation to a process if information is not carefully considered for normal vs. special cause variation.

Flowcharts. A flowchart, or project map, is another basic quality tool, not included in the classic list of 7. Flowcharts document

organizational structures and process flows, so they are ideal for identifying bottlenecks and inefficiencies in a system.

Considerations for Medical Quality Improvement

The evaluation and improvement of medical quality of care is unique with regard to considerations for confidentiality and liability. The long-standing practice of clinical peer review allows providers to give feedback on the medical care provided to individual patients. Naturally, sensitive information is routinely discussed and medical decision-making is often critiqued. Rising from concerns that civil liability might impair high-quality review, legislation has created legal protections for peer review participants in the domains of immunity, confidentiality, and privilege. Immunity is protection from retaliatory lawsuits, privilege prevents the discoverability or admissibility of evidence in a legal proceeding, and confidentiality prohibits the release of information outside of the judicial context.

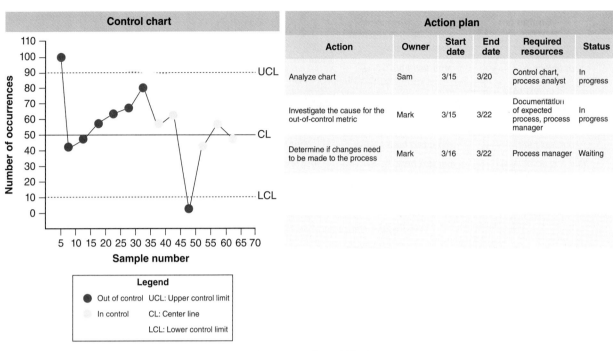

• **Figure 22.7** Control Chart.

- One point beyond the three-sigma control limit.
- Eight or more points on one side of the centerline without crossing.
- Four out of five points outside of one-sigma from the centerline.
- Six points or more in a row steadily increasing or decreasing.
- Two out of three points outside the two-sigma distance from the centerline.
- 14 points in a row, alternating up and down.
- Any noticeable/predictable pattern, cycle, or trend.

The federal government, all 50 states, and the District of Columbia have enacted peer review legislation. The level of protection and eligibility vary considerably. In almost all states, peer review is not protected if the information is relevant to criminal or disciplinary complaints. The most common of the other exclusions relate to review meeting structure, voluntary discussions outside of organizationally convened and properly attended meetings, and exclusions if the provider under review attends the peer review meeting. Very importantly, peer review protection is generally written for physicians in healthcare systems. The application to other providers and to emergency medical service and transport systems is more variable and, often, less clear. Transport programs must understand the regulations in the jurisdiction(s) in which they operate to assure that providers and enterprises are adequately protected.

Medical quality review sometimes engenders questions about information access under the limitations of the Health Insurance Portability and Accountability Act (HIPAA) Privacy Rule. The statutes (45 CFR 164.501 and 506) specifically permit information access for "conducting quality assessment and improvement activities" as long as "each entity either has or had a relationship with the individual ... and the protected health information pertains to the relationship."

There are nonliability interests in confidentiality and the atmosphere of peer review meetings, as well. Meetings must be fair,

sensitive to the feelings of participants, respectful, and trustworthy. Clinical peer review must be approached from a fundamental assumption that providers are well intentioned, striving for good patient outcomes, and interested in learning.

Conclusion

Robust attention to evaluating continuously the performance of all elements of the transport program will improve business performance, team environment, and clinical outcomes. The approach is best aligned with Deming's classic principles of managerial commitment, employee empowerment, and fact-based decision-making and is best accomplished when deeply integrated into the values of the organization. Accomplishing the change is built on standard tools, a little math, and rapid cycles of the Find, Organize, Clarify, Understand, and Select (FOCUS)-PDCA process.

References

Duffy GL, Furterer SL. *The ASQ Certified Quality Improvement Associate Handbook.* 4th ed. ASQExcellence; 2020.

Lindor RA, Campbell RL, Reddy S, Hyde RJ. State variability in peer review protections heightens liability risks. *Mayo Clin Proc Innov Qual Outcomes.* 2021;5(2):476–479. (In Eng). doi: 10.1016/j.mayocpiqo.2020.10.011

Office of the Federal Register, National Archives and Records Administration. 45 CFR § 164.501 (2023) – Definitions. Office of the Federal Register, National Archives and Records Administration.

Pelletier LR, Beaudin CL. *HQ Solutions: Resource for the Healthcare Quality Professional.* 4th ed. Wolters Kluwer; 2018.

Joshi M, Ransom ER, Nash DB, Ransom SB. *The Healthcare Quality Book: Vision, Strategy, and Tools.* 5th ed. AUPHA/HAP Book; 2022.

Spath P. *Introduction to Healthcare Quality Management.* 3rd ed. Health Administration Press (HAP); Association of University Programs in Health Administration (AUPHA); 2018.

23

Accreditation for Air and Ground Medical Transport

RHONDA REEDER

COMPETENCIES

1. Discuss the historical background of accreditation in the transportation industry.
2. Discuss the value of accreditation for transport programs.
3. Discuss the future challenges to accreditation.

Accreditation means to give authority or reputation; to trust; to accept as valid or credible. Most medical professionals are familiar with the term accreditation because of the organization that accredits hospitals, the Joint Commission. The history of accreditation for hospitals is an interesting one that laid the foundation for other accrediting agencies to follow.

History of the Joint Commission

In 1915, the American College of Surgeons (ACS), recognizing the need to standardize patient care in hospitals, allocated $500.00 to establish standards to promote quality patient care.[1] Hospitals in 1915 were not necessarily places patients went to be cured; instead, they were places patients went to die. Medical knowledge was minuscule compared with today's world. Penicillin had not yet been discovered, and although aseptic technique was used in surgery, no effective medications were available to manage postoperative infections.[2]

By 1917, the ACS developed a one-page list of requirements called Minimum Standards for Hospitals. An on-site inspection was developed by the ACS in 1918 to determine whether hospitals with more than 100 beds could meet compliance with the Minimum Standards for Hospitals. More than 700 hospitals throughout the United States were evaluated in the first year, and only 89 (13%) met the minimum standards requirements. Although these results were dismal, the inspection raised the awareness of the medical community, who were ready to accept the need for standardization and a verification process to improve quality.

More than 3000 hospitals were voluntarily surveyed by 1951. With the growth and overwhelming success of voluntary accreditation for hospitals, the ACS organization became overwhelmed and invited other organizations to participate. The Joint Commission on Accreditation of Hospitals (JCAH) was chartered in 1951 with the ACS and the following participating organizations: The American College of Physicians, the American Medical Association, the Canadian Medical Association, and the American Hospital Association.[3]

Later in the 1950s, the Canadian Medical Association withdrew to form its own national organization, and JCAH expanded to include healthcare outside the hospital environment, such as home health, mental health, and ambulatory healthcare. This expansion eventually resulted in a name change to the Joint Commission on Accreditation of Healthcare Organizations or JCAHO, known as *the Joint Commission* today.[2]

The White Paper Calls for Improved Emergency Medical Services

The Joint Commission was well established before standards even existed for medical transport. In fact, problems in transport were not even identified until 1966 when the white paper titled "Accidental Death and Disability: The Neglected Disease of Modern Society"[4] was published by the National Academy of Science. At that time, helicopter transport for the civilian population was unheard of, and standardization did not exist for ground transport vehicles or for the medical attendants who accompanied patients. Untrained personnel in the back of a mortician's vehicle did 50% of the ground transports, whereas fire, police, or volunteer groups performed the other 50%.[1]

The white paper triggered legislation that specifically addressed Emergency Medical Services and even suggested the use of helicopters.[1]

The Maryland State Police Aviation Division developed the earliest known public service helicopter system in 1969. A few hospital-based helicopter programs were seen by the mid-1970s, but the growth of these types of services did not really peak until the mid-1980s. At this time, hospitals were regionalizing, with specific hospitals recognized as centers of excellence in one or more specialty areas. Trauma center designation often included a helicopter program or access to a helicopter program, which was an added impetus to the growth in the number of helicopter services.

Also, the Vietnam experience proved a sharp decrease in mortality rates because of the rapid response of helicopters in transporting the injured from the field to definitive care. From a civilian perspective, the Golden Hour theory by Dr. R. Adams Cowley of the Shock Trauma Unit of Baltimore proposed that a critically injured patient had a precious 60 minutes to obtain definitive surgical treatment after an injury to survive.[5] The Golden Hour theory and the Vietnam experience[1] were frequently touted as reasons for a hospital, especially a trauma center, to start a helicopter service.

In 1980, a new organization, the Association of Hospital Based Emergency Air Medical Services (ASHBEAMS; the name was later changed to the Association of Air Medical Services [AAMS]), was formed. This organization started as a forum for administrators and personnel to get together and network with other hospital-based helicopter programs. No standards were available at this time, so those assigned to start up a hospital-based helicopter program usually had no air transport experience, no pattern to follow, and no awareness of the potential hazards and managers who understood the risks even less. The aviation component (aircraft, pilots, and maintenance) was contracted from an aviation vendor. Pilots were usually Vietnam veterans who were still operating under the oath they practiced in the military – complete the mission. Care providers were thrust into the unfamiliar aviation environment without standardized transport training and with the ingrained attitude that the patient, not safety, always comes first. Clearly, all were well-intentioned, but as more and more accidents began to occur, it was recognized that the profession needed standardization, not unlike the ACS recognized the need for standards in hospitals in the early 1900s.[4,6]

In 1985, 16 air medical accidents with 12 fatalities occurred.[3] The Federal Aviation Administration (FAA) was concerned, and the press began to alert the public. At the time, ASHBEAMS had minimal guidelines addressing patient care issues, but when the press started to focus on the number of air medical accidents, ASHBEAMS began to meet with other national groups, such as the Helicopter Association International (HAI), the National Flight Nurses Association (NFNA), National Flight Paramedics Association (NFPA), and the National EMS Pilots Association (NEMSPA), to develop consensus standards on safety and operational practices.

In 1986, the ASHBEAMS Safety Committee started a peer review safety audit called Priority One, with use of the safety guidelines that had been developed through the consensus process of the organizations listed previously. Priority One was beta-tested at Duke University in Durham, North Carolina and at the Staff for Life Program in Columbia, Missouri. As a result of these visits, the Safety Committee found that patient care standards specific to the transport environment were needed as well as safety guidelines to make the process complete. Therefore a feasibility study was performed to determine the need and viability of an accreditation program specifically for air medical transport.

Part of the feasibility study involved dialog with the Joint Commission and other accrediting bodies. Many organizational leaders felt that the Joint Commission should incorporate transport standards into its accreditation process and then layer in the air medical profession, which would negate the expense and effort needed to create another accrediting agency. However, the Joint Commission was not interested in responsibility for standards addressing the aviation environment, and stated that it was completely out of their field of expertise. Also, in the late 1980s, helicopter services were starting to be outsourced or privately owned and no longer sponsored or based at hospitals. Typically, fixed-wing medical transport services were privately owned and operated by an aviation company with no connections to hospitals. Both types of services were completely outside the realm of the Joint Commission.

Accreditation Organization Founded for Air Medical Transport

In 1989, with the feasibility study completed and presented, ASHBEAMS members voted to fund start-up costs for an air medical accreditation agency. Conceptually, this organization would be separate and independent of ASHBEAMS and would be made up of member organizations so that each member organization had equal representation on the Board of Directors.

The following seven organizations met on July 13, 1990, in Kansas City, Missouri, to form the Commission on Accreditation of Air Medical Services (CAAMS): the American College of Emergency Physicians, the AAMS, the National Association of Air Medical Communication Specialists, the National Association of EMS Physicians (NAEMSP), the NFNA (now called Air & Surface Transport Nurses Association [ASTNA]), and the NFPA (now called the International Association of Flight and Critical Care Paramedics [IAFCCP]).

CAAMS was formally incorporated in Pennsylvania as a nonprofit organization. The mission of CAAMS was and is to improve the quality of patient care and safety of the transport environment. Along with the tools for the new organization's foundation, such as the articles of incorporation, policies, and bylaws, the most important task for the new board was to develop the accreditation standards.

All accrediting organizations have a similar process of site visits that usually occur every 3 years to verify compliance with standards. However, the standards are what define the site survey process. Medical transport services that apply for accreditation are awarded or are withheld from accreditation based on compliance with the accreditation standards. Therefore the standards must be attainable, measurable, and consistent with current practice.

Accreditation Standards

To gain acceptance of the accreditation standards, CAAMS used guidelines and standards from many of the organizations mentioned previously (ASHBEAMS, HAI, NFNA, NEMSPA, and NFPA) to begin the process. In an attempt to create a document that would address both safety and patient care issues, the CAAMS board studied the National Transportation Safety Board's accident reports to determine whether a standardized practice, policy, or procedure could have prevented an accident. The CAAMS board also worked with officials from the FAA who were specifically assigned to be a liaison with the air medical profession.

In some cases, the accreditation standards exceeded FAA regulations, and in some cases, the regulation was copied into a standard to provide needed emphasis on a particular issue. For example, an FAA regulation is that personnel and passengers must be seat-belted for all takeoffs and landings.[6] However, during site visits, medical personnel would often tell site surveyors that if they were busy with the patient on liftoff or landing, they did not bother with the seatbelts. Indeed, in some of the survivable air medical accidents, several medical attendants received serious back and spinal injuries because they were not secured in their seatbelts on liftoff.

Before the first edition of *Accreditation Standards* was published in 1991, numerous drafts were mailed to organizations and individuals affiliated with the air medical transport profession. CAAMS also held a public hearing at the air medical transport conference in September 1990 in Nashville, Tennessee, to gather opinions and suggestions for the draft of standards that were distributed.

Accreditation standards are revised every 3 years to keep abreast of current practice. It is important to note that the standards are developed through comments and suggestions of professionals who provide medical transport every day. In order to measure a program's quality, each standard is supported by measurable criteria. The following broad topics included in the Accreditation Standards are comprehensive with a focus on quality patient care, safety, and competency (Box 23.1).

Site Surveyors

Several accrediting agencies in related healthcare fields were willing to share copies of their policies and qualifications for site surveyors when CAAMS was developing its new accrediting agency. One of those organizations, the Commission on Accreditation of Rehabilitation Facilities (CARF), was very generous and allowed the Executive Director of CAAMS to participate in its site surveyor training course. Subsequently, the course developed by the CAAMS Site Surveyor Selection Committee was based on the principles of CARF's program. Originally, in 1991, there were 35 applicants for the 12 site surveyor positions. Applicants were chosen based on the requirements and on their level of experience.

Applicants were required to have a minimum of 4 years of experience and a background in two of the four following categories: aviation, communications, medical, and management, with a heavy emphasis on management experience. The first site surveyor training class was held in 1991, with classes repeated every 2 to 3 years to keep up with attrition and site-visit demands. Site surveyors must complete a minimum of 1 survey each year to maintain survey skills and involvement. If the surveyor is not available or if CAMTS is unable to utilize a surveyor during that time period, they may be required to attend another class.

Past and Future Challenges

In 1997, CAAMS changed its name to the Commission on Accreditation of Medical Transport Systems (CAMTS) to capture a wider range of potential applicants and to accommodate the need for standards and accreditation for critical care ground services. Many of these grounds mobile intensive care unit (MICU) services consisted of pediatric and neonatal specialty teams, and many were part of an already existing air service. The services needed to be able to have their entire transport program accredited. Although the Commission on Accreditation of Ambulance Services exists for ground emergency services, it does not have standards that specifically address critical care. Therefore, CAMTS developed the ground standards (critical care standards were already in place) and began to fill this void in 1997 when it offered accreditation for ground critical care services as well as air medical services. In 2000 CAMTS also included basic life support (BLS) and advanced life support (ALS) ground standards to accommodate the transport services that either provided air or critical care ground services and provided BLS and ALS ground transport.[2,5] In 2004, CAMTS added a section to provide standards for accreditation of medical escorts on commercial airlines and ground vehicles.

As mentioned previously, most medical professionals understand accreditation because of exposure to the hospital accrediting

---

• BOX 23.1   Commission on Accreditation of Medical Transport Systems Accreditation Standards

General Standards*

Management and Staffing
Management/Policies
Staffing
Physical Well-being
Meeting and Records

Quality Management
Quality Management Program
Utilization Management
Safety Management System

Medical Section (Patient Care)
Medical Mission and Professional Licensure
Medical Direction, Clinical Supervisor, and Program Director
Training
Community Outreach
Medical Configuration of Aircraft/Ambulance
Infection Control

Communications
Rotor-Wing Standards
Certificate of the Aircraft Operator
Weather and Weather Minimums

Pilot Staffing and Training
Maintenance
Helipad and Refueling

Fixed-Wing Standards
Certificate of the Aircraft Operator
Aircraft

Weather and Weather Minimums
Pilot Staffing and Training
Maintenance

Ground Interfacility Standards
Vehicles
Driver Qualifications
Maintenance and Sanitation
Mechanic
Policies

Medical Escorts
Management/Staffing
Quality Management
Patient Care
Communications

*Apply to all modes of transport.

agency (the Joint Commission). However, in developing an air medical accreditation process, aviation professionals had to be educated on the purpose and goals of accreditation. Although the aviation component was accustomed to regulations, the aviation professionals were not familiar with accreditation and did not understand the need for yet another process when most believed they were already overregulated by the FAA. The fixed-wing community was particularly baffled. Most fixed-wing transport services were owned and managed by private aviation operators who were totally unfamiliar with the term accreditation. CAMTS worked through the NEMSPA, as one of its member organizations, to try to gain wider acceptance and developed a formal Aviation Advisory Committee to involve the fixed-wing community, managers from the major EMS Aviation Operators, and the FAA. The purpose of the Aviation and Safety Advisory Committee, which meets annually, is to provide updated information and to provide a forum for gathering input from the aviation professionals.

Another challenge facing the accreditation of air medical programs through CAMTS was the volatile healthcare market of the 1990s. Hospitals were closing, merging, or buying up other hospitals, and if transport was part of hospital's system, it suddenly needed to show a positive financial outlook or cease to exist, which was quite a turnaround from the 1980s when hospitals did not worry about what the helicopter cost as long as it brought patients into the hospital and was available as a visible marketing tool. Therefore, when the focus shifted to the bottom line of the budget, many hospital-based helicopter programs were fighting for survival and had difficulty justifying the cost of accreditation.

Since the year 2000, CAMTS has been meeting the demands of a rapidly changing air medical and ground transport community. A simple one-helicopter program based at one specific hospital is no longer the norm. With private business and aviation companies hiring their own medical teams and outsourcing communication centers, scheduling a site visit has become much more complicated. In many cases, a team of three or more site surveyors is necessary to visit all the satellite bases, maintenance centers, and communication centers that may be a part of a single program.

An increase in the number of applicants for accreditation has also been experienced as state and local EMS agencies move toward requiring CAMTS accreditation. There are some states that require CAMTS accreditation and some that have adopted the patient care standards. The Department of Defense (DOD) requires CAMTS accreditation for civilian contracts. CAMTS is placed in a potentially litigious position, especially if a medical transport service does not meet the standards and does not receive accreditation. The CAMTS Board of Directors prefers that states provide "deemed status" to CAMTS-accredited services for accredited programs that have met or exceeded higher standards than the minimal standards usually required by government agencies. In addition, there are legal challenges to states that require CAMTS accreditation based on the 1978 Airline Deregulation Act.[7] The primary focus was on the competitive market environment for air carriers. To ensure that states would not undo federal deregulation with regulation of their own, Congress included a preemption provision as follows: "A State, political subdivision of a state, or political authority of at least two states, may not enact or enforce a law, regulation, or other provision having the force or effect of law related to *price, route, or service* of an air carrier that may provide air transport." Because some of the CAMTS Accreditation Standards exceed Federal Aviation Regulations regarding pilot training and certain operating criteria, such as higher weather minimums, states that require CAMTS accreditation are being

challenged in federal court. For this reason, states that previously required CAMTS accreditation are moving away from this requirement in their regulations. The Commission can either grant full accreditation for 3 years or probational accreditation which holds a 2-year status after a survey is completed.

Many services apply for accreditation and reaccreditation not because they are required to do so by state regulations or by contracts but for the obvious benefits of accreditation such as outside auditing, accreditation as a marketing tool, competitive edge, and reimbursement advantages as well as discounted insurance premiums for liability and medical malpractice policies.[8,9]

Many medical transport services also find several intangible benefits as a result of going through the accreditation process, such as more cohesive working relationships, team building, a revitalized pride, and professionalism among personnel. Along with these benefits, the program receives a listing of the contingencies or areas that do not meet the intent of the accreditation standards or are not in compliance with the accreditation standards. This list of concerns and deficiencies is used for performance improvement that is reported back to CAMTS in follow-up reports (see Boxes 23.1 and 23.2).

Today, twenty-one member organizations are involved, with each sending one representative to serve on the board of directors. Board members make all the accreditation decisions, create and update policies, and revise the Accreditation Standards. In addition to the founding organizations listed earlier, CAMTS is proud to include the following member organizations:

Aerospace Medical Association (AsMA)
Air Medical Operators Association (AMOA)
Air Medical Physicians Association (AMPA)
Air & Surface Transport Nurses Association (ASTNA)
American Academy of Pediatrics (AAP)
American Association of Critical Care Nurses (AACN)
American Association of Respiratory Care (AARC)
American College of Emergency Physicians (ACEP)
American College of Surgeons (ACS)
Association of Air Medical Services (AAMS)
Association of Critical Care Transport (ACCT)
Emergency Nurses Association (ENA)
European HEMS @ Air Ambulance Committee (EHAC)
International Association of Flight & Critical Care Paramedics (IAFCCP)
International Association of Medical Transport Communications Specialists (IAMTCS)

• BOX 23.2 Commission on Accreditation of Medical Transport Systems Frequently Cited Areas of Weakness

The quality management or performance improvement program lacks follow-up and loop closure.
Medical director is not involved in the interviewing and hiring process for the medical personnel.
Skills maintenance program documentation is weak.
Initial orientation is not well documented.
Continuing clinical experiences are not documented.
No designated Safety Management System exists.
Safety committee does not have representation from communications and maintenance.
No annual drill exists for the postaccident/incident plan.

National Air Transportation Association (NATA)
National Association of EMS Physicians (NAEMSP)
National Association of Neonatal Nurses (NANN)
National Association of State EMS Officials (NASEMSO)
National EMS Pilots Associations (NEMSPA)
United States Transportation Command (USTRANSCOM)
Ad-hoc Board Members

Since 2017 CAMTS has been accredited by the American National Standards Institute (ANSI) Accreditation Standards Developer (ASD). The ANSI is a private, nonprofit organization that administers and coordinates the United States voluntary standards and conformity assessment system.

In the fall of 2018, CAMTS published its 11th edition of *Accreditation Standards* that reflect changes in current healthcare and transport practices. This edition also addresses international medical transport services as appropriate to the country of residence and the specific regulator of that country as referenced by the term "Authority Having Jurisdiction." These standards were in development for 3 years, and various drafts and town hall meetings were held to discuss the changes and suggestions from constituents. Types of care are specifically defined by the qualifications of the medical team along with equipment, medications, interventions, and quality metrics in the 11th edition. Although the Patient Care section of the standards is more specific, the scope of this edition has been broadened to address other modes of medical transport. The term "surface vehicle" used throughout the document refers to vehicles such as ground ambulance, boat, snowmobile, all-terrain vehicle, and so forth being used for patient care and transport. CAMTS also added a category titled "Special Operations." These are services that provide medical care and/or potential medical transport that do not necessarily fit within the previous sections of these standards. Some examples include medical coverage at sporting, concert, or special events; special public safety operations (such as tactical rescue or "SWAT" callouts); and citizen recovery from potentially unstable environments (programs that provide this coverage were eligible to apply for accreditation under the 2018 Special Operations Accreditation).[9] In 2022, CAMTS introduced the first edition accreditation standards for mobile integrated healthcare programs.

In November 2015, CAMTS registered CAMTS EU in Europe and Switzerland. CAMTS EU is a stand-alone nonprofit organization that is based in Switzerland with the same mission, vision, and values as CAMTS. CAMTS EU was created to serve constituents outside of North America recognizing not only cultural differences but government restrictions and laws of other countries while maintaining the integrity of the process in the United States and Canada. In 2019, CAMTS EU was changed to CAMTS Global to better reflect the mission as an accreditation body for medical transport companies from all continents outside of North America.

Internationally, there is more interest and applications for accreditation and a heightened interest with the CAMTS Global presence. There are four CAMTS-Global Accreditation Services which are in Saudi Arabia, the UK, Thailand, and Switzerland. In addition, there are two programs that hold dual accreditation in both CAMTS-global and CAMTS which are in Thailand and the United States.

CAMTS has trained several European site surveyors and will be adding more international medical transport professionals and Canadian site surveyors. Site surveyors represent all disciplines involved in medical transport so that a site visit is planned with surveyors who have the appropriate experience and background.

TABLE 23.1	Examples of Other Accrediting Bodies for Medical Transport	
Association	**Accreditation Offered**
National Accreditation Alliance Medical Transport Applications	Air and ground transport
Commission on Accreditation on Ambulance Services	Ground transport
European Airmedical Institute (EURAMI)	Air Ambulance accreditation

None of the current site surveyors has less than 10 years of experience in medical transport.

It is the diversity and wealth of experience of the site surveyors and board members that provide CAMTS with the strength and integrity to offer accreditation to medical transport services in North America and abroad and to continually improve medical transport services for patients now and in the future.

CAMTS has a variety of resources that are available. On-site consultative services are available to program that want to measure the quality of their services in comparison to the CAMTS standards. They can also participate in consult to prepare for an accreditation site visit. In addition, CAMTS completes several workshops such as how to prepare for accreditation each year. There are also webinars to include preparing for an accreditation and reaccreditation that are available on the CAMTS website.

CAMTS has several publications including a textbook, Safety and Quality Medical Transport Systems, the CAMTS Accreditation Standards, and Hazards of Helicopter Shopping. There is also a Best Practice publication that includes a collection of best policies, education, quality, safety, and other documents shared by services that are CAMTS accredited. CAMTS is a transparent organization and there are various documents and resources available at CAMTS.org.

Other Accreditation Bodies

CAMTS serves as the primary accreditation body for medical transport systems. However, several other agencies have come into the transport market over the years. These accreditation bodies provide accreditation processes for air or ground or both. Table 23.1 contains examples of some of these other bodies.

Summary

Accreditation provides a framework for program evaluation and improvement. It also demonstrates to the public and the patients that a transport program complies with specific standards to ensure safe and competent patient transport.

References

1. Helicopter Association International. *Helicopters 1948–1998: A Contemporary History HAI*. Helicopter Association International; 1998.
2. Duffy M, Joint Commission on Accreditation of Healthcare Organizations. *An Introduction to the Joint Commission: Its Survey and Accreditation Processes, Standards, and Services*. Chicago, IL: Joint Commission on Accreditation of Healthcare Organizations; 1988.

3. Frazer R. Air medical accidents: 20-year search for information. *Air Med.* 1999;5(5):34.

4. Samuels D, Bock H; Department of Transportation, US, et al. *Air Medical Crew National Standard Curriculum.* ASHBEAMS; 1988.

5. Rhodes M, Perline R, Aronson J, Rappe A. Field triage for on-scene helicopter transport. *J Trauma.* 1986;26(11):963–969.

6. AIM/FAR. *§91,105 Flight Crewmembers at Stations.* Washington, DC: Federal Aviation Administration; 2017.

7. Richardson JG. *Health and Longevity.* Home Health Society; 1914.

8. Commission on Accreditation of Air Medical Systems. *Accreditation Standards of the Commission on Accreditation of Medical Transport Systems.* 7th ed. CAAMS; 2006.

9. Commission on Accreditation of Medical Transport Systems. *2015 Accreditation Standards of the Commission on Accreditation of Medical Transport Systems.* 10th ed. CAMTS; 2015.

24

Mental Health and Wellness for the Provider

JAMES C. BOOMHOWER

COMPETENCIES

1. Normalize the emotional and psychological challenges associated with critical care medicine.
2. Recognize common symptomology of stress responses including acute stress reactions and posttraumatic stress disorder (PTSD).
3. Identify lifestyle components that can aid in stress management, maintaining mental health and well-being in the short and long term.
4. Identify moderators of stress, including resources available to clinicians in need.

Introduction

As a transport provider, you will often be subjected to a variety of stress and trauma throughout your career. Transport providers are part of a unique branch of medicine that is utilized both in and out of the hospital setting. In collaboration with prehospital Emergency Medical Services (EMS) teams and a variety of medical professionals throughout many branches of medicine, along with, at times, being the sole care provider for patients in austere and resource-limited environments. Transport professionals are often called to assist in management and resuscitation of some of the sickest, most complex, injured patients; and are often at the front line between members of the community and the trauma, sickness, and suffering of the community.

In this edition of the ASTNA text, the editors express the importance of this topic to be a dedicated chapter, rather than a footnote, in recognition of the severity of the mental health epidemic within the healthcare industry. The unique stressors the paramedics and nurses are asked to manage in this tremendously rewarding and challenging work demands purposeful attention, recognition, and support. Critical Care Transport Professionals carry higher rates of suicide, depression, and posttraumatic stress than any other branch of healthcare professions. This is an homage to the understanding that our awareness of mental health, how to recognize when we need assistance, how to provide fundamental psychological first aid (PFA), and where to find additional resources for further assistance is no less important than understanding how vasoactive medications work, how to safely operate a mechanical ventilator, or how to interpret an ABG. We hope this chapter encourages you to treat your mental health and wellness with the same fury and passion as you treat the physical health of those you have taken a pledge to serve. Throughout this

chapter, we will illustrate tools and techniques to help you recognize and mitigate stress. We would also encourage you to remember: your responses to stressful events are not abnormal, they are normal responses to an abnormal event.

Critical care transport providers are asked to perform work in a variety of externally stimulating environments in scenarios and places where their own physical well-being is frequently at risk. This combination of factors creates a perfect storm of stressors that are unique to those in the aeromedical and critical care transport community. These stressors generate multiple forms of strain, including anxiety, depression, compassion fatigue, and burnout, to name a few. The barrage of mental and physical stressors, and the strains that they manifest can lead to poor mental health, which has the potential to impact not only the transport provider but also their families, the patients they care for, and the teams with which they work. Simply put, these strains occur when expectations exceed resources, and in which there are a variety of stressors.[1]

In addition to the individual and personal cost of poor mental health, burnout has been associated with increased medical mistakes and increased risk of litigation.[2] It has been established that decreased well-being in first responders decreased the safety of the professionals and resulted in increased medical mistakes, and increased distraction while on shift. Burnout is often seen as the result of high job demands and low job resources. Burnout decreases the performance of employees and increases turnover rates.[3]

The 2017 CDC census data reports one first responder dies by suicide every 4 days in the United States of America. The rates of severe psychological distress are over 27% in ambulance personnel, more than three times the rate of similar symptoms in the general population.[4] It is imperative that medical professionals commit to caring for their own mental health and emotional wellness with the same tenacity and determination as they do when caring for the patients who entrust their lives to them every day.

Making your own mental health a priority requires a departure from the classic ideology of the "Stoic" healthcare provider. This was best expressed by Dr. Rachel Naomi Remen *"The expectation that we can be immersed in suffering and loss daily and not be touched by it is as unrealistic as expecting to be able to walk through water without getting wet."*[5] As transport professionals, it is accepted that the direct exposure to suffering and trauma of our patients can affect our own well-being. We encourage you to have the same tools and foresight for your emotional needs as you would have a rain jacket when you know it's going to rain. Personal wellness must be a priority for the transport provider in order to allow those providers to care for their patients, and enjoy a long and fruitful career.

Over the past 30 years, the reporting of symptoms of psychological distress has become more accurate and consistent. This creates a more precise picture of the mental health of emergency workers. First responders cultivate feelings of purpose through work, however, a disproportionately high number of first responders experience psychological and emotional distress when compared to the general public.[6-8] First responders are exposed to chronic stressors that alter the appraisal and differentiation of stimuli.[9] As a transport professional, these stimuli become even more intense. The frequency, duration, and severity of transports, coupled with the physiological effects of flight or ground transport for extended periods of time can worsen the effects of these stimuli.

First responders share certain personality traits which alter their perception of success and failure, thus altering their appraisal of emotional load associated with an event.[8] Conversely, exposure to chronic traumatic events influences the first responder's perception of stressors and experience of strain. First responders are exposed to specific job stressors such as lack of social support, shift work, and unpredictable professional environments that generate emotional, physical, and cognitive strain.[10]

Transport professionals often suffer an interesting dichotomy in the lack of social support. Our profession is very small, and there is tremendous variation in practice from one transport program to the next. Furthermore, only a small number of people truly understand the work that critical care clinicians are asked to do, and even fewer can acknowledge its unique set of stresses and concerns. Oftentimes well-meaning individuals unintentionally alienate those clinicians who are looking for support by reminding us how "cool" or "unique" the work that we do is, and in doing so invalidate the stresses and trauma that is being expressed. Long-term exposure to environmental stressors in ambulance personnel correlated positively with anxiety, depression, burnout, and compassion fatigue.[4] It has been found that critical care healthcare workers had high rates of burnout that were correlated with variation of workload (84.1%), overload (76.8%), responsibility for peoples' lives (69.5%), and lack of perceived control (63.4%).[11]

Critical care transport providers are a specific subset of the larger first responder population and are called upon to care for the most severely ill and injured patients. While the increased autonomy associated with critical care providers has its benefits, it also has its share of emotional and cognitive burden on top of what already exists for other first responders around the world. First responders are under increasing time pressures both internationally[12] and in the United States.[13,14] Challenges are diverse and involve physical demands such as heavy lifting, frequent interruptions and disturbances, and violence at work.[15] First responders face greater physical demands, greater patient expectations, increased exposure to death

and physical harm, and have lower decision authority than professionals working in other areas such as nursing, home health, or respiratory therapy.[11] First responders are increasingly exposed to aggressive behavior and patient violence,[4] additionally, critical care air medical providers are exposed to additional stressors in the form of vibration, noise, turbulence, temperature, weather, mission compatibility, and the inherent risk of mortality.[16]

Importance of Wellness

Mental health and wellness impact a variety of aspects of the professional and personal life of healthcare providers. Positive mental health has been correlated with improved performance, job satisfaction, and job retention. While poor mental health has been correlated with depression, substance abuse, marital distress, anxiety, suicide, compassion fatigue, and burnout.[17] Poor mental health has been found in all first responder populations, including Law Enforcement Officers, Emergency Medical Technicians and Paramedics, Fire Fighters, Nurses, Respiratory Therapists, and Physicians.[17] In addition to the individual and personal cost of poor mental health, burnout has been associated with increased medical mistakes and increased risk of litigation.[2] Decreased well-being in first responders, and decreased safety of the professionals have resulted in increased medical mistakes and increased distraction while on shift.[14] Burnout is significantly influenced by high job demands and low job resources and has been found to decreased performance of employees and increased turnover rates.[3]

Acutely traumatic events such as the death of a patient, the injury of a coworker, or a vehicle crash while on duty increase emotional distress in first responders transiently,[18] and chronic exposure to stressors such as sleep deprivation through shift work, financial strain, and feeling underappreciated in the community also impact mental health.[19] The nature and frequency of exposure of first responders to traumatic events increases the risk of mental health consequences,[14] and chronic work-related stressors increase burnout in first responders, even if the responders had not been exposed to a major disaster.[20] Exposure to stress and stressors leads to short-term responses, such as cardiovascular activation, negative affect, and fatigue, as well as longer-term outcomes such as burnout or PTSD.

Types of Stressors

Acute Stressors. Acute stressors are high-intensity, short-duration situations that may lead to strain. Acute job stressors include interpersonal conflict, work overload, inadequate recognition, inadequate resources, and poor interaction with colleagues.[3,21] The unique job stressors of the critical care transport professional such as time pressure in the setting of Cerebrovascular Accident (CVA) intervention and trauma cases to name just a few, along with interpersonal conflicts impacted individual well-being within organizations on a day-to-day level.[22] The unique organizational restraints of the programs within critical care transport may also play a role as an acute stressor. Differences in training, levels of equipment, and mission profile of the provider and the team can greatly impact stress levels and a provider's ability to provide care in stressful situations.

Chronic Stressors. Chronic stressors are often low-intensity incidents that occur repeatedly over a long duration. Chronic job stressors include time away from home and family, financial trouble, feeling unappreciated by management, inadequate resources, and lack of community.[3,21] Some stressors may be either chronic or acute depending on the setting. For example, time away from home may act as an acute stressor if a project requires a worker to spend more time at work for a few days, or may be chronic if the job has long work hours as a baseline scheduling pattern.[23] Just as is true within a disease process, the idea of "acute on chronic" stress holds true as well. For example, chronically getting off shift late and delaying time with family and loved ones off shift, patients that are rude and/or violent to transport staff, and the chronic use of a critical care transport for calls of which no such severity exists all create a chronically stressful environment, making the "trigger" for the stress response harder to find, but the need for support just as paramount. A bullet point reference showing common stress symptomology is seen in Box 24.1.

Types of Strain

Behavioral Strain. Behavioral strains describe changes in behavior following exposure to stressors. Behavioral strains in the workplace may take the form of disloyalty (from supervisory staff), work withdrawal (unwillingness to take on extra shifts or projects within the agency), distraction, decreased performance (struggling with complex patient care, not meeting time metrics), and intention to quit.[24] Behavioral strains are the most obvious manifestation of strain in stressor-strain relationships. Individuals alter their behavior based on the strains and the anticipated outcomes of their related tasks.[25] This can make unexpected outcomes all the more daunting; for example, if a patient has an unexpected deterioration or death while in transport.

Psychological Strain. Psychological strain is a general term that describes unpleasant emotions, including sadness, anxiety, and distraction, that may or may not impact the ability to function.[26] Burnout is a state of emotional, mental, and physical exhaustion generated by prolonged exposure to stressors or decreases in support that results in alienation from activities and reduced performance.[13] Compassion fatigue is the emotional withdrawal experienced by those who care for the sick or injured, sometimes referred to as vicarious traumatization or secondary traumatization.[27] Compassion fatigue is distinct from burnout in that compassion fatigue results from the provider taking on the emotional burden of patient. Whereas burnout is a general psychological strain that can affect members of any profession, compassion fatigue is more specific to individuals in helping professions, such as those in healthcare.

Causes of Stress

The Critical Care Transport Professional is called upon to manage complex patient loads, long shifts, demanding and dangerous scenarios, and a fast-paced environment. Critical Care Transport Providers are exposed to the acute and first stages of illness and injury and are paramount in resuscitating patients.[28] In many instances, especially within specialty teams (neo/peds, high-risk OB), transport professionals are also tasked with being an agent of calm within the sending institutions that they are called to as they are often the subject matter expert on infrequently seen patient populations.

Moderators of Stress

Resiliency Training. As data increasingly supports a preventative approach to PFA and resiliency training, more programs are supporting a "teach first" approach to mental health and wellness alongside reactive support platforms including peer support programs and Critical Incident Stress Management (CISM) teams. Foundational training in PFA includes awareness of stress, stress responses, and crisis mitigation techniques (i.e., therapeutic ventilation [Fig. 24.1]), alongside local resource awareness (Box 24.2).

Peer support platforms are run at either the local agency level or a regional area. These teams are primarily staffed by fellow first responders (if not HEMS/CCT clinicians specifically) and receive clinical oversight by a chaplain, or licensed therapist/psychologist. Many teams hold a variety of certifications in crisis intervention and are experts in describing and understanding emotional strain (affective communication). These teams can play a pivotal role in the prevention of PTSD by working with individuals in the days and weeks after stressful and traumatic events.

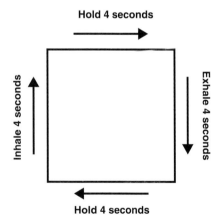

• **Figure 24.1** Box Breathing, Also Known as Therapeutic Ventilation.

• BOX 24.1   Symptoms of Stress

Common reactions to a stressful event include the following:
- Disbelief and shock
- Tension and irritability
- Fear and anxiety about the future
- Difficulty making decisions
- Being numb to one's feelings
- Loss of interest in normal activities
- Loss of appetite
- Nightmares and recurring thoughts about the event
- Anger
- Increased use of alcohol and drugs
- Sadness and other symptoms of depression
- Feeling powerless
- Crying
- Sleep problems
- Headaches, back pains, and stomach problems
- Trouble concentrating

• BOX 24.2   Crisis Hotlines

If you or someone you know needs immediate help, please contact one of the following crisis hotlines:
- Disaster Distress Helpline: 1-800-985-5990
- The national suicide hotline and crisis text line have now merged. They can be reached by phone or text as "988"

Critical Incident Stress Management

The American Psychological Association[29] highlights the commonalities in experiences of those who qualify an event as traumatic.

Those experiences include:

- A real or perceived threat to an individual
- A scenario that is overwhelming
- A scenario that creates feelings of fear
- A scenario that creates feelings of a lack of or loss of control
- A scenario that creates a feeling of helplessness
- A scenario that changes the way you see yourself or others. (Otherwise known as changing an individual's worldview).

Tools to Mitigate Stress (Box 24.3)

Critical Incident Stress Management

CISM is an interventional protocol designed to help deal with major traumatic events.[30] CISM is highly structured and requires specific standardized training for individuals involved in the processes after a major event. The seven components of CISM are preincident education, individual crisis or peer support, demobilization, defusing, debriefing, family support, and referral services. Grief and loss sessions are included when deaths are involved.

Grief and loss sessions are provided after the death of an individual involved in a critical incident. These sessions help those involved to work through the grief process and deal with the sense of loss involved in the critical incident.[31]

Crisis management briefings are used to keep participants informed: "before, during and after crisis, to present facts, facilitate a brief, controlled discussion" and provide information about the critical incident. These briefings may be adjusted as information about the critical incident changes.

Hydration and Nutrition

A balanced diet is important to help counteract the effects of stress and to help maintain a healthy body.[32] Nutritionists specializing in shift workers advocate for combining proteins and carbohydrates into together into meals[33] as this is an especially useful tactic for healthier snacks while on shift (see Box 24.4) for suggestions. Caffeine appears to be a favorite among transport professionals; however, caffeine is a strong stimulant that is known to produce a stress reaction in the body. The avoidance of caffeine

---

helps individuals feel more relaxed and improves sleep patterns.[4] Caffeine is found in coffee, tea, soda, and chocolate. If used, it is best consumed before lunch and with a balanced meal. Alternatives to caffeine, such as green or herbal teas, are acceptable and often healthier.[3]

Hydration is also a key component of wellness and overall health. While not always practical in the transport setting, it is imperative to stay hydrated as much as possible. Water is the best fluid you can consume to maintain hydration, clear the body of toxins, and maintain essential minerals within normal levels; other fluids including sports drinks, coffee, tea, and alcohol do not provide optimal hydration and have other nutritional consequences as well.

Sleep

Although inadequate sleep periods may not solely produce stress among transport professionals, sleep deprivation is associated with increased risk for accident and injury.[10,13,15,21,34,35] Disruption in circadian rhythm and shortened sleep cycles have been found to increase stress and increase the risk for injury and accident in transport professionals.

Most experts agree that 6 to 8 hours of sleep per day is required for optimal health and wellness. However, rest can also be achieved by taking breaks throughout the day. Many agencies have options for clinicians that require a rest period for a small portion of their shift, while other agencies have mandated rest periods built into their workday. It is important, whenever possible, to be well rested, and emotionally and physically prepared for work when you arrive. However, with complex schedules and the sleep-wake cycles of medical providers, this may not always be possible. Resting in place of sleep has been shown to mitigate the effects of fatigue in the short term, allowing providers to potentially obtain more restful sleep when they are able. Transport professionals can minimize the effects of shift work by minimizing secondary jobs, maintaining a consistent sleep pattern when not on duty, and avoiding activities that can disrupt sleep patterns (such as alcohol, caffeine, and exposure to electronic screens before sleep).

Promoting Wellness

Many of the strategies that work to mitigate stress can also be used to promote wellness more generally and to help the transport professional manage exposure to stressors and symptoms of strain. Among some of the strategies are exercise, laughter, talking to others, and scheduling appropriate sleep patterns and duration of sleep.

Exercise

Exercise mitigates stress in several ways. Exercising releases endorphins that chemically make an individual feel better. Exercise also

---

stops the production of the chemicals that are produced during the fight-or-flight phase of stress.[5]

Exercise does not have to be extremely strenuous or take a long time. Any movement that engages the cardiovascular and musculoskeletal systems produces positive effects.[27] Team sports or activities with a partner also add to the benefits of exercise. Walking during a break or using the stairs can accomplish exercise. There are many ways to monitor progress and track goals or create a competitive game out of it. Associated weight loss can also prove beneficial, as well as strength-building exercises that improve work performance and reduce the risk of on-the-job injuries.

Laughter

Laughter has been found to be an effective stress management tool.[36] Laughter allows for the release of endorphins that produce feelings of euphoria and relaxation. Laughter has been proven to benefit both neuroendocrine and cardiac systems and has shown improved clinical courses for chronically and acutely ill individuals.[37] Watching a funny movie, visiting a comedy club, or joking with friends can help relieve stress through humor. Sharing dark or morbid humor may facilitate stronger emotional bonds among crews but may alienate or isolate crews from other friends and family who do not work in the healthcare industry. In this way, laughter can act as both a positive coping mechanism and avenue by which an individual may feel more alone.

It is important to remember that some individuals may find certain stress management techniques helpful while others may not find the benefit from the same option. Laughter at the expense of others or humor that makes others uncomfortable often leads to increased isolation and worsening emotional state over the long term. Laughter has shown physiological, psychological, social, spiritual, and quality-of-life benefits.[38] Adverse effects are very limited, and laughter is practically lacking in contraindications. Therapeutic efficacy of laughter is mainly derived from spontaneous laughter (triggered by external stimuli or positive emotions) and self-induced laughter (triggered by oneself at will), both occurring with or without humor.[38] The brain is not able to distinguish between these types, so it is possible that even spontaneous laughter with no true source is still beneficial. Although there is not enough data to demonstrate that laughter is an all-around healing agent, there exists sufficient evidence to suggest that laughter has some positive, quantifiable effects on certain aspects of health.

The Importance of Expressing Thoughts and Feelings

Individuals often keep feelings of stress internalized for fear of showing weakness or loss of control.[39] When sharing feelings that involve stress, individuals should not minimize their feelings or the feelings of others. Transport professionals should share their concerns with others but must also be willing to seek professional help if these feelings begin to jeopardize their sense of well-being.

Even if the transport professional is not ready or willing to share feelings verbally, the goal can be accomplished through nonverbal mechanisms, such as drawing, coloring, singing, playing a musical instrument, gardening, or journaling. Communication happens through both verbal and nonverbal means, so sharing feelings can happen even if words are not actually spoken. The transport professional should make an effort to find a method of expressing themselves in order to prevent the internalization of negative emotions. It is important to allow time and space for the release of emotional pressure, which can look very different depending on the particular interests and skills of the individual.

Summary

Maintaining good mental health and wellness may be one of the most elusive portions of the transport provider's career. The transport provider is often self-motivated, diligent, and perseverant type, as they are accustomed to achieving a goal by overcoming ever-changing obstacles. While we care for our patients, it is also important to care for ourselves. Small steps on a day-to-day basis may help lead to a long, healthy life and rewarding career.

References

1. Kerlin MP, McPeake J, Mikkelsen ME. Burnout and joy in the profession of critical care medicine. *Crit Care*. 2020;24:98. doi:10.1186/s13054-020-2784-z

2. Hamilton S, Tran V, Jamieson J. Compassion fatigue in emergency medicine: The cost of caring. *Emerg Med Australas*. 2016;28(1):100–103. doi:10.1111/1742-6723.12533

3. Demerouti E, Bakker AB, Nachreiner F, Schaufeli WB. The job demands-resources model of burnout. *J Appl Psychol*. 2001;86(3):499. doi:10.1037/00219010863499

4. Petrie K, Milligan-Saville J, Gayed A, et al. Prevalence of PTSD and common mental disorders amongst ambulance personnel: A systematic review and meta-analysis. *Soc Psychiatry Psychiatr Epidemiol*. 2018;53(9):897–909. doi:10.1007/s00127-018-1539-5

5. Supportive Care Coalition. *Leaning in Supportive Care*. March 3, 2019. https://supportivecarecoalition.org/cultivating-professional-resilience/2018/7/10/leaning-in

6. Martin CE, Tran JK, Buser SJ. Correlates of suicidality in firefighter/EMS personnel. *J Affect Disord*. 2017;208:177–183. doi:10.1016/j.jad.2016.08.078

7. Newland C, Barber E, Rose M, Young, A. Data suggests ways to reduce the impact of critical stress on EMTs and paramedics. *J Emerg Med Serv*. 2015. https://www.jems.com/special-topics/survey-reveals-alarming-rates-of-ems-provider-stress-and-thoughts-of-suicide/

8. McIntosh WL, Spies E, Stone DM, Lokey CN, Trudeau ART, Bartholow B. Suicide rates by occupational group – 17 states, 2012. *MMWR Morb Mortal Wkly Rep*. 2016;65(25):641–645. doi:10.15585/mmwr.mm6525a1

9. Scherer KR, Moors A. The emotion process: Event appraisal and component differentiation. *Annu Rev Psychol*. 2019;70:719–745. doi:10.1146/annurev-psych-122216-011854

10. Greinacher A, Derezza-Greeven C, Herzog W, Nikendei C. Secondary traumatization in first responders: A systematic review. *Eur J Psychotraumatol*. 2019;10(1):1562840. doi:10.1080/20008198.2018.1562840

11. Elshaer NSM, Moustafa MSA, Aiad MW, Ramadan MIE. Job stress and burnout syndrome among critical care healthcare workers. *Alexandria J Med*. 2018;54(3):273–277. doi:10.1016/j.ajme.2017.06.004

12. Arble E, Arnetz BB. A model of first-responder coping: An approach/avoidance bifurcation. *Stress and Health*. 2017;33(3):223–232. doi:10.1002/smi.2692

13. Freudenberger HJ. Staff burn-out. *J Soc Issues*. 1974;30(1):159–165. doi:10.1111/j.1540-4560.1974.tb00706.x

14. Jones S, Nagel C, McSweeney J, Curran, G. Prevalence and correlates of psychiatric symptoms among first responders in a Southern State. *Arch Psychiatr Nurs*. 2018;32(6):828–835. doi:10.1016/j.apnu.2018.06.007

15. Goudreau J, Edmondson G, Conlin M. Dispatches from the war on stress. *Bus Week.* 2007;4045:74.

16. Thomas F, Hopkins RO, Handrahan DL, et al. Sleep and cognitive performance of flight nurses after 12-hour evening versus 18-hour shifts. *Air Med J.* 2006;25(5):216–225.

17. Rodríguez-Rey R, Palacios A, Alonso-Tapia J, et al. Burnout and posttraumatic stress in paediatric critical care personnel: Prediction from resilience and coping styles. *Aust Crit Care.* 2019;32(1):46–53. doi:10.1016/j.aucc.2018.02.003

18. Santa Maria A, Wörfel F, Wolter C, et al. The role of job demands and job resources in the development of emotional exhaustion, depression, and anxiety among police officers. *Police Q.* 2018;21(1):109–134. doi:10.1177/1098611117743957

19. Wolter C, Santa Maria A, Wörfel F, et al. Job demands, job resources, and well-being in police officers – a resource-oriented approach. *J Police Crim Psychol.* 2019;34(1):45–54. doi:10.1007/s11896-018-9265-1

20. Van der Ploeg E, Kleber RJ. Acute and chronic job stressors among ambulance personnel: Predictors of health symptoms. *Occup Environ Med.* 2003;60(suppl 1):i40–i46. doi:10.1136/oem.60.suppl_1.i40

21. Frakes MA, Kelly JG. Off-duty preparation for overnight work in rotor wing air medical programs. *Air Med J.* 2005;24(5):215–217.

22. Sonnentag S. The recovery paradox: Portraying the complex interplay between job stressors, lack of recovery, and poor well-being. *Res Organ Behav.* 2018. doi:10.1016/j.riob.2018.11.002

23. Marjanovic NS, Teiten C, Pallamin N, L'Her E. Evaluation of emotional excitation during standardized endotracheal intubation in simulated conditions. *Ann Intensive Care.* 2018;8(1):117. doi.org:10.1186/s13613-018-0460-0

24. Cavanaugh MA, Boswell WR, Roehling MV, Boudreau JW. An empirical examination of self-reported work stress among US managers. *J Appl Psychol.* 2000;85(1):65. doi:10.1037/0021-9010.85.1.65

25. Valencia C, Currier K, Lindsay S, Lemperis P, Hughes T, Sowers J. Levels of arousal in positive moods: Effects on motor performance. *Open J Occup Ther.* 2018;6(3):11. doi:10.15453/2168-6408.1447

26. Burton I. Cultural and personality variables in the perception of natural hazards. In: Wohlwill JF, Carson DH, eds. *Environment and the Social Sciences: Perspectives and Applications.* American Psychological Association; 1972:184–195. https://psycnet.apa.org/doi/10.1037/10045-016

27. Figley CR, ed. *Compassion Fatigue: Coping With Secondary Traumatic Stress Disorder in Those Who Treat the Traumatized. Brunner.* Mazel Psychological Stress Series, No. 23. Brunner/Mazel; 1995.

28. Hsieh CC, Yu CJ, Chen HJ, Chen YW, Chang NT, Hsiao FH. Dispositional mindfulness, self-compassion, and compassion from others as moderators between stress and depression in caregivers of patients with lung cancer. *Psychooncology.* 2019;28:1498–1505. doi:10.1002/pon.5106

29. American Psychological Association. Building Your Resilience. 2020. https://www.apa.org/topics/resilience/building-your-resilience

30. Mitchell JT. Critical Incident Stress Management. 2008. http://www.info-trauma.org/flash/media-e/mtichellCriticalIncidentStressManagement.pdf

31. Mitchell JT. Critical Incident Stress Debriefing (CISD). http://www.info-trauma.org/flash/media-f/mitchellCriticalIncidentStressDebriefing.pdf

32. Blackwood A. Food + stress. body + soul. *Nutrition.* 2007;24(20):64.

33. Beugelink, Raina RD. The shift fix. *Shift Work Nutrition.* 2022;06.

34. Frakes MA, Kelly JG. Sleep debt and outside employment patterns in helicopter air medical staff working 24-hour shifts. *Air Med J.* 2007;26(1):45–49.

35. Frakes MA, Kelly JG. Shift length and on-duty rest patterns in rotor-wing air medical programs. *Air Med J.* 2004;23(6):34–39.

36. Folkman S, Lazarus RS, Dunkel-Schetter C, DeLongis A, Gruen RJ. Dynamics of a stressful encounter: Cognitive appraisal, coping, and encounter outcomes. *J Pers Soc Psychol.* 1986;50(5):992. doi:10.1037/0022-3514.50.5.992

37. Sahakian A, Frishman WH. Humor and the cardiovascular system. *Altern Ther Health Med.* 2007;13(4):56–58.

38. Mora-Ripoll R. The therapeutic value of laughter in medicine. *Altern Ther Health Med.* 2010;16(6):56.

39. North C, Wraa C. *Stress: Taming Your Shadow 2000.* Critical Care Transport Medicine Conference; April 18, 2000.

25

Post-Incident and Emergency Response Planning

DONNA YORK, KRISTA HAUGEN, J. HEFFERNAN, TOM BALDWIN, AND TODD DENISON

Introduction

This chapter is designed to assist medical transport program providers and leaders in preparing for, and progressing through, the critical functions before and after incidents or accidents. The goal is effectively to set team members, survivors, family members, the entire organization, and the community on a path toward recovery, healing, and growth. It is highly recommended that leaders engage in further study on each topic, as the depth and breadth of knowledge and experience required to mount an effective response exceeds the scope of this text.

Development and exercising of a robust, thoughtfully developed Post-Accident Incident Plan (PAIP) and an Emergency Response Plan (ERP) are essential to assuring effective, impactful responses to untoward events. This chapter will identify key elements and factors to be considered in plan development and drafting, with the understanding that there is no one-size-fits-all approach to this process.

Since 1972, in the United States, there have been over 1100 individuals involved in helicopter emergency medical services (HEMS) accidents serious enough to warrant National Transportation Safety Board (NTSB) investigation. Approximately one-third of these individuals lost their lives in crashes.[1] Data for ground ambulances, overall, and for ground critical care ambulances, in particular, is difficult to find. Older data suggest that there are at least 1500 ambulance crashes with injuries and 29 fatal crashes annually.[2,3] It appears that 9-1-1 ambulances crash at a rate of 5 events per 100,000 incidents. When the human impact of these incidents and accidents is considered, there are thousands of people affected. The individuals involved, their families, friends, colleagues, and communities are all impacted by the trauma, stress, and grief these events produce.

Emergency Response Plan and Post-Accident and Incident Plan

An ERP provides an opportunity to prepare for a medical transport program's response to emergencies, to manage the emergency, and to provide a path to recovery for all involved parties. While the ERP should be comprehensive and will likely be complex, the forward-facing plan and resources should be as simple to follow as possible to all event managers to follow it effectively while operating under stressful conditions.

The program's initial phase response plan, the PAIP is the road map for everyone and sets the tone for much of the experience moving forward. The PAIP must include the communications center staff and leadership who are responsible for initiating the immediate critical steps that enhance crew survival and ensure an organized response. The plan should include a notification flowchart with up-to-date contact information for leadership and those designated to respond.

Preparedness is paramount to effectively managing crises and disasters. The limited medical transport industry data on survivors and surviving family members' experiences post-incident/accident, as well as their long-term trajectories, also presents barriers to determining how best to respond. One study on the experiences of air medical crash survivors noted that industry planning for "post-accident response was identified to be lacking in scope and quality."[4]

Plan development, documentation, and execution require concentrated coordination involving many parties. Federal Aviation Administration (FAA) Federal Aviation Regulation (FAR) Part 135 vendors for medical transportation services are federally regulated entities that have specific roles and guidance dictated for their conduct following an accident. Programs and suppliers have innumerable contractual relationships, and the program may be part of a larger entity. For these reasons, it is essential that the ERP and PAIP are very clear about responsibility, action, and assignment of duties. For example, use of the term "company" in reference to any of the participating organizations can cause confusion and misplaced expectations. It is essential that all entities review, approve and participate in exercises of these plans to assure the necessary clarity and definitions to promote effective initial action, recovery, and even as it affects subsequent litigation.

It is important to ensure that all response team members are trained and proficient in their assigned roles. Periodic tabletop and live exercises help to maintain proficiency, build team member expertise, and drive continuous improvement. It can be helpful to plan these exercises so that participants gain experience in their roles, and also in cross-covering for the likelihood that some members of the leadership structure may be delayed or unavailable early in an event.

The Incident/Accident – Immediate Response

Types of Incidents/Accidents

The National Transportation Safety Board (NTSB) broadly defines aviation incidents and accidents (see Box 25.1). There are no similarly specific references for ground vehicles. Program PAIPs and ERPs often provide more detailed triggers for plan activation (see Box 25.2). Whether the event is classified as an incident or accident, and regardless of the trigger, the humans involved will likely need to be responded to and receive support.

- It is also helpful to plan and prepare for other types of events that may not generate a vehicle PAIP activation, but warrant a response from the company and activation of the ERP, including support and resources for teams and families, such as:
- Team member suicides
- Team member loss of life off duty
- Violence against any team member while at work (during a transport or not)
- Other events that deeply impact team members

Incident: An occurrence other than an accident, associated with the operation of the aircraft, which affects or could affect the safety of operations.

Accident: An occurrence associated with the operation of an aircraft which takes place between the time any person boards the aircraft with the intention of flight and all such persons have disembarked, and in which any person suffers death or serious injury, or in which the aircraft receives substantial damage.

Program Leadership

Before an incident, the program leadership team is accountable for developing sufficient organizational processes and personnel to support the ERP, PAIP, and organizational recovery. Once an incident has occurred, the leadership team ensures that those structures are followed, makes key decisions, keeps the organization aligned with its values, and facilitates collaboration and communication with internal and external stakeholders. The provision of medical care to the victims of the accident should be the highest priority. Key principles for crisis leadership are described in Box 25.3.

Response Structure

All team members and plan participants must be well-versed in Incident Command Systems (ICS) and utilize this structure for incidents and accidents (see Fig. 25.1). Each role should be clearly outlined, and individuals should be assigned to these roles ahead of time and know the functions for which they are responsible. Premade checklists outlining roles and tasks are helpful. As some

• BOX 25.3 Leading in Disaster Recovery[5]

- Having a noble purpose – people are the purpose
- Being ethical – it takes courage to do the right thing
- Being intentional – hope is not a method
- Making decisions – perfect is the enemy of good
- Keeping perspective – seek wise counsel
- Leading with empathy – it's about real connection
- Being innovative – because you have to
- Supporting the team – people ... not human resources
- Prioritizing self-care – to be effective

• BOX 25.2 Sample PAIP Triggering Events

Aircraft Accident:
- Declaration of emergency or "Mayday" calls
- Emergency landings in which the aircraft is damaged and/or team members are injured
- Fatality or serious injury to team members on aircraft or bystanders
- Unaccounted for or missing aircraft

Aircraft Incident:
- Minor aircraft damage (bird strikes, lightning strikes, damage on ground)
- Minor injuries to team members on aircraft or bystanders
- Emergency landings that do not result in damage to aircraft or injuries to team members
- Unplanned landings resulting in minor aircraft damage or minor injuries

Aircraft Unplanned Landings:
- Weather abort with patient loaded
- Non–weather-related aborts
- Aircraft divert resulting in unplanned landing
- Precautionary landing

Visual Flight Rules (VFR) Aircraft Overdue or Contact Lost:
- VFR aircraft missed their position check call and communications specialist is unable to reach crew
- VFR aircraft is overdue at destination and communications specialist is unable to reach crew

Instrument Flight Rules (IFR) Aircraft Overdue at Destination:
- IFR aircraft overdue at destination and communications specialist is unable to reach crew

Other Events:
- Inadvertent Instrument Meteorological Conditions (IIMC) events
- Wire strikes
- Wheels up landings
- Any landing where airport or Landing Zone (LZ) emergency response teams are present because of an aircraft issue/malfunction

Ambulance Emergencies:
- Any fatality resulting from an ambulance accident or other emergency
- Serious injuries resulting from an accident during a ground ambulance operation
- Ambulance involved in serious accident
- Crew requires emergency assistance

Ambulance Crew in Distress:
- Ambulance crew is under duress (i.e., taken hostage, life-threatening situations)
- Ambulance is carjacked or stolen

Ambulance Incident:
- Minor injuries or minor vehicle/property damage sustained during ambulance operation
- Transport terminated due to vehicle mechanical malfunction
- Any urgent but nonemergent event

Ambulance Crew Overdue:
- Crew has not reported in as required by predetermined schedule
- Communications specialist is unable to reach crew to verify their location and welfare
- Welfare of the crew is in question

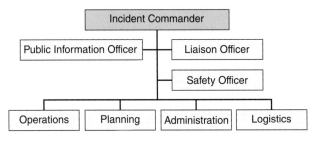

• **Figure 25.1** Incident command structure.

responses to events last multiple days and even weeks, it is important to have more than one individual prepared to manage any given role to allow for substitution and to permit emergency response team members a reprieve.

Information Flow and Communication

The entire responding group should have predetermined platforms, processes, and strategies for initial notifications, both internally and externally. Ongoing informational updates should occur at regular intervals to multiple groups including, but not limited to: leadership, company staff, partners, external customers, and families. Off-duty team members must be notified of the event and invited to come to the designated program site where resources are available and factual information can be shared. Use of a team roster to ensure that no team members are inadvertently overlooked during the notification process will help avoid issues post-accident – the importance of this detail cannot be overly stressed.

Messaging should be factual, accurate, timely, and compassionate, with a high degree of sensitivity and maintaining appropriate privacy/confidentiality.

Standing Down and Returning to Service

Standing down a program is entirely appropriate and likely necessary post incident or accident. There are initial operational safety considerations related to remaining in service across all operational domains – clinical staff, pilots, ground vehicle operators, communications specialists, and maintainers. The functionality of the communication center and the communications specialists, although a nexus to managing the PAIP, needs to be considered. Communications staff have close relationships with transport team members and likely had temporal communication with the involved vehicle, perhaps triggering the emergency response. Options could include transferring phones to a neighboring program's communication center, reducing the staffing level, or utilizing appropriately trained program leadership or other program communications specialists to backfill positions.

Neighboring medical transport programs should be contacted and informed that transport requests may be referred to their programs. Neighboring programs can provide resources and support to assist with the event and may care for injured team members. Individual programs need internal policies about how safely to respond to requests to respond to incidents and accidents involving their own, or neighboring, programs within the contexts of blinded decision-making, conservative response, and safe operations.

Decisions regarding standing down and returning to service should be clearly communicated to customers and partners in a timely manner and updated at regular intervals.

Team members need time to understand and process the event and aftermath. It is recommended that all team members be given compensated time off because losing pay creates pressure to return to service prematurely. The program administrator will need to assess whether return to service is appropriate without exerting any pressure to return on team members.

Media Considerations

An appropriate individual must be assigned to deal with the media, preferably one that has received Public Information Officer (PIO) training. It may be helpful to provide basic training and practice for program leaders and incident commanders on how to interact effectively with the media.

Predesignated a media staging area away from the crash site and team members. The predesignated media area should contain, at a minimum, a work area, chairs, work-table space, cell phone, and computer connectivity, if possible separate from the hospital network, electrical access for computer and phone charging, appropriate food and drink, and access to restroom facilities.

A proactive approach to information sharing helps to limit speculation on the part of the media, as well as the public. When possible, one of the program leaders should be designated as a liaison for information sharing with the public relations official. Provide factual information to the media, public, and stakeholders, while assuring that this communication occurs in concert with applicable investigative or regulatory agencies. The public needs to know that victims are being cared for, the transport team is being supported, and that the program will continue. Providing the human side of this situation to the media may cause a shift in focus from the negative aspects of the event. It is essential to assure that survivors and family members are given visibility on any messages formulated for public consumption before they are disseminated.

The media are likely to cover the event daily for several days to weeks, depending on the nature of the incident or accident. Program staff need to expect this so that they are not overwhelmed by the media coverage and should be encouraged to limit exposure to media and social media. Positive media relationships developed before an event facilitate more effective interactions after an event happens.

Notifications and People Support

When a medical transport vehicle accident or incident occurs, the timeliness and quality of information conveyed may vary depending on the circumstances. Notification of a crash or incident may come to the communications center via scene witnesses, from the media or from the team themselves. With the advent of the 24-hour news cycle and social media, team members or family may receive information directly before official notification from a program representative occurs. It is important to ensure teams and their families understand this, so they are not disappointed, frustrated, or angry when reality does not meet their expectations regarding notification.

Those impacted both directly and indirectly will require varying levels of support. This may include psychological, emotional, and spiritual support. Needs will vary by social and workplace groups, by individual, by time, and are difficult to predict. Depending on the degree of traumatic impact and grief response, people may need assistance with activities of daily living and reminders to eat, to remain hydrated, and to rest. They may need transportation, child or elder care assistance, and/or help with managing or canceling planned activities. Be sensitive to cultural norms, whether they are geographical, ethnic, organizational, or historical. It is not possible to plan for every set of circumstances, so peer leaders, managers, and program leaders need to be watchful for needs and adapt to address them as they arise.

Family Member Notification and Support

Family members of the onboard crew should be notified as soon as possible, both the families of those who perish and those who survive. Ideally, this notification should occur in person, but, due to the rapid dissemination of information over social media, this may not be possible. It definitely should be done verbally; video calls offer one option when in-person communication is not possible.

Assign appropriate family liaisons to help identify and meet the needs of the family members. Identify a private area at the facility for family members to gather. Family liaisons and program leaders should compassionately communicate facts only and avoid speculation. There are four primary objectives families that need to be covered initially:
1. Primary needs: food, beverages, and comfort items
2. Emotional support
3. Accurate, factual, and timely information, initially and with regular updates
   • What happened?
   • Where is their loved one?
   • Where are their loved one's belongings?
   • What is happening now?
   • What to expect?
4. Practical and logistical support, including financial resources[6]

Each locality likely has specialty resources that can provide mental health professionals and grief specialists to assist family members. It is not appropriate for program peer support teams to be expected to provide support to family members, as this requires specialized training and experience.

The makeup of families and their locations are widely variable. For example, a team member may have parents who live across the country, a nontraditional family structure, a language barrier for family members, and declared or functional dependents. It is important to drill different scenarios ahead of time, know the team members, determine potential needs, and know local resources. Local hospitals may have resources like Child Life Services who may be able to assist with children who have lost a loved one. There are also multiple crisis response organizations across the country that have comfort dogs and crisis-trained handlers. While external organizations can be very helpful, it is important to thoroughly vet these organizations and ensure they are appropriately trained, insured, and legitimate.

For air medical accidents, a family liaison from the Transportation Disaster Assistance (TDA) Department of the NTSB may be available to help provide information on the investigative process to family members as well as prepare them for the length, complexity, and limits to receiving specifics about the investigator's findings. Your organization may need to facilitate the connection between families and the liaison depending on the nature of the accident.

Site Visits

Families of those lost in accidents, as well as accident survivors, often wish to travel to the accident site. This can be a beneficial experience, if managed well, in helping those involved and impacted process what happened. It is important to coordinate with authorities to ensure the timing of the visit is appropriate, should investigators still be on scene or if there are other circumstances that may impact the timing of the visit. The NTSB Family Liaison can be a helpful resource in advising on arranging site visits.

Organizing site visits can take significant logistical planning. Timing of the visit, safety, funding, supplies, resources, and emotional support for those visiting are all important aspects of site visits that need to be considered. It is critical that the site be inspected for any remaining aircraft pieces/parts or human remains prior to any site visits. Encountering such items can be highly traumatizing for families and survivors. There are third-party vendors who may be enlisted to ensure sites are appropriately cleared.

Personal Effects

For those who may respond to the scene of an incident or accident, or who may come into contact with personal effects of those involved, it is important not to dispose of or disregard these items. Even the most seemingly small item may have importance and meaning to family members after losing a loved one. An organization should strongly consider enlisting the assistance of third-party vendors who specialize in cleaning/decontaminating and returning personal effects.

The Ripple Effect

The ripple effect of incident or accident extensively impacts a large number of people. The center of the ripple is those directly involved – those on the vehicle and communicating with them, including patients. The next ring extends to the families of the living and the dead. Another ripple includes the operational team members and administrative team in the organization, who are colleagues of those involved. It is important to think broadly about the work team, including on- and off-duty staff, clinicians, communications specialists, dispatchers, pilots, ground vehicle operators, maintainers, physicians, leadership, administrative, and support staff. Next, operational community partners, including first responders at the event site, clinicians caring for the patient before the event, and medical providers or institutions who work regularly with the transport teams. All of those impacted by the accident would benefit from support and resources tailored to meet their unique needs.

Returning Team Members

The impact of an accident on team members not directly involved should not be underestimated. People can be vicariously traumatized and experience significant stress and grief reactions. Immediately available resources and support services, streamlined and affordable access to qualified mental health professionals, and clear, open, honest, and regular communication from leadership can set team members on a path to healthy healing and recovery. Responses to incidents and accidents are highly individual, as is the desire to return to service (see Box 4).

When returning to service, team members will respond individually and according to their own readiness and their personal timelines, variability should be expected. It is likely that some team members will feel ready to return to service before others – casting any judgment or creating pressure on other team members should be avoided. The decision to return to service MUST put

• BOX 25.4   Focus on Healing

"The healing process may require a continuous effort to realize and re-realize that our trauma exposure response is not going away unless we give it proper attention. The sooner the better for this realization, since we are hoping to consider this from a preventative standpoint when possible, and, as those who are savvy in the ways of the human body will tell you, 'By the time you are thirsty, you're already dehydrated.'"[7]

safety first, along with the health and well-being of returning team members. While it is reasonable for the team members themselves to ultimately dictate when they return to service, it is also important to objectively screen team members for readiness.

Programs should consider offering re-familiarization flights to staff before returning to first full shift. Often, this option is reserved for survivors or those impacted directly by an event/incident. However, programs should consider this as an option for other team members by request. Leadership should make clear that, if team members thought they were ready to return to service but become uneasy and change their minds, they are free to communicate these concerns and accommodation plans will be explored and implemented. Support and resources should be readily available and accessible, and leadership should maintain open communication.

Survivors

Of the 1100-plus people who have been involved in helicopter accidents since 1972, two-thirds survived with varying degrees of injuries.[1] There has been minimal research or data collected on the nature of these injuries or on the outcomes of survivors. There is little information on survivors of fixed-wing accidents and scattered information on survivors of ground accidents. One study specific to survivors of air medical transport (AMT) survivors, concluded that the "personal and professional impact of surviving an AMT accident is far-reaching and poorly understood."[4] Recommendations from the study included further research, emphasizing:

- Development of strategies to help survivors recover. Psychological and financial recoveries were emphasized.
- Education for medical transport organization leadership on how to respond to survivors. Transparency and avoiding minimization of the accident were items of focus.
- Preplanning for accidents as organizations and individuals.
- Determining how to use the "learned experience" of survivors to help improve responses and the industry. The Survivors Network for the Air Medical Community maintains a website that serves as a venue for survivors to tell their stories and share lessons learned, available at: www.survivorsnetwork-airmedical.org.

The costs, both economic and noneconomic, experienced by accidents survivors and their families have not been quantified and even "a conservative estimate of [the impact of injuries and fatalities that have resulted from helicopter emergency medical services crashes] is staggering."[8] Surviving with debilitating injuries such as traumatic brain injuries, spinal cord injuries, and burns can cost millions over the course of the survivor's lifetime. Unmitigated traumatic stress, pain, suffering, loss of livelihood, and often, loss of purpose, can be devastating for survivors and the far-reaching effects are immeasurable.

Families of Survivors

Families of survivors will have many of the same needs as families of the fallen, depending on the nature of the incident/accident and the effects on their loved ones. There is no limit to the variety of potential scenarios when it comes to survivors and the impact on their lives, families, livelihood, and future.

Families of Returning Team Members

The families of team members not directly involved in an accident may have angst about their loved ones returning to service. Some may pressure team members to leave the medical transport industry, others may be supportive of continuing to work in the industry, and some may be ambivalent. As team members return to service, it is important to remain sensitive to the fact that they may be dealing with family members at home who may be struggling with their decision to continue to work. Providing resources for families and team members to help address these difficult questions may help ease concerns and open the door to communicating about fears families may have.

Community Partners and First Responders

Medical transport organizations often have close relationships with hospitals, specialty teams, and the first responder community. Those who respond to the incident or accident and those who care for survivors may know them. This adds an extra layer of stress and presents an opportunity to bring community partners and first responders into the fold as support and resources are being offered.

Leadership

To perform during an overwhelmingly emotional event, the leader may deny his or her own feelings of fear, grief, and anger to allow the program to move forward. Although this denial may be necessary initially, if this progresses for too long, the program may move on and leave the program leadership emotionally destitute and dysfunctional. Program leadership must set aside some time to go through their formal grieving process and recognize the impact the event has on them, as individuals. Peer support, as in connecting with others in similar positions who have been through similar experiences, may be helpful. Professional counseling resources should be available for all individuals involved. Without this assistance, unhealthy methods of dealing with the stress may eventually impair long-term effectiveness. The help of a professional counselor should be sought in a confidential setting, preferably away from the work environment. Time away from work with family and friends may also promote healing.

Incident Response Team Members

Serving on the incident response team can be emotionally intense, grief-producing, and exhausting. Assigning qualified people to assist the team in ensuring their primary needs are being met during the response and allowing them time to debrief and decompress is essential. Professional counseling may also be an invaluable resource for incident response team members as they may be exposed to wreckage, human remains, and raw human emotions that can be highly traumatic and difficult to process.

Near-Term Considerations

Human Resources

The human resources (HR) department professionals are essential in assisting with meeting the needs of survivors and families post incident or accident. They may guide the processing of forms for injured and deceased employees. HR staff may assist survivors and family members with understanding and navigating company benefits. For public and not-for-profit agencies, families may be eligible to receive Public Safety Officers' Benefits (PSOB). HR staff also help with the process for team members to return to work. Involve the HR team early in developing the PAIP and in keeping it current (see Box 25.5).

Funeral Planning

Families may plan their own private funerals which may or may not include invitations to those outside of the family. Death in the line of duty often translates to a public funeral, a ritual observed by firefighters, EMS personnel, and police officers. Families may or may not wish to be involved with the public funeral and their wishes should be respected. The EMS community is likely to communicate a desire for a public funeral early, and often there is an outpouring of community support including offers to assist or be involved with the public funeral. A trusted member of the EMS community who has experience in planning public funerals, often a member of a local fire department, should be identified. This person may be invaluable in planning with the family and program leadership an otherwise overwhelming event. Involve spiritual representatives in the planning with the family so that the funeral plans are culturally sensitive to meet the needs of the family and those of the community at large. Honor guards are often invaluable additions to funerals and memorial services.

In addition, regular meetings with the designated individuals planning the public funeral are necessary to ensure that the medical transport program and staff needs are met and information is flowing. Municipal and state police involvement may be necessary to ensure that a processional of rescue vehicles can occur.

The medical transport service leadership should consider taking their teams out of service to allow attendance at the funerals. Mental health professionals support participation in these rituals as an essential part of the healing process. Neighboring transport programs can be called to cover transport requests that come in during the funeral. Several hours of downtime after each funeral may be needed before team members are capable and prepared to return to service.

Programs should develop a written funeral plan/template in advance of a catastrophic event. Having a plan that includes checklists of actions, funeral day templates, and an overall organized plan can reduce the stress programs and individuals will face. Additionally, it can give the family options if they are unsure how to proceed.

• BOX 25.5 Supporting Victims

"How people respond after a disaster makes a difference in the trajectory ahead for those who have been personally marked. The way family members, friends, colleagues, and those whose job it is to support victims behave – including what words they use and what actions they take – are more important than outsiders might realize ..."[9]

Memorial Services

Other memorial services may occur in addition to public and private funerals. The crisis response experts can provide advice regarding the appropriate timing for the memorial service. The service should provide an opportunity for team members to share personal remarks and eulogies. This service can provide team members with an opportunity to move forward in the recovery process. Participation in the funeral and memorial service can be healing for team members but should not be required. The program may be taken out of service for this time, and coverage by other transport services may be requested. This coverage reduces the chance of transport team members missing the service and conveys to the community the program's commitment to provide service.

While well-intended, numerous memorial services and funerals may result in memorial fatigue, especially for family members who may hold their own funeral, attend the public service, state services, and national services. It is important for the medical transport community to be mindful of and sensitive to the families' experiences as they navigate post-accident life.

While the investigative and operational duties for medical transport companies to engage in post-incident or accident are generally well-outlined, the response to the people who may be impacted has not been well-developed across the industry.

Monetary Donations – Crowdfunding

Crowdfunding is a popular way to show support in current society. Media messaging around crowdfunding is important to consider. While the program or owner entities may be providing robust financial support to those impacted by an accident, the public's perception around crowdfunding requests may be that the individuals are not getting the support they need. In reality, crowdfunding is an indication that people just want to help in some way. Crowdfunding should not be discouraged, however, the messaging around crowdfunding is important to consider.

Learning From History – Commercial Aviation

The commercial aviation industry experienced several crashes involving various major airlines in the 80s and 90s in which responses to surviving family members were less than effective. These responses added further pain to the families' experiences. In her book, *In the Wake of the Storm: Living Beyond the Tragedy of Flight 4184*, Theresa Ann Severin describes her experience:

> *"This account examines my own journey down the road to recovery and the regaining of hope, as I chronicle my battle to overcome the shock and loss I suffered, not only from the immediate impact of my sister's and nephew's deaths, but also American Airlines' mishandling of the post-crash situation. While I direct a great deal of criticism at this corporation for the ongoing pain we were all forced to endure, such inconsistent and flawed approaches for dealing with the families of victims of air disasters were not isolated to American Airlines; rather, **their lack of knowledge, sensitivity, and understanding on this issue was reflective of an industry-wide problem**. I came to realize the terrible management of the overall situation was not the product of individuals, or even of one specific company, but of a misdirected and outdated corporate*

*system that allowed for the human cost in this tragedy to be over-looked. Thus, my goals became directed toward exposing the flaws inherent in the corporate mentality, so that others never have to undergo the same **perpetual trauma** that all those associated with the crash of Flight 4184 have come to know."*[10]

The lack of effective, appropriate responses from commercial airlines at the time led groups of survivors and surviving family members to join and advocate for what became the Aviation Disaster Family Assistance Act of 1996 (ADFAA) and the development of the Transportation Disaster Assistance (TDA) Department of the National Transportation Safety Board (NTSB). While this legislation is specific to Part 121 aviation operators, it provides a model based on lessons learned which includes assurances, many of which are likely beneficial for the medical transport industry to consider for all transport modalities (see Box 25.6).

While there are no guarantees, if supported and managed well, surviving individuals and families, teams, and organizations can potentially be guided to a trajectory of healing, recovery, and even post-traumatic growth, as opposed to enduring "perpetual trauma." The medical transport industry has a prime opportunity to learn from commercial aviation and make every attempt to meet the

---

• BOX 25.6 Guidelines to Assist Air Medical Transport Companies in Responding to Aviation Accidents[11]

1. **Definition of "family member" for purposes of notification and provision of airline services.**
   - The company, in choosing its definition of "family member" for the purposes of notification and assistance for travel to and accommodations at the site of crash or memorial services, should recognize that today's families may not have traditional boundaries and every attempt must be made to be inclusive and culturally sensitive.
   - When companies make initial notification to a family that a loved one was a passenger on an aircraft involved in an aviation accident, the company should inquire if there is another family member who should also receive formal company notification. These secondary contacts would be notified after initial notification to families of all passengers.
   - Families should designate a point of contact for purposes of information sharing in the aftermath of the disaster.

2. **Guidelines for the initial notification of family members by the company in the immediate aftermath of an aviation accident, including the use of third parties to assist in the notification process.**
   - Companies should establish systems and procedures to establish communication with family members as soon as possible.
   - Companies, through changes to their procedures, as well as with the assistance of the media, should take measures to limit phone inquiries to the company following an aviation accident as much as possible through the use of public service announcements, media broadcasts, and internet sites.
   - Once a company determines a point of contact for a passenger, the company should establish and continue contact periodically with that family, even if it is just to inform the family that the company has no new information to provide.
   - Companies should consider contracting the notification process to a third party if the air company cannot meet those needs on its own.
   - Companies should provide family members with all passenger information that they have as quickly as possible. Accuracy is essential.
   - Companies should strongly consider adopting policies to ascertain the financial needs of families in the immediate aftermath of aviation accidents, and provide assistance as appropriate.
   - Notification by the company to family members of their loved one's involvement in an accident, death, or injury should be followed promptly by a person-to-person contact from either the company, the American Red Cross, or an official entity, if requested by family members.
   - Upon notification, the company should advise family members that the name of their loved one will not be publicly released by the company until the family has personally notified other family members.

3. **Company assistance to family members with travel and accommodations at accident sites and memorial services.**
   - If a company chooses to provide transportation and accommodations to the family assistance center or any memorial service, the company should endeavor to provide transportation and accommodation in the timeliest manner possible.
   - If a company chooses to provide transportation and accommodations to the family assistance center or to any memorial service, the company should offer such assistance to more than one person per family.

4. **Guidelines for training of company personnel who interact with family members.**
   - Company employees or third-party contractors will be adequately trained to meet the needs of survivors and family members in the event of an aviation disaster.
   - There should be an emotional awareness component to the training curriculum.
   - Companies should consider utilizing various methods of instruction during the training process.
   - Company training plans should include an assurance that the company and the American Red Cross will coordinate on training.
   - Companies should continually work to improve overall training standards. Training should include, at a minimum, communication skills, logistical support, emotional support, stress response, and the roles of the parties at the accident site.
   - A team comprised of company employees, family members and survivors, regulators, the American Red Cross, and mental health professionals should be created to develop protocols standardizing training content for company employees.
   - All company training programs should include information for managers about employee stress and the need for critical incident stress management for family assistance personnel.

5. **Return of personal effects (property) to the family members by the company.**
   - The company should make available to all families in a readily accessible manner the unassociated personal effects from an accident, as quickly as possible. Return of pilot's personal effects must be cleared by the NTSB.
   - The company should strongly consider utilization of a third party with experience in return of personal effects associated with aviation accidents.

6. **Guidelines for companies and American Red Cross interaction in assisting the victims of aviation disasters.**
   - The company and the American Red Cross, at both the national and local levels depending on the scope of the company, should meet to understand their respective roles and interactions in the aftermath of aviation accidents.

7. **Recommendations to ensure that families of non-US citizens involved in an aviation disaster receive appropriate assistance from both the airline and the US government (for international transport services or for patients/families involved in an accident).**
   - Upon receipt of notification that a foreign-citizen victim was involved in an aviation accident occurring within the United States or its territories, the State Department should assist in establishing an appropriate liaison between the company and the foreign government of the victim.
   - Initial notification of any of the families of foreign-citizen victim who reside in the United States should be carried out by the company.
   - The Department of State should assist directly when a company advises that it is having difficulty notifying the family of a US-citizen victim because that family resides, or is currently located, outside the United States.

Continued

• **BOX 25.6** **Guidelines to Assist Air Medical Transport Companies in Responding to Aviation Accidents—cont'd**

- When the company publicizes a toll-free number or other means for contacting the company following an aviation accident, it should also publicize a non-toll-free number for use by persons calling from outside the United States, if applicable.
8. **Recommendations to improve the passenger manifests (or other systems) used by the company to establish points of contact with families of passengers.**
   - The Task Force recommends that companies should have readily available for every flight the following data: the full name of each passenger, a contact phone number of each passenger, and an emergency contact name of each passenger.
   - Companies should be provided with the option of collecting this information either through an automated process or a manual process.
   - Each passenger should be encouraged to provide the information that companies would be required to request under any improved passenger manifest system.
   - Information provided to the company for manifest reasons must only be used in the case of an emergency.
9. **Recommendations on uniform guidelines for medical examiners and coroners on the identification of the remains of victims.**
   - The victims of an aviation accident should be positively identified.
   - DNA testing should be utilized by medical examiners or coroners to identify the victims of an aviation accident who cannot otherwise be identified through conventional means.
   - All extensive conventional efforts should be employed to identify the victims and associate all separated remains. It should not be required that DNA testing be utilized to identify unassociated remains. Any unassociated remains should be interred in a proper ceremony coordinated in conjunction with the families of the victims and the American Red Cross.
   - When extensive conventional efforts have failed to identify all victims of an aviation accident, DNA testing should be utilized in an effort to identify those victims still unidentified. DNA testing should not be mandatory, however, for associating remains to victims previously identified.
   - If there is a possibility of additional remains being associated with a victim following identification, the family should be informed of such a possibility at the time the remains are returned. (For example, a victim might be identified during the early stages of the recovery effort. Additional remains of that victim might then be identified by conventional means in the latter phases of the recovery effort.) Families should be

given the opportunity to decide whether they want to be informed of additional remains being identified as belonging to their family member. The medical examiner or coroner should honor that decision.
10. **Recommendations on methods to improve the treatment of families and survivors by the legal community, including methods to ensure that attorneys do not intrude on the privacy of survivors and families of passengers involved in an aviation accident.**
    - A solicitation prohibition is recommended to be 45 days to include attorney's associate, agent, representative, or "runners."
11. **Recommendations on methods to ensure that representatives of media organizations do not intrude on the privacy of survivors and families of passengers involved in an aviation accident.**
    - Those who work in the media are in the best position to address instances of insensitive treatment that survivors and family members have received following an aviation accident. The Task Force calls upon members of the media to respect the privacy of survivors and family members after an air crash. The Task Force also calls upon each media organization, as well as professional trade associations, to establish standards respecting the rights of survivors and families.
    - The company should designate a liaison between survivors and family members and the press during the initial days following an aviation accident.
    - The company should work with survivors, families, and the media to appropriately limit media contact so that survivors and families can decide in advance whether they wish to speak with the media. The company should inform survivors and families that it is their choice if they want to interact with the media.
    - Survivors and family members should have time to cope with the tragedy prior to having any names publicly released and should be provided an opportunity to personally notify other loved ones of their family member's involvement in an aviation accident.
12. **Findings and recommendations on the availability of information from cockpit voice recorders.**
    - The right to privacy of those recorded on the audio portion of the CVR should not be violated for any reason, other than for its use as an accident investigation tool.
    - The same should apply to photographs, videos, or any other information from the scene which may be upsetting to survivors and family members.

assurances put forward by the task force. This requires commitment and preparedness at all levels of an organization.

Preparation

Personal Preparedness

When developing action plans related to disaster or crisis preparedness, there is shared accountability between the organization and team members. While the organization is responsible for preparing, building, and executing the ERP, PAIP, and tactical response to an incident or accident, there are many things that team members and their families can do to also prepare themselves (see Box 25.7).

While it is difficult to consider one's own morbidity and mortality, preparing for either eventuality can make life significantly easier for survivors and surviving family members should an accident occur. When people think of preparing in the event of an accident, they may prepare their affairs with their death in mind. It is critical to also plan for the case of surviving with potentially disabling injuries. Having robust insurance policies, short and

long-term disability, and gap insurance may help ease the financial burden in the event of on-the-job injury. Workman's compensation alone may be insufficient, especially for those who have more than one job. Financial planning can significantly ease the burden of the financial stress that frequently accompanies incidents and accidents.

Organizational Preparedness

Clearly, while preventing incidents and accidents during all modes of medical transportation is an over-arching goal, it is essential to prepare should an incident or accident occur. Team members and organizations need to strongly overcome the "it won't happen to me" or "it won't happen here" mindset. The medical transport realm is complex and carries risk. Incidents and accidents can happen to anyone.

It is essential for organizations to be trauma-informed. Trauma-informed organizations are those that recognize what potentially traumatizes people and how to identify and respond effectively to those who may be traumatized. While it seems obvious that crashes in the medical transport community are highly traumatizing, other

• BOX 25.7 Individual and Family Preparedness Recommendations

- Plan and prepare in case of injury or line-of-duty-death with appropriate family members
- Ensure communication centers/dispatchers have correct duty staff listed each shift – it is critical that aircraft manifests and duty/shift rosters are accurate
- Ensure emergency contact information is up to date
- Keep financial affairs in order
- Create a Will, Advanced Directives, and Power of Attorney
- Write letters of instruction
- Ensure life insurance, long-/short-term disability policies, and gap insurance policies will meet your/your families' needs
- Ensure beneficiary statuses on all accounts are up to date
- Keep secure records of accounts, digital assets, and business records with usernames and passwords
- Designate guardians for children/dependents
- Designate guardians for pets
- Create a savings account in case of disaster
- Know your organization's plan for financial assistance and support post incident/accident
- Participate in tabletop exercises with the organization and learn what to potentially expect
- Research estate planning or get professional assistance

• BOX 25.8 Impact of Trauma

"As human beings we belong to an extremely resilient species ... but traumatic experiences do leave traces, whether on a large scale (on our histories and cultures) or close to home, on our families, with dark secrets being imperceptibly passed down through generations. They also leave traces on our minds and emotions, on our capacity for joy and intimacy, and even on our biology and immune systems."[11]

impactful events that may be highly traumatizing are often overlooked. These events include incidents with little or no vehicle damage or minor to no injuries to vehicle occupants, near-misses, and clinical or social situations with interpersonal violence. These and other similar occurrences in which team members express such sentiments as, "I thought I was going to die" are impactful and result in various degrees of trauma. Resources and qualified support are critical elements to appropriate response and should be available, accessible, affordable, and offered to all team members. Chapter 24 offers a more detailed discussion of this information.

Responses to trauma are highly individualized and depend on a wide variety of variables so it is essential to have resources, processes, and qualified professionals in place to meet each team member where they are in their individual response to trauma.

Critical Incident Stress, Traumatic Stress Injury, and Grief

The nature of the work in medical transport may lead team members to carry chronic or accumulated stress. It is highly recommended that organizations develop and maintain trauma-informed resources and systems to allow for, and normalize, the discussion and management of stressors to promote health and well-being. This proactive management of stress and organizational response better positions the organization and employees should a catastrophic event occur. Preplanning and system development will foster teams to be in a healthier place to manage the significant trauma and grief that accompanies these types of tragedies. Unless individuals and organizations have made concerted efforts to maintain health and well-being, team members may face crisis, such as an incident or accident, already carrying a heavy load of stress (see Box 25.8).

Responses to crisis and trauma are highly individualized. There is no black-and-white approach or cookie-cutter program to meet the needs of those involved in a completely standardized fashion. Qualified response team members must meet the affected individuals

where they are, constantly assessing their individual needs and determining how to best meet them as issues arise. That said, planning a response amid a crisis will only serve to exacerbate traumatic stress for all involved. The response plan, qualified responders, resources, and processes should be well-established, trained, and practiced before a crisis arises and serve as guidelines for the response. There are a number of initial needs[8]:

1. Primary needs (food – with healthy options, water, tissues, and comfort items)
2. Emotional support and resources, including financial resources
3. Education on stress responses and healthy coping
4. Communication: Accurate, factual, and timely information, along with regular updates
   - What happened?
   - Where are the people directly involved and how are they?
   - What is happening now?
   - What to expect?
5. Practical and logistical support
6. Impacted people may not remember what is said – written reminders are helpful

Being prepared to offer psychological first aid (PFA) and potentially critical incident stress management (CISM) strategies is helpful in the initial phases of a response. Note that CISM is controversial and there is disparity in the literature regarding the overall benefit of CISM.[13] Those conducting CISM should be highly trained using a standardized curriculum taught under the supervision of a certified instructor of that curriculum.

Trained peer support teams who are overseen by a mental health professional are a helpful resource. If the event occurred within their organization, however, they may be impacted personally and therefore not available to provide peer support. Building relationships with local first responder agencies and organizations who have trained peer support teams can create mutual aid opportunities when one organization is overwhelmed by an incident or accident. Fire departments, law enforcement agencies, and local hospitals may have chaplains who may be of great assistance.

Streamlined, affordable, and confidential access to trauma-informed counselors and therapists who understand first responders is essential. There are numerous tools to combat traumatic-stress injury, such as eye-movement desensitization and reprocessing (EMDR) and cognitive behavioral therapy (CBT)[12]. These treatments and methods can significantly shorten treatment time and enhance team member recovery significantly. Specialists such as grief counselors may be warranted, depending on the nature of the incident or accident. Costs of these treatments should be considered in the budgeting process for all organizations. Ideally, the organization would cover all costs for team members seeking professional help. Recovering these individuals in the healthiest way possible sets them up for success in returning to service and effectively managing the complexities of the work.

Chapter 24 provides additional insight into wellness and mental health for transport team members.

Longer Term Considerations

Evaluate Program Safety

How an organization addresses safety and factors that contributed to an incident or accident is critical. Modern risk management has demonstrated that there is typically not a singular "root cause" and that systems approach in the context of a Just Culture should be utilized to fully understand an event. Chapter 9 speaks to risk management and Just Culture in more depth.

Review of these processes is a necessary step in providing reassurance for survivors, family members, and all members of the transport medical team, administration, and risk management offices, regarding the program's commitment to safety. The team, operator, and administration should all be involved. An independent safety audit may be useful to ensure objectivity. The effectiveness of the ERP/PAIP should also be evaluated and revised as necessary. A timetable for implementation of recommendations for process improvement should be developed.

A plan to evaluate the program's safety program should minimally include a review of:

- Safety and operational policies and procedures
- Safety education for staff
- Quality and effectiveness of crew resource management (CRM) training
- Community outreach safety education
- Quality of the program's safety culture (see Box 25.9).

Vehicle and Equipment Replacement

Plans to replace a damaged or destroyed vehicle must be considered during planning for return to service. All equipment on board the crashed vehicle may need to be replaced; the use of an equipment list should ease the process of identification of capital purchases required. When possible, an individual in the purchasing department should be designated to handle the process of timely equipment replacement. Equipment vendors may be able to provide loaner units to facilitate reestablishment of service in a timely manner. Equipment that was on board the vehicle may not be able to be used even if it appears serviceable, as the impact of the crash is not easily assessed. Expert vendor and biomedical resources can assist with this decision-making.

Some team members may be interested in the symbolic and practical work of moving the program forward and be interested in tasks such as ordering and restocking the replacement vehicle. Other team members may be uneasy with the notion of moving forward and so every attempt should be made to identify and support each team member in their unique responses.

In air medical accidents, identification of the tail number for the replacement aircraft may become a sensitive issue for team members. Retiring and honoring the tail number of the accident aircraft and starting anew is often wise.

Request for Physical Memorials

Individuals or groups in the community may find a need to memorialize the accident site and deceased team members. These issues may raise sensitivities with family members and the team, especially if suggestions are not consistent with the wishes of the respective groups. Decisions dealing with these requests require sensitivity, excellent communication, and patience. The result can be a beautiful tribute to those who were lost and a symbol of hope for those who remain.

Formal Investigation

As the formal investigation continues, announcements of findings should be shared with key personnel in a timely manner in concert with investigative and/or regulatory agencies, such as the NTSB, FAA, OSHA, and the state health department. The program leader may need to adopt a strategy to relay information to transport teams before media reports. Ongoing regular meetings with the staff may be beneficial.

NTSB Reports

A factual NTSB report is generally produced shortly after an AMT accident. Probable cause reports may take years. Establishing communication with the TDA Family Liaison allows the liaison an opportunity to provide notice when an NTSB report is about to be released. This provides survivors, family members, and organizations a cue to muster resources, as the release of reports may increase stress and reproduce trauma. As pilot actions or inactions are often listed in the probable cause section of NTSB reports, it is essential to help provide resources and support to surviving pilots and families.

Legal Issues

The legal consequences of a crash quickly become apparent. Attorneys, risk managers, and the insurance carrier should be notified as early as possible. Leadership should be prepared to share the ERP and PAIP, as well as steps taken to mitigate the event.

Even within this litigious society, the number and nature of suits filed may be surprising. The news of such suits may become a significant distraction to team members as they work to re-enter the transport environment. Some issues to keep in mind are:

- Insurance subrogation, the legal doctrine of substituting one creditor for another, can lead to litigation involving customers, which could become an image problem for the program if the insurance provider sues the customer in the name of the operator or vehicle owner. Working closely with the legal department to support and reassure customers may be essential to preserve a positive working relationship.
- Filing deadlines and statutes of limitations should be anticipated so that the flight team and public relations director can be prepared to manage the media. Often, announcements of lawsuit filings appear in the press. Knowledge of lawsuits may generate an emotional response from team members. Because safety policy, procedures, and communications logs are likely to be subpoenaed, such documents may be archived as manuals are updated.

Several years are often necessary to settle lawsuits that result from medical transport accidents. This possibly may be reported in the media. A relationship should be developed with legal counsel regarding their commitment to communication with the program when legal activity is likely to attract the media's interest. Keeping survivors, families, and team members informed is essential.

Anniversaries

The anniversary of a crash is a time of special recognition for the team and family members. The program leader should be prepared to deal with special requests for time off and recognize that the staff may need to be together. A meeting of the staff with an opportunity to talk about feelings may be beneficial and should be offered to the flight team. Mental health workers should be available if team members need to speak in confidence about their feelings around the anniversary.

Each anniversary is acknowledged in various ways by the staff. If the psychologic needs of the staff and program leadership are regarded as a high priority, it is easier to deal with each anniversary.

After-Action Reviews – Initial and Recurrent

Program leadership and response team members will likely be emotionally and physically exhausted after responding to an event. It is valuable, after allowing time for recovery, to engage in after-action reviews of the response, taking into consideration the perspectives of those who responded, along with those who were on the receiving end of the response. Evaluating what went well and what could be improved upon can help shape future responses. Recurrent reviews occurring over time can help the response team understand the longer-term impacts post-incident/accident.

Survivors, family members, and returning team members may have important observations regarding the incident-/accident-response to consider. The feedback may be immediate, occur over time, or both. As they have potentially experienced high levels of trauma and grief, depending on the nature of the event, those involved may be highly emotional in sharing feedback. While the feedback may be difficult to hear, it's essential that their message

is not lost in the delivery. Hard conversations are necessary if we are to learn and improve future responses.

Conclusion

Responding effectively to incident/accident survivors and family members in the medical transport industry is paramount in setting people on the road to recovery and post-traumatic growth. A robust plan, preparation, quality resources, and practice are essential in managing and supporting people after incidents and accidents.

References

1. Blumen I. Wizard of Odds: A Statistical Analysis of HEMS Accidents and Risk. AMTC Presentation; 2019.
2. NHTSA. Fatality Analysis Reporting System (FARS) 1992–2010 Final and 2011 Annual Report File (ARF).
3. NHTSA. National Automotive Sampling System (NASS) General Estimates System (GES), 1992–2011.
4. Jaynes CL, Valdez A, Hamilton M, et al. Survivors perceptions of recovery following air medical transport accidents. *Prehosp Emerg Care*. 2014;19(1):44–52. doi:10.3109/10903127.2014.923075
5. McNaughton E, Willis J, Lallemant D. New Zealand Red Cross; 2015. Leading in Disaster Recovery: A Companion Through the Chaos.
6. Mutlow M. When Accidents Happen: Managing Crisis Communication as a Family Liaison Officer. Independently published; 2020.
7. Van Dernoot Lipsky L, Burk C. Trauma Stewardship: An Everyday Guide to Caring for Self While Caring for Others. 1st ed. Berrett-Koehler Publishers; 2009.
8. Haugen KM. A Shot in the Dark. Vertical Mag. February 24, 2016. https://verticalmag.com/features/a-shot-in-the-dark/
9. Brataas K. Managing the Human Dimension of Disasters. 1st ed. Routledge; 2021.
10. Severin T. In the Wake of the Storm: Living Beyond the Tragedy of Flight 4184. 1st ed. North Cross Press; 2008.
11. Slater RE, Hall JE. Task Force on Assistance to Families of Aviation Disasters FINAL REPORT. October, 1997.
12. Van der Kolk B, MD. The Body Keeps the Score: Brain, Mind, and Body in the Healing of Trauma. Reprint ed. Penguin Publishing Group; 2015.
13. Conn SM. Increasing Resilience in Police and Emergency Personnel: Strengthening Your Mental Armor. 1st ed. Routledge; 2018.

Index

A

AAMS. *see* Association of Air Medical Services
Abandonment, 335
Abbreviated Injury Scale (AIS), 255, 255b
ABCDEFGHI approach, 166–167
Abdominal cavity, 289, 290
Abdominal evisceration, 291
Abdominal trauma, 289
  abdominal vascular injuries and, 291
  colon and small intestine, 290
  liver, 290
  pancreas and duodenum, 290
  spleen, 290
Abdominal vascular injuries, 291
Abduction, 299b
Absolute temperature, 54
Absolute ventilators, 221
Absorptive atelectasis, 211–212
Acceleration, 62, 63t, 246
"Accidental Death and Disability: The Neglected
  Disease of Modern Society," 349
Accidents, 362. *see also* Post-Accident Incident Plan
  (PAIP)
  air medical, 125–126
  ground ambulance, 129–132, 129f, 130f
  types of, 362
Accreditation, for air and ground medical transport,
  349–354
  accreditation standards and, 350–351, 351b
  benefits of, 352
  Joint Commission on Accreditation of Hospitals
    (JCAH) and, 349
  other bodies for, 353, 353t
  past and future challenges in, 351–353
  site surveyors and, 351
  White Paper, 349–350
Accreditation standards, 350–351, 351b
Acid injuries, 310
Acidosis, 253
Active shooter situations, 85–86, 86f
Acute anterior cervical cord syndrome, 275–276
Acute cardiac tamponade, 285
Acute epidural hematoma, 263
Acute hemolytic transfusion reactions, as adverse
  effect of blood transfusion, 238b
Acute Physiology and Chronic Health Evaluation
  (APACHE), 164
Acute stressors, 356
Acute stress, responses to, 110–111
Acute subdural hematomas, 263
Adam's apple, 191
Adaptive support ventilation, 219
Additive ventilators, 221
Adduction, 299b
Adenoid, 192f
Administrative law, 333
Adult learning principles, 20–21
Adult respiratory distress syndrome (ARDS), 209
  management of, 224–225
  ventilation strategy for, 225

Advanced airway management techniques, 190–197
Advanced practice registered nurse (APRN), 16
AE Control Team (AECT), 45
Aerodontalgia. *see* Barodontalgia
Aerodynamics, factors affecting, 27–28, 27f
  aircraft weight, 28
  density altitude, 28
  environmental factors, 27–28
Agricultural emergencies, 81–82, 81f
Air and Surface Transport Nurses Association
  (ASTNA), 8–9
  continuing education/staff development, 22b
  recommended competencies for transport nurses,
    21b
Airbags, 75–76, 76b
Aircraft accidents, 76–79, 78f
Aircraft decompression, 64
Aircraft fire emergencies, 143–144
Aircraft instruments, 34–36
  attitude indicator (artificial horizon), 35–36, 36f
  other gauges, 36
  pitot-static system, 34–35
Aircraft maintenance regulations, 30–31
Aircraft mechanical emergencies, 143
Aircraft motion, 63, 63t
Aircraft pressurization system, 64
Aircraft safety
  fixed-wing, 140
  training for, 137
Aircraft survival kit, 146b, 151
Airfoil function, 27f
Air medical accidents, 125–126, 125t
  fixed-wing, 126–127, 127f, 128f
  risk mitigation, 132–135
  safety technologies in, 135–136, 135b
Air Medical Journal, 145
Air Medical Physician Association (AMPA), 10, 17,
  125
Air medical program models, 5–6
Air Medical Resource Management (AMRM), 36,
  132–135
Air Medical Safety Survey, 124
Air medical transport
  accreditation for, 349–354
    accreditation standards and, 350–351, 351b
    benefits of, 352
    Joint Commission on Accreditation of
      Hospitals (JCAH) and, 349
    other bodies for, 353, 353t
    past and future challenges in, 351–353
    site surveyors and, 351
    White Paper and, improved emergency medical
      services and, 349–350
  fixed-wing, 3
  guidelines to assist, in accidents, 367–368b
  by helicopter, 2f, 3–5, 5f, 6f
  origins of, 2–6
Airmen's Meteorological Information
  (AIRMET), 32
AIRMET. *see* Airmen's Meteorological Information

Airport patterns, aviation and, 25–26, 26f
Airspeed indicator, 35, 35f
Airway
  adult and infant, 199f
  laryngoscopic view of, 192f
  management, 169
  primary assessment, 158, 158b
  sagittal view of, 192f
Airway management, 185–208
  advanced techniques, 190–197
  basic life support airway interventions, 189–190
  complications of intubation, 193b
  end-tidal carbon dioxide detection, 203–204,
    203f, 204f
  indications for, 186
  intervention for, 189–190
  laryngeal mask airway, 195–196, 196f
  medication-assisted, 200–203
  needle cricothyrotomy, 197–198, 198b
  neuromuscular blocking agents, 201, 201f, 202t
  orotracheal intubation, 194b
  patient assessment in, 185–189
  pediatric, 199–200, 199f
  physical examination in, 186–187
  physiologic examination and considerations
    associated with, 187–189
  postintubation management, 204
  pulse oximetry, 188f, 204
  rapid four-step cricothyrotomy, 198b, 199, 199f
  Seldinger technique, 199b
  surgical airway, 197–199
  surgical cricothyrotomy, 198–199, 198b
  video-assisted intubation, 195
Airway obstruction, 283
Airway pressure release ventilation, 222
AIS. *see* Abbreviated injury scale
Alert patient, 266, 266b
A-level of decibel (dBA), 61
Alkali injuries, 310
Allergic reactions, 240f
  as adverse effect of blood transfusion, 238b
Alloimmunization, as adverse effect of blood
  transfusion, 238b
Allow natural death, 172
Altered mental status (AMS), causes for, 160, 160b
Alternating current (AC), 308
  exit wound from, 309f
Altimeter (Altitude indicator), 35, 35f
Altitude
  aviation and, 24, 25f
  operating at, 29
Altitude hypoxia, 56
Altitude indicator, 35, 35f
Alveolar cytotoxicity, 223
Alveolar overdistension, 211
Ambient temperature, 33
Ambulance volante, 1
Ambus, 46t
American Association of Respiratory Care, 17
American Red Cross, 6

AMPA. *see* Air Medical Physician Association
Amperage, 307–308, 308t
Amputations, 297
AMRM. *see* Air medical resource management
Analgesia, for traumatic brain injury, 272
Anaphylactoid reactions, 239
Anaphylaxis, 239–240, 240f
Anatomical dead space, 212
Anechoic, 320
Ankle dislocations, 296t, 301
Ankle fractures, 301
Ankylosis, 299b
Anniversary, of crash, 371
Anterior arch of atlas, 192f
Anterior arch of cricoid cartilage, 192f
Anterior cord syndrome, 274
Anterior dislocation, 301
Anterior jugular vein, 197f
Anterior subluxation, 275–276, 276f
Antibiotic therapy
    for burn trauma, 317–318
    for traumatic brain injury, 271
Anticoagulation reversal therapy, for TBI, 270–271, 271t
Aortic ultrasound, 327, 327f
APACHE. *see* Acute Physiology and Chronic Health Evaluation
Apical four chamber (A4C) view, of heart, 325, 325f
APRN. *see* Advanced practice registered nurse
Arc burns, 309, 312
Armored Brigade Combat Team (ABCT), 45–46
Armored Personnel Carrier Ambulance (M113A3), 45–46
Arterial injury, 297
Artificial horizon, 35–36, 36f
Aryepiglottic fold, 192f
ASHBEAMS. *see* Association of Hospital Based Emergency Air Medical Services
ASOS. *see* Automated Surface Observing System
Assault, 334
Assertiveness, in teamwork, 108
Assessment of patient, 157
    diversity assessment, 164–165
    equipment assessment, 164
    history in, 161–163
    pain assessment, 164
    prehospital assessment, 157
    scene assessment, 157–165, 157b
    scoring systems for, 164
    secondary assessment, 161–164, 163b
    sedation assessment, 164
    during transport, 175
    trauma history in, 162–163
Assist-control ventilation, 218–219
Association of Air Medical Services (AAMS), 8, 19
Association of Hospital Based Emergency Air Medical Services (ASHBEAMS), 350
Asthma, ventilation strategies for, 224
ASTNA. *see* Air and Surface Transport Nurses Association
Atelectasis
    absorptive, 211–212
    cyclic, 211
ATIS. *see* Automatic Terminal Information Service
Atlas and Database of Air Medical Services, 126–127
Atlas fracture, 276–277
Atracurium, 202t
Atropine, 201
Attitude indicator, 35–36, 36f
Authority, in teamwork, 101
Automated Surface Observing System (ASOS), 31–32
Automated Weather Observing System (AWOS), 31–32

Automatic Terminal Information Service (ATIS), 31–32
Autonomic dysreflexia (AD), 280
Auto-PEEP, 215–216
Aviation
    fundamentals, 26–29
    for medical personal, 24–37
    physics of, 26–27, 27f
    regulations, 29–31
        Federal Aviation Regulations, 29–31
    terminology, 24–26
        airport patterns, 25–26, 26f
        altitude, 24, 25f
        distance and speed, 26
        relative directions, 25, 25f
        time, 24, 24t
Aviation Disaster Family Assistance Act of 1996 (ADFAA), 367
Aviation fuel, 77
Aviation sectional map, 95
Aviation Weather Service (AWS), 31–33
AVPU mnemonic, 159
AVPU scale, 256–258
AWOS. *see* Automated Weather Observing System
Axis fracture, 276–277

B
Bag-valve-mask ventilation, 186–187
Balanced diet, for stress, 358
Balloon tubing, 107
Bariatric patient transport, 173–175
    assessment and intervention differences in, 174
    comorbid factors in, 174t
    preparation for, 174–175
    vehicle selection for, 173–174
Barodontalgia, 59
Barometric pressure changes, 58–59
    barodontalgia, 59
    barosinusitis, 59
    barotitis media, 58
    delayed ear block, 59
    gastrointestinal changes, 59
    middle ear, 58–59
Barosinusitis, 59
Barotitis media, 58
Barotrauma, 209
Barton, Clara, 6
BAS. *see* Battalion Aid Stations
Base deficit, 236
Basic life support airway interventions, 189–190
Basilar skull fractures, 262
Battalion Aid Stations (BASs), 42, 42f
Battery, 334
BCCTPC. *see* Board for Critical Care Transport Paramedic Certification
BCI. *see* Blunt cardiac injury
Bees insignia, 7f
Behavioral strains, 357
Bends, 65
Berlin Definition, 210t, 224–225
Bilaterally constricted pupils, 266–267
Bilaterally dilated pupils, 266–267
Bilaterally small pupils, 266–267
Bilateral wrist fractures, 250
Bi-level positive airway pressure (BiPAP), 221
Bladder rupture, 292
Bladder trauma, 292, 293f
Blast-related TBI, 265
Blood transfusion, adverse effects of, 238b
Blue Threat, 117
Blunt cardiac injury (BCI), 286–288
Blunt head injury, 261–274
Blunt thoracic aortic injuries (BTAI), 288
Blunt trauma, 282
B-mode, 321, 321f

Board for Critical Care Transport Paramedic Certification (BCCTPC), 9, 17
Body mass index (BMI), 173
Bone, 295
    demineralization, 295
Boots, 139
Boyle, Robert, 52–53
Boyle's law, 27–28, 52–53, 53t
Brainstem reflexes, 267
Breathing
    primary assessment, 158–159, 158b
    tactical, 111, 112f
Brown-Séquard syndrome, 274
Bullet wounds, 250
Burn trauma, 307–319
    airway/breathing/inhalation injury and, 314–315
    antibiotics for, 317–318
    assessment of, 310–314
    causes of, 307f
    chemical burn injuries and, 314
    in children, 313
    circulation/fluid resuscitation for, 315–316
    electrical injuries and, 307, 312–313, 313f
    etiology and epidemiology of, 307
    evaluation of, 318
    impact of transport in, 318–319
    lightning injuries and, 313–314, 313f
    Lund and Browder chart in, 310, 312f
    management of, 314–317
    pain management of, 317
    pathophysiology of, 307–310
    primary survey of, 314
    radiation burn injuries and, 314
    rule of nines of, 310, 311f
    scene safety for, 314
    transport considerations of, 317
    vital signs of, 318
    wound management of, 316
Burn unit referral criteria, 319b

C
CAAMS. *see* Commission for the Accreditation of Air Medical Service
Cabin differential pressure, 64
Cabin pressurization, 63–66
Caffeine, 358
Caisson disease, 65
Calcaneus fractures, 250
Calcium content, of bone, 295
CAMTS. *see* Commission on Accreditation of Medical Transport Systems
Canadian C-Spine Rule, 279
Capnography, 203
Capnometry, 203
Carbon monoxide poisoning, 311
Cardiac arrest, 328–329
    causes of, 328t
Cardiac FAST exam, 323–324, 324f
Cardiac output (CO), 230
    factors affecting, 231f
Cardiac tamponade, 241, 285–286, 286f, 326–327
Cardiac ultrasound, 324
    apical four chamber view, 325, 325f
    inferior vena cava, 325–326, 326f
    parasternal long axis view, 324, 325f
    parasternal short axis view, 325, 325f
    pathology, 326–327
        left ventricular systolic function, 326
        right ventricular size and function/pulmonary embolism, 326–327
    subxiphoid view, 325, 325f
Cardiogenic shock, 240–241
Cardiopulmonary arrest, during transport, 172
CARESOM, 5
Care Under Fire (CUF), 39

CARF. *see* Commission on Accreditation of Rehabilitation Facilities
Case law, 333
Case study
  for flicker vertigo, 66b
  on teamwork, 100b, 102b, 103b, 105b
  for transport physiology, 66b, 67b
  for trauma, 259b
CASEVAC *vs.* MEDEVAC, 44
Casualty evacuation, 44
Causation, 334
Cause-and-effect diagram, 346, 347f
Cave rescue, 84–85, 85f
Cavitation, 251
Ceiling and visibility, 33
Cell phones, for signaling, 148
Cellular ischemia, micropathophysiologic changes during, 234f
Cellular phones, 91
Cellular respiration, 230, 231f
Cement injury, 310
Central cord syndrome, 274
Cerebral autoregulation, loss of, 270, 270f
Cerebral contusion, 264–265
Cerebral perfusion pressure (CPP), 269
Cerebrospinal fluid (CSF)
  drain, 272–273
  in traumatic brain injury, 261
Certification, critical care, 339
Certified Flight Registered Nurse (CFRN), 15
Certified in Neonatal Pediatric Transport (C-NPT), 15
Certified Registered Nurse Anesthetist (CRNA), 50
Certified Transport Registered Nurse (CTRN), 15
Cervical spinal injuries (CSIs), 275–276
CFRN. *see* Certified Flight Registered Nurse
Change management, 345, 345b
Channel guard, 92–93
Charles, Jacques, 54
Charles' law, 27, 53t, 54
Check sheet (tally sheet), 346
Chemical burn injuries, 307
  assessment of, 314
  management of, 318
Chemicals, as railway hazards, 81
Chemical Transportation Emergency Center (CHEMTREC), 71
CHEMTREC. *see* Chemical Transportation Emergency Center
Chest escharotomy sites, 316f
Chest x-ray (CXR), interpretation of, 165–167, 166f
Children
  burn trauma in, 313, 313f
  orthopedic injuries, 299
  urinary output in, 318
Chokes, 65
Chronic stressors, 356–357
Circulation, primary assessment, 159, 159b
Circumferential burns, 316
CIS. *see* Critical incident stress
CISM. *see* Critical incident stress management
Citrate toxicity, as adverse effect of blood transfusion, 238b
Citric acid cycle, 230
Civil injury law, 334
Civil tort law, 334
Clavicle, 197f
  fractures, 296t, 300
Clavicular head dislocation, 296t
Clinical care, critical phases of, 121
Clinical decision-making, 22, 22f
Clinical error, human faces of, 113b
Clinical risk management
  human performance in, 117
  organizational underpinnings of, 114, 114b

Clinical safety training, 137
Closed fracture, 297
Closed head injury, 314
Clothing
  fire-resistant, 139
  as survival basics, 146
CMV-assist, 218
Coagulation cascade, 235f
Coagulopathy, 237, 253
COBRA. *see* Consolidated Omnibus Budget Reconciliation Act
Cockpit, 34, 36
Cold caloric test, 267f
Cold weather survival, 151
Cold zone, 72, 74f
Colon, injury of, 290
Color Doppler ultrasound, 321, 321f
Coma, 266
Comatose state, 266, 266b
Combitube, 195
Commercial aviation, 366–368
Commercial medical escorts, 180–181
  air carrier regulations and, 181
  documentation of, 181
  electrical power and adapters and, 181
  in nonstop flight, 181
  oxygen adapters and, 181
  oxygen requirements and, 181
  privacy and, 181
Commercial motor vehicle accidents, 76, 77f
Comminuted fractures, 298f
Commission for the Accreditation of Air Medical Service (CAAMS), 9, 350
Commission on Accreditation of Medical Transport Systems (CAMTS), 9–10, 351–353
  frequently cited areas of weakness by, 352b
  initial training program requirements, 20b
  recommendations, 22
  securing patients and equipment, 142
  weather minimums, 132
Commission on Accreditation of Rehabilitation Facilities (CARF), 351
Committee on Tactical Combat Casualty Care (CoTCCC), 39
Common carotid artery, 197f
Communication, 88–98
  aircraft radios for, 96–97
    effectiveness of, 96
    with media, 97
    medical direction in, 97
    sensitive radio traffic in, 96–97
    telephones and, 97
  air medical personnel resources and, 178
  barriers to, 107
  centers. *see* Communication centers
  Crew Resource Management and, 106–107, 107f
  electronic, 97, 97b
  emergency, 144
  for emergency procedures, 97–98
  language and, 95–96
  operations, 90–95
    alternative sites/backup equipment for, 91
    closed-circuit television/web cameras in, 96
    computer-aided dispatch systems in, 93–94, 94f
    computers and peripherals in, 93
    control centers, 90
    headsets and foot switches in, 93
    maps in, 94–95
    pagers in, 93
    radios in, 91–93, 92b
    recorders in, 93
    telephones in, 91
    weather radar in, 94
  optimize, 107–108

Communication (*Continued*)
  policies and procedures in, 95
  in preparing patient for transport, 155–156
  satellite, 97
  speaking and, 95–96
Communication and Optimal Resolution (CANDOR) approach, 122
Communication centers, 88, 89b, 89f
Communication recorders, 93
Communications center manual, 95
Communications specialist, 88–90
  roles and responsibilities of, 88–89
  selection of, 89
  training of, 90, 90b
Community partners, 365
Compartment syndrome, 303–304
Compassion fatigue, 357
Compass radial overlay, 95
Compensated shock, 233f
Compensatory stage, 56
Competency-based education, 21
Complete cord transection, 274
Complete dislocation, 298
Compound dislocation, 298
Compression, 246
Compression cervical spine injuries, 276
Compression fractures, 250
Computed tomography (CT)
  for acute subdural hematomas, 263
  interpretation of, 167–168, 168f, 169f
  subarachnoid hemorrhage, 264f
Computer-aided dispatch systems, 93–94, 94f
Concussion, 265
Confined spaces, 81
Consciousness, 266, 266b
Consent, 156–157
  issues, 335–336
Consolidated Omnibus Budget Reconciliation Act (COBRA), 154, 176, 337
Contaminated wastes, disposal of, 177
Continuing professional development, 21
Continuous mandatory ventilation, 218
Continuous positive airway pressure (CPAP), 220–221
Continuous quality improvement (CQI), 18
Continuous tone-controlled subaudible squelch (CTCSS), 92–93
Control chart, 347, 348b, 348f
Controlled flight into terrain, 127
Contusion
  myocardial, 286–287, 287f
  pulmonary, 289
Conus elasticus, 197f
Convective SIGMETs, 32
Cormack-Lehane scale, 193f, 195
Corniculate cartilage, 192f
COVID-19, 49, 337–338
  helmet-based ventilation for, 222
  mechanical ventilation in, 225
CPAP. *see* Continuous positive airway pressure
CQI. *see* Continuous quality improvement
Cranial nerves, extraocular, 267
Craniectomy, for traumatic brain injury, 273–274
Crashworthy aircraft and vehicle systems, 136
Credentialing, 339
Creeps, 65
Crew Resource Management (CRM), 36, 103, 118, 132
  origins of, 102–103
  problems in, 103–107
    availability of resources, 109
    communication, 106–107, 107f
    delegation, 103–105
    leadership, 109

Crew Resource Management (Continued)
    recognizing decision-making hazards, 109
    situational awareness, 105–106
    workload management and delegation,
        103–105, 104f
Crew responsibilities, 145
Cricoid cartilage, 191, 197f
Cricothyroid membrane, 191, 192f
Cricothyrotomy
    difficult, 187
    needle, 197–198, 198b
    rapid four-step, 198b, 199, 199f
    Seldinger technique, 199b
    surgical, 198–199, 198b
Crime, 334
Criminal acts, 334
Criminal law, 334
Critical care equipment, 155, 156b
Critical care paramedics, members of transport
        team, 16
Critical care transport, 1, 333
    decisions, 339–340
    diversion policies, 337–338
    ethical issues, 339
    family considerations in, 340–341
    interfacility patient transfers, medical direction
        during, 338
    legal issues in, 335–338
    litigation, 341
    medicine, 339
    nursing in, 6–7, 6f, 7b, 7f
    orders and giving report, 340–341
    paramedics in, 7–8
    patient- and family-centered care, 340
    professional issues in, 333–342
    use of hospital helipads, 337
Critical incident stress, 369–370
Critical incident stress management (CISM), 98,
        357, 358, 369
Critical stage, 56
CRM. see Crew Resource Management
Crowdfunding, 366
Crush injuries, 304
Crush syndrome, 304
CTCSS. see Continuous tone-controlled subaudible
        squelch
CTRN. see Certified Transport Registered Nurse
Cuffed ETTs, 200
Cumulonimbus (CB), 33
Cuneiform cartilage, 192f
Current pathway, 308–309
Curvilinear probe, 320–321, 321f
Cutaneous injuries, electrical, 312
Cyclic atelectasis, 211

D
DAI. see Diffuse axonal injuries
Daily shift safety procedures, 140–143
Dalton's law, 53–54, 53t
Damage control resuscitation, 258
Damages, 334
DCR. see Damage control resuscitation
D-Dimer testing, 241
Dead space, 212–213
    anatomical, 212
    mechanical, 213
DEATH mnemonic, 62b
Deceleration, 246
Decerebrate posturing, 267–268
Decibels (dBs), 60, 61t
Decompression, 64–65, 64b
Decompression sickness, 65–66, 65b
Decontamination, 73–74
Delayed ear block, 59
Delayed sequence intubation, 200

Delegation, Crew Resource Management and,
        103–105
Deming's 14 points, 343, 343b
Dens fracture, 276–277
Density altitude, 28
Department of Transportation (DOT), hazardous
        materials defined by, 71
Depressed skull fracture, 262
Dermatome map, 278, 278f
Dermis, 308
Descriptive communication, 107
Desert survival, 150–151
Dewpoint, 33
Diagnostic tests, 165–168
Diaphragmatic injury, 288–289
Diaphragmatic tear, 288
Diastatic fracture, 262
Differential pressure, 64
Diffuse axonal injuries (DAI), 265
Direct-contact burns, 312, 313f
Direct current, 307
    exit wound from, 309f
Directive communication, 107
Direct laryngoscopy, 193–195, 194f
    difficult, 187
Direct pressure, 246
Dislocated elbow, 301
Dislocated finger, 301
Dislocated hip, 301
Dislocated wrist, 301
Dislocations, 298
    orthopedic injuries, 296t
    upper extremities, 301
Dispatch/communications, 140–141
Dispatcher, 88–89
Distal femoral shaft fractures, 296t
Distance and speed, aviation and, 26
Distributive shock, 239–240
Disturbance stage, 56
Diversity assessment, 164–165
Documentation
    of commercial medical escorts, 181
    of evidence, 86
    in international transport, 179
    legal issues in, 336
    of orders regarding patient care, 340–341
    in patient transport, 173, 173b
Doll's eye, 267, 267f
"Do not resuscitate," 172
DOPE, 228, 228b
Doppler ultrasound, 321, 321f
Dorsiflexion, 299b
Drills, 98
Driving pressure, 214
D sign, 326
Duodenum, injury of, 290
Duty times, pilot and air medical personnel, 180
Dynamic hyperinflation, 211

E
Ear block, 59
Early shock, 252–253t
Earmuffs, 139
Earplugs, 139
Education
    competency-based, 21
    continuing, 21
    for transport team members, 339
Effective performance time (EPT), 57, 57t
Elbow fractures, 300
Electrical emergencies, 81
Electrical hazards, in railway, 80
Electrical injuries, 307
    arc burns, 312
    assessment of, 312–313, 313f

Electrical injuries (Continued)
    cutaneous, 312
    direct-contact burns, 312, 313f
    flame burns with, 309
    management of, 317
    pathophysiology of, 308–310
Electronic communication, 97, 97b
ELM. see External laryngeal manipulation
Emergencies
    agricultural, 81–82, 81f
    aircraft mechanical, 143
    communication, 144
    electrical, 81
    explosive materials, 87
    fire, 143–144
    ground vehicle, 145
    hazardous materials, 71–72
    in-flight, 143–145
    landings, 144
    radioactive material, 72–73
    transportation, 74–81
Emergency egress, 144
Emergency locator transmitter (ELT), 144
Emergency medical technician-paramedic (EMT-P), 7
Emergency Medical Treatment and Active Labor Act
        (EMTALA), 154, 337
Emergency notification system, 79, 80f
Emergency rescue, in a railway incident, 79–80
Emergency Response Guidebook (ERG), 71–72
Emergency Response Plan (ERP), 361
    information flow and communication, 363
    legal issues in, 370–371
    organizational preparedness, 368–369
    personal preparedness, 368, 369b
    program leadership team, 362, 362b
    program safety evaluation, 370
    vehicle and equipment replacement, 370
Emergency vehicle operators (EVOs), 19
Emotional awareness, stress and, 111
EMTALA. see Emergency Medical Treatment and
        Active Labor Act
EMT-P. see Emergency medical technician-paramedic
Endotracheal intubation (ETI), 191
    indications for, 220b
Endotracheal tube (ETT), 191
Endotracheal tube introducer (ETI), 194
End-tidal carbon dioxide (EtCO$_2$), 236
    detection, 203–204, 203f, 204f
    shark-fin morphology, 226–227, 227f
    waveform
        curare cleft type, 226f
        to show hypercapnia, 226f
Energy forces, 247f
En route critical care, 48–50, 49f
En Route Critical Nurses (ECCNs), 46
En Route Patient Staging System (ERPSS), 49–50
Environmental hazards, 157, 157b
Epidermis, 308
Epidural hematoma, 169f, 263–264, 263f
Epiglottis, 191, 192f
Epinephrine, 189, 236
    for anaphylactic shock, 240
Equipment
    assessment, 164
    critical care, 155, 156b
    immobilization, 177–178
    personal protective, 138–139
    survival, 151
ERG. see Emergency Response Guidebook
Escharotomies, 316
Escharotomy sites, 317b
    chest, 316f
    on finger, 316f
Escort flight, 180–181
Esophageal injuries, 288

Esophagus, 191, 192f
EtCO₂ waveform capnography, for traumatic brain injury, 272
Ethical decision-making, in transport environment, 339
Ethical issues, in critical care transport, 339
ETI. see Endotracheal tube introducer
Etomidate, 201
ETT. see Endotracheal tube
Eustachian tube, 58
Eversion, 299b
Evidence preservation, 86
Evisceration, abdominal, 291
EVO. see Emergency vehicle operators
Exercise, for stress, 358–359
Exhaled tidal volume, 213
Exit wound
    from alternating current, 309f
    from direct current, 309f
Explosive materials emergencies, 87
Explosive projectiles, 251
Exposure assessment, 161, 161b
Expressed consent, 335
Extended FAST exam, 324, 324f
Extension, 299b
    injuries, 276
Extension-rotation injuries, 276
Extension teardrop fracture, 276
External laryngeal manipulation (ELM), 191, 194
External rotation, 299b
External ventricular drainage (EVD) catheter, 272
External ventricular drain (EVD) collection system, 273f
Extraglottic devices, 195
    difficult, 187
Extrication, 249–250, 249f

F
Face-to-face communication, 107
Falls, 250
Family
    notification and support, 364
    in patient preparation, 172
    of returning team members, 365
    of survivors, accident, 365
Family-centered care, during transport, 340
FAR. see Federal Aviation Regulations
FAST. see Focused Assessment with Sonography in Trauma
Fat embolism, 303
Fatigue, 62
    compassion, 357
    on human performance, 110
Fatigue policies, 138
Febrile nonhemolytic transfusion reactions, as adverse effect of blood transfusion, 238b
Federal Aviation Administration (FAA), 31
    medical helicopter accident, 126f
    procedure for aircraft accidents, 77–79
    regulations, 132, 135b
Federal Aviation Regulations (FARs), 29–31, 178–179
Federal KKK-A-1822F (KKK) standard, 129
Femoral shaft fractures, 301
Fentanyl, 270
Fetal Evaluation for Transport by Ultrasound (FETUS) exam, 328
Fetal heart rate (FHR), POCUS evaluation of, 328
Fibula fractures, 301
Fick's law, 53t, 55
Field triage, 256, 256f
Fingerprints, 86
Firearm injuries, 250–251

Firearms, 251
    situations, 86–87
Fire building, 148, 149f
Fire emergencies, 143–144
Fire-resistant clothing, 139
First-degree burn, 311
First responders, 365
Fitness standards, 138
Fixed-wing aircraft
    safety, 140
    vibration, 61
Fixed-wing air medical accidents, 126–127, 127f, 128f
Fixed-wing patient transport, 3, 175–181
    air medical personnel resources in, 178
    bedding and linens in, 177
    COBRA and, 176
    contaminated wastes, disposal of, 177
    escort and medical assist transports in, 180–181
    Federal Aviation Regulations (FARs), 178–179
    ground ambulance capabilities in, 177
    immobilization equipment in, 177–178
    in-flight factors in, 178
    international transport issues in, 179–180
    loading considerations in, 177
    nutrition and fluid requirements in, 177
    oxygen requirements in, 176
    patient care supplies and medications in, 176–177
    patient medical equipment requirements in, 176
    patient "packaging" in, 177–178
    preflight preparation in, 175
    preparation for, 175–177
    safety and emergency procedures in, 178–179
Fixed wing transport, 48, 48t
Flaccid, patient, 267–268
Flail chest, 285, 286f
Flame burns, 309
Flashlight, for signaling, 148
Flat-terrain rescues, 83
Flexion, 299b
    injuries, 275–276
Flexion-rotation injuries, 276
Flicker vertigo, 66, 66b
Flight data monitoring system, 29
Flight following, 141
Flight level, 60
Flight operations, 90
Flight pressure altitude, 64
Floating tagline, 84, 84f
Flowchart, 347
Flow pattern, in mechanical ventilation, 216
Flow rate, in mechanical ventilation, 216
Flow triggering, 216
Focused Assessment with Sonography in Trauma (FAST) exam, 321–322
    cardiac view, 323–324, 324f
    extended, 324, 324f
    left upper quadrant, 322, 322f, 323f
    limitations of, 324
    pelvic view, 323, 323f
    right upper quadrant, 322, 322f
Followership, in teamwork, 101
Food, during survival, 149
Foot dislocation, 301
Footwear, 139
Force, 246
Forced water landings, 144–145
Foreseeability, 334
Four-step cricothyrotomy, 198b, 199, 199f
Fractional concentration of oxygen, in inspired gas, 214
Fractures, 297–298, 298f
    atlas, axis, and dens, 276–277
    extension injuries, 276
    flexion injuries, 275–276

Fractures (Continued)
    lower extremities, 301
    open/closed, 297
    orthopedic injuries, 296t
    pelvic, 296t, 301–303
    radiographic appearance, 298f
    skull, 262
    splinting, 299–300
    thoracic and lumbar spine injuries, 277
    upper extremities, 300
    vertical compression, 276
Fragmentation, 251
    injuries, 87
Frank-Starling curve, 236
Freight trains, 79
Frequency, 320–321
Front-to-side method, 141
Fuel, as railway hazards, 80
Fuel vapors, 66
Full duplex system, 92
Full Outline of UnResponsiveness (FOUR) Score, 160, 160t
Full-thickness/third-degree burn injuries, 311
Funeral planning, 366

G
Gas exchange, 56
Gas laws, 52–55, 53t
    Boyle's law, 52–53
    Charles' law, 54
    Dalton's law, 53–54
    Fick's law, 55
    Gay-Lussac's law, 54
    Graham's law, 55
    Henry's law, 54–55
    variables, 52
Gastric decompression, 170
Gastroesophageal trauma, 291
Gay-Lussac's law, 53t, 54
GCS. see Glasgow Coma Scale
General damages, 334
Genital trauma, 292–293
Genitourinary trauma, 291
G force, 62
Glasgow Coma Scale (GCS), 160, 254–255, 263, 268–269, 268t
    adult, 160t
    pediatric, 160t
Global oxygen consumption (VO₂), 230
Glycolysis, 230
Golden Hour theory, 350
Graham's law, 53t, 55
Gravitational force, 62–63
"Great masquerader," 241
Greenstick fractures, 298f
Grief, 369–370
Ground ambulance accidents, 129–132, 129f, 130f, 131b
Ground ambulance capabilities, 177
Ground ambulance resources, 180
Ground ambulance safety, 140
    recommendations, 131b
    training, 137
Ground MEDEVAC, 45–46, 46t
Ground medical transport, accreditation for, 349–354
    accreditation standards and, 350–351, 351b
    benefits of, 352
    Joint Commission on Accreditation of Hospitals (JCAH) and, 349
    other bodies for, 353, 353t
    past and future challenges in, 351–353
    site surveyors and, 351
    White Paper and, improved emergency medical services and, 349–350

Ground-to-air signals, 148
Ground transport times, 180
Ground vehicle emergencies, 145
Groupthink, 109
Gunshot wounds, 265

H
Half-duplex system, 92
Handguns, 251
Hand injuries, 300
Hangman's fracture, 276
Hard palate, 192f
Hare traction splint, 300
Hazardous materials (HAZMAT), 143
   definition of, 71
   emergencies, 71–72
      decontamination in, 73–74
      radioactive, 72–73
      transport vehicle or container for, 72
   incident, safety zones for, 74f
   warning placards and labels, 73f
Hazards, environmental, 157, 157b
Head injuries
   closed, 314
   from explosions, 87
Head-on collisions, 247–248, 248f, 250, 250f
Healthcare environments, 343, 344f
Health Insurance Portability and Accountability Act
      (HIPAA), 336–337, 348
   regulations, 162–163
Hearing protection, 139
Heart
   apical four chamber view of, 325, 325f
   parasternal long axis view of, 324, 325f
   parasternal short axis view of, 325, 325f
   subxiphoid view of, 325, 325f
Heart and lung team, 49
Heart rate, stress and, 111, 111f
Heat escape-lessening posture (HELP), 150, 150f
Heavily armored ground ambulance (HAGA),
      45–46
Helicopter
   accidents
      EMS and non-EMS fatal, 125, 127f
      FAA, 126f
   patient transport by, 2f, 3–5, 5f, 6f
   safety, 139–140, 140f
   shopping, 135
   vibration, 61
Helicopter air ambulance (HAA), 29
Helicopter Air Ambulance Regulations, 29, 29t,
      30b
Helicopter Emergency Medical Service (HEMS), 10,
      125
   Federal Aviation Administration (FAA) regulations
      for, 135b
Helicopter shopping, 154
Helicopter terrain awareness and warning system
      (HTAWS), 29
Helipad/airport safety, 141
Helium-oxygen mixture (Heliox), 223
Helmet-based ventilation, 222
Helmets, 138–139
HELP. see Heat escape-lessening posture
Hemorrhage, 237
   intracranial, 262–265
   massive, 158, 158b
Hemorrhagic contusions, 264
Hemothorax, massive, 284–285, 284f
HEMS. see Helicopter Emergency Medical Service
Henry's law, 53t, 54–55, 65
Hertz (Hz), 60
HFNC. see High-flow nasal cannula
High-flow nasal cannula (HFNC), 221–222
High-frequency jet ventilation (HFJV), 223

High-frequency oscillatory ventilation, 223
High-frequency ventilation, 222–223
High-pressure alarm, 227–228
High-reliability organizations (HROs), 115
HIPAA. see Health Insurance Portability and
      Accountability Act
Hip dislocation, 301
Hip fracture, 301
Histogram, 346, 346f
History
   of nursing, 6–7
   of paramedics, 7
   of patient assessment, 161–163
   of patient transport, 1–11
      in 20th and 21st centuries, 8, 8t
HMMWV (M996), 45–46
Hospital helipads, use of, 337
Hot loading, 139
HOTSAW mnemonic, 142, 142b
Hot zone, 72, 74f
HTAWS. see Helicopter terrain awareness and
      warning system
Human error
   causes of, 119f
   combating, 100
   problem of, 99–100
Human factors, 117
   engineering, 118
   managing, 118
   risk assessment, 118b
   support, 118b
Human Factors Analysis and Classification System
      (HFACS), 115–116, 116f
Human-made disasters, 85
Human & Organizational Performance (HOP),
      117
Human performance, 109–111
   in clinical risk management, 117
   fatigue on, 110
   improvement of, 111
   noise on, 110
   stress and, 109–111, 109f
   workload on, 110
Human resources (HR), 366
Humerus fractures, 296t, 297–298
Humidity, 60
Hydration, 148, 150f
   for stress, 358
Hydraulics, 83
Hydrofluoric acid, 310
Hydrogen cyanide, 311
Hyoid bone, 192f, 197f
Hyperbaric oxygen therapy (HBOT), 311
Hypercapnia, 55
   EtCO$_2$ waveform, 226f
   permissive, 224
Hyperechoic, 320
Hyperextension, 299b
Hyperextension fracture-dislocation injuries, 276
Hyperextension injuries, 276, 277f
Hyperkalemia, succinylcholine-induced, 202
Hyperosmolar therapy, for traumatic brain injury,
      272
Hyperthermia, in traumatic brain injury, 271
Hypertonic saline (HTS), for traumatic brain injury,
      272
Hyperventilation, 57–58
   traumatic brain injury and, 271–272
Hypoechoic, 320
Hypotension, 188–189
   in traumatic brain injury, 270
Hypothermia, 237, 251–253
Hypoventilation, 226, 226f
Hypovolemic shock, 237–239, 238b
Hypoxemia, 55, 187–188

Hypoxia, 55–57
   major organ system changes associated with,
      233f
   signs and symptoms of, 56–57, 56t
   stages of, 56
   treatment of, 57
   types of, 56–57
Hypoxic hypoxia, 56

I
IAFCCP. see International Association of Flight and
      Critical Care Paramedics
IAMTCS. see International Association of Medical
      Transport Communications Specialists
IBSC. see International Board of Specialty
      Certification
ICS. see Incident command system
Ideal gas law, 27, 28f
IFR. see Instrument flight rules
I-gel, 196–197
Immobilization equipment, 177–178
Immunoglobulin E (IgE), 239
Impacted fractures, 298f
Impact injuries, 87
Implied consent, 335
Inadvertent instrument meteorologic conditions
      (IIMC), 30
Incident, 362
   mass casualty, 256–258
   response team members, 365
   types of, 362
Incident commander, 68
Incident Command System (ICS), 68, 69f, 142,
      362–363, 363f
Independent Duty Medical Technician (IDMT),
      40–41
Indifferent stage, 56
Industrial emergency scenes
   agricultural emergencies, 81–82, 81f
   electrical emergencies, 81
   trench collapse, 82
Inferior dislocation, 301
Inferior turbinate, 192f
Inferior vena cava, coronal view of, 325–326, 326f
In-flight emergencies, 143–145
In-flight safety, 141–142
Informed consent, 335
Infraglottic injury, 312, 313f
Inhalation injuries
   management of, 314–315
   with thermal burns, 311–312
Inhaled nitric oxide (iNO), 223
Initial training program requirements, 20b
Injury
   dynamics, 245–247
   mechanism of, 246–247
   orthopedic, 295
Injury Severity Score (ISS), 255–256, 255t
Insertion, of laryngeal mask airway, 196f
Inspiratory time, 216
Inspiratory-to-expiratory time ratio, 216
Instrument flight rules (IFRs), 30, 136
Instrument meteorologic conditions (IMCs), 30
Integrated quality systems, 344–345
Intensity, of sound wave, 60
Intentional explosions, 87
Intentional torts, 334
Interfacility patient transfers, medical direction
      during, 338
Internal jugular vein, 197f
Internal rotation, 299b
International Association of Flight and Critical Care
      Paramedics (IAFCCP), 9
International Association of Medical Transport
      Communications Specialists (IAMTCS), 10

International Board of Specialty Certification (IBSC), 17
International survival concerns, 151
International transport issues, 179–180
Intertheater patient movement request, 45
Intracerebral hematoma, 264, 264f
Intracranial hematomas, gunshot wounds and, 265
Intracranial hemorrhage, 262–265
Intracranial pressure (ICP), 261, 269
  monitoring of, 272
Intraparenchymal fiberoptic catheter, 272
Intraparenchymal hematomas, 264
Intratheater patient movement requests, 45
Intratheater *vs.* intertheater transport and activation, 44–45, 46t
Intubation
  complications of, 193b
  endotracheal, 191
  orotracheal, 191, 194b
  tracheal, 191–193
  video-assisted, 195
Inversion, 299b
Isobaric-differential system, 64
Isobaric system, 64
ISS. *see* Injury Severity Score
Isthmus of thyroid gland, 197f

J
Jackson's zones of injury, 310
JCAH. *see* Joint Commission on Accreditation of Hospitals
Jefferson fracture, 276
Joint Commission, 349
Joint Commission on Accreditation of Hospitals (JCAH), 349
Joint Medical Augmentation Unit (JMAU), 50
Joint Trauma Service (JTS), 39, 50
Judicial law, 333
Just Culture, 115

K
Kehr's sign, 290
Kendrick Traction Device, 300
Ketamine, 201
KIAS. *see* Knots of indicated airspeed
Kinematics of trauma, 245, 247–251
Kinetic energy, 246
Kink-resistant catheter, 197–198
Knee dislocation, 296t, 298
Knee fractures, 301
Knots of indicated airspeed (KIAS), 35
Knowledge-based errors, 99–100
Krebs cycle, 230, 231f
Kyphosis, 299b

L
Laboratory tests, 165, 165t
Lactic acidosis, 317
Landing zone selection and safety, 69, 70f, 142
Landstuhl Regional Medical Center (LRMC), 44
Language barriers, 179
Lapses, definition of, 99
Laryngeal mask airway, 195–196, 196f
Laryngoscopic view of airway, 192f
Larynx, 191, 192f
Late shock, 252–253t
Laughter, for stress management, 359
Law enforcement-related situations, 85–87
Law of gaseous diffusion (Graham's law), 55
Law of partial pressure (Dalton's law), 53–54
Law, overview of, 333–334
Leadership
  Crew Resource Management and, 109
  Post-Accident Incident Plan, 365
  in teamwork, 101

Lean, 345–346
Lean "DOWNTIME" wastes, 346b
Lean-to shelter, 147f
Learning, culture of
  building, 115
  communication within, 121
  operationalizing, 121
Le Fort fractures, 303–304, 304f
Left upper quadrant (LUQ), FAST exam, 322, 322f, 323f
Left ventricular systolic function, 326
Legal issues, 333
  in critical care transport, 335–338
    abandonment, 335
    consent, 335–336
    Consolidated Omnibus Budget Reconciliation Act, 337
    documentation, 336
    Emergency Medical and Active Labor Act, 337
    Health Insurance Portability and Accountability Act, 336–337
  in incidents/accidents, 370–371
Lethargic patient, 266, 266b
Level of consciousness (LOC), 266, 266b
Licensure, 339
Lidocaine, 270
Lightning injuries, 313–314, 313f
  management of, 317–318
Linear acceleration, 62
Linear probe, 320–321, 321f
Linear skull fracture, 262
Linear stellate fractures, 262
Litigation, 341
Liver injuries, 290
LMA. *see* Laryngeal mask airway
LOC. *see* Level of consciousness
Locomotives, of train, 80, 80f
Long bone fractures, 297–298
Long-duration negative acceleration, 63
Long-duration positive acceleration, 63
Long-duration transverse acceleration, 63
Lordosis, 299b
Low-angle rescue, 83
Lower extremities
  dislocations, 301
  fractures, 301
  testing for neurologic function in, 302f
Low minute ventilation alarm, 228
Low-pressure alarm, 228
Lumbar drainage catheter, 272
Lumbar spine injuries, 277
Lund and Browder chart, 310, 312f
Lung ultrasound, 327, 327f
  extended FAST exam, 324, 324f

M
MacIntosh, 194
Mallampati classes, 186, 187f
Mallampati score, 187
Malpractice, elements of, 334, 334b
Mandible, 192f
Mannitol
  for burn trauma, 317
  for traumatic brain injury, 272
MAP. *see* Mean arterial pressure
Mapping software, 94–95
Maps, 94–95
Marine Corps En Route Care System (ERCS), 47
Marvingt, Marie, 6, 6f
Mass, 62
Mass casualty incidents (MCIs), 68, 256–258
Mass casualty triage, 71, 72f
Massive hemorrhage, 158, 158b
Massive hemothorax, 284–285, 284f
MAST. *see* Military Assistance to Safety and Traffic

Maxillofacial trauma, 303–304
Mayday, 144
McConnell's sign, 326
Mean arterial pressure (MAP), 235–236
Mechanical dead space, 213
Mechanical emergencies, aircraft, 143
Mechanical ventilation, 209–229
  advanced ventilatory modes of, 222–223
    airway pressure release ventilation in, 222
    high-frequency ventilation, 222–223
  classification of positive pressure ventilation in, 217–219
    adaptive support ventilation, 219
    assist-control ventilation in, 218–219
    pressure-synchronized intermittent mandatory ventilation plus, 219
    pressure ventilation in, 218
    synchronized intermittent mandatory ventilation in, 219
    synchronized intermittent mandatory ventilation plus, 219
    volume ventilation in, 217–218
  gases used in, 223
    helium-oxygen mixture, 223
    inhaled nitric oxide, 223
  noninvasive positive pressure ventilation in, 219–223
  terminology related to, 210t
  troubleshooting in, 226–228
    monitoring, 226–227, 226f, 227f
    ventilator alarms, 227, 227t
    ventilator asynchrony, 228
  ventilation strategies in, 224–226
    ARDS patient, management of, 224–225
    asthmatic patient, management of, 224
    COVID-19, 225
    metabolic acidosis, 225–226
    obstructive lung disease, 224
    proning, 225
  ventilator-induced lung injury in, 209–212
    absorptive atelectasis, 211–212
    barotrauma, 209
    cyclic atelectasis, 211
    oxygen toxicity, 211
    volutrauma, 211
  ventilator settings in, 212–217
    auto-PEEP, 215–216
    breaths per minute in, 212
    dead space, 212–213
    driving pressure, 214
    exhaled tidal volume in, 213
    flow pattern in, 216
    flow rate in, 216
    fractional concentration of oxygen, in inspired gas, 214
    frequency in, 212
    inspiratory time, 216
    inspiratory-to-expiratory time ratio in, 216
    minute ventilation, 212
    peak inspiratory pressure in, 213–214
    plateau pressure, 214
    positive end-expiratory pressure in, 214–215
    rate in, 212
    rise time, 217
    tidal volume in, 212
    trigger sensitivity in, 216–217
Mechanical ventilator protocol card, 215f
Mechanism, Glasgow, age, and arterial pressure (MGAP), 255, 255t
MED channels, 91–92, 92b
MEDEVAC, 44
MEDEVAC helicopters, 46
Medevac status, 31
Median glossoepiglottic fold, 192f
Medical assist transports, 180–181

Medical control, air medical personnel resources and, 178
Medical control physicians, 18
Medical direction, 17
Medical protocols, 17
Medical quality improvement, 347–348
Medical Transport Leadership Institute, 19
Medication-assisted airway management, 200–203
Members of transport team, 12–23
  communication specialists as, 18
  critical care paramedics as, 16
  emergency vehicle operators as, 19
  nurse as, 13–16
  paramedics as, 16–17, 16b
  physicians as, 17–18
  pilots as, 18
  respiratory therapist as, 12, 17
  respiratory therapists as, 17
  team definitions, 13–15t
Memorial services, 366
Mental health and wellness, for providers
  importance of wellness, 356
  promoting wellness, 358–359
Mental model, sharing of, teamwork and, 108
Metabolic acidosis
  mechanical ventilation in, 225–226
  severe, 189
METARs. see Meteorological Aerodrome Reports
Meteorological Aerodrome Reports (METARs), 31–32, 32f, 32t
Methemoglobinemia, 223
MH-47 Chinook, 50
Microphones, 93
Middle cricothyroid ligament, 197f
Middle ear, 58–59
Middle turbinate, 192f
Military Assistance to Safety and Traffic (MAST), 5
Military patient transport, 38–51, 51f
  en route critical care, 48–50, 49f
  fixed wing transport, 48, 48t
  Ground MEDEVAC, 45–46, 46t
  intratheater vs. intertheater transport and activation, 44–45
  Joint Trauma Service and, 50
  Navy/Marine Corps en route care, 47–48
  patient movement and, 44
  point of injury and, 39–41, 40f
  role 1 and, 41, 41f
  role 2 and, 41–43, 43t
  role 3 and, 43, 44f
  role 4 and, 43–44
  roles of care and, 38–44
  rotary wing transport, 46–47, 47f, 47t
  special operations and, 50
Miller blade, 194
Mine-resistant ambush protected vehicle (MRAP), 45–46
Minimum equipment list, 31
Minimum Standards for Hospitals, 349
Minor injuries, in lightning, patients with, 314
Minute ventilation, 212
Missing or overdue aircraft or ground vehicle procedure, 145
Mivacurium, 202t
M-mode, 321, 321f
Moderate injuries, in lightning, patients with, 314
Motorcycle, 250f
  crashes, 250
Motor examination, 267–268
Motor strength, muscles, 275b
Motor vehicle accidents and extrication, 74–76, 75b, 75f
Motor vehicle collisions (MVC), orthopedic injuries in, 300

Motor vehicle crashes, 247–250, 248f
  extrication, 249–250, 249f
  head-on collisions, 247–248, 248f
  injury patterns by, 162, 162b
  rear-end collisions, 248
  rollovers, 249, 249f
  side impact, 248–249, 250
Mountains, air rescue in, 83f
Multiple aircraft response, 143
Multiplex system, 92
Muscles, motor strength of, 275b
Musculoskeletal system, 295
Musculoskeletal tissue trauma, 295–306
Mushrooming effect, 251
MVC. see Motor vehicle collisions
Myocardial contusion, 286–287, 287f
Myoglobinuria, 317

N
NAACS. see National Association of Air Communication Specialists
Nasopharyngeal airway, 189, 190f
National Aeronautics and Space Administration (NASA) Beginner's Guide to Aerodynamics, 26
National Association of Air Communication Specialists (NAACS), 10
National Emergency Medicine Service Pilots Association (NEMSPA), 10
National Emergency X-Radiography Utilization Study (NEXUS), 279
National Fire Protection Agency, 72
National Flight Nurses Association (NFNA), 8–9
National Highway and Transportation Safety Administration (NHTSA), 5
National Highway Traffic Safety Administration, 129
National Oceanic and Atmospheric Administration (NOAA), 31–33
National Traffic Safety Board, 25–26
National Transportation Safety Board (NTSB), 31, 361
  incidents and accidents defined by, 362, 362b
  report, 370
National Weather Service (NWS), 31–33
Natural disasters, 85
Natural shelter, 147f
Navy/Marine Corps en route care, 47–48
Neck, 197f
Needle cricothyrotomy, 197–198, 198b
Negligence, 334
NEMSPA. see National Emergency Medicine Service Pilots Association
Neonatal Resuscitation Program (NRP) guidelines, 211–212
Neurogenic shock, 239
Neurologic assessment, 159–161
Neurologic trauma, 261–281
  blunt head injury, 261–274
  spinal cord injury, 274–280
    atlas, axis, and dens fractures, 276–277
    cervical spine injuries, 275–276
    etiology and incidence rate, 274
    extension injuries, 276
    extension-rotation injuries, 276
    flexion injuries, 275–276
    flexion-rotation injuries, 276
    initial assessment of, 274
    interventions and treatment of, 279–280
    neurologic examination, 278
    secondary assessment of, 274–276, 275b
    sensory examination, 278
    thoracic and lumbar spine injuries, 277
    vertebral artery dissection, 277
    vertical compression, 276
    without radiographic abnormality, 278
  traumatic brain injury, 261

Neurologic trauma (Continued)
  blast-related, 265
  brainstem reflexes and extraocular cranial nerves, 267
  complications, 265
  Glasgow Coma Scale in, 268–269, 268t
  interventions and treatment of, 269–274, 269b, 270f
  intracranial hemorrhage, 262–265
  level of consciousness, 266, 266b
  management guidelines for, 269b
  motor examination in, 267–268
  pathologic and clinical considerations in, 262–265
  penetrating injuries, 265
  physical assessment of, 266–269, 266b, 266t
  pupils and, 266–267
  reexamination in, 269
  respiratory pattern in, 268
  skull fracture, 262
  types of, 262–265
Neuromuscular blocking agents, 201, 201f, 202t
Never events, 122
Newton's first law of motion, 62, 246
Newton's second law of motion, 62
Newton's third law of motion, 62
NFNA. see National Flight Nurses Association
NHTSA. see National Highway and Transportation Safety Administration
Nightingale, Florence, 6
Night vision goggles, 136
Night vision imaging systems (NVIS), 125
NiPPV. see Noninvasive positive pressure ventilation (NiPPV)
NOAA. see National Oceanic and Atmospheric Administration
Noise
  hearing protection for, 139
  on human performance, 110
  stress of transport, 00014#s0915
Nondepolarizing agents, 202–203
Noninvasive positive pressure ventilation (NiPPV), 219–223
  absolute ventilators, 221
  additive ventilators, 221
  bi-level positive airway pressure, 221
  continuous positive airway pressure, 220–221
  helmet-based ventilation, 222
  high-flow nasal cannula, 221–222
  oxygen consumption in, 221
Norepinephrine, 236
Norms, group, 102
NOTAMs. see Notices to Air Missions
Notices to Air Missions (NOTAMs), 31
NTSB. see National Transportation Safety Board (NTSB)
Nurses
  advanced practice registered, 16
  transport. see Transport nurse
Nursing, in critical care transport, 6–7, 6f, 7b, 7f
NVIS. see Night vision imaging systems
NWS. see National Weather Service

O
Oblique fractures, 298f
Obstetric hemorrhage, 237
Obstetric ultrasound, 327–328
Obstructive lung disease, 224
Obstructive shock, 241
Obtunded patient, 266, 266b
Occupational and workplace safety training, 138
Oculocephalic reflex, 267
Oculovestibular reflex, 267
Oliguria, 318
On-scene safety, 143

OODA loop, 105, 106f
Open fracture, 297
Open pneumothorax, 283–284, 283f
Open water survival, 150
Operating at altitude, 29
Operational control, 90
Operational safety training, 137
Operations Compliance Form, 133f
OPQRST, 162, 171
Optic nerve sheath diameter, 273, 273f, 274f
Oral commissure burns, 313, 313f
Orbital blowout fracture, 262
Organizational preparedness, 368–369
Oropharyngeal airway, 189, 190f
Oropharynx, 192f
Orotracheal intubation, 191, 194b
Orthopedic injuries, 295
    assessment of, 298–299
    classification of, 297–298
    common terms, 300
    compartment syndrome, 303–304
    complications of, 296t
    fat embolism, 303
    hemorrhage management, 296–297
    management of, 299–301
    mechanisms of, 296
    soft tissue wound management, 297
    splinting, 299–300
    traumatic amputations, 297
Outreach safety education, 138
Overpressure injuries, 87
Oxygen
    airline, requirements and, 181
    consumption, in NiPPV, 221
    toxicity, 211
Oxygen adapters, 181
Oxygen cylinder duration calculation, 176, 176t
Oxygen delivery (DO₂), 230
Oxygen-hemoglobin dissociation curve, 188f, 232f
Oxygen saturation, 204

P
Pagers, 93
Pain assessment, 164
PAIP. see Post-Accident Incident Plan (PAIP)
Palatine tonsil, 192f
Pancreas, injury of, 290
Pancuronium, 202t
Paramedics
    in critical care transport, 7–8
    transport. see Transport paramedics
Pararescue jumpers (PJ), 50
Parasternal long axis (PSLA) view, of heart, 324, 325f
Parasternal short axis (PSSA) view, of heart, 325, 325f
Pareto chart, 346, 347f
Parkland formula, 315
Paroxysmal sympathetic hyperactivity (PSH), 280
Partially compensated metabolic acidosis, 225–226
Partial pressure of oxygen (PaO₂), 56
Partial-thickness injury, 311
Passive leg raise (PLR), 236
Passive process, 58
Patella fractures, 301
Patient assessment, 153–184
    in airway management, 185–189
    communication in, 155–156
    consent in, 156–157
    fixed-wing patient transport. see Fixed-wing patient transport
    preparation for transport, 153
Patient care
    in survival situation, 151
    during transport, 340

Patient Evacuation Center (PEC), 45
Patient location, international transport and, 179–180
Patient movement, 44
    types of, 45–50
Patient safety, 113–123, 139–140
    data collection and analysis, 122
    engineering principles, 118b
    event classification, 122
    family efforts toward, 113b
    managing events, 121–122
    maximizing accessibility, 121
    minimizing anxiety, 121, 121b
    PESTLE Analysis, 116–117, 117b
    priorities, 122b
    process improvement, 122
    report management, 121
Patient Safety and Quality Improvement Act (PSQIA), 113–114
Patient transport
    assessment and reassessment during, 175
    bariatric, preparation for, 173–175
    challenge, twenty-first-century, 157
    decision to, 154–155
    history of, 1–11
        associations, 8–10
        origins, 1–2, 2f
    indications for, 153–157
    interfacility considerations, 154
    preparing for, 168–172
    specialty patient populations, 154
PEA. see Pulseless electrical activity
Peak inspiratory pressure (PIP), 213–214
Pediatric airway management, 199–200, 199f
PEEP. see Positive end-expiratory pressure
Pelvic binder, placement for, 302–303, 302f
Pelvic FAST exam, 323, 323f
Pelvic fractures, 296t, 301–303
Penetrating trauma, 250–251, 282
Pericardiocentesis, 286, 286f, 329
Peritoneal cavity, 292
Permanent cavity, 251, 251f
Permissive hypercapnia, 224
Personal effects, of incident/accident, 364
Personal flotation device (PFD), 144–145
Personal preparedness, 368, 369b
Personal protective equipment (PPE), 72, 138–139
    for cave exploration and rescue, 84
Personal safety, 138
Personal survival equipment, 146b
PESTLE Analysis, 116–117, 117b
PFD. see Personal flotation device
Phased array probe, 320–321, 321f
Phenylephrine, 189
Phone-radio patch, 92
Phonetic alphabet, 96b
Physical examination
    in airway management, 186–187
    secondary, 163, 163b
Physician medical director, 17–18
Physicians, 17–18
Physics of aviation, 26–27, 27f
Physiologically deficient zone, 63
Physiologic zone, 56, 63
PIC. see Pilot-in-command
Pillow splint, 301
Pilot and air medical personnel duty times, 180
Pilot error, 132
Pilot-in-command (PIC), 132
    qualifications, 18–19
Pilot Reports (PIREP), 32
Piriform recess, 192f
Pitot-static system, 34–35
Plan–do–check–act (PDCA), 343, 345f

Plantar flexion, 299b
Plateau pressure, 214
Pleural effusions, 327, 327f
PLR. see Passive leg raise
Plug-type emergency exit, 78, 78f
Pneumocephalus, 262
Pneumothorax, 165–166, 166f
    closed, 283
    open, 283–284, 283f
    tension, 241, 284, 284f
Point-of-care ultrasound (POCUS), 168, 320–332
    aortic ultrasound, 327, 327f
    cardiac ultrasound, 324
    fundamentals of, 320–321
    lung ultrasound, 327, 327f
    obstetric ultrasound, 327–328
    in prehospital and transport medicine, 321
    RUSH exam, 329, 329t
    in trauma, 321–322
Poisoning
    carbon monoxide, 311
    tissue, 56–57
Positive end-expiratory pressure (PEEP), 214–215
Post-Accident Incident Plan (PAIP), 98, 145, 361
    anniversaries, 371
    crowdfunding, 366
    formal investigation, 370
    funeral planning, 366
    human resources in, 366
    information flow and communication, 363
    legal issues in, 370–371
    media considerations in, 363
    memorial services, 366
    notifications and people support, 363–365
        community partners and first responders, 365
        families of survivors, 365
        family member, 364
        leadership, 365
        personal effects, 364
        returning team members, 364–365
        ripple effect, 364
        site visits, 364
        survivors, 365
    NTSB report, 370
    organizational preparedness, 368–369
    personal preparedness, 368, 369b
    program leadership team, 362, 362b
    program safety evaluation, 370
    request for physical memorials, 370
    response structure, 362–363, 363f
    reviews, 371
    standing down and returning to service, 363
    triggering events, 362b
    vehicle and equipment replacement, 370
Postcrash responsibilities, 145
Postdescent collapse, 65
Posterior dislocation, 301
Posterior elbow dislocation, 296t
Posterior hip dislocation, 296t
Posterior lamina of cricoid cartilage, 192f
Postintubation management, 204
Postoperation debriefings, 143
Potassium, disorders of, as adverse effect of blood transfusion, 238b
PPE. see Personal protective equipment
PQRST, 162, 171
Preflight briefing, 143
Preflight preparation, 175
    and logistics, 179
Pregnancy
    personal safety and, 138
    point-of-care ultrasound, 328
    thermal burns and, 308
Premedications, airway management and, 200–201
Preoxygenation, 188, 200
Preparation of practice, 19–20

Preparedness, 361
    organizational, 368–369
    personal, 368, 369b
Preparing patient for transport, 168–172
    airway management in, 169
    circulation management in, 170
    documentation in, 173, 173b
    family in, 172
    fixed-wing patient transport. *see* Fixed-wing
        patient transport
    gastric decompression in, 170
    pain management in, 171
    safety in, 171–172
    ventilation management in, 169–170
    wound care and splinting in, 171
Pressure (P), 52
Pressure-controlled ventilation, 218
Pressure-control plus (PCV+) ventilation, 218–219
Pressure differential, 58, 64
Pressure ratio, 64
Pressure-regulated volume-controlled ventilation,
    218
Pressure-synchronized intermittent mandatory
    ventilation plus, 219
Pressure-time histories, 60
Pressure triggering, 217
Prevention, principles of, 114
Primary airway assessment, 158, 158b
Primary assessment, 157–161
    in airway management, 185–186
Primary breathing assessment, 158–159, 158b
Primary circulation assessment, 159, 159b
Primary disability assessment, 159b
Primary prevention, 114
Priority One, 350
Privacy Rule, 336
Private line, 92–93
Processes, 343–344
Professional issues, in critical care transport,
    333–342
Program manager, 19
Pronation, 299b
Proning, 225
Propofol, 201
Prospective scoring, 254–255
Protective footwear, 139
Proximal tibia shaft fractures, 296t
Pseudo-PEA, 328
"5 Ps," with compartment syndrome, 316
Psychological strains, 357
Pulmonary contusion, 289
Pulmonary edema, 318
Pulmonary embolism, 241, 326–327
Pulseless electrical activity (PEA), 328
Pulse oximetry, 188f, 204
Punitive damages, 334
Pupils, 266–267
Push-dose pressor, 189
Push-to-talk (PTT) method, 93

Q
qSOFA. *see* Quick Sequential Organ Failure
    Assessment
Quality, 343–348
    domains of, 343–344
    improvement frameworks, 345–346
    integrated quality systems, 344–345
    medical quality improvement, 347–348
    tools, 346–347
Quasi-intentional torts, 334–335
Quick Sequential Organ Failure Assessment
    (qSOFA), 239

R
RAAA. *see* Ruptured abdominal aortic aneurysms
Radial acceleration, 62

Radiation burn injuries, 307
    assessment of, 314
    management of, 318
Radioactive material emergencies, 72–73
Radio Altimeter, 35
Radio bands, 91–93, 92b
Radio-phone patch, 92
Radios
    aircraft, 96–97
    in communication operations, 91–93, 92b
    communication via, 95–96
    phone-radio or radio-phone patch in, 92
    portable units of, 96
    for signaling, 148
    squelch control in, 92–93
    use of, 92
Radio traffic, 96–97
Railway incidents, 79–81, 80f
    recommendations for, 80b
Railway yard, hazards of, 81
Rapid four-step cricothyrotomy, 198b, 199, 199f
Rapid sequence induction, 173
Rapid Ultrasound for Shock and Hypotension
    (RUSH) exam, 329, 329t
Rear-end collisions, 248
Reassessment, during patient transport, 175
Red lights and siren (RLS), 137
Reflective practice, 22
Refusal of care, 335–336
Relative directions, aviation and, 25, 25f
Relative mass of gas/number of molecules (n), 52
"Renal-dose" dopamine, 236–237
Renal trauma, 291–292
Repeater system, 92
Rescues
    cave, 84–85, 85f
    whitewater, 83–84, 84f
    wilderness, 83
Resiliency training, 357
Resistance, 308
Respiration, abnormal patterns of, 268f
Respiratory pattern, 268, 268f
Respiratory therapist (RT), 12, 17
Rest, for air medical personnel, 180
Resuscitative endovascular balloon occlusion of the
    aorta (REBOA), 259, 289, 289f
Retroglottic devices, 197, 197b
Retroperitoneal space, 290
Retrospective scoring, 255–256
Revised Trauma Score, 254–255, 255t
Richmond Agitation and Sedation Scale, 164,
    164t, 204
Right upper quadrant (RUQ), FAST exam, 322,
    322f
Rigid splint, 300
Ripple effect, of incident/accident, 364
Rise time, 217
Risk assessment tool, 132, 133f
RLS. *see* Red lights and siren
Rocuronium, 202t
Rollover motor vehicle crash, 249, 249f
Rolodex, 93
Rotary wing transport, 46–47, 47f, 47t
Rotation, 299b
Rotor wash, 139–140
Rotor wing, 26, 34, 35
Royal Flying Doctor Service, 3
RT. *see* Respiratory therapist
Rule-based errors, 100
Rule of nines, 310, 311f
Rule of threes, 146
Run chart, 347
Rupture
    of bladder, 292
    of small intestine, 290
Ruptured abdominal aortic aneurysms, 327

S
Safety
    definition of, 124–136
    in fixed-wing patient transport, 178–179
    patient, 113–123
    in preparing patient for transport, 171–172
    survival and, 124–152
        air medical accidents and, 125–126
        ASTNA position paper for, 138
        attitude, 145
        daily shift procedures, 140–143
        dispatch/communications in, 140–141
        emergency egress and, 144
        fitness standards in, 138
        fixed-wing aircraft safety, 140
        forced water landings and, 144–145
        ground ambulance, 140
        helicopter, 139–140
        helipad/airport, 141
        in-flight, 141–142
        missing or overdue aircraft or ground vehicle
            procedure, 145
        patient, 139–140
        personal, 138
        personal protective equipment for, 138–139
        postcrash responsibilities for, 145
    survival basics. *see* Survival basics
Safety assurance, 137
Safety committee, 137
Safety management, 136–138
Safety management system (SMS), 114
    CAMTS elements of, 137b
    components of, 114, 114f, 136f
Safety policy, 136–137
Safety promotion, 137
Safety risk management, 137
Safety training, 137–138
Safety zones, for hazardous materials incident, 74f
Sager splint, 300
Sagittal view of airway, 192f
SAH. *see* Subarachnoid hemorrhage
SAMPLE, 162
Satellite communications, 93, 97
Satellite phones, 91
Satellite tracking, 136
Scanning, 141
Scatter diagram, 346–347, 347f
Scattered burns, 310
Scene assessment, 157–165, 157b
Scene management, 69–74
    guidelines for, 71b
Scene operations and safety, 68–87
    cave rescue, 84–85, 85f
    human-made disasters, 85
    in industrial emergency scenes
        agricultural emergencies, 81–82, 81f
        electrical emergencies, 81
        trench collapse, 82
    in law enforcement-related situations, 85–87
        active shooter situation, 85–86, 86f
        evidence preservation in, 86
        explosive materials emergencies, 87
        weapons, 86–87
    natural disasters, 85
    scene management in, 69–74
        approach to scene in, 69, 70f
        guidelines for, 71b
        hazardous materials emergencies, 71–72, 73f,
            74f
        mass casualty triage, 71, 72f
        on-scene considerations, 69–71, 70f
        prearrival/en route considerations for, 69
        radioactive material emergencies, 72–73
    thunderstorms, 85
    in transportation emergency scenes, 74–81
        aircraft accidents, 76–79, 78f

Scene operations and safety (*Continued*)
    commercial motor vehicle accidents, 76, 77f
    motor vehicle accidents and extrication, 74–76, 75b, 75f
    railway incidents, 79–81, 80b, 80f
    whitewater rescue, 83–84, 84f
    wilderness emergency medical services, 82–83, 83f
    in wilderness emergency scenes, 82–83
Scene safety, 142–143
Schimmoler, Laureate M., 6
Scoliosis, 299b
Scope of practice, 338–339
Scoring, 254–256
    systems, 164
Scottish Ambulance Service (Air Wing), 3
Search and rescue (SAR), 83
Secondary assessment, 161–164, 163b
    in airway management, 185–186
Secondary prevention, 114
Second-degree burns, 311
Second Victim Experience, 121
Security Rule, 336
Sedation
    airway management and, 201
    assessment, 164
    for traumatic brain injury, 272
Seizures, posttraumatic, 271
Seldinger technique, 194–195, 199b
Self-contained breathing apparatus (SCBA), 77
Sellick maneuver, 191
Sentinel events, 122
Septic shock, 239
Serum lactate, 236
Severe lightening injuries, 314
Shared accountability, 117
Shark-fin morphology, EtCO$_2$, 226–227, 227f
Shearing, 246
Shelter, 147–148, 147f
Shiley tracheostomy tube, 198
Shock, 230–244
    cardiogenic, 240–241
    compensated, 233f
    distributive, 239–240
        anaphylaxis, 239–240, 240f
        neurogenic, 239
        septic, 239
    early and late, 251, 252–253t
    hypovolemic, 237–239
    major organ system changes associated with, 233f
    management of, 236–237
    obstructive, 241
    pathophysiologic changes in, 252t
    physiology of, 230–241
        cellular respiration, 230, 231f
        diagnosis, 232–236
        oxygen-carrying capacity and delivery, 230, 231f, 232f
        physiologic response, 231–232, 233f, 234f, 235f
    signs and symptoms of, 252–253t
    uncompensated, 234f
Shock index (SI), 235–236, 255
    values, 159, 159t
Shoulder dislocation, 301
SIGMET. *see* Significant Meteorological Information
Signaling, 148
Signal mirror, for signaling, 148
Significant Meteorological Information (SIGMET), 32
Sikorsky, Igor, 4
Simplex system, 92
Sinus block, 59
Site visits, 364
Situational awareness, 141
    Crew Resource Management and, 105–106

Six-Sigma, 345–346
Skin, 308
Skull fracture, 262
Sleep, 138
    stress and, 358
Slips, definition of, 99
Small intestine, injury of, 290
Smoke and fire, for signaling, 148
Snag tag, 84, 84f
Snow trench shelter, 147f
Soar Flight Medic/Flight Surgeon Team, 50
Society for the Recovery of Drowned Persons, 1
Sodium bicarbonate, 317
Soft palate, 192f
Soft splint, 300
Soft tissue trauma, 295–306
    wound management, 297
Sort, assess, lifesaving interventions, and treatment/transport (SALT) triage, 71, 72f
Sound, 60
Sound waves, 60
Space, 63
Space blanket, 60
Space-equivalent zone, 63
Spatial disorientation, 66
Special damages, 334
Special Operations Critical Care Evacuation Team (SOCCETT), 49
Special Operations Independent Duty Corpsman (SOIDC), 50
Spectrum, of sound wave, 60
Speed, 62
Sphenoidal sinus, 192f
Spinal cord injury, 274–280
    atlas, axis, and dens fractures, 276–277
    cervical spine injuries, 275–276
    etiology and incidence rate, 274
    extension injuries, 276
    extension-rotation injuries, 276
    flexion injuries, 275–276
    flexion-rotation injuries, 276
    initial assessment of, 274
    interventions and treatment of, 279–280
    neurologic examination, 278
    secondary assessment of, 274–276, 275b
    sensory examination, 278
    thoracic and lumbar spine injuries, 277
    vertebral artery dissection, 277
    vertical compression, 276
    without radiographic abnormality, 278
Spinal cord syndromes, 274, 275f
Spiral fractures, 298f
Spleen injuries, 290
Splinting, 299–300
    dislocations
        lower extremities, 301
        upper extremities, 301
    fractures
        lower extremities, 301
        upper extremities, 300
    objectives of, 299
    principles of, 299, 300b
    rigid splint, 300
    Sager splint, 300
    soft splint, 300
    traction splint, 300
Sprain, 295, 301
Squelch control, 92–93
Stab wounds, 250, 251f
Staggers, 65
Stagnant hypoxia, 56
Standards of care, 338–339
START adult triage, 256–258, 257f
Statutes, 333
    of time limitations, 334

Step-by-step procedure
    needle cricothyrotomy, 198b
    orotracheal intubation, 194b
    rapid four-step cricothyrotomy, 198b
    Seldinger technique, 199b
    surgical cricothyrotomy, 198b
Sterile cockpit, 141
Sternocleidomastoid muscle, 197f
Sternothyroid muscle, 197f
Sternum, 197f
"Stoic" healthcare provider, 356
Strains, 247
    behavioral, 357
    psychological, 357
Stratification, 346
Street map, 95
Stress
    causes of, 357
    critical incident, 369–370
    emotional awareness and, 111
    heart rate and, 111, 111f
    human performance and, 109–111, 109f
    inoculation of, 111
    mitigation tools, 358, 358b
        exercise, 358–359
        hydration and nutrition, 358, 358b
        laughter, 359
        sleep, 358
    moderators of, 357–358, 357b, 357f
    responses to, 110–111
    symptoms of, 357b
    tactical breathing and, 111, 112f
    thermal, 110
    thoughts and feelings and, 359
Stresses of transport, 55–66
    barometric pressure changes as, 58–59
    decreased humidity as, 60
    fatigue as, 62
    flicker vertigo as, 66
    fuel vapors as, 66
    gravitational force as, 62–63
    hyperventilation as, 57–58
    hypoxia as, 55–57
    noise as, 60–61
    spatial disorientation as, 66
    thermal changes as, 60
    vibration as, 61–62
Stressors
    acute, 356
    chronic, 356–357
    external, responses to, 110
Stryker Medical Evacuation Vehicle (M1133), 45–46
Stuporous state, 266, 266b
Subacute epidural hematomas, 263
Subarachnoid hemorrhage, 169f, 264, 264f
Subatmospheric decompression sickness, 65
Subdural bolt, 272
Subdural hematoma, 169f, 262–263, 263f
Subglottic injury, 312
Subluxated dislocation, 298
Submerged snag tag, 84f
Subspecialty teams, 48–49
Subxiphoid view, of heart, 325, 325f
Succinylcholine, 201–203, 202t
Sucking chest wound, 283, 283f
Superficial injury, 311
Superior thyroid artery, 197f
Superior turbinate, 192f
Supination, 299b
Supraglottic airway devices, 195–197
Supraglottic injury, 312
Surgical airway, 197–199
Surgical cricothyrotomy, 198–199, 198b
Survival basics, 145–151
    clothing as, 146

Survival basics *(Continued)*
  on cold weather, 151
  on desert, 150–151
  equipment, 151
  fire building in, 148, 149f
  food as, 149
  hydration as, 148, 150f
  international survival concerns and, 151
  open water survival, 150
  overland travel and navigation and, 149–150
  patient care, 151
  personal equipment, 146
  physical preparation as, 146
  priority setting and, 146
  psychological preparation as, 146
  rule of threes in, 146
  shelter as, 147–148, 147f
  signaling as, 148
  water landing in, 150
Survival equipment, 151
Survival kits, 146, 146b
Survival skills, 146–150
Survivors, accident, 365
  families of, 365
Swiss Air-Rescue (REGA), 3, 4f
Swiss Cheese Model, 115, 115f
Synchronized continuous mandatory ventilation
    plus, 219
Synchronized intermittent mandatory ventilation
    plus, 219
Syncope, 65
Systems, 343–344

T
Tactical breathing, 111, 112f
Tactical Combat Casualty Care (TCCC) guidelines,
    39, 40t, 296
Tactical Critical Care Evacuation Team
    (TCCET), 49
Tactical Evacuation Care (TACEVAC), 39
Tactical Field Care (TFC), 39
TAF. *see* Terminal Aerodrome Forecast
Task fixation, teamwork and, 108
Task saturation, teamwork and, 104
Team culture, 101
Team members
  families of returning, 365
  health and wellness, 117–118
  incident response, 365
Teamwork, 100–101
  assertiveness in, 108
  authority in, 101
  barriers to communication in, 107
  case studies on, 100b, 102b, 103b, 105b
  character and, 101
  clear leader intent, 101
  Crew Resource Management in, 103. *see also*
      Crew Resource Management
  followership in, 101
  group norms in, 102
  leadership in, 101
  managing boundaries in, 101
  rank and experience difference, 108
  sharing of mental model and, 108
  task fixation in, 108
  value of, 100–101
Teardrop hyperflexion fracture dislocations, 275–276
Technical error, 99
Telephones, 91, 97
Temperature (T), 52
Temporal bone fractures, pneumocephalus from, 262
Temporary cavity, 251, 251f
Temporary flight restrictions (TFRs), 31
Tension pneumothorax, 241, 284, 284f
Terminal Aerodrome Forecast (TAF), 32, 32t

Terrain awareness and warning systems (TAWS),
    125, 136
Tertiary prevention, 114
TFRs. *see* Temporary flight restrictions
Theater Patient Movement Requirements Center
    (TPMRC), 45
Thenar eminence technique, 189–190, 190f
Thermal burn injury
  assessment of, 310–311
  inhalation injuries with, 311–312
  pathophysiology of, 308
  pregnancy and, 308
Thermal stress, on human performance, 110
Third-degree injuries, 311
Thoracic spine injuries, 277
Thoracoabdominal trauma, 282–294
  bariatric considerations in, 293
  causing airway obstruction, 283
  causing cardiac tamponade, 285–286, 286f
  causing diaphragmatic injury, 288–289
  causing esophageal injuries, 288
  causing flail chest, 285, 286f
  causing massive hemothorax, 284–285, 284f
  causing open pneumothorax, 283–284
  causing pulmonary contusion, 289
  causing tension pneumothorax, 284, 284f
  causing tracheobronchial injuries, 288
  resuscitative endovascular balloon occlusion, 289,
      289f
Thromboelastography (TEG), 238–239
Thunderstorms, 85
Thyroid cartilage, 191, 192f
Tibia fractures, 301
Tidal volume, 212
  exhaled, 213
Time, aviation and, 24, 24t
Time of useful consciousness, 57, 57t
Tinnitus, 61
Tissue poisoning, 56–57
Toe dislocation, 301
Tongue, 192f
Topographic maps, 95
Torsion, 299b
Tort law, 334
Torts
  intentional, 334
  quasi-intentional, 334–335
Total body surface area (TBSA) burns, 315
Towering cumulus (TCU), 33
Trachea, 192f
Tracheal intubation, 191–193
Tracheobronchial injuries, 288
Track and rails, as railway hazards, 81
Traction splint, 300
Traffic collision avoidance system, 136
Traffic control zone, at roadway accident scene,
    69–71, 70f
Training, 18
  for transport team members, 339
Train, locomotives of, 80, 80f
Tranexamic acid (TXA), 238, 297
Transaction and Code Set Rule, 336
Transfusion-associated circulatory overload, as
    adverse effect of blood transfusion, 238b
Transfusion-associated immunomodulation, as
    adverse effect of blood transfusion, 238b
Transfusion-related acute lung injury, as adverse
    effect of blood transfusion, 238b
Translaryngeal jet ventilation, 198
Transport
  decisions, 339–340
  family members, 340, 341b
Transportation Disaster Assistance (TDA), 364
Transportation emergency scenes, 74–81
  aircraft accidents, 76–79, 78f

Transportation emergency scenes *(Continued)*
  commercial motor vehicle accidents, 76, 77f
  motor vehicle accidents and extrication, 74–76,
      75b, 75f
  railway incidents, 79–81, 80b, 80f
Transport environment, safety in, 138–140
Transport nurse, 13–16
  ASTNA recommended competencies for, 22b
  qualifications of, 15b
Transport paramedics, 16–17, 16b
Transport physiology, 52–67
  cabin pressurization in, 63–66
  case studies, 66b, 67b
  decompression in, 64–65
  decompression sickness in, 65–66, 65b
  gas laws in, 52–55
  stresses of transport in, 55–66. *see also* Stresses
      of transport
Transport providers, mental health and wellness for,
    355–360
Transport team members. *see* Members of transport team
Transpulmonary pressure, 209
Transverse fractures, 298f
Trauma
  abdominal, 289. *see also* Abdominal trauma
  assessment of, 253–254
  bladder, 292, 293f
  blunt, 282
  burn, 307–319. *see also* Burn trauma
  care, trends in, 258–259
  case study for, 259b
  definition of, 245
  field triage in, 256, 256f
  gastroesophageal, 291
  genital, 292–293
  genitourinary, 291
  injury dynamics, 245–247
  kinematics of, 245, 247–251
  management of, principles of, 245–260
  mass casualty incidents, 256–258
  maxillofacial, 303–304
  mechanism of injury, 246–247
  neurologic, 261–281
  pathophysiologic factors of, 251–253
  penetrating, 250–251, 282
  point-of-care ultrasound in, 321–322
  renal, 291–292
  scoring of, 254–256
  thoracoabdominal, 282–294. *see also*
      Thoracoabdominal trauma
  triage patient transport in, 258, 258f
  ureter, 291–292
  urethral, 292, 293f
Trauma and Injury Severity Score, 256
Trauma-informed organizations, 368–369
Trauma Score, 254–255, 254f
Traumatic amputations, 297
Traumatic brain injury (TBI), 261
  blast-related, 265
  brainstem reflexes and extraocular cranial nerves, 267
  complications, 265
  Glasgow Coma Scale in, 268–269, 268t
  interventions and treatment of, 269–274, 269b, 270f
  intracranial hemorrhage, 262–265
  level of consciousness, 266, 266b
  management guidelines for, 269b
  motor examination in, 267–268
  pathologic and clinical considerations in, 262–265
  penetrating injuries, 265
  physical assessment of, 266–269, 266b, 266t
  pupils and, 266–267
  reexamination in, 269
  respiratory pattern in, 268
  skull fracture, 262
  types of, 262–265

Traumatic pneumocephalus, 262
Traumatic-stress injury, 369–370
Trauma triage decision making, 256f
Trench collapse, 82
Triad of death, 237, 238f
Triage, mass casualty, 71, 72f
Triage patient transport, in trauma, 258, 258f
Triger, M., 65
Trigger sensitivity, 216–217
Tripler Army Medical Center (TAMC), 44
Tubercle of epiglottis, 192f
Tumbling, 251
Tunnels/bridges, as railway hazards, 81
T wave progression, 304, 305f
Two-challenge rule, 108
Two-way paging, 93

U
Ultrasound, 168
Uncompensated shock, 234f
Unconsciousness, 269b
Undercut, 83
Unilaterally affected pupil, 266–267
Unilaterally dilated pupil, 266–267
Unilateral small pupil, 266–267
Unmanned aerial systems (UAS), 141
Unmanned aerial vehicles (UAVs), 141
Upper extremities
    dislocations, 301
    fractures, 300
        testing for neurologic function in, 300f
Ureter trauma, 291–292
Urethral trauma, 292, 293f
Urinary output (UO), in children/adults, 318
USAISR Burn Flight team, 49
US Army Burn Flight Team, 49–50

V
Vaginal bleeding, 293
Valgus, 299b
Vallecula, 192f
Varus, 299b
Vasopressin, 189
Vasopressors, for shock, 236–237

Vecuronium, 202t
Vehicle crashes, injury patterns by, 162, 162b
Vehicle rollovers, 249, 249f
Velocity, 62
Venous injury, 291
Ventilation. *see* Mechanical ventilation
Ventilation management, 169–170
Ventilator alarms, 227, 227t
Ventilator asynchrony, 228
Ventilator-induced lung injury (VILI), 209–212
Ventricle of larynx, 192f
Vertebral artery dissection, 277
Vertical compression, 276
Vertical speed indicator, 35, 36f
Vertigo, flicker, 66, 66b
Vestibular fold, 192f
Vestibule, 192f
VFR. *see* Visual flight rules
Vibration, 61–62
Vicarious liability, 335, 335b
Video-assisted intubation, 195
Viscoelastic properties, of tissues, 247
Visibility, ceiling and, 33
Visual flight rules (VFRs), 30
Visual illusions, 66
Visual meteorologic conditions (VMCs), 30
Visual *vs.* instrument rules, 30
Vocal cord, 192f
Vocal process of arytenoid cartilage, 192f
Voice box, 191
Voice over Internet Protocol (VoIP) radio
    communication, 93
Voltage, 308
Volume (V), 52
Volume-cycled pressure-variable ventilation,
    217–218
Volutrauma, 211

W
Warm zone, 72, 73–74, 74f
Waterfalls, 84
Water landings, 150
    forced, 144–145
Weapons, 86–87

Weather
    cameras, 32–33
    considerations, 31–34
    reporting sources, 31–33
    trends, 34
Weather minimums, 30, 132
Weather radar, 94
Wedge fracture, simple, 275
Weight, 62
    and balance considerations, 30
Wellness
    importance of, 356
    promoting, 358–359
Whistle, for signaling, 148
White Paper, improved emergency medical services
    and, 349–350
Whitewater, 83
    rescues, 83–84, 84f
Wilderness emergency medical services, 82–83, 83f
Wilderness rescues, 83
Wind, 33–34
    gusts, 34
    shear, 34
Withdrawal of consent, 335–336
Workload
    Crew Resource Management and, 103–105, 104f
    on human performance, 110
Wound care and splinting, 171
Wreckage, as railway hazards, 80–81
Wrist, dislocated, 301
Wrist fractures, 300
Written communication, 107

Y
Yaw, 251

Z
Zone of coagulation, 311
Zone of hyperemia, 310
Zone of stasis, 310